IN DEFENSE OF THE BRAIN: CURRENT CONCEPTS IN THE IMMUNOPATHOGENESIS AND CLINICAL ASPECTS OF CNS INFECTIONS

edited by

PHILLIP K. PETERSON, MD

Director
Division of Infectious Diseases
Hennepin County Medical Center
Professor of Medicine
University of Minnesota Medical School
Minneapolis, Minnesota

JACK S. REMINGTON, MD

Professor of Medicine
Division of Infectious Diseases and Geographic Medicine
Stanford University School of Medicine
Stanford, California
Marcus A. Krupp Research Chair
Chairman, Department of Immunology and Infectious Diseases
Research Institute
Palo Alto Medical Foundation
Palo Alto, California

b
Blackwell
Science

BLACKWELL SCIENCE

Editorial offices:

350 Main Street, Malden, Massachusetts 02148, USA
Osney Mead, Oxford OX2 0El, England
25 John Street, London WC1N 2BL, England
23 Ainslie Place, Edinburgh EH3 6AJ, Scotland
54 University Street, Carlton, Victoria 3053, Australia

Other Editorial Offices:

Blackwell Wissenschafts-Verlag GmbH Kurfürstendamm 57, 10707 Berlin, Germany
Zehetnergasse 6, A-1140 Vienna, Austria

Distributors:

USA
Blackwell Science, Inc.
Commerce Place
350 Main Street
Malden, Massachusetts 02148
(Telephone orders: 800-215-1000 or 617-388-8250; Fax orders: 617-388-8270)

Canada
Copp Clark Professional
200 Adelaide Street, West, 3rd Floor
Toronto, Ontario M5H 1W7
(Telephone orders: 416-597-1616
1-800-815-9417
fax: 416-597-1617

Australia
Blackwell Science Pty., Ltd.
54 University Street
Carlton, Victoria 3053
(Telephone orders: 03-9347-0300; fax orders 03-9349 3016)

Outside North America and Australia
Blackwell Science, Ltd.
c/o Marston Book Services, Ltd.
P.O. Box 269
Abingdon
Oxon OX14 4YN
England
(Telephone orders: 44-01235-465500; fax orders 44-01235-465555)

Acquisitions: Christopher Davis
Production: Ellen Samia
Manufacturing: Lisa Flanagan
Typeset by The Composing Room of Michigan, Inc.
Printed and bound by Braun-Brumfield, Inc.

Printed in the United States of America
97 98 99 00 5 4 3 2 1

Notice: The indications and dosages of all drugs in this book have been recommended in the medical literature and conform to the practices of the general medical community. The medications described do not necessarily have specific approval by the Food and Drug Administration for use in the diseases and dosages for which they are recommended. The package insert for each drug should be consulted for use and dosage as approved by the FDA. Because standards of usage change, it is advisable to keep abreast of revised recommendations, particularly those concerning new drugs.

Library of Congress Cataloging-in-Publication Data

In defense of the brain: current concepts in the immunopathogenesis and clinical aspects of CNS infections / edited by Phillip K. Peterson and Jack S. Remington
p. cm.
Includes bibliographical references and index.
ISBN 0-86542-555-8 (c)
1. Nervous System—Infections—Immunological aspects.
2. Neuroimmunology I. Peterson, Phillip K. II. Remington, Jack S., 1931- .
[DNLM: 1. Central Nervous System Diseases—etiology. 2. Central Nervous System Diseases—immunology. WL 300 I349 1997]
RC346.5.I5 1997
616.8′ 047—dc21
DNLM/DLC 97-4121
for Library of Congress CIP

Contents

Preface

The brain has a high opinion of itself, and rightfully so, since the very essence of being human is defined by the brain. "I think, therefore, I am." Even "human" emotions arise from subcortical areas within the brain, both feelings that give life its meaning (love, joy, and appreciation of beauty, for example) and those in need of cortical control (such as hatred, anger, and violent urges.)

Given the enormity of its importance, it should not be surprising that the brain evolved an elegant strategy for its defense, restricting entry not only of foreign invaders, but also elements of the immune system that could provoke a disturbance. Early observations demonstrating a poor alloreactive response to tissue engraftment within the central nervous system (CNS) led to the concept of the brain as "immunologically privileged." Characteristics of the normal brain that supported this concept included: 1) the presence of a blood-brain barrier composed of highly specialized endothelial cells that limit the passage of immunocytes and molecules, such as immunglobulins and cytokines, from the circulation into the CNS, 2) a lack or low level of expression of proteins with immunologic properties, such as adhesion molecules and class I and class II major histocompatibility complex (MHC) antigens, on the cells of the CNS (neurons and glia), 3) the lack of a lymphatic drainage, and 4) an absence of resident lymphocytes within the parenchyma of the brain.

More recent scientific evidence, however, has revealed that the immune privilege of the brain is incomplete. The contributors to this book, in the delineation of these recent discoveries, make it clear that the brain is not that exclusionary after all. Activated T cells traffic through the CNS for the purposes of immune surveillance. A lymph-like system is present in the brain. The cerebral cortex itself is composed predominantly of cells (astrocytes and microglia) which when activated upregulate the expression of MHC and adhesion molecules and release immune mediators, such as cytokines and toxic free radicals, that can be injurious to foreign invaders and to neighboring neurons alike. And, in the face of certain types of microbial challenge, the troops (neurophils, monocytes, and lymphocytes) can be called in.

Also made clear by the authors of this book are important reasons for a system of immune defense of the brain. A number of infectious agents have evolved properties that favor their survival within the CNS. Some of the most common, the most life-threatening, and the most debilitating conditions which plague our species are caused by these agents. Cerebral malaria, which kills over one million children each year in sub-Saharan Africa alone, rabies, a historically frightening disease that remains uniformly fatal, and Creutzfeldt-Jacob disease, a fatal neurodegenerative disease caused by a most unusual infectious agent (i.e., PRIONS), are but three such examples.

It was shared interest in mechanisms of host defense and a particular interest in two forms of brain infection (CNS toxoplasmosis and HIV encephalopathy), that inspired the editors to develop this book. We asked the contributors to provide the reader a current understanding, at a molecular level, of the strategies used by the host to defend the brain. In some chapters, new concepts of the treatment and prevention of CNS infections are highlighted, especially in those instances where understanding of the immunopathogenesis is limited. The result of this collaboration has been a collection of outstanding dissertations on the complex interplay between infectious agents and host responses involved in CNS infections as well as directions for future research on immunopathogenesis and therapy of these infections.

We are particularly grateful to the contributors to this volume, to Chris Davis and Blackwell Science for expeditious publication, and to Doug Webb and Pfizer, Inc. for an educational grant that supported this endeavor. It is our hope that the discussions herein will stimulate new discoveries about the immunopathogenesis and ultimately the treatment of CNS disorders that are known or are likely to be caused by infectious agents.

PHILLIP K. PETERSON, MD
JACK S. REMINGTON, MD

Contributors

Ann Arvin, MD
Professor of Pediatrics, Microbiology, and Immunology
Stanford University School of Medicine
Chief, Infectious Diseases Service
Lucile Packard Children's Hospital
Stanford, California

John E. Bennett, MD
Head, Clinical Mycology Section/Laboratory of Clinical Investigation
National Institute of Allergies and Infectious Diseases
National Institutes of Health
Bethesda, Maryland

Joanne Burke, PhD
Department of Veterinary Clinical Studies
School of Veterinary Medicine
University of Glasgow
Glasgow, United Kingdom

Chun C. Chao, PhD
Neuroimmunobiology and Host Defense Laboratory
Minneapolis Medical Research Foundation
Associate Professor of Medicine
University of Minnesota Medical School
Minneapolis, Minnesota

Blanche L. Curfman, MD
Senior Molecular Biologist
Laboratory of Molecular Medicine and Neuroscience
National Institutes of Health
Bethesda, Maryland

Bernhard Dietzschold, DVM
Professor
Department of Microbiology
Thomas Jefferson University
Philadelphia, Pennsylvania

John N. Galgiani, MD
Chief, Section of Infectious Diseases
Medical Service
VA Medical Center
Tucson, Arizona

Genya Gekker, MD
Research Scientist
Neuroimmunobiology and Host Defense Laboratory
Minneapolis Medical Research Foundation
Minneapolis, Minnesota

Howard E. Gendelman, MD
Professor of Medicine
Department of Microbiology and Pathology
University of Nebraska Medical Center
Omaha, Nebraska

Anuja Ghorpade, MD
Instructor, Department of Microbiology and Pathology
University of Nebraska Medical Center
Omaha, Nebraska

William F. Hickey, MD
Professor
Department of Pathology
Dartmouth Medical School/D.H.M.C.
Lebanon, New Hampshire

Shuxian Hu, MD
Research Scientist
Neuroimmunobiology and Host Defense Laboratory
Minneapolis Medical Research Foundation
Minneapolis, Minnesota

Christopher A. Hunter, PhD
Assistant Professor
Department of Pathobiology
School of Veterinary Medicine
University of Pennsylvania
Philadelphia, Pennsylvania

Young S. Kim, MD
Postdoctoral Researcher
Division of Infectious Diseases
San Francisco General Hospital
Department of Medicine
University of California at San Francisco
San Francisco, California

Hilary Koprowski, MD
Professor, Department of Microbiology and Immunology
Director, Center for Neurovirology
Thomas Jefferson University
Philadelphia, Pennsylvania

Dr. Dominic Kwiatkowski
Internal Child Health Group
University Department of Paediatrics
John Radcliffe Hospital
Oxford, United Kingdom

Stephen L. Leib, MD
Postdoctoral Fellow
Division of Infectious Diseases
University Hospital
Basel, Switzerland

Eugene O. Major, MD
Chief, Laboratory of Molecular Medicine and Neuroscience
National Institutes of Neurological Disorders and Stroke
National Institutes of Health
Bethesda, Maryland

George H. McCracken, Jr., MD
Professor of Pediatrics
The Sarah M. & Charles E. Saey Chair in Pediatric Infectious Diseases
University of Texas Southwestern Medical Center
Dallas, Texas

Jose G. Montoya, MD
Acting Assistant Professor of Medicine
Division of Infectious Diseases and Geographic Medicine
Stanford University School of Medicine
Stanford, California

Theodore E. Nash, MD
Chief, Gastrointestinal Parasites Sections
Laboratory of Parasitic Diseases
National Institute of Allergy and Infectious Diseases
National Institutes of Health
Bethesda, Maryland

Michael B.A. Oldstone, MD
Professor
Department of Immunology
Scripps Clinic & Medical Foundation
La Jolla, California

Yuri Persidsky, MD
Instructor, Department of Microbiology and Pathology
University of Nebraska Medical Center
Omaha, Nebraska

Phillip K. Peterson, MD
Director
Division of Infectious Diseases
Hennepin County Medical Center
Professor of Medicine
University of Minnesota Medical School
Minneapolis, Minnesota

Stanley B. Prusiner, MD
Professor of Neurology
Department of Neurology
University of California at San Francisco
San Francisco, California

Glenn F. Rall, PhD
Associate Member
Division of Basic Science
The Fox Chase Cancer Center
Philadelphia, Pennsylvania

Jack S. Remington, MD
Professor of Medicine
Division of Infectious Diseases and Geographic Medicine
Stanford University School of Medicine
Stanford, California
Marcus A. Krupp Research Chair
Chairman, Department of Immunology and Infectious Diseases
Research Institute
Palo Alto Medical Foundation
Palo Alto, California

Axel Ring, MD
Postdoctoral Fellow
Laboratory of Molecular Infectious Diseases
Division of Infectious Diseases
The Rockefeller University
New York, New York

Xavier Saez-Llorens, MD
Professor of Pediatrics
University of Panama School of Medicine
Head, Pediatric Infectious Diseases Division
Hospital del Nino
Panama City, Panama

W. Michael Scheld, MD
Professor of Medicine and Neurosurgery
Division of Infectious Diseases
University of Virginia Health Sciences Center
Charlottesville, Virginia

Yasuhiro Suzuki, PhD, DMSc
Senior Research Associate
Department of Immunology and Infectious Diseases
Research Institute
Palo Alto Medical Foundation
Palo Alto, California

Martin G. Täuber, MD
Professor and Chief, Infectious Diseases
Co-Director, Institute for Medical Microbiology
University of Berne
Berne, Switzerland

Gregory C. Townsend, MD, MACP, FAAP
Assistant Professor of Research
Department of Internal Medicine and Pediatrics
University of Virginia Health Sciences Center
University of Virginia
Charlottesville, Virginia

Elaine I. Tuomanen, MD
Head of Laboratory of Molecular Infectious Diseases
Division of Infectious Diseases
The Rockefeller University
New York, New York

Richard J. Whitley, MD
Loeb Eminent Scholar Chair in Pediatrics
Professor of Pediatrics, Microbiology, and Medicine
Children's Hospital
Birmingham, Alabama

To Karin and Françoise

1 Pathophysiology of Alterations in the Blood-Brain Barrier During Bacterial Meningitis

GREGORY C. TOWNSEND
W. MICHAEL SCHELD

Bacterial meningitis remains a significant health problem worldwide, particularly in developing countries and also in the United States. Data from recent comprehensive surveys on the epidemiology and outcomes of bacterial meningitis in the United States, collected in the late 1970s to early 1980s, suggest that approximately 18,000 to 25,000 people are affected yearly (1,2). Although the introduction and widespread use of the *Haemophilus influenzae* type b vaccine have dramatically reduced the incidence of bacterial meningitis among children in this country, the outcome for victims of bacterial meningitis has not changed appreciably in the last 15 years. The mortality associated with bacterial meningitis is approximately 10%, and long-term sequelae such as hearing loss, seizures, and mental retardation are seen in up to 30% to 50% of survivors. A greater understanding of the mechanisms that lead to the consequences of bacterial meningitis will be required if improvements in these grim statistics are to be made.

The pathophysiology of bacterial meningitis has been the focus of a great deal of investigation during the last 20 years. It has become apparent from results of studies using experimental animal models and from clinical trials that the pathophysiologic sequelae of bacterial meningitis are due, in large part, to the response of the host to the presence of bacteria within the subarachnoid space (3–5). These host responses may be elicited by intact bacteria or by bacterial products, including lipopolysaccharide (LPS) and lipoteichoic acids. The inflammatory response includes the entry of leukocytes into the subarachnoid space and the release of soluble inflammatory mediators such as cytokines, prostaglandins, platelet-activating factor (PAF), proteolytic enzymes, and reactive nitrogen and/or oxygen species. The presence of leukocytes and inflammatory mediators within the subarachnoid space results in alterations in the homeostatic mechanisms operating within the central nervous system (CNS).

The blood-brain barrier (BBB) is a unique functional part of the vasculature within the CNS that contributes to the maintenance of homeostasis. The choroid plexus, arachnoid membrane, and cerebral microvascular endothelium represent the structural correlates of the BBB. The primary site of breakdown of the BBB during bacterial meningitis appears to be the microvascular endothelium. The endothelial cells of the cerebral microvasculature exhibit properties not observed in the general circulation, such as intercellular tight junctions, rare plasmalemmal vesicles, and high electrical resistance (Table 1-1). Ordinarily these unique properties allow this endothelium to restrict the passage of circulating cells, macromolecules, and ions from the vascular space into the subarachnoid space or into the interstitium of the cerebral parenchyma.

During bacterial meningitis, the permeability of the BBB increases. In the clinical setting, this can be observed by comparison of concentrations of specific proteins (e.g., albumin, immunoglobulin) in the cerebrospinal fluid (CSF) and blood. In animal models, more direct measurements can be made by calculating entry into the CSF or brain tissue of a systemically administered radiolabeled molecule (6,7). It is likely that the increased permeability contributes to the generation of cerebral edema and thus to increased intracranial pressure. Ultimately these pathophysiologic changes lead to neuronal dysfunction and death, and are therefore responsible for some of the acute clinical manifestations and long-term complications associated with bacterial meningitis. Understanding the processes that contribute to alterations in the BBB during bacterial meningitis, and the mechanisms responsible for these processes, may lead to the development of adjunctive therapeutic methods that will improve the outcome of the disease.

As noted already, the cells of the cerebral microvasculature that comprise the BBB possess several unique and interesting features (8,9). Cerebral microvascular endothelial cells have few plasmalemmal vesicles and rarely demonstrate pinocytosis. Cytoplasmic fenestrations or channels are also lacking in these cells. Cell-cell connections possess continuous five-layer tight junctions that demonstrate high electrical resistance. The tight junction, or zonula occludens, is characterized by the presence of specialized proteins such as zonula occludens–associated protein 1 (ZO-1).

Table 1-1. Representative Differences Between Properties of Microvascular Endothelium of the Blood-Brain Barrier and of Most Other Vascular Beds

Property	*Blood-Brain Barrier Vasculature*	*Other Vasculature*
Tight junctions	Present	Generally absent
Pinocytosis	Rare	Abundant
Fenestrae	Rare	Abundant
Electrical resistance	High (~2000 $\Omega \cdot cm^2$)	Low (< 100 $\Omega \cdot cm^2$)
Perivascular space	Small	Extensive
Specific enzymes such as		
Alkaline phosphatase	Present	Absent
γ-Glutamyl transpeptidase		
Monoamine oxidase		
Specific glucose transporter	Present	Absent
Specific receptors for proteins such as		
Transferrin	Present	Absent
Insulin		
Cellular mitochondrial content	~10%	< 5%

Because of these properties, and although lipid-soluble molecules cross the BBB readily, there is little transcellular or intercellular transport of other macromolecules or ions, except those facilitated by specific transport mechanisms. These characteristics are influenced by associated CNS cells, such as astrocytes, and by the underlying basement membrane. It must be noted that regions of the brain involved in neuroendocrine feedback, generally termed *circumventricular organs,* lack a complete barrier. Cerebral microvascular endothelial cells in these regions exhibit open intercellular junctions and fenestrations. The barrier function in these areas is augmented by differentiation of ependymal cells into barrier-forming cells.

The ability of the BBB to restrict the passage of macromolecules is compromised during bacterial meningitis in association with structural and functional alterations in the cerebral microvasculature. Examination of cerebral microvascular endothelial cells obtained after the induction of experimental meningitis in rats reveals an increase in the density of cytoplasmic plasmalemmal vesicles. Complete separation of the intercellular tight junctions is also observed. These findings are consistent among animal models in which meningitis is induced by *H. influenzae, Streptococcus pneumoniae,* or *Neisseria meningitidis* (7). In situ perfusion of colloidal gold-albumin complexes demonstrates that the venular segments of the pia-arachnoid microvasculature represent the primary site of albumin passage. The albumin passes by a paracellular route through open intercellular junctions. Albumin is taken up by plasmalemmal vesicles of meningeal arterioles, but there is little transendothelial passage by this route (10).

Although the localization of BBB disruption and the ultrastructural changes associated with this process have been identified, it is not entirely clear how the bacteria or bacterial products exert their effects on cerebral microvascular endothelial cells (or other sites of the BBB) to disrupt the BBB in bacterial meningitis. Establishing a possible direct causal relationship between bacteria and BBB disruption is difficult for two main reasons. First, the only animal models in which systemically administered bacteria have been demonstrated to elicit meningitis involve infant rats, pigs, and primates. These models are impractical because of the small sample sizes obtained (in the former) or the expense (in the latter two). In all of the other models, in which most of the research has been conducted, the bacteria or other test substances must be inoculated directly into the CSF, bypassing the cerebral circulation. This does not permit examination of the effects of circulating bacteria on cerebral microvascular endothelial cells. Second, in intact in vivo models, it is not possible to eliminate the contributing effects of other host cells and of the many endogenous mediators that might be produced in response to the significant concentrations of bacteria within the cerebral circulation. Therefore, these models do not provide information regarding the direct effect of bacteria within the intravascular space on cerebral microvascular endothelial cells.

The most direct evidence, then, for a possible direct causal effect of bacteria on increased BBB permeability in meningitis comes from in vitro studies. In vitro studies have demonstrated that adherence of some strains of N. *meningitidis* and of S. *pneumoniae* to human umbilical vein endothelial cells in culture may result in disruption and widening of intercellular junctions (11,12). While these findings cannot be extended to cerebral microvascular endothelial cells with certainty, they suggest the possibility that the bacteria associated with meningitis may be able to disrupt the BBB.

More specific evidence supporting this possibility has come from studies performed with cultured cerebral microvascular endothelial cells. In one study, monolayers of rat cortical cerebral microvascular endothelial cells were exposed to *H. influenzae* LPS (or more properly, lipo-oligosaccharide (LOS)) for 4 hours. This resulted in a significant increase (approximately 2.0–2.5-fold) in the permeability of the cell layer to radioactive albumin during a 1-hour measurement interval. This increase was not associated with cell death as assessed by release of lactate dehydrogenase into the tissue culture medium (13).

In another study, monolayers of bovine cortical cerebral microvascular endothelial cells were exposed to live *H. influenzae*, killed *H. influenzae*, a cell-free filtrate of *H. influenzae* culture medium, or *H. influenzae* LPS. The endothelial cells thus exposed exhibited rounding up, detachment, fragmentation, and death, resulting in disruption of the monolayer. In experiments with live *H. influenzae*, these changes were maximal after 4 to 6 hours of exposure. The same effects were also achieved with exposure of the monolayer to *Escherichia coli* LPS, and were blocked by pretreatment with polymyxin B, an antibiotic that binds to and inactivates the lipid A component of LPS (14). These results, occurring in the absence of host cell mediators, suggest a direct effect of these bacterial components on the permeability of the BBB.

The study just described (14) also demonstrated that the presence of serum is necessary for *H. influenzae* to disrupt the bovine cerebral microvascular endothelial cell monolayer; endothelial monolayers remained confluent and intact when incubated with LPS or with live *H. influenzae* in serum-deficient medium. Cytopathic effects of LPS on cerebral microvascular endothelial cells were also blocked by the addition of a monoclonal antibody against CD14; CD14 is a protein found on leukocytes (monocytes, macrophages, and polymorphonuclear leukocytes) and in serum that participates in the responses of cells to LPS.

Results of other studies also suggest that CD14 mediates the effects of LPS on cerebral microvascular endothelial cells. The cytotoxic effects of *H. influenzae* LOS on bovine cerebral microvascular endothelial cells were blocked by incubation of the cells in serum containing a monoclonal antibody against CD14, or in medium depleted of serum. The addition of soluble CD14 to serum-free medium restored the cytotoxic effects (15). In another experiment, LPS-induced protein tyrosine phosphorylation in human and bovine cerebral microvascular endothelial cells was inhibited by pretreatment with anti–human CD14 monoclonal antibody (16). One study demonstrated that the cytotoxic effects of *H. influenzae* LPS on human umbilical vein endothelial cells can be blocked by anti-CD14 antibody or by immunodepletion of serum of CD14. The cytotoxic responses were restored by addition of soluble CD14 (17). Thus, the deleterious effects of bacteria on the BBB depend at least in part on some factor(s) present in the serum that may act by facilitating binding of bacterial components such as LPS to the endothelial cells.

The results of the above-mentioned experiments, performed in the absence of eukaryotic cells other than endothelial cells, suggest that other host cells are not necessary for disruption of the BBB to occur during bacterial meningitis. However, it is possible that in vivo the increased BBB permeability observed in bacterial meningitis is mediated largely by adherent activated leukocytes and by circulating host-derived inflammatory mediators.

Among the many endogenous proinflammatory mediators that may contribute to disruption of the BBB during bacterial meningitis is nitric oxide. Nitric oxide is a ubiquitous intercellular messenger that causes vascular endothelial cell relaxation and is responsible for the maintenance of vascular tone. Nitric oxide also acts as a neurotransmitter.

After release from the cell that generates it, nitric oxide diffuses into neighboring target cells, where it interacts with specific molecular targets such as heme iron, iron-sulfur complexes, and DNA. Many of the effects of nitric oxide are probably mediated by activation of the heme iron–containing enzyme guanylate cyclase, which produces cyclic guanosine monophosphate (cGMP), which in turn activates other cellular processes. The interaction of nitric oxide with iron-sulfur complexes may affect enzymes associated with DNA replication and mitochondrial respiration. Among its potential pathologic effects is its apparent ability to inhibit mitochondrial respiration (18).

Nitric oxide may contribute directly or indirectly to the increased BBB permeability observed in bacterial meningitis. It is possible that relaxation of the vascular smooth musculature in response to nitric oxide is accompanied by increased width of the intercellular junction, such as is observed in bacterial meningitis. Inactivation of enzymes associated with mitochondrial respiration (18) and with DNA replication by chelation of iron cofactors may lead to cellular dysfunction.

Nitric oxide may also contribute indirectly through its derivatives. Nitric oxide and superoxide (O_2^-), an oxygen-derived free radical produced by phagocytes and endothelial cells, may combine to form peroxynitrite (ONOO–), a powerful oxidant (19–21). Peroxynitrite or one of its decomposition products, hydroxyl radical (HO·) (22,23), may cause oxidation of amino acid moieties or lipid peroxidation (24,25), thus interfering with normal cellular function and membrane integrity. Peroxynitrite may also inhibit mitochondrial respiration (26). These effects may in turn lead to destabilization of the BBB, as well as to neuronal dysfunction and death.

That nitric oxide contributes to the disruption of the BBB during bacterial meningitis is supported by data from animal models. One study demonstrated increased concentrations of nitrite, one of the metabolites of nitric oxide, in the CSF of rats with experimental *H. influenzae* meningitis. This study also revealed a correlation between CSF nitrite concentrations and an increase in percent BBB permeability to systemically administered radiolabeled albumin (27). In another study, inhibition of nitric oxide synthase reduced CNS nitric oxide production and resulted in attenuation in increases in BBB permeability (28). These studies suggest strongly that nitric oxide production contributes to alterations of the BBB during bacterial meningitis.

Other endogenous mediators that may contribute directly or indirectly to alterations in BBB permeability include prostaglandins, PAF, toxic oxygen intermediates, and proteolytic enzymes. Although data regarding the relevance of these to BBB disturbance during bacterial meningitis are lacking, the known characteristics of all of these molecules point to the possibility that they may cause endothelial cell dysfunction and thus compromise the integrity of the BBB. Some data from experiments involving PAF support this. Intracisternal inoculation of large doses of PAF in one animal model resulted in increased CSF concentrations of protein, an indirect measure of BBB permeability (29). In another model, smaller doses of PAF inoculated intracisternally were synergistic with *H. influenzae* LOS in eliciting increased BBB permeability to systemically administered radiolabeled albumin (30).

All of the above-mentioned molecules proposed to be potential mediators of BBB disruption are products of leukocytes, particularly polymorphonuclear neutrophils. There is a great deal of evidence that leukocytes contribute significantly to the generation of increased BBB permeability during bacterial meningitis. For example, a few studies demonstrated that cyclophosphamide-induced neutropenia protects against increases in BBB permeability in animal models of *H. influenzae* meningitis (31–33). An important step in the appearance of leukocytes at the site of infection is the increased expression and avidity of adhesion molecules that facilitate binding of leukocytes to endothelial cells. Several studies showed that antagonism of leukocyte–endothelial cell adhesion (by proteins that mimic ligands for leukocyte–endothelial cell adhesion molecules or by monoclonal antibodies directed against adhesion molecules) attenuates increases in CSF protein concentrations or in permeability to systemically administered radiolabeled albumin, in association with reduced CSF pleocytosis (29,34–38).

Other leukocyte-derived factors that may contribute to increased permeability of the BBB are the cytokines, particularly interleukin (IL)-1 and tumor necrosis factor (TNF). In vitro models of the BBB demonstrated that these cytokines are capable of inducing decreased electrical resistance across a cell culture monolayer (39). In animal models, intracisternal (but not intravenous) inoculation of these cytokines results in increases in many of the indices of subarachnoid space inflammation, including BBB permeability, and administration of anticytokine antibodies reduces BBB permeability (40–42). In addition, BBB permeability in patients with bacterial meningitis correlates with CSF TNF concentrations (43).

Importantly, it must be noted that the effects of administration of these cytokines can be blocked by preinduction of neutropenia in animal models (41) or by exposure to indomethacin (a cyclo-oxygenase inhibitor) in vitro (39). Taken together, these results suggest that IL-1 and TNF contribute to alterations in BBB permeability. To some extent, these alterations depend on the presence of leukocytes, and in the absence of leukocytes, are mediated at least in part by the generation of phospholipid derivatives. It is likely that in vivo the effects of these cytokines are mediated largely by leukocyte products (as noted already) whose synthesis is increased in response to cytokine stimulation.

Regardless of the nature of the stimulus for BBB damage, the ultrastructural and functional changes observed result from changes at the cellular and subcellular level. To date, little research has been performed to investigate this issue as it relates specifically to bacterial meningitis (e.g., stimulation of cerebral microvascular endothelial cells with LPS or with cytokines). In general, it is known that a variety of stimuli promote increased endothelial cell adenylate or guanylate cyclase activity, which results in increased intracellular concentrations of cyclic adenosine monophosphate (cAMP) or cGMP, respectively. These are in turn associated with calcium influx into the endothelial cells and activation of phospholipases and protein kinases. Although the precise mechanisms are unknown, it is thought that these changes induce the formation of pinocytotic vesicles and result in cytoskeletal changes that cause opening of the tight junctions. Indeed, infusion of lipid-soluble derivatives of cAMP or cGMP, or infusion of histamine (a potent activator of adenylate cyclase), is associated with increased pinocytosis and macromolecular transport in cultured cerebral microvascular endothelial cells (44).

A few investigators extended this research to areas relevant to bacterial meningitis. In one study, exposure of rat cerebral microvascular endothelial cells to *H. influenzae* LPS resulted in the production of cAMP and cGMP. Production of cAMP, but not of cGMP, was observed prior to increases in the permeability of the monolayer (13).

A study referenced earlier (16) examined the role of protein tyrosine phosphorylation in endothelial cells stimulated by LPS. Exposure of human or bovine cerebral microvascular endothelial cells to LPS or to lipid A resulted in rapid and dose-dependent tyrosine phosphorylation of several proteins. These changes were detectable within 15 minutes of exposure, were maximal by 30 minutes, and declined by 60 to 90 minutes. Pretreatment of endothelial cells with a tyrosine kinase inhibitor inhibited LPS-stimulated protein tyrosine phosphorylation, lactate dehydrogenase release, and IL-6 release.

A study of the effects of TNF on bovine cerebral microvascular endothelial cells demonstrated that after 1-hour exposure of the luminal membrane to recombinant hu-

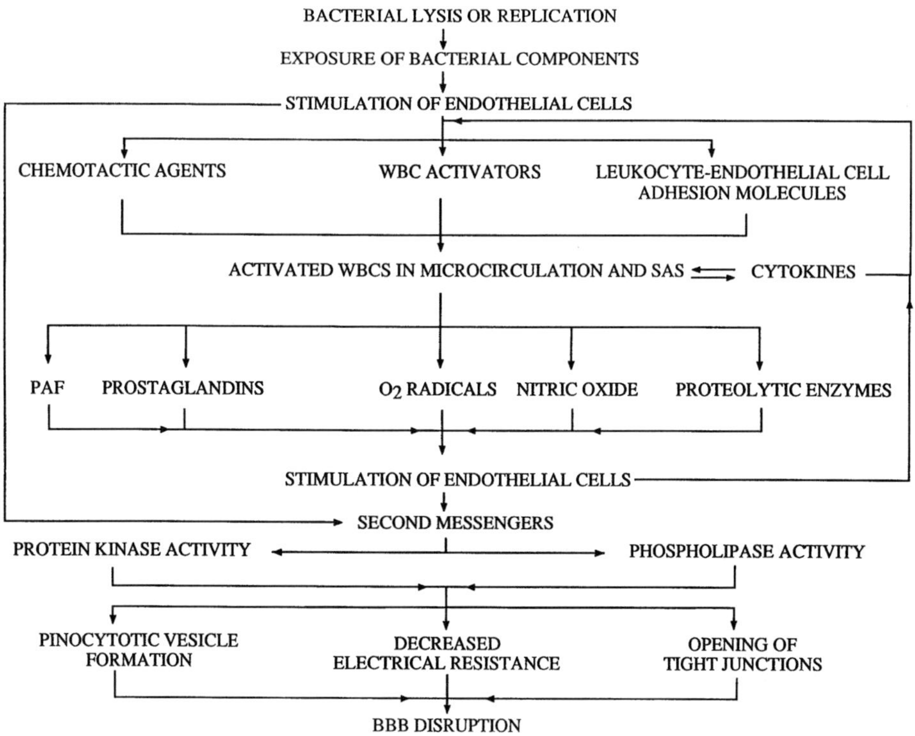

Figure 1-1. Hypothetical scheme of the pathophysiology of alterations in the blood-brain barrier (BBB) during bacterial meningitis. WBC = white blood cell; SAS = subarachnoid space; PAF = platelet-activating factor.

man TNF-α, there was no increase in the transendothelial passage of either sucrose or inulin for up to 4 hours. However, at 16 hours after the 1-hour exposure, there was a significant increase in the permeability of the cerebral microvascular endothelial cell monolayers for both markers. These increases in permeability were associated with reorganization of F-actin filaments into stress fibers (45).

The results of these studies indicate that stimulation of cerebral microvascular endothelial cells with LPS or with endogenous inflammatory mediators may result in the generation of intracellular second messenger systems. This likely initiates a cascade of intracellular events that result in loosening of the tight junctions and increased pinocytosis, thus compromising the integrity of the BBB.

In summary, alterations in the BBB during bacterial meningitis are the result of a complex interplay of processes involving bacterial and host components. A hypothetical scheme of these processes is outlined in Figure 1-1. Because of the crucial role played by the BBB in CNS homeostasis, and because of the proposed contribution of increases in permeability of the BBB to the pathophysiologic consequences of bacterial meningitis, it is possible that an understanding of these processes may help to identify targets to which effective adjunctive therapies for bacterial meningitis can be directed.

REFERENCES

1 Schlech WF III, Ward JI, Band JD, et al. Bacterial meningitis in the United States, 1978 through 1981: the National Bacterial Meningitis Surveillance Study. *JAMA* 1985;253:1749–1754.

2 Wenger JD, Hightower AW, Facklam RR, et al, the Bacterial Meningitis Study Group. Bacterial meningitis in the United States, 1986: report of a multistate surveillance study. *J Infect Dis* 1990;162:1316–1323.

3 Quagliarello V, Scheld WM. Bacterial meningitis: pathogenesis, pathophysiology, and progress. *N Engl J Med* 1992;327:864–872.

4 Pfister H-W, Fontana A, Täuber MG, et al. Mechanisms of brain injury in bacterial meningitis: workshop summary. *Clin Infect Dis* 1994;19:463–479.

5 Sáez-Llorens X, Ramilo O, Mustafa MM, et al. Molecular pathophysiology of bacterial meningitis: current concepts and therapeutic implications. *J Pediatr* 1990;116:671–684.

6 Boje KM. Cerebrovascular permeability changes during experimental meningitis in the rat. *J Pharmacol Exp Ther* 1995;274:1199–1203.

7 Quagliarello VJ, Long WJ, Scheld WM. Morphologic alterations of the blood-brain barrier with experimental meningitis in the rat: temporal sequence and role of encapsulation. *J Clin Invest* 1986;77:1084–1095.

8 Betz AL. An overview of the multiple functions of the blood-brain barrier. *NIDA Res Monogr* 1992;120:54–71.

9 Bradbury MWB. The blood-brain barrier. *Exp Physiol* 1993;78:453–472.

10 Quagliarello VJ, Ma A, Stukenbrok H, Palade GE. Ultrastructural localization of albumin transport across the cerebral microvasculature during experimental meningitis in the rat. *J Exp Med* 1991;174:657–672.

11 Geelen S, Bhattacharyya C, Tuomanen E. The cell wall mediates pneumococcal attachment to and cytopathology in human endothelial cells. *Infect Immun* 1993;61:1538–1543.

12 Virji M, Kayhty H, Ferguson DJP, et al. The role of pili in the interactions of pathogenic *Neisseria* with cultured human endothelial cells. *Mol Microbiol* 1991;5:1831–1841.

13 Tunkel AR, Rosser SW, Hansen EJ, Scheld WM. *Haemophilus influenzae* type b lipopolysaccharide (LPS)-induced formation of cAMP and cGMP in cerebral microvascular endothelial cells (MECs). In: *30th Interscience conference on antimicrobial agents and chemotherapy*. Atlanta, GA: 1990.

14 Patrick D, Betts J, Frey EA, et al. *Haemophilus influenzae* lipopolysaccharide disrupts confluent monolayers of bovine brain endothelial cells via a serum-dependent cytotoxic pathway. *J Infect Dis* 1992;165:865–872.

15 Arditi M, Zhou J, Dorio R, et al. Endotoxin-mediated endothelial cell injury and activation: role of soluble CD14. *Infect Immun* 1995; 61:3149–3156.

16 Arditi M, Zhou J, Torres M, et al. Lipopolysaccharide stimulates the tyrosine phosphorylation of mitogen-activated protein kinases p44, p42, and p41 in vascular endothelial cells in a soluble CD14-dependent manner. Role of protein tyrosine phosphorylation in lipopolysaccharide-induced stimulation of endothelial cells. *J Immunol* 1995;155:3994–4003.

17 Frey EA, Miller DS, Jahr TG, et al. Soluble CD14 participates in the response of cells to lipopolysaccharide. *J Exp Med* 1992;176: 1665–1671.

18 Cleeter M, Cooper J, Darley-Usmar V, et al. Reversible inhibition of cytochrome c oxidase, the terminal enzyme of the mitochondrial respiratory chain, by nitric oxide: implications for neurodegenerative diseases. *FEBS Lett* 1994;345:50–54.

19 Kooy N, Royall J. Agonist-induced peroxynitrite production from endothelial cells. *Arch Biochem Biophys* 1994;310:352–359.

20 Ischiropoulos H, Ling Z, Chen J, et al. Peroxynitrite-mediated tyrosine nitration catalyzed by superoxide dismutase. *Arch Biochem Biophys* 1992;298:431–437.

21 Blough N, Zafiriou O. Reaction of superoxide with nitric oxide to form peroxynitrite in alkaline aqueous solution. Inorg Chem 1985;24: 3502–3504.

22 Beckman JS, Beckman TW, Chen J, et al. Apparent hydroxyl radical production by peroxynitrite: implications for endothelial injury from nitric oxide and superoxide. *Proc Natl Acad Sci USA* 1990;87:1620–1624.

23 Hogg N, Darley-Usmar VM, Wilson MT, Moncada S. Production of hydroxyl radicals from the simultaneous generation of superoxide and nitric oxide. *Biochem J* 1992;281:419–424.

24 Radi R, Beckman JS, Bush KM, Freeman BA. Peroxynitrite-induced membrane lipid peroxidation: the cytotoxic potential of superoxide and nitric oxide. *Arch Biochem Biophys* 1991;288:481–487.

25 Radi R, Beckman JS, Bush KM, Freeman BA. Peroxynitrite oxidation of sulfhydryls. *J Biol Chem* 1991;266:4244–4250.

26 Radi R, Rodriguez M, Castro L, Telleri R. Inhibition of mitochondrial electron transport by peroxynitrite. *Arch Biochem Biophys* 1994; 308:89–95.

27 Buster BL, Weintrob AC, Townsend GC, Scheld WM. The potential role of nitric oxide in the pathophysiology of experimental bacterial meningitis in the rat. *Infect Immun* 1995;63:3835–3839.

28 Boje KM. Inhibition of nitric oxide synthase partially attenuates alterations in the blood-cerebrospinal fluid barrier during experimental meningitis in the rat. *Eur J Pharmacol* 1995; 272:297–300.

29 Cabellos C, MacIntyre DE, Forrest M, et al. Differing roles for platelet-activating factor during inflammation of the lung and subarachnoid space: the special case of *Streptococcus pneumoniae*. *J Infect Dis* 1992;90:612–618.

30 Townsend GC, Scheld WM. Platelet-activating factor augments meningeal inflammation elicited by *Haemophilus influenzae* lipooligosaccharide in an animal model of meningitis. *Infect Immun* 1994;62:3739–3744.

31 Wispelwey B, Lesse AJ, Hansen EJ, Scheld WM. *Haemophilus influenzae* lipopolysaccharide-induced blood brain barrier permeability during experimental meningitis in the rat. *J Clin Invest* 1988;82:1339–1346.

32 Wispelwey B, Hansen EJ, Scheld WM. *Haemophilus influenzae* outer membrane vesicle-induced blood-brain barrier permeability during experimental meningitis. *Infect Immun* 1989;57:2559–2562.

33 Lesse AJ, Moxon ER, Zwahlen A, Scheld WM. Role of cerebrospinal fluid pleocytosis and *Haemophilus influenzae* type b capsule on blood brain barrier permeability during experimental meningitis in the rat. *J Clin Invest* 1988;82:102–109.

34 Granert C, Raud J, Xie X, et al. Inhibition of leukocyte rolling with polysaccharide fucoidin prevents pleocytosis in experimental meningitis in the rabbit. *J Clin Invest* 1994;93:929–936.

35 Rozdzinski E, Jones T, Burnette WN, et al. Antiinflammatory effects in experimental meningitis of prokaryotic peptides that mimic selectins. *J Infect Dis* 1993;168:1422–1428.

36 Rozdzinski E, Sandros J, van der Flier M, et al. Inhibition of leukocyte-endothelial cell interactions and inflammation by peptides from a bacterial adhesin which mimic coagulation factor X. *J Infect Dis* 1995;172:785–793.

37 Townsend GC, Musso GF, Starzyk RM, Scheld WM. *Bordetella pertussis* filamentous hemagglutinin peptide F20 reduces subarachnoid space inflammation in experimental *Haemophilus influenzae* type b bacterial meningitis. In: *34th Interscience conference on antimicrobial agents and chemotherapy*. Orlando, FL, 1994: Abstract G59.

38 Tuomanen EI, Saukkonen K, Sande S, et al. Reduction of inflammation, tissue damage, and mortality in bacterial meningitis treated with

monoclonal antibodies against adhesion-promoting receptors of leukocytes. *J Exp Med* 1989;170:959–969.

39 de Vries HE, Blom-Roosemalen MC, van Oosten M, et al. The influence of cytokines on the integrity of the blood-brain barrier in vitro. *J Neuroimmunol* 1996;64:37–43.

40 Kim KS, Wass CA, Cross AS, Opal SM. Modulation of blood-brain barrier permeability by tumor necrosis factor and antibody to tumor necrosis factor in the rat. *Lymphokine Cytokine Res* 1992;11:293–298.

41 Quagliarello VJ, Wispelwey B, Long WJ, Scheld WM. Recombinant human interleukin-1 induces meningitis and blood-brain injury in the rat: characterization and comparison with tumor necrosis factor. *J Clin Invest* 1991;87:1360–1366.

42 Megyeri P, Abraham CS, Temesvari P, et al. Recombinant human tumor necrosis factor alpha constricts pial arterioles and increases blood-brain barrier permeability in newborn piglets. *Neurosci Lett* 1992;148:137–140.

43 Sharief MK, Ciardi M, Thompson EJ. Blood-brain barrier damage in patients with bacterial meningitis: association with tumor necrosis factor-alpha but not interleukin-1 beta. *J Infect Dis* 1992;166:350–358.

44 Joó F, Lengyel I, Kovács J, Penke B. Regulation of transendothelial transport in the cerebral microvessels: the role of second messenger-generating systems. *Prog Brain Res* 1992;91:177–187.

45 Deli MA, Descamps L, Dehouck MP, et al. Exposure of tumor necrosis factor-alpha to luminal membrane of bovine brain capillary endothelial cells cocultured with astrocytes induces a delayed increase of permeability and cytoplasmic stress fiber formation of actin. *J Neurosci Res* 1995;41:717–726.

2

Leukocyte Migration into the Central Nervous System

WILLIAM F. HICKEY

Many pathologic conditions of the central nervous system (CNS) develop when leukocytes of various types enter the brain or spinal cord in response to a variety of stimuli. Diseases ranging from viral encephalitis and brain abscess to multiple sclerosis (MS) and Wallerian degeneration are defined by the influx of granulocytes, T cells, B cells, and macrophages into the brain parenchyma associated with tissue damage of varying extent and severity. Yet, in the development of these inflammatory processes, the "immunologic privilege" of the CNS must be overcome.

Immunologic privilege of the nervous system is a phenomenon defined by a number of experimental observations and physiologic features. In a healthy state, the CNS is devoid of identifiable leukocytes (1–4). Neutrophils and plasma cells are never encountered, and T cells and macrophages are very rare but detectable. The major histocompatibility complex (MHC) molecules required for presentation of antigen to $CD4^+$ and $CD8^+$ T cells are virtually undetectable (4–6). Moreover, allogeneic and in some circumstances even xenogeneic tissue grafts survive when placed in the brain, but would be rapidly rejected if placed elsewhere in the body (7,8). Finally, there is the phenomenon of the blood-brain barrier (BBB) (9). This is the physiologic result of the anatomic structure of the cerebral capillaries. In the CNS small blood vessels are characterized by endothelial cells with tight junctions at their borders. Also, the endothelial cells are not fenestrated; that is, they do not have the transcellular pores found in capillary endothelial cells of other organs. The immunologic consequence of this endothelial barrier is that there is no simple diffusion of soluble substances from the plasma into the tissue fluid of the CNS. Thus, serum proteins, including elements of the complement and coagulation systems and all classes of antibodies, are effectively excluded from the nervous system environment. Finally, the vascular surface of the endothelial cells expresses fewer types of adhesion molecules at lower levels than what is found on comparable cells in other bodily sites; these are the molecules required by leukocytes to cross the endothelium and enter the tissue. Thus, as a result of all this the CNS exists in a condition that is not readily induced to become inflamed. Yet, inflammation does develop and cells and proteins from the blood find their way into the nervous system. How does this occur?

Leukocyte migration across an endothelial cell layer is a carefully controlled process (3,4,6,10). The state of the endothelial cell is critical in permitting or inhibiting this occurrence. The interaction of hematogenous cells with the endothelium, and ultimately their extravasation into an organ, involves a process currently believed to involve three general steps: a) loose interaction between the leukocyte and the endothelium, b) firm binding to the endothelial cell, and c) emigration from the vascular lumen and penetration of or crossing the endothelial basement membrane (6,11–15). While it remains possible that such "homing receptors" or "molecular addressins" will be discovered, it appears that the CNS endothelium employs the same adhesion molecules that function on leukocytes and activated endothelial cells (e.g., high endothelial venules (HEVs) in lymphoid organs) elsewhere in the body.

Adhesion molecules belonging to three broad classes function in this process: a) selectins (12,13,16–18), b) integrins (19,20), and c) molecules belonging to the immunoglobulin supergene family (20,21). The mechanism of leukocyte attachment and movement out of a vessel has been the subject of a number of reviews (11,18,20–22). When emigration occurs, leukocytes make loose contact with the endothelium via C-type lectins, or "selectin" molecules producing a "rolling" motion (11–13,18). E-selectin seems to be involved in both neutrophil and $CD4^+$ T-cell adhesion; L-selectin seems to be more specifically related to T-cell homing to lymph nodes (18). The transient interaction between leukocytes and endothelial cells producing the phenomenon of leukocyte rolling along the endothelium is dictated in part by E- and P-selectins (6,11,12,16,18). However, because some circulating activated leukocytes can interact with endothelial cells that have not themselves been activated, it is probable that some lectin-like molecules are constitutively expressed by the endothelium of a noninflamed organ.

The leukocyte slows and sticks to the endothelial cell in a process mediated by a diverse collection of adhesion molecules including PECAM, vascular cell adhesion molecule-1 (VCAM-1), very late antigen-4 (VLA-4), (lymphocyte function–associated antigen-1 (LFA-1), Mac-1, and the intercellular adhesion molecules (ICAMs) (18,23–25). During this step the leukocyte firmly attaches to the endothelium using molecules of the integrin and immunoglobulin supergene family groups (6,18,26). It is possible that a nervous system–specific addressin exists, although there is no current evidence for it. Addressins are complex glycoproteins on the vascular surface of specific endothelial cells that are believed to confer leukocyte homing properties to the sites where they are expressed. While no molecules with this role are present on normal CNS endothelial cells, they can be detected in inflamed areas (27–32).

Once firmly attached, leukocytes pass through the endothelium, degrade the basement membrane focally, and enter the parenchyma. These later steps are not as completely defined as is the attachment phase, but involve elaboration of appropriate basement membrane degrading enzymes and vectorial movement out of the vessel lumen (6,33–36). The role of basement membrane degrading enzymes might prove critical; administration of exogenous sulfated polysaccharides has proved effective in blocking the development of experimental allergic encephalomyelitis (EAE), possibly by preventing T-cell access to the CNS by competitive inhibition of these enzymes (34,36). Willenborg et al. (36) showed that the mannose-6-phosphate receptor potentially plays a role in this process. Whether this receptor actually interacts with phosphorylated sugar moieties on cell surface molecules, or anchors enzymes to the cell's surface for membrane attachment is still being studied; however, blockage of the mannose-6-phosphate receptor inhibits cell migration into the CNS and blocks clinical EAE (36).

It should be noted that these numerous analyses of the interaction of leukocytes with vascular endothelium were performed under a wide variety of in vitro and in vivo conditions. Such studies frequently differ with respect to the state of the endothelium used (activated or nonactivated), the cytokines used to activate the endothelium (typically tumor necrosis factor (TNF)-α or interferon (IFN)-γ, or both), the source of the endothelium, the species from which the endothelium and leukocytes were derived, the type of leukocyte being investigated for migration, and the activation state and culture conditions for the leukocyte. The available data, therefore, demonstrate a wide variation of "critical molecules" both for the slowing and "rolling" of cells on vessels and for the adhesion to vessels walls (11,12,37–39).

Most endothelial cells in the body, especially those of the CNS, are not normally stimulated. They can be activated by strong systemic immune responses (graft-versus-host disease (GVHD)) or by circulating cytokines (IFN, TNF). When inflammation develops in the CNS, the endothelial cells can develop a phenotype resembling HEVs of immune tissues with respect to their adhesion molecule expression (27–30). Moreover, recent evidence also suggests that the interaction or mutual ligation of adhesion molecules between lymphocytes and endothelial cells may initiate signal transduction, augmenting or perpetuating their activation (19,40). Thus, a complete understanding of the in vivo migration of leukocytes into the CNS must take into account not only the adhesion molecules typically used by specific types of leukocytes under in vitro conditions, but also the relative activation states of the leukocyte and endothelium, the cytokines to which the cells have been exposed, and the presence of a preexisting inflammatory focus in the area. The importance of these variables will be made obvious hereafter.

T CELLS

The mechanism of T-lymphocyte entry into the CNS is of central importance to a number of neurologic conditions. Unlike granulocytes and macrophages, T cells are highly antigen specific. In addition to the ability of these cells to perform immunologic surveillance of the body's constituents in search of foreign or altered self-antigens, T cells initiate many of the inflammatory conditions of the CNS. These include the viral encephalitides, chronic meningitis, some paraneoplastic conditions, and autoimmune disorders such as MS, to name a few. Understanding the parameters governing the passage of these cells across the CNS endothelium might provide therapeutic opportunities to inhibit or modify the natural course of some severe neurologic conditions.

One research model that has provided numerous insights into T-cell traffic into the CNS is EAE. This autoimmune condition has been used for decades in MS research because it mimics certain features of MS, especially the early phases of the initiation of inflammation (41). EAE as a system is now very well analyzed. It is initiated by $CD4^+$, $CD8^-$, Th1 phenotype T cells specific for myelin or other nervous system antigens (42–45). These T cells must recognize their antigen in the context of MHC class II molecules after arriving in the CNS. The disease can be induced by actively immunizing the test animal with a neural antigen (typically a myelin derivative protein) in emulsion, or by adoptively transferring neural antigen–specific T cells to the animal. After a period of time, chronic inflammation appears in the neural parenchyma and the animal develops a transient, paralytic illness that may relapse thereafter. Since it is a strictly T cell–dependent system, it has proved to be most useful in analyzing how such cells penetrate the nervous system.

In the late 1970s, investigators studying the adoptive transfer of EAE noted that the T cells to be injected were far more effective in initiating the condition when they were activated prior to injection (46,47). Whether the antigen for which the T cells were specific was employed in this activation, or whether a mitogenic lectin was used did not appear to be critical (47). These findings led Wekerle et al. (4) to hypothesize that T cells might be empowered to gain entry to the CNS when they are in the activated state, but not as resting or naive cells.

A subsequent study more extensively delineated the parameters governing T-cell entry into the CNS (48). It appears that activation of a T cell embues it with an ability to enter the CNS rapidly and with ease (48). Moreover, activation is a sine qua non for T cells penetrating the normal, noninflamed neural parenchyma. Naive cells or cells in the resting phase are excluded. However, when activated, cells of both the $CD4^+$ and $CD8^+$ phenotype can enter the CNS regardless of their antigen specificity (i.e., the antigen they seek does not have to be a CNS constituent) or even their MHC compatibility with the host. Thus, cognate recognition of antigen at the endothelial barrier is not required, nor does it play any role in the T cells' passage into the brain or spinal cord. In systems in which such antigen recognition cannot occur because the antigen sought is not a CNS constituent or because the endothelium being crossed is not MHC compatible with the T cells' requirements, the T cells still reach the nervous system (48–50). One additional feature of activated T cells appears to be their apparently random distribution throughout the body following intravenous injection (48). Cells specific for a CNS antigen do not merely go to the CNS; they are found throughout all the organs and tissues of the body. This pattern of distribution also occurs with cells specific for an irrelevant antigen not located in the host into which the cells are injected. Such cells are found in the CNS, peripheral nervous system, eyes, and all sites believed to have some degree of immunologic privilege, including the medulla of the thymus. This apparently random scatter of activated T lymphoblasts would be ideal for the detection of foreign antigens associated with invading pathogens; the antigen would be sought throughout the organism, permitting the inciting antigen no place to "hide" from the host's sensitized T cells. Yet, most organs would not be subjected to the passage of naive, nonstimulated T cells, which are abundant in the circulation.

The rate of entry and accumulation of rat T lymphoblasts in the CNS following infusion differs somewhat between studies. In studies from this laboratory, the T cells were detected in the CNS within 2 hours following infusion (48,50). The concentration of

T cells specific for a non-CNS antigen appeared to peak in the CNS between 9 and 12 hours after injection and thereafter decreased so that by 24 to 48 hours, the concentration had returned to baseline. When the cells were CNS antigen specific, they appeared in the nervous system with the same kinetics, but persisted there in concentrations slightly lower than peak values until inflammation and disease appeared some days later. Work from the laboratory of Willenborg (51) revealed the same rapid entry into the rat nervous system of CNS antigen–specific T lymphoblasts; however, the data suggest a slow, progressive accumulation of such cells in the neural parenchyma until inflammation appears. While both studies (48,51) demonstrated the rapid entry and retention of T cells in the CNS following infusion, they differed with respect to relative levels of T cells found therein during the days before clinical disease becomes obvious. This may be a by-product of the two distinct methods employed to quantify the T cells in the neural parenchyma during this period. Nevertheless, the important features of the rapid entry and persistence of activated T cells in the organ in which they find their antigen, culminating in fully developed chronic inflammation, were common to both studies.

It was known that activated, encephalitogenic T cells rapidly entered many tissues including the thymus (48,52). But with respect to T-cell entry into the CNS, one critical distinction must be made relative to the concept of lymphocyte homing. This phenomenon is associated with the selective traffic of lymphocytes to specific lymphoid compartments in the body by T cells expressing specific homing receptors that have ligands on selected vascular beds—typically the HEVs of lymph nodes or gut-associated lymphoid tissue (31,32,53). Cross et al (54), and previously Trotter et al. (55), noted the accumulation of CNS antigen–specific T cells in the nervous system following intravenous injection. Their observations are completely consonant with the work noted in the previous paragraph; however, the designation of this phenomenon as homing could be challenged somewhat. Homing, to the extent it exists, relates to the passage of naive or memory T cells into selected tissues of the immune system in a nonrandom, preferential manner. These cells are involved in the typical recirculation pattern for lymphocytes that takes them from the blood to immune system tissue, to the lymph, and again to the blood. The movement of activated T cells, at this time, appears to be a random process of antigen seeking that involves all tissues of the body in a near-random process. In both of the studies (54,55) in which homing to the nervous system appeared to be occurring, the animals were killed, and the cells were sought at a time when the disease was evident or inflammation was just beginning. The time points studied were already days after the initial T cells would have entered the CNS to start the process of inflammation; however, infused cells are detected in increased numbers in a nonrandom distribution at this phase of the process. Thus, it appears beneficial to make some distinctions relative to T-cell trafficking into the CNS.

Activated T cells (and not resting lymphocytes) enter the CNS in a nonselective manner regardless of their antigen specificity or MHC restriction requirements. The *entry* is not selective in any manner currently discernible. The antigen-specific part of the process occurs after the antigen has been recognized. The *retention* of activated T cells in the tissue in which they find their antigen is highly selective and specific (48,50). T lymphoblasts specific for the encephalitogenic antigen myelin basic protein rapidly enter and persist in a CNS in which they are able to recognize their antigen in an MHC-compatible environment; they enter with the same kinetics but rapidly disappear from a CNS in which they cannot recognize their antigen due to MHC incompatibility, even though their antigen is there in abundance (48,49). Thus, it must be that persistence in a tissue is a post–antigen recognition event, while the initial entry is not.

Another useful distinction relative to T-cell penetration into the CNS relates to the phase of the inflammatory process at which the T cells are observed there. In the adoptively transferred rat EAE system, the antigen-specific T cells enter the neural parenchyma within a few hours of injection, but disease does not appear for approximately 3 more days. During this time, focal areas of the CNS undergo changes culminating in inflammation and clinically evident paralysis (Fig 2-1). Many, if not most, of the changes occurring immediately before the disease is evident are not antigen specific. The endothelium is changing its phenotype from that of a quiescent, nonactivated state to a fully activated state. Many adhesion molecules that are expressed normally at very low levels are enhanced or their distribution is altered, and other such moieties are expressed de novo, the end result being a transformation of the vasculature to a phenotype noted by some to resemble HEVs (27–30). This alteration of the endothelium is not itself antigen specific, although it occurs only after specific antigen recognition has occurred, permitting inflammation to develop. During the phase of leukocyte accumulation preceding and accompanying the appearance of disease, the attraction of hematogenous cells to the neural parenchyma is not itself antigen specific. It occurs in EAE whether the inciting antigen is myelin basic protein, proteolipid protein, or a nonmyelin antigen. Thus, the *initial entry phase* and antigen recognition—the antigen-specific part of the process of inflammation induction—should be distinguished from the *recruitment phase* during which leukocytes are attracted from the circulation by virtue of the novel adhesion molecule expression and chemokine production occurring at the site of nascent inflammation in the nervous system (56–59). In the rat EAE model, this initial phase must be complete within 24 to 48 hours; the antigen nonspecific recruitment begins with the arrival of natural killer (NK) cells, additional T cells (predominantly memory T cells), and large numbers of monocytes/macrophages.

Distinguishing the initial entry phase from the recruitment phase may be of great use in defining the mechanism by which certain modes of blocking EAE development function. Yednock et al. (60) and Baron et al. (61) showed that EAE can be inhibited by blocking the T-cell activation antigen VLA-4 or its endothelial ligand VCAM-1. In their studies, it was possible to inhibit EAE development by administering monoclonal antibodies to block these molecules even 2 days *after* the encephalitogenic T cells were injected. The same could be said for the work of Archelos et al. (62) who blocked EAE with anti–ICAM-1 antibody. It appears that antibodies against VLA-4, VCAM, or ICAM function by inhibiting the recruitment phase of EAE, that is, blocking the arrival and accumulation of additional leukocytes from the blood, not by stopping the initial entry of T cells or their antigen recognition in the CNS. This may be a very useful therapeutic concept as it may not be necessary to stop the penetration of antigen-specific T lymphoblasts in order to abrogate disease; merely preventing the continued accumulation of hematogenous effector cells may be sufficient.

To understand how T cell–mediated inflammation begins in the CNS, it would be very helpful to know the specific adhesion molecules involved during the initial entry phase

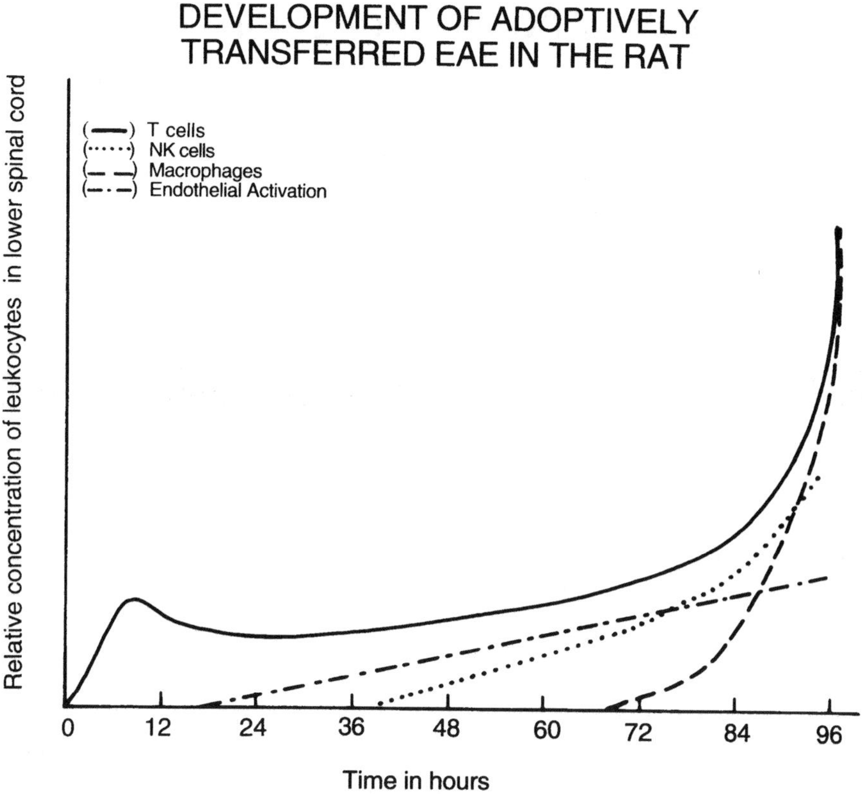

Figure 2-1. The graph shows the relative abundance of leukocytes found in the spinal cord of a rat as experimental autoimmune encephalitis (EAE) develops. Encephalitogenic T cells were injected at 0 hours. T cells persist in the cord until histologic inflammation and clinical disease become evident at 96 hours. At about 48 hours, NK cells begin to accumulate in the CNS. They continue to accumulate as inflammation develops. Activated macrophages are first noted admixed with some T cells about small parenchymal blood vessels during the third day. The augmentation, redistribution, and de novo expression of adhesion molecules on the parenchymal vessel endothelium begin for some molecules as early as 24 to 48 hours, but most changes occur between 48 and 96 hours.

versus the recruitment phase of the process. Unfortunately, the molecule(s) governing the initial penetration remain to be defined (Fig 2-2). Antibodies against VLA-4 and ICAM-1 do not appear to interfere with this process (Hickey WF, Yednock TA, unpublished data). However, during the recruitment phase, VLA-4, ICAM-1, CD11b/CD18 (Mac-1), LFA-1, and possibly the mannose-6-phosphate receptor may play a role (36,60–64). One molecule that does not appear to have any role in the EAE induction process, although its expression is constitutive on CNS endothelium and it is augmented during the induc-

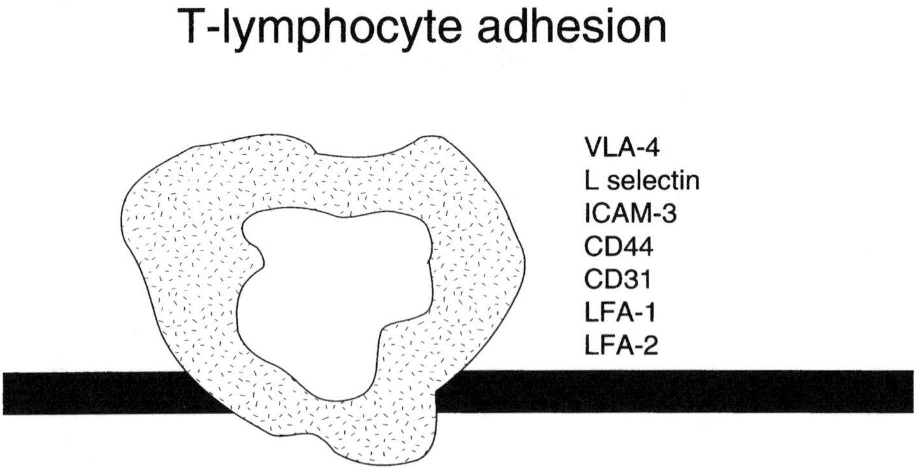

Figure 2-2. Cartoon of a T lymphocyte crossing the endothelium. Listed at the right are a number of adhesion molecules possibly involved in such migration. However, the actual molecules required may vary with the activation state of the endothelium and the T cell itself, and may involve molecules currently undefined. VLA-4 = very late antigen-4; ICAM-3 = intercellular adhesion molecule-3; LFA = leukocyte function–associated antigen.

tion of EAE, is PECAM-1 (CD31) (65), and the significance of ICAM-1 in the process is questioned (64).

There must be additional uninvestigated, if not undefined, adhesion molecules that are active in the initial entry process. Molecule(s) critical to the initial entry of T cells would seem to be required to meet certain conditions. Since only activated T cells enter the CNS, the critical activation-related molecule(s) must not be expressed, or must be expressed in inactive forms or at subfunctional levels, on resting T cells. Also, because T lymphoblasts enter all organs, the molecule(s) must bind to a ligand that is constitutively expressed on the resting, nonactivated capillary and venule endothelium of virtually all tissues and organs. No previously studied adhesion molecule fully meeting these requirements and tested in the EAE model has been demonstrated to block the ability of activated T cells to enter the target organ. However, numerous new molecules probably exist. Studies with B-cell hybridomas produced from hamsters repeatedly immunized with encephalitogenic rat T lymphoblasts have identified more than 20 activation-related cell surface molecules that do not appear to conform to the staining patterns for currently known T-cell activation molecules (Zhao, Hickey WF, unpublished data). Thus, there may be a sizable group of such adhesion molecules that await characterization and functional studies.

While activated T cells enter the CNS readily, what happens to them thereafter is also a subject of interest relative to T-cell trafficking in the nervous system. On this topic investigations over the last 5 years have been very illuminating. Pender et al. (66–68) initially documented the phenomenon of apoptosis of T cells occurring in the CNS of animals with EAE after the disease had become fully established. Thus, there may be a control mechanism that is activated in the nervous system and holds the inflammatory process in check once it has been initiated. T cells entering the CNS that are specific for a myelin antigen causing EAE appear to be selectively targeted for apoptotic death (66–68). Coinjection of cells specific for myelin basic protein with cells specific for ovalbumin (OVA) (not found in the rat CNS) demonstrates that the cells able to recognize their antigen in the CNS become apoptotic to a far greater extent than do cells that cannot find their antigen, although both are present in the CNS inflammatory infiltrate (68). A recent report from Sedgwick's laboratory proposed a probable mechanism for this (69). T cells that recognize their antigen on the surface of parenchymal microglial cells become "terminally differentiated." They are induced to secrete IFN-γ and TNF-α, but their ability to make interleukin (IL)-2 is abrogated (69); without this cytokine they die. This would explain why the neural antigen–specific, inflammation-inducing cells die, but cells not recognizing antigen in the CNS survive. Also, it might provide a regulatory mechanism whereby T cells arriving at a site of inflammation in the nervous system that might recognize their antigen there and widen the destructive process are selectively culled from the responding T-cell repertoire.

In this light it is interesting to note the early arrival of NK cells in the CNS as the recruitment phase of inflammation begins. NK cells produce abundant IFN-γ (70), which is a potent stimulator of MHC class II on microglial cells. This would potentiate the ability of the parenchymal microglial cells to interact with MHC class II–restricted T cells, and doom them to apoptosis as the inflammatory process heats up. The exact role of these early-arriving NK cells is undefined (Zhao, Sedgwick JD, Hickey WF, unpublished data); however, a preliminary report revealed that depletion of NK cells in the EAE model makes the condition a bit more severe (71)—an observation that is consonant with the above-described mechanism of inflammatory regulation by microglial cells. The molecules used by these NK cells to cross the endothelium, and the signals to which they are responding in the preclinical phases of EAE, remain obscure.

B CELLS

B lymphocytes and the plasma cells they differentiate into are the other cells of the immune system embued with a high degree of antigen specificity. While they appear in the CNS in the course of numerous inflammatory conditions, and may be the principal immune cell functioning in conditions like brain abscess and subacute sclerosing panencephalitis (SSPE), very little is known of the mechanisms or parameters controlling their arrival. However, a system developed by Helen Cserr promises to be useful in this regard (72).

If a fine cannula placed in the rat forebrain is permitted to remain in place for 2 weeks or longer, the BBB becomes re-established (72–74). This provides the investigator with a "window" behind the BBB through which specific substances can be infused in minute amounts. Cserr and Knopf (72–74) and subsequently Weller et al. (75) demonstrated that solutes in the fluid of the CNS drain to deep cervical or paravertebral lymph nodes. However, the immunologic consequences of the arrival of this material in immune tissues are not fully defined.

A study using rats with a cannula implanted in the brain examined the traffic of B cells to the CNS (76) (Knopf PM, Cserr HF, Basu D, Hickey WF, unpublished data). When animals are hyperimmunized by subcutaneous injection of OVA in complete Freund's adjuvant, significant circulating titers of anti-OVA antibodies are achieved. However, in the CNS there is only a normal partition of the antibody into the cerebrospinal fluid (CSF). The location and distribution of anti-OVA antibodies can be delineated by using OVA directly coupled to fluorescein isothiocyanate (FITC). Along the cannula track in the brain, macrophages bind the anti-OVA antibodies to their membrane via their Fc receptor. Neither inflammation nor anti-OVA B cells or plasma cells can be detected. If saline solution or an irrelevant antigen is infused through the cannula, there is no significant change in the findings in the brain. However, if a small amount of OVA is injected through the cannula into the CNS, the situation alters dramatically. In the vicinity around the cannula track, a focus of inflammation characterized by scattered leukocytes develops. Moreover, in addition to the anti-OVA antibody–coated macrophages, now B cells and plasma cells specific for OVA can be detected. The area of immunoglobulin positivity of the CNS no longer remains in the immediate vicinity of the cannula; the entire hemisphere shows the presence of IgG. Microglial cells become activated to express MHC molecules and scattered T cells are present. Away from the cannula, around small blood vessels, plasma cell groups binding OVA-FITC are found. Most dramatically, the CSF is now shown to contain oligoclonal bands of anti-OVA IgG, demonstrating production of antibody against this antigen within the CNS itself.

In this paradigm, it appears that if the host has memory B cells specific for a given antigen, then leakage of this antigen from the CNS is sufficient to activate them and, seemingly like T cells, the B cells seek their antigen. When they locate it in the CNS, they have the ability to arrest and differentiate into plasma cells. A number of critical questions relative to this system persist. Are the B cells dependent on T cells initially locating the antigen and then summoning them? Is antigen recognition on the endothelial cell critical to the B-cell entry? Is this migration truly homing to where the antigen is, or is it a random process of entry? And, of course, what adhesion molecules are required to permit B-cell entry? While the answers to these questions are elusive, the system itself promises to be most manipulable and should permit the answers to be determined. Regardless of the specifics, it does appear that B cells have the ability to enter the CNS in search of antigen and perform their effector functions when the antigen is located.

MONOCYTE/MACROPHAGE ELEMENTS

While cells of the monocyte/macrophage lineage are not in themselves antigen specific, they play a critical role in most inflammatory processes, and are key participants in a myriad of CNS inflammatory diseases. However, the members of this group of cells continuously entering the CNS are phenotypically diverse and may subserve distinct functions.

Radiation bone marrow chimeras have been very helpful in studying this group of cells in the nervous system. In bone marrow chimeras an animal of genotype "B" is lethally irradiated and then rescued by intravenous administration of bone marrow from a partially allogeneic animal of genotype $(AxB)F_1$. After the marrow has been infused, the appearance of cells in various tissues that bear the markers of type "A" of necessity indicates that these cells have a bone marrow origin. The normal parenchymal cells in all organs will remain only of the "B" type, while cells ultimately derived from the bone marrow will express both "A" and "B" molecules. Such chimeric animals can be exceptionally useful in following the kinetics of the appearance of certain types of cells in the normal, uninflamed CNS tissue, or systems can be constructed to depend on the function of the "A" molecules expressed on the donor marrow cells but not on the "B" host's own cells.

A careful study of the CNS of rat bone marrow chimeras demonstrated that a number of cells of the monocyte/macrophage family enter the CNS from the bone marrow as part of normal physiology (49,77–80). At least five distinct varieties can be defined by their morphology, location, and the cell surface molecules they express.

Tissue macrophages, as normally noted in other tissues, can be recognized as the macrophages of the arachnoid and pial membranes. These cells enter from the marrow into the brain's coverings in a relatively rapid manner. In 60 to 90 days, more than 60% of these cells will become of the phenotype of the donated bone marrow. As such, they are the monocytic cell type exhibiting the most rapid turnover. They express low levels of MHC class I and II molecules and have CD4 (in rats and humans) on their membranes. Moreover, they have a low but constitutive expression of a variety of adhesion molecules (e.g., ICAM-1). While it has long been known that these macrophages become activated and dramatically increase in number during meningeal inflammatory processes, especially those producing chronic inflammation, such as *Mycobacterium tuberculosis* and cryptococcal infections, their function in normal homeostasis is undefined. The molecules governing their entry into the meninges, or the tissue signals to which they are responding remain to be defined. However, since these monocytic cells turn over as part of normal physiology, it must be concluded that they are directed by normal homeostatic mechanisms. In the state of health, there is no evidence that they function as anything more than tissue resident phagocytes.

Another incompletely understood cell of this group is the macrophage of the Virchow-Robin space. These macrophages appear to be closely related to the meningeal macrophages, although they are not immunophenotypically identical. They come from the bone marrow in a slower manner than do the meningeal macrophages, about half of them being replaced in 2 to 3 months of chimerism. Morphologically they resemble their meningeal counterparts at the light microscopic and ultrastructural level; however, they do not express detectable levels of MHC class II or CD4 in the normal state. They may represent the same cell as the meningeal macrophage, but comprise a subgroup that has to a greater extent come under the immunoinhibitory influence of the neural parenchyma. To date, no specific or unique function that the meningeal macrophages are not capable of has been attributable to them.

Two monocytoid cells, possibly closely related although they differ in location and morphology, are the perivascular cells and the choroid plexus macrophages. Both cell types lie adjacent to the endothelial cells of small venules and capillaries throughout the CNS, immediately beyond the basement membrane. These cell types are located in the perivascular space wherein they have long, branching cytoplasmic processes extending along and embracing the small vessels against which they rest (49,77,80). Being this closely associated with a blood vessel, they are ideally situated to sense changes in the endothelium and in BBB permeability and to encounter cells crossing into the tissue from the blood. The monocytes/macrophages of this group arrive in the CNS more slowly than do the previously noted cells. Approximately 30% of them turn over from the marrow in 2 to 3 months. After a year of marrow chimerism, virtually 100% express the donor marrow–derived phenotype. Again, these cells enter the CNS as part of normal physiology, not requiring inflammation to attract them (49,77). While we know little that specifically applies to this cell type in the choroid plexus, the perivascular cells of the CNS parenchyma have distinct and important functions. Indeed, from an immunologic standpoint they may be one of the most important cells in the CNS.

In both rats and humans, the perivascular cells are phenotypically distinct from regular tissue histiocytes, and are capable of performing specific immunologic functions. In mice, rats, and humans, the cell surface molecules these cells express constitutively, or can be induced to elaborate, are varied (2,30,81,82). They certainly can express MHC antigens, CD4, and a variety of adhesion molecules if the stimuli are correct (2,30,77,81,82). When chimeras of body type "B" with a marrow of $(AxB)F_1$ type are given encephalitogenic T cells that must recognize their antigen in the context only of "A" MHC class II molecules, the chimeras develop EAE. Only the marrow-derived perivascular cells of the CNS are appropriately situated and have the ability to elaborate the required MHC molecules to be the antigen-presenting cells in this system (49,50). Likewise, isolated choroid plexus macrophages are competent antigen-presenting cells in vitro (83).

Perivascular cells appear to be able to sense or transduce signals from the blood to the neural parenchyma. If bacterial lipopolysaccharide (LPS) is injected into the systemic circulation, perivascular cells in the brain respond (84). Within 6 hours after LPS injection, perivascular cells have synthesized the enzyme cyclo-oxygenase II, the rate-limiting enzyme in the production of proinflammatory eicosanoids. As such, the perivascular cell might serve as a rapid response mechanism alerting the nervous system of an immunologic challenge to the organism. Since inflammation does not occur in the CNS itself following LPS infusion (although the CNS physiology is markedly changed), the exact role of this activation of the perivascular cells remains to be explained.

Another aspect of the physiologic entrance of members of the monocyte/macrophage family into the nervous system merits attention. Members of this cell group are suspected of serving as a "Trojan horse," transporting human immunodeficiency virus type 1 (HIV-1) and possibly other CNS viruses (85).

Perivascular cells are capable of taking up and holding soluble material placed in the CNS parenchyma (86). As such, they are ideally situated and suited to be antigen-presenting cells. They sample the proteins and other soluble materials in the brain fluid, process it, and are evidently ready to present it to T cells when they pass by. This accumulation of CNS substances may have importance in the maintenance of tolerance for self neural antigens.

A final feature—currently attributed principally to the perivascular cells, but possibly a feature of other monocyte/macrophage family cells—relates to their fate when their CNS residence ends. They do not appear to die in situ; there is no evidence for that. In a study of neural grafting in which tissue from the forebrain of a neonatal Lewis rat was placed in the frontal lobe of an MHC-mismatched Brown Norway rat, evidence of cellular emigration from the CNS appeared (87). After graft placement, when the recipient animal's cervical lymph nodes and spleen were studied for the presence of cells bearing the donor MHC molecules, such cells were found in both locations, although they were rare. Since members of the monocyte/macrophage family almost exclusively express MHC molecules in CNS tissue, and since the grafts contained no meninges (hence no meningeal macrophages), the cells found in the recipients' immune tissue were most probably derived from the perivascular cell pool. While this experiment does not replicate the physiologic condition, it does bespeak a potential two-way traffic of monocytic cells into and out of the CNS. In addition, it suggests an answer to questions concerning what happens to the meningeal and perivascular cells as they are replaced from the bone marrow.

Parenchymal microglial cells constitute up to 10% of the CNS parenchymal cells in some brain areas. They are found in both white and gray matter putting out arborizing processes to touch the dendritic tips of the adjacent microglia, establishing a continuous web that invests the whole CNS (81,88). In the healthy animal, these parenchymal cells are very quiescent immunologically. They express no detectable MHC molecules, they show low levels of or no adhesion molecules, and their CD4 expression is not detectable (1,2,5,81,89). However, in a state of activation, as would occur following cytokine exposure or in a zone of inflammation, they rapidly become positive for all of the above (77,81,82,89).

Microglia form part of the glia limitans, the true boundary of the CNS parenchyma. Ultrastructural, immunohistochemical analyses of the CNS demonstrated that between 5% and 13% of the foot processes extending from the CNS parenchyma to abut on CNS vessels are derived from microglia (90). Thus, a subset of these cells also is immediately available to any cell or material crossing the BBB from the circulation. However, these cells are extremely slow in their turnover from the bone marrow. In 2 to 3 months, less than 1% of these cells will be replaced from the bone marrow; even after a year of bone marrow chimerism, only a few percent of the parenchymal microglial cells will exhibit the donor marrow–derived phenotype (77,78). While their entrance from the bone marrow is believed to occur mostly in fetal life, and can be described as physiologic, which adhesion molecules or chemokines govern it is unknown.

It appears that these microglial cells are relatively poor antigen-presenting cells, at least when freshly isolated from the adult rat CNS (69,91,92). In mammals, parenchymal microglial cells can be distinguished from the perivascular cells and other hematogenously derived leukocytes by their level of CD45 (91,92). These CD45-low microglia do possess some antigen-processing and -presenting functions, but they appear defective when compared to the perivascular cells. As noted above in the discussion of T-cell apoptosis, antigen presentation by parenchymal microglial cells may target the T cell responding to MHC-bound antigen to terminal differentiation and death (68,69).

Parenchymal microglial cells can become fully competent macrophages. Del rio Hortega (93) detailed this transformation over half a century ago. In the inflammatory infiltrates associated with EAE, a few microglia become phagocytes to engulf tissue and inflammatory cell debris (78,79). At the edge of CNS infarctions or traumatic contusions, selected microglia are induced to become macrophages, also to remove necrotic and injured tissue (Horner HA, Hickey WF, unpublished observations). However in all these situations, the large majority of the macrophages that appear are not derived from microglia; they are freshly recruited hematogenous cells of the circulating monocyte/macrophage group (78,79,81).

There appears to be very little interconversion between subpopulations of monocytes/macrophages. While some parenchymal microglial cells can become macrophages, it appears to be a one-way process. Investigations in chimeric rats showed that macrophages responding to an inflammatory focus in the CNS do not remain after the inflammation subsides (78,79). Moreover, phagocytic cells of the donor marrow type certainly assume the morphology of parenchymal microglial cells. Perivascular cells do not become either parenchymal microglial cells or phagocytic macrophages in areas of inflammation (78,79). Thus, this cell type appears to have a narrowly defined repertoire that does not overlap with some of the other CNS resident monocytic elements. How much interconversion actually does occur between specific CNS macrophage/monocyte cell phenotypes remains to be fully elucidated; however, the data to date suggest that these conversions might be very limited and governed by factors unknown at this time.

There is no question that of all the leukocytic cell types found in the CNS in health or disease, the monocyte/macrophage family members are the most complex, and the parameters controlling the entry of each type into the CNS must reflect this (Fig 2-3). In the nervous system members of this group have distinct phenotypes; whether this reflects the existence of distinct lineages in the marrow or merely the differentiating effects of the local environment cannot be specified at this time. Some enter as part of normal physiology while others arrive during the inflammatory process. Their function may vary dramatically between what they do in the normal CNS and what they are capable of in the inflamed tissue. While the investigation of chemokines (56–59) may greatly enlarge our understanding of the migrations of cells in this group, it will take a long time to understand this group because of the complexity.

CONCLUSIONS

Leukocyte entry into the CNS and the immunologic surveillance of that tissue are critical features of the interaction of the immune and nervous systems. However, the production of severe and damaging inflammation is occasionally a by-product of the process. Based on what is currently known about the interaction of these two systems, it appears that leukocytes must come from the periphery in order to initiate inflammation. Certainly T and B cells can and do enter the CNS, but their antigenic specificity

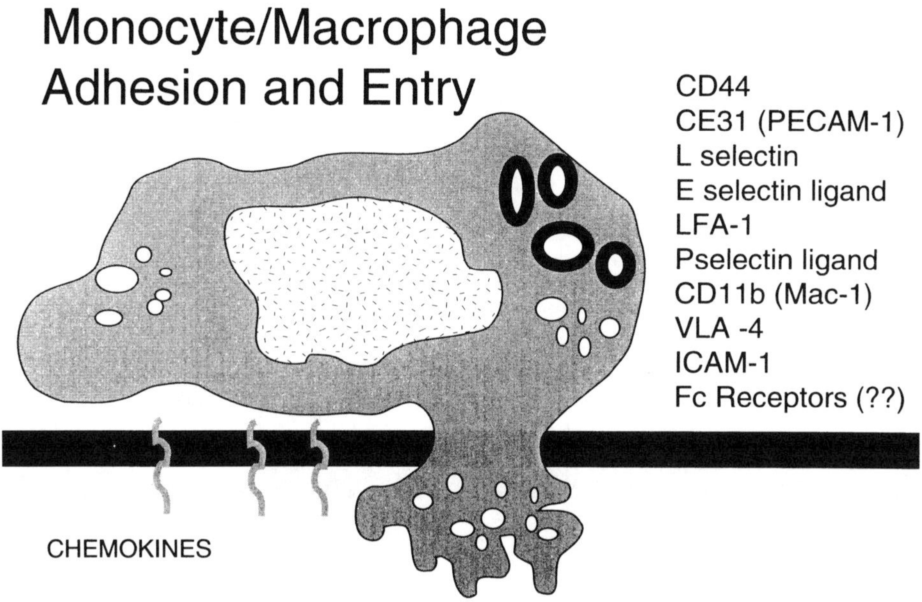

Figure 2-3. Cartoon of a monocyte cell crossing the endothelium. A number of adhesion molecules known in experimental systems to be active in such interactions are shown at the right. As with lymphocytes, which molecules actually play critical roles in the migration almost certainly varies with a) the endothelial activation state, b) the nature of the response to which the monocyte is responding (i.e., the physiologic entry of CNS resident monocyte/macrophage/microglial cells versus a pathologic recruitment of inflammatory cells), c) the activation state or predetermined function of the monocytic cell entering, and d) the chemokine signals being generated from the CNS parenchyma.

and their clonal expansion appear to already have occurred in tissues of the immune system before they arrive in the nervous system. It is therefore important to develop as complete an understanding as possible of the chemical signals and adhesion molecules used to attract or permit leukocytes to enter the brain and spinal cord in both health and disease.

The factors controlling the entry of leukocytes into the CNS must be exceptionally complex (Fig 2-4). Because there are numerous types of leukocytes, many of which can exist as resting or activated forms, and because the CNS endothelium itself can vary from a basal, quiescent to a highly activated state, there are numerous permutations of leukocyte–endothelial cell combinations. Since it appears that the adhesion molecules active in each type of interaction might be distinct (or at least not totally coextensive), there must be both specific and unique sets of such cell surface molecules to regulate when and which leukocyte types will be permitted in. Yet, it might not be a complexity that precludes manipulation.

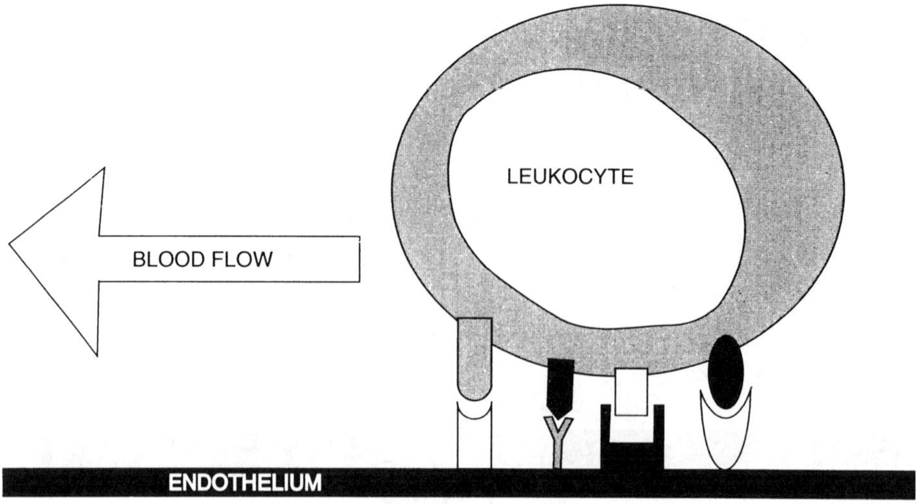

- One molecular interaction is not sufficient; many must occur for leukocyte entry to be effective.
- For each leukocyte class the specific molecular interactions are distinct, but leukocytes may share adhesion molecules.
- Disruption of one molecular interaction may block entry of all leukocytes using that molecule.

Figure 2-4. General parameters governing leukocyte entry into the CNS.

If an analogy is drawn between the complex leukocyte–endothelial interactions and a group of combination locks, the situation can be more readily perceived. While the combination needed to open each lock is distinct, many combinations can share certain numbers. Likewise, there may be certain adhesion molecules that are employed by many leukocyte types in their penetration of the nervous system. For therapeutic purposes, it might not be necessary to know the complete "combination" for each leukocyte–endothelial pair. As one omitted or incorrect number in a combination will prevent opening of the lock, similarly blocking one required adhesion molecule on a leukocyte of the endothelial membrane may inhibit its appearance in the CNS. Certainly, this is consistent with the ability of single antibodies to one adhesion molecule to prevent the complex cascade involved in the evolution of EAE. Therefore, it is possible that the types of cells that participate in nervous system inflammation (as well as inflammation elsewhere) could be manipulated to minimize the deleterious effects or to shunt the reaction to a more beneficial outcome. In order for this to become more than a theoretical possibility, it will be necessary to develop a far more complete understanding of the molecules and signals used by T cells, B cells, and monocytes/macrophages to enter the nervous system as part of normal physiology and in disease.

REFERENCES

1 Hauser SL, Bhan AK, Gilles FH, et al. Immunohistochemical staining of human brain with monoclonal antibodies that identify lymphocytes, monocytes and the Ia antigen. *J Immunol* 1983;5:197–205.

2 Hickey WF, Kimura H. Elicitation of MHC gene products and T-lymphocytes in the CNS of rats by graft-versus-host disease. *Proc Natl Acad Sci USA* 1987;84:2082–2086.

3 Williams KC, Hickey WF. Migration of hematogenous cells through the central nervous system. *Curr Top Microbiol Immunol* 1995;202:221–245.

4 Wekerle H, Linnington C, Lassmann H, Meyermann R. Cellular immune reactivity within the CNS. *Trends Neurosci* 1986;9:271–277.

5 Lampson LA, Hickey WF. Monoclonal antibody analysis of MHC expression in histologically normal and glioma containing human brain biopsies. *J Immunol* 1986;136:4054–4062.

6 Sloan DJ, Wood MJ, Charlton HM. Leukocyte recruitment and inflammation in the CNS. *Trends Neurosci* 1982;15:276–280.

7 Barker CF, Billingham RE. Immunologically privileged sites. *Adv Immunol* 1977;25:1–6.

8 Nicholas MK, Stefansson K, Antel JP, Arnason BG. An in vivo and in vitro analysis of systemic immune function in mice with histologic evidence of neural transplant rejection. *J Neurosci Res* 1987;18:245–257.

9 Rapoport SI. Blood brain barrier in physiology and medicine. New York: Raven, 1976:43–127.

10 Williams KC, Ulvestadt E, Hickey WF. The immunology of multiple sclerosis. *Clin Neurosci* 1995;2:229–245.

11 Butcher EC. Leukocyte-endothelial cell recognition: three (or more) steps to specificity and diversity. *Cell* 1991;67:1033–1036.

12 Lawrence MB, Springer TA. Leukocytes roll on a selectins at physiologic flow rates: distinction from and prerequisite for adhesion through integrins. *Cell* 1991;65:859–873.

13 McEver RP. Selectins. *Curr Opin Immunol* 1994;6:75–84.

14 Shimizu Y, Newman W, Tanhka Y, Shaw S. Lymphocyte interactions with endothelial cells. *Immunol Today* 1992;13:106–112.

15 Cross AH. Immune cell traffic control and the central nervous system. *Semin Neurosci* 1992;4.

16 Bevilaqua MP. Endothelial-leukocyte adhesion molecules. *Annu Rev Immunol* 1993;11:767–804.

17 Bevilacqua MP, Nelson RM. Selectins. *J Clin Invest* 1993;91:379–387.

18 Harlan JM, Liu DY. *Adhesion: its role in inflammatory disease.* New York: WH Freeman, 1992.

19 Hynes RO. Integrins: versatility, modulation, and signaling of cell adhesion. *Cell* 1992; 69:11–25.

20 Stoolman LM. Adhesion molecules controlling lymphocyte migration. *Cell* 1989;56:907–910.

21 Springer TA. Adhesion receptors of the immune system. *Nature* 1990;346:425–434.

22 Springer TA. Traffic signals for lymphocyte recirculation and leukocyte emigration. *Cell* 1994;76:301–314.

23 Butcher EC, Scollay RG, Weissman IL. Organ specificity of lymphocyte migration: mediation by highly selective lymphocyte interaction with organ specific determinants on high endothelial venules. *Eur J Immunol* 1980;10:556–561.

24 Carlos TM, Harlan JM. Leukocyte-endothelial cell adhesion molecules. *Blood* 1994;84: 2068–2101.

25 Stephan BJ, Butcher EC, Engelhardt B. Evidence for the involvement of ICAM-1 and VCAM-1 in lymphocyte interaction with endothelium in EAE in the CNS of the SJL/J mouse. *Am J Pathol* 1994;145:189.

26 Boyd AW, Wawrk SO, Burns GF, Fecondo JV. Intercellular adhesion molecule 1 has a central role in cell-cell contact-mediated mechanism. *Proc Natl Acad Sci USA* 1988;95:3095–3099.

27 Cannella B, Cross AH, Raine CS. Upregulation and coexpression of adhesion molecules correlate with relapsing autoimmune demyelination in the central nervous system. *J Exp Med* 1990;172:1521–1524.

28 Cannella B, Cross AH, Raine CS. Adhesion related molecules in the central nervous system: upregulation correlates with inflammatory cell influx. *Lab Invest* 1991;65:23–31.

29 Cannella B, Raine CS. The adhesion molecule and cytokine profile of multiple sclerosis lesions. *Ann Neurol* 1995;37:424–435.

30 Lassmann H, Zimprich F, Rossler K, Vass K. Inflammation in the nervous system. *Rev Neurol* 1991;147:763–781.

31 O'Neil JK, Butter C, Baker D, et al. Expression of vascular addressins and ICAM-1 by endothelial cells of the spinal cord during relapsing EAE in the Biozzi AB/H mouse. *Immunology* 1991;72:520.

32 Kraal G, Weissman IL, Butcher EC. Differences in *in vivo* distribution and homing of T cell subsets to mucosal *vs.* non-mucosal lymphoid organs. *J Immunol* 1983;130:1097–1102.

33 Ihrcke NS, Wrenshall LE, Lindman BJ, Platt JL. Role of heparin sulfate in immune system-blood vessel interactions. *Immunol Today* 1993;14:500–505.

34 Naparstek Y, Cohen IR, Fuks Z, Vlodavsky I. Activated T lymphocytes produce a matrix degrading heparin sulphate endoglycosidase. *Nature* 1984;310:241–244.

35 Willenborg DP, Parish CR. Inhibition of allergic encephalomyelitis in rats by treatment with sulfated polysaccharides. *J Immunol* 1988;140:3401–3405.

36 Willenborg DO, Parish CR, Cowden WB. Phosphosugars are potent inhibitors of central nervous system inflammation. *FASEB J* 1989; 3:1968–1971.

37 Granert C, Raud J, Xie X, et al. Inhibition of leukocyte rolling with polysaccharide fucoidin prevents pleocytosis in experimental meningitis in the rabbit. *J Clin Invest* 1994;93:929–936.

38 Pizcueta P, Luscinskas FW. Monoclonal antibody blockade of L-selectin inhibits mononuclear leukocyte recruitment to inflammatory sites in vivo. *Am J Pathol* 1994;145:461–469.

39 Silber A, Newman W, Sasseville VG, et al. Recruitment of lymphocytes during cutaneous delayed hypersensitivity in nonhuman primates is dependent on E-selectin and vascular cell adhesion molecule 1. *J Clin Invest* 1994;93:1554–1563.

40 Rosales C, Juliano RL. Signal transduction by cell adhesion receptors in leukocytes. *J Leukoc Biol* 1995;57:189–198.

41 Alvord EA Jr, Kies M, Suckling A. *Experimental allergic encephalomyelitis: a useful model for multiple sclerosis.* New York: Alan R. Liss, 1984.

42 Miller SD, Karpus WJ. The immunopathogenesis and regulation of T cell mediated demyelinating diseases. *Immunol Today* 1994; 15:356–361.

43 Merrill JE, Kono DH, Clayton J, et al. Inflammatory leukocytes and cytokines in peptide induced experimental allergic encephalomyelitis in SJL/J and B10.PL mice. *Proc Natl Acad Sci USA* 1992;89:574–578.

44 Kuchroo VK, Das MP, Brown JA, et al. B7-1 and B7-2 costimulatory molecules activate differentially the Th1/Th2 development: application to autoimmune disease. *Cell* 1995;80:707–718.

45 Chen Y, Kuchroo VK, Inobe J, et al. Regulatory T cell clones induced by oral tolerance: suppression of allergic encephalomyelitis. *Science* 1994;265:1237–1240.

46 Pantich HS. Adoptive transfer of EAE with activated spleen cells: comparison of in vitro activation by concavalin A and myelin basic protein. *Cell Immunol* 1980;56:163–171.

47 Holda JH, Welch AM, Swanborg RH. Autoimmune effector cells I. Transfer of EAE with lymphoid cells cultured with antigen. *Eur J Immunol* 1980;10:657–659.

48 Hickey WF, Hsu BL, Kimura H. T-lymphocyte entry into the central nervous system. *J Neurosci Res* 1991;28:254–260.

49 Hickey WF, Kimura H. "Perivascular microglia" are bone marrow derived and present antigen in vivo. *Science* 1988;239:290–293.

50 Hickey WF. Migration of hematogenous cells through the blood brain barrier and the initiation of CNS inflammation. *Brain Pathol* 1991;1:97–102.

51 Ludowyk PA, Willenborg DO, Parish CR. Selective localisation of neuro-specific T lymphocytes in the central nervous system. *J Neuroimmunol* 1992;37:237–245.

52 Naparstek Y, Holoshitz J, Eisenstein S, Cohen IR. Effector T lymphocyte cell lines migrate to the thymus and persist there. *Nature* 1982;300:262–265.

53 Woodruff JJ, Clarke LM. Specific cell adhesion mechanisms determining migration pathways of recirculating lymphocytes. *Annu Rev Immunol* 1987;5:201–222.

54 Cross AH, Cannella B, Brosnan CF, Raine CS. Homing to central nervous system vasculature by antigen specific lymphocytes. I. Localization of ^{14}C-labeled cells during acute, chronic and relapsing experimental allergic encephalomyelitis. *Lab Invest* 1990;63:162–170.

55 Trotter J, Steinman L. Homing of Lyt2+ and Lyt2− T cell subsets and B lymphocytes to the central nervous system of mice with acute experimental allergic encephalomyelitis. *J Immunol* 1984;132:2919–2923.

56 Baggiolini M, Dewald B, Moser B. Interleukin 8 and related chemotactic cytokines CXC and CC chemokines. *Adv Immunol* 1994;55:97–179.

57 Flurie MB, Randolph GJ. Chemokines and tissue injury: a review. *Am J Pathol* 1995;146: 1287–1293.

58 Godiska R, Chantry D, Dietsch GN, Gray PW. Chemokine expression in murine experimental allergic encephalomyelitis. *J Neuroimmunol* 1995;58:167–175.

59 Karpus WJ, Lukacs NW, McRae BL, et al. Prevention and treatment of PLP peptide induced EAE by anti-MIP-1α administration. *J Neuroimmunol* 1994;54:171–179.

60 Yednock TA, Cannon C, Fritz LC, et al. Prevention of experimental autoimmune encephalomyelitis by antibodies against α4β1 integrin. *Nature* 1992;356:63–66.

61 Baron JL, Madri JA, Ruddle NH, et al. Surface expression of alpha4 integrin by CD4 T cells is

required for their entry into brain parenchyma. *J Exp Med* 1993;177:57–68.

62 Archelos JJ, Jung S, Maurer M, et al. Inhibition of experimental autoimmune encephalomyelitis by an antibody to the intercellular adhesion molecule ICAM-1. *Ann Neurol* 1993;34:145–154.

63 Willenborg DO, Simmons RD, Tamatani T, Miyasaka M. ICAM-1 dependent pathway is not critically involved in the inflammatory process of EAE or in cytokine induced inflammation of the CNS. *J Neuroimmunol* 1993; 45:147–155.

64 Willenborg DO, Staykova MA, Miyasaka M. Short term treatment with soluble neuroantigen and anti-CD11a (LFA-1) protects rats against autoimmune encephalomyelitis. *J Immunol* 1996;157:1973–1980.

65 Williams KC, Zhao RW, Ueno K, Hickey WF. PECAM-1 (CD31) expression in the CNS and its role in EAE in the rat. *J Neurosci Res* 1996;45:747–757.

66 Pender MP, Nguyen KB, McCombe PA, Kerr JFR. Apoptosis in the nervous system in experimental allergic encephalomyelitis. *J Neurol Sci* 1991;14:81–87.

67 Schmied M, Breitschopf H, Gold R, et al. Apoptosis of T lymphocytes in experimental autoimmune encephalomyelitis. *Am J Pathol* 1993;143:446–452.

68 Tabi Z, McCombe PA, Pender MP. Antigen specific down regulation of myelin basic protein reactive T cells during recovery from EAE: further evidence of apoptotic deletion of autoreactive T cells in the CNS. *Int Immunol* 1995;7:967–973.

69 Ford AL, Foulcher E, Lemckert FA, Sedgwick JD. Microglia induce CD4 T lymphocyte final effector function and death. *J Exp Med* 1996; 184:1737–1745.

70 Trinchieri G. Biology of natural killer cells. *Adv Immunol* 1989;47:187.

71 Matsumoto Y, Aikawa Y, Shin T, et al. Role of NK and TCRγδ cells in rat acute EAE. *J Neuropathol Exp Neurol* 1996;55:641. Abstract.

72 Cserr HF, DePasquale M, Harling-Berg CJ, et al. Afferent and efferent arms of the humoral immune response to CSF-administered albumins in a rat model with normal blood-brain barrier permeability. *J Neuroimmunol* 1992;41:195–202.

73 Cserr HF, Knopf PM. Cervical lymphatics, the blood-brain barrier and the immunoactivity of the brain: a new view. *Immunol Today* 1992;13:507–512.

74 Harling-Berg CJ, Knopf PM , Merriam J, Cserr HF. Role of cervical lymph nodes in the systemic humoral immune response to human serum albumin microinfused into the rat CSF. *J Neuroimmunol* 1989;25:185–193.

75 Kida S, Weller RO, Zhang ET, et al. Anatomical pathways for lymphatic drainage of the brain and their pathological significance. *Neuropathol Appl Neurobiol* 1995;21:181–184.

76 Knopf PM, Basu D, Sirulnick E, et al. B cell traffic and intra-thecal antibody synthesis in normal brain. *FASEB J* 1994;8:A248.

77 Hickey WF, Vass K, Lassmann H. Bone marrow derived elements in the central nervous system: an immunohistochemical and ultrastructural survey of rat chimeras. *J Neuropathol Exp Neurol* 1992;51:246–256.

78 Lawson LJ, Perry VH, Gordon S. Turnover of resident microglial in the normal adult mouse brain. *Neuroscience* 1992;48:405–415.

79 Lassmann H, Schmied M, Vass K, Hickey WF. Bone marrow derived elements and resident microglia in brain inflammation. *Glia* 1993;7:19–24.

80 Rinner WA, Bauer J, Schmidts M, et al. Resident microglia and hematogenous macrophages as phagocytes in adoptively transferred EAE: an investigation using rat radiation bone marrow chimeras. *Glia* 1995;14:257–266.

81 Perry VH. *Macrophages and the nervous system*. Austin, TX: RG Landes, 1994.

82 Vass K, Lassmann H. Intrathecal application of interferon gamma. Progressive appearance of MHC antigens within the rat nervous system. *Am J Pathol* 1990;137:789–798.

83 Nathanson JA, Chun LLY. Immunological function of the blood CSF barrier. *Proc Natl Acad Sci USA* 1989;86:1684–1688.

84 Elmquist JK, Breder CD, Sherin JE, et al. Intravenous lipopolysaccharide induces cyclooxygenase 2-like immunoreactivity in rat brain perivascular microglia and meningeal macrophages. *J Comp Neurol* 1997 (in press).

85 Dickson DW, Mattiace LA, Kure K, et al. Biology of disease: microglia in human disease, with an emphasis on acquired immune deficiency syndrome. *Lab Invest* 1991;64:135–156.

86 Kida S, Steart PV, Zhang ET, Weller RO. Perivascular cells act as scavengers in the cerebral perivascular space and remain distinct from pericytes, microglia and macrophages. *Acta Neuropathol (Berl)* 1993;85:646–652.

87 Broadwell RD, Baker BJ, Ebert PS, Hickey WF. Allografts of CNS tissue possess a blood brain barrier: III. Neuropathological, methodological and immunological considerations. *Microsc Res Tech* 1994;27:471–494.

88 Perry VH, Gordon S. Macrophages and microglia in the nervous system. *Trends Neurosci* 1988;11:273–276.

89 Flaris NA, Densmore TL, Molleston MC, Hickey WF. Characterization of microglia and macrophages in the central nervous system of rats. *Glia* 1993;7:34–40.

90 Lassmann H, Zimprich F, Vass K, Hickey WF. Microglial cells are a component of the perivascular glia limitans. *J Neurosci Res* 1991;28:236–243.

91 Ford AL, Goodsall AL, Hickey WF, Sedgwick JD. Normal adult rat microglia separated from other CNS macrophages by flow cytometric sorting: phenotypic differences defined and direct ex vivo antigen presentation to myelin basic protein reactive CH4+ cells compared. *J Immunol* 1995;154:4309–4321.

92 Sedgwick JD, Schwender S, Imrich H, et al. Isolation and direct characterization of resident microglial cells from the normal and inflamed central nervous system. *Proc Natl Acad Sci USA* 1991;88:7438–7442.

93 del rio Hortega P. Microglia. In: Penfield W, ed. *Cytology and cellular pathology of the nervous system*. New York: Hoeber, 1932:481–524.

3

Microglia: A "Double-Edged Sword"

PHILLIP K. PETERSON
GENYA GEKKER
SHUXIAN HU
CHUN C. CHAO

"The pathological substratum of many nervous diseases is in a large measure characterized by the existence and intensity of the intervention of the microglia."
Pio del Rio-Hortega (1)

Migratory granular cells were identified within the nervous system well over 100 years ago, and studies on the nature of these neuroglial elements were carried out by a number of eminent, and often enthusiastic scientists of the late nineteenth and early twentieth century. Nevertheless, the undisputed father of microglial cell biology was the Spanish neuroanatomist, Pio del Rio-Hortega. In his treatise on microglia published in 1932 (1), del Rio-Hortega presented a strong argument for a mesodermal origin of the microglia (a matter of controversy to this day). He also characterized the diverse morphologic features of these cells (ranging from motile, ameboid shapes to elongated, resting forms), described their distribution within the nervous system, and proposed three functional states: ameboid state in the fetus, stable and resting state in the mature brain, and a third state in which they recover their ameboid features "for active discharge of their macrophagic properties" (1).

After a prolonged eclipse, due in part to the loss of del Rio-Hortega's staining techniques, scientific interest in microglial cells has rebounded sharply in the past 10 years. The reawakening of interest in microglia has been fueled both by technical advancements, such as the development of specific monoclonal antibodies and techniques for culturing highly purified populations of microglia, and by mounting evidence that microglia play an important pathogenetic role in two of the most devastating neurodegenerative diseases of the late twentieth century, acquired immunodeficiency syndrome (AIDS) dementia and Alzheimer's disease.

Microglial cells have been the subject of recent reviews (2,3). Like del Rio-Hortega and his predecessors, contemporary authorities share the view that microglia contribute essential scavenger functions, both within the developing brain and following brain injury. Being the resident macrophages of the brain, microglia are also regarded as defenders of the nervous system. However, a concept that has received increased attention in recent years is that of microglia as a "double-edged sword." On the negative side, activated microglia are capable of damaging neurons, and by harboring intracellular pathogens, microglia in some instances seem to favor the parasite over the host. The principal aim of this chapter is to review current and emerging concepts about both the positive and the negative sides of these remarkable cells.

DEFINITIONS, DISTRIBUTION, AND DERIVATION

Long recognized as the resident macrophages of the brain parenchyma, microglia have been distinguished from macroglia (astrocytes and oligodendrocytes) by their avid phagocytic potential. Like other types of mononuclear phagocytes, which can adopt a range of forms depending on their location in a given tissue, microglia appear to provide an extreme example of such specialization (4). This fundamental characteristic of microglia, termed *plasticity*, applies both to their ability to change shape and to their capacity to upregulate or downregulate their functional activities (5).

Three basic subtypes of microglia are currently recognized: ameboid, ramified, and reactive (Fig 3-1). All three subtypes are considered to be different forms of a single cell type, with the ameboid form being an active macrophage during brain development and the precursor of inactive ramified cells, which can in turn be transformed in adult tissue and become reactive or ameboid microglia. Ameboid microglia are present in prenatal and early postnatal brain tissue and possess a broad flat morphology with pseudopodia. Ramified microglia, which are found in the mature brain, have a small cell body (5–10 mm) and emanating thin branching processes. With their dendritic morphology, microglial cells have been likened to dendritic antigen-presenting cells (APCs) as well as to macrophages (6). Reactive microglia arise in adult brain tissue following traumatic injury, inflammation, or infection. In the early stages of reactivation, microglia may assume bushy or elongated, rodlike forms. Fully reactive microglia are distinguished from their downregulated ramified precursors by a lack of protruding processes, by expression of markers of cell activation, and by their phagocytic potential. Furthermore, reactive microglia have the capacity to proliferate, another feature that distinguishes microglia from other types of tissue macrophages.

The timing of the transformation from the ameboid to the ramified microglial cell form in the human brain has not been fully delineated. Our laboratory found that 16-week-old, fresh fetal human cortical brain is populated by ramified microglia, which are similar in appearance to the ramified microglia in normal adult brain (Fig 3-2A). In the rat brain, the ameboid form predominates in the area of the corpus callosum until about the fifteenth postnatal day when the transformation from ameboid to ramified microglia is complete (7). The environmental factors that determine the transition from ameboid to ramified forms are largely unknown, although astrocytes have been proposed to play a key role in this process (8,9). Most studies of cultured microglial cells have been carried out with cells isolated from fetal or neonatal brain tissue, and in the process of isolating and culturing microglia they convert to an ameboid morphology (Fig 3-2B). Thus, the results of studies with cultured microglia are most relevant to understanding ameboid microglial cell biology. After a week in culture, some ameboid mi-

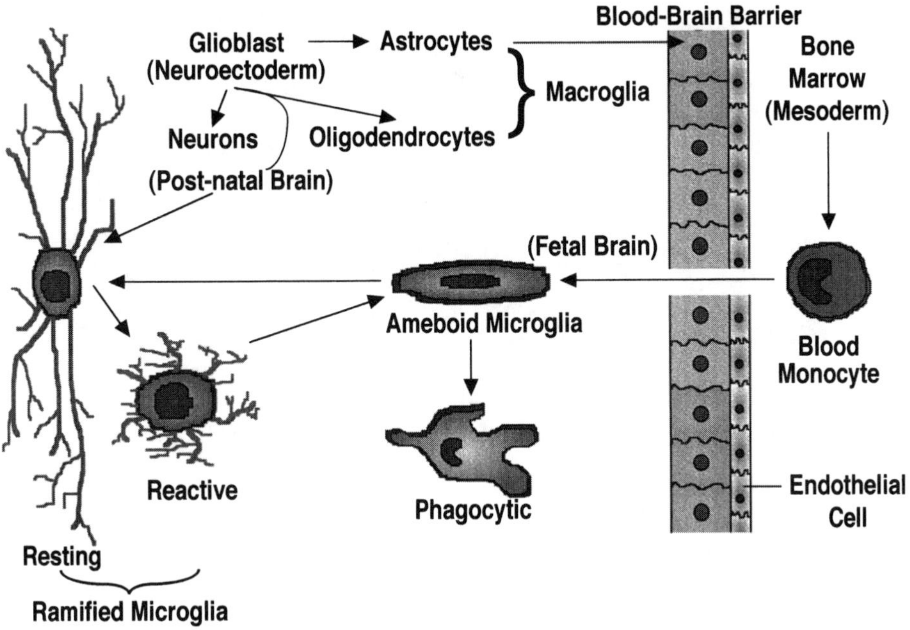

Figure 3-1. Scheme of the types and proposed origins of the microglia. Ameboid microglia are normally present in the fetal and early postnatal brain, whereas resting ramified microglia are the only subtype found in the healthy mature brain. Ameboid microglia can differentiate into ramified forms, and following a variety of CNS insults, ramified microglia transform into reactive, ameboid, and phagocytic subtypes. Blood monocytes, derived from mesodermal stem cells in the bone marrow, are the likely source of microglia in the developing brain. Ramified microglia, however, have been proposed to arise from blood monocytes or from a neuroectodermal stem cell, which is also the progenitor of all other types of brain cells.

croglia begin to assume a ramified-type morphology (Fig 3-2C), and special cell culture techniques that have been described appear to promote the development of ramified forms in vitro (10).

The percentage of microglial cells in the entire nervous system glial cell population ranges from 5% to 20%, and because there are 10 times as many glial cells as neurons in the central nervous system (CNS), it has been estimated that there are at least as many microglia as there are neurons (2). Although they are present in large numbers in all major divisions of the CNS, microglia are not uniformly distributed. More microglia are found in the gray matter than the white matter, and particularly densely populated areas include the hippocampus, olfactory telencephalon, basal ganglia, and substantia nigra. Also, considerable morphologic heterogeneity of microglia exists within different brain regions.

While all microglial cells are by definition brain macrophages, not all macrophage-

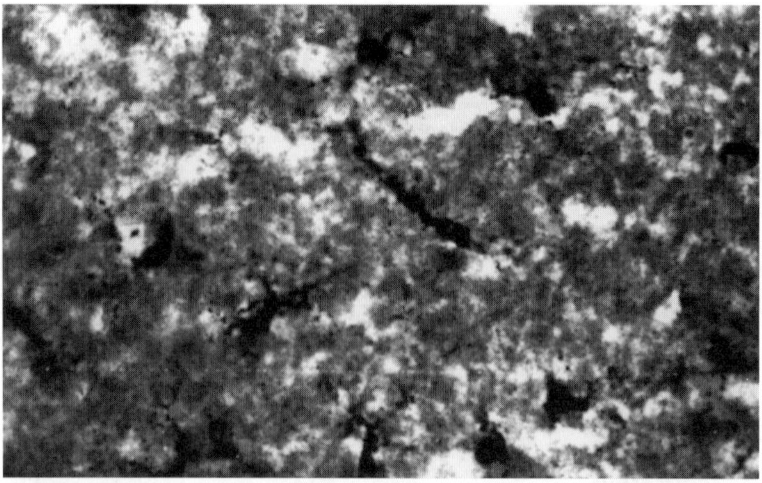

(A)

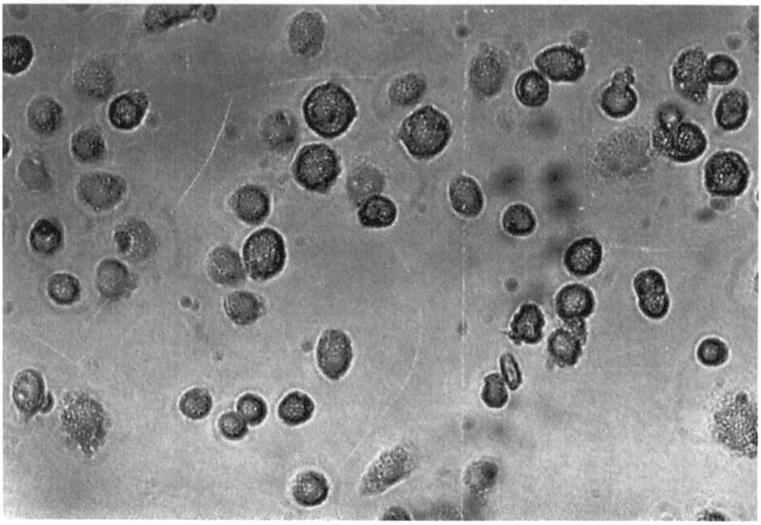

(B)

Figure 3-2. Human microglial cell subtypes. (A) Ramified microglial cells stained with antibodies specific for human macrophages in cerebral cortical tissue of an adult. (B) Ameboid microglia in cell cultures derived from an 18-week-old fetus. (C) Some fetal microglia assume a ramified morphology after 7 days of culture. (Light microscopy, × 400.)

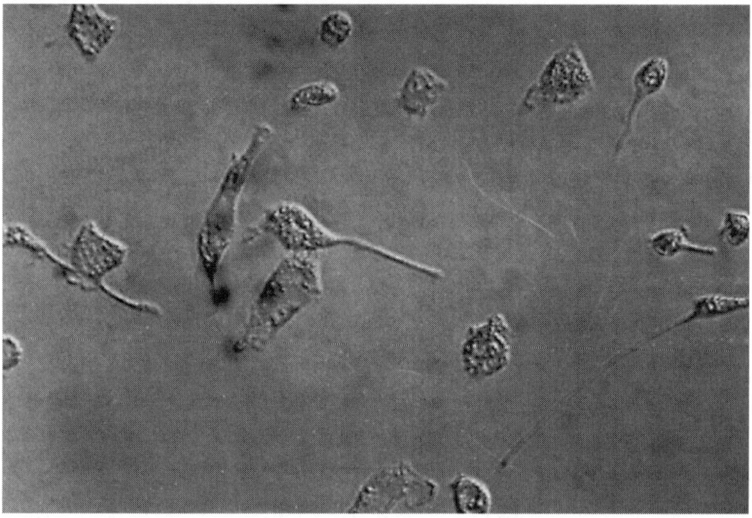

(C)

Figure 3-2. *(continued)*

like cells in the brain are microglial cells. Two other types of brain macrophages are the perivascular cells, which are associated with blood vessels throughout the brain but lie outside the brain parenchyma, and macrophages found in the choroid plexus and circumventricular organs, where there is no blood-brain barrier (BBB).

The most hotly debated issue regarding microglial cell biology has been their cellular origin (11). As already mentioned, del Rio-Hortega strongly favored the argument that microglia, which he regarded as the reticuloendothelial system of the brain, are derived during fetal development from blood monocytes (1). In late fetal and early neonatal stages of brain development, before the BBB is fully formed, monocytes were thought to invade the brain in certain areas such as the cingulum and the supraventricular corpus callosum. While he agreed that microglia could eventually arise from other (neuroectodermal) elements, del Rio-Hortega believed the evidence pointed only to a mesodermal origin.

del Rio-Hortega's concept of bone marrow–derived blood monocytes as the ontogenetic source of microglia is consistent with the unifying hypothesis of a "mononuclear phagocyte system" and is supported by the weight of contemporary experimental data and opinion (12–14). Currently, there seems to be little argument that the colonizing cells of the developing brain are of mesodermal origin. However, there is emerging evidence pointing to a neuroectodermal stem cell as the progenitor of postnatal ramified microglia (15–18), as well as to neurons and the macroglia (see Fig 3-1). Some of the most convincing evidence of a different lineage of ramified microglia has come from experiments with radiation bone marrow chimeras (16). The results of these studies suggest that while bone marrow–derived monocytes readily populate the meninges and the perivascular brain macrophage pool, parenchymal microglia are rarely derived from hematopoietic cells. In contrast to an earlier report that blood monocytes differentiate into microglial cells when they are cultured on monolayers of astrocytes (9), a more recent study showed that ameboid microglia are the only type of mononuclear phagocyte capable of transformation into quiescent ramified cells when they are placed in contact with astrocytes (18). Thus, it now appears that microglia in the parenchyma of the mature brain may be a distinct class of mononuclear phagocyte that does not belong to the mononuclear phagocyte system.

FUNCTIONS

Scavenger Activities

Some controversy exists about exactly how much cell loss occurs in the developing CNS. Nevertheless, a recent report suggested that at least 50% of the cells in the neocortex die in the course of normal remodeling of the fetal brain (19). Ameboid microglia are believed to serve a key function in this remodeling process by phagocytizing dead and damaged cells. In an in situ model for studying ameboid microglia in the developing brain, these cells were shown by time-lapse video microscopy to quickly migrate to the surface of a cortical brain slice where they contacted dead and damaged cells with velum-like processes followed by rapid phagocytosis (20).

Although this scavenger activity of ameboid microglia in the normal developing brain has long been recognized, the function of microglia in the CNS of the healthy mature brain is unknown. These ramified cells, which surround the neurons and are intermingled among other glia, are considered to be "resting" but poised to respond to internal disturbances provoked by any number of external agents (e.g., head trauma, stroke, microbial invaders, or inflammation).

Immunologic Properties

The process of reactivation of ramified microglia is accompanied by characteristic morphologic changes as well as by the upregulation of one or more properties that are generally associated with "activated" macrophages. These activation markers include the upregulated expression of certain membrane receptors (Table 3-1), the generation of a wide variety of secretory products (Table 3-2), or an increased chemotactic, phagocytic, or antimicrobial capacity. Although the understanding of each of these immunologic properties of microglia has accelerated in recent years, knowledge in this area is still evolving.

Antigen Processing and Presentation The healthy CNS traditionally has been considered an immunologically privileged site in that the BBB is able to exclude components of the immune system, and brain cells express unusually low levels of the major histocompatibility complex (MHC) class I and class II antigens. However, inflammatory responses are mounted in the brain against both autoantigens and infectious agents. A series of studies carried out during the past decade clearly demonstrated that

Table 3-1. Microglial Cell Membrane Receptors*

- Cell adhesion molecules
  - Immunoglobulin (Ig) superfamily
    - Ig Fc receptors
    - MHC class I glycoproteins
    - MHC class II glycoproteins
    - CD4 receptors
    - Intercellular adhesion molecule 1 (ICAM-1)
  - Integrins
    - Leukocyte function–associated antigen 1 (LFA-1; CD11a/CD18; CR1)
    - Mac-1 (CD11b/CD18; CR3)
    - p150, p95 (CD11c/CD18; CR4)
- Complement receptors: C1q, C5a
- Cytokine/chemokine receptors
  - Interferon (IFN)-α, IFN-γ
  - Interleukin (IL)-1, IL-8
  - Tumor necrosis factor (TNF)-α
  - Macrophage colony-stimulating factor (M-CSF), granulocyte-macrophage colony-stimulating factor (GM-CSF)
- CD14 receptors
- Mannose receptors
- Opioid receptors (μ, κ)
- Benzodiazepine receptors

*Receptors reported in the literature, the expression of which may be influenced by the state of activation as well as by the anatomic location, age, and animal species from which the microglia are derived.

such inflammatory responses within the CNS are associated with marked upregulation of both class I and class II MHC molecules on microglia (21–23). Cytokines are known to play a key role in the upregulation of the expression of these plasma membrane glycoproteins, with interferon (IFN)-γ being the most potent inducer, and transforming growth factor (TGF)-β downregulating IFN-γ–induced effects. While the MHC antigens generally have been thought to be expressed only by reactive microglia, studies of histologically normal human brain tissue demonstrated strong constitutive MHC class II (HLA-DR) antigen expression on ramified microglia (24).

Autoantigens and microbial products are generally recognized by T lymphocytes in the context of MHC molecules on APCs. Although cytokine-stimulated astrocytes also can express MHC molecules, microglial cells are presently regarded as the principal APCs within the brain. However, results of recent studies using radiation bone marrow chimeras suggest that nonmicroglial brain macrophages are the effective APCs for experimental autoimmune encephalomyelitis–inducing $CD4^+$ myelin basic protein–re-

Table 3-2. Secretory Products of Microglia*

Cytokines
IL-1α, IL-1β, IL-6, IL-10, TNF-α, transforming growth factor (TGF)-β
Chemokines
Monocyte chemoattractant protein (MCP)-1, macrophage inflammatory protein (MIP)-α, MIP-1β
Free radicals: superoxide, nitric oxide
Eicosanoids: prostaglandin D_2, leukotriene C_4
Growth factors: nerve growth factor, fibroblast growth factor
Proteases: elastase, plasminogen
Cathepsins B and L
Quinolinic acid, glutamate
Amyloid precursor protein
Complement factors: C1, C3, C4

*Secretory products reported in the literature, the generation of which is influenced by the state of activation as well as by the anatomic location, age, and animal species from which the microglia are derived.

active T cells (25). Thus, the capacity of adult CNS microglia to interact with and to stimulate CD4+ T lymphocytes is open to question.

Secretory Products

Cytokines and Chemokines In concert with general scientific interest in cytokines as the principal communication signals of the immune system, the field of neuroimmunology is replete with reports demonstrating that activated microglia produce a variety of cytokines (see Table 3-2) (26). Most extensively studied have been the proinflammatory cytokines, interleukin (IL)-1, IL-6, and tumor necrosis factor (TNF)-α, all of which are released by ameboid microglia upon stimulation with the gram-negative bacterial cell wall component lipopolysaccharide (LPS) (27–30). LPS-stimulated astrocyte cultures from rodent brain specimens also produce these cytokines (26). Results of studies of human fetal glial cell cultures, however, suggest that microglia are substantially more responsive to LPS than are astrocytes (30). In contrast to microglia within adult brain tissue (31), ameboid microglial cells express CD14 receptors, which are the main plasma membrane binding site for LPS-induced cytokine expression (32). CD14 receptors also appear to be involved in the uptake of nonopsonized *Mycobacterium tuberculosis* (33), and may function as the microglial cell receptor for mycobacterial lipoarabinomannan-induced TNF-α production (34).

The production of TNF-α by human fetal microglial cells is downregulated by the anti-inflammatory cytokines IL-10 and TGF-β (35), whereas TNF-α upregulates IL-10 production (36) and mediates the release of TGF-β (37). Also, microglial cell production of IL-1 and TNF-α is regulated by a number of neurotransmitters and endogenous as well as exogenous opioids (38–40), indicating the potential for considerable "cross talk" between neurons and activated microglia. Receptors for many proinflammatory and anti-inflammatory cytokines have been identified on microglial cells (see Table 3-1) (41), and recent studies in our laboratory demonstrated that human fetal microglia constitutively express κ (42) and μ (42a) opioid receptors.

The intense interest in microglial cell cytokine production reflects the emerging concept that these immune mediators not only contribute to normal neural development and defense of the CNS, but also have the potential when overexpressed to injure and even to kill neurons (43). The topic of microglia-mediated neurotoxicity is addressed later in this chapter and is also reviewed in Chapters 5 and 8. The neuropathogenic effects of cytokines have been implicated in a wide range of CNS disorders including traumatic brain injury (44), autoimmune diseases (45), Alzheimer's disease (46), human immunodeficiency virus (HIV)–associated dementia (47) (see Chapter 18), and bacterial meningitis (see Chapter 7). Also, cytokines serve a key messenger function in the bidirectional communication between the brain and the immune system (48,49), and they appear to be the principal mediators of the symptoms of "sickness" (50) that often accompany infectious and autoimmune diseases.

Although del Rio-Hortega and his contemporaries recognized that microglia migrate to areas of brain injury or inflammation (1), only recently have studies been carried out to identify the signals that direct the movement of these cells. In addition to TGF-β and the complement protein C5a (51), monocyte chemoattractant protein (MCP)-1, a member of the β (C-C) subfamily of chemokines, stimulates the chemotactic responsiveness of rodent microglia (52). Recent in vitro studies in our laboratory showed that human fetal microglia also migrate toward MCP-1, as well as toward two other β chemokines, namely, macrophage inflammatory protein (MIP)-1α and MIP-1β (unpublished observation). Additionally, LPS- and cytokine-stimulated human microglia produce MCP-1, MIP-1α, and MIP-1β (52a). These findings suggest that β chemokines released from activated microglia could serve as chemotactic signals for the recruitment of ameboid microglia into inflammatory foci within the CNS, and if produced in the vicinity of the BBB, these chemotactic peptides could also play a role in the trafficking of monocytes or T lymphocytes into the brain (see Chapter 2).

Free Radicals A study in 1987 showed that primary microglial cell cultures derived from neonatal rat brain specimens release superoxide anion (O_2^-) on stimulation with phorbol myristate acetate or opsonized zymosan (53). Because O_2^- is metabolized to more toxic reactive oxygen intermediates (ROIs), which can have both antimicrobial and cytotoxic activities, it was suggested that this "respiratory burst" activity of microglia could play a dual rule in defense and injury of the CNS. Subsequent in vitro studies of murine (54), swine (55), and human (56) microglia demonstrated that activated cells from all three species have the capacity to generate O_2^-. While IFN-γ and TNF-α prime ameboid microglia for enhanced O_2^- production, TGF-β antagonizes the stimulatory effect of these cytokines (57).

In recent years, attention has focused on the reactive nitrogen intermediate nitric oxide (NO), which like ROIs, can both inhibit the growth of intracellular microorganisms and kill neighboring cells. Although primary neonatal murine and rat microglial cell

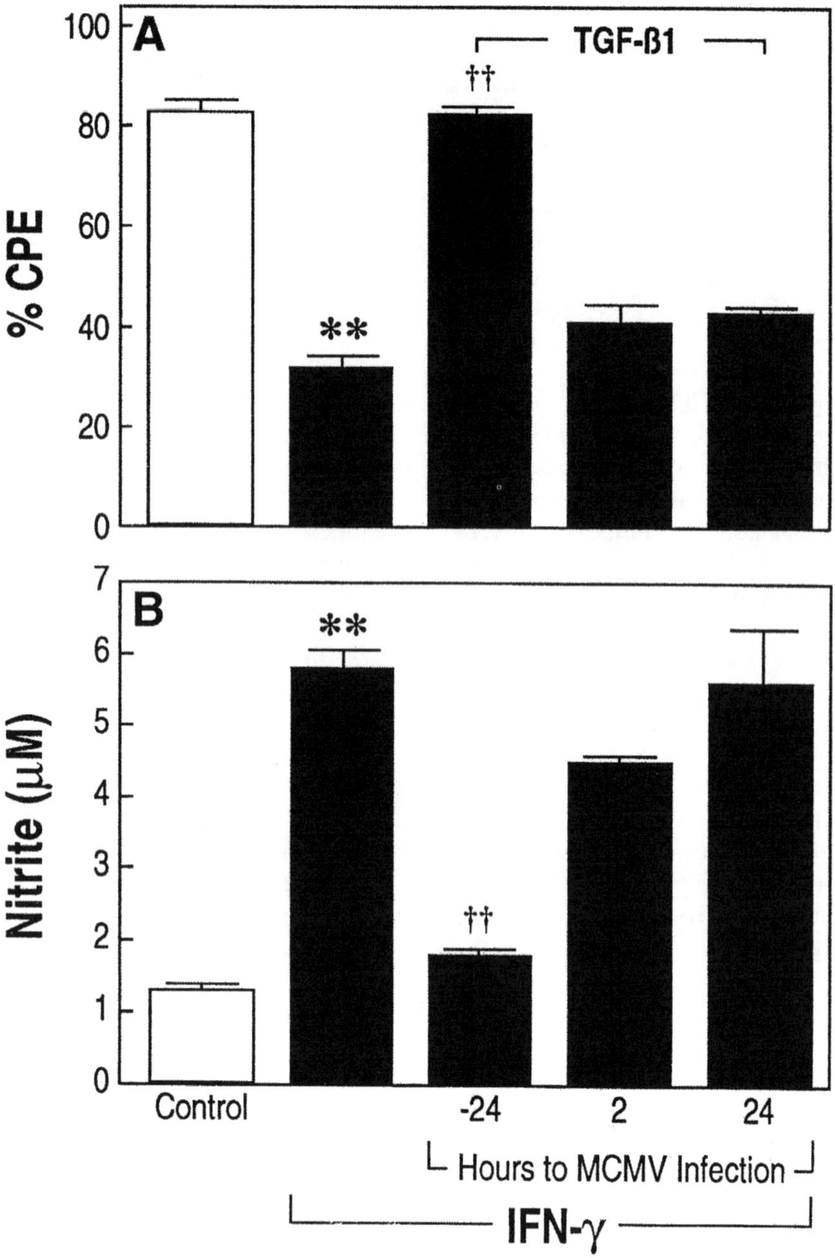

Figure 3-3. The role of cytokines and nitric oxide (NO) in the regulation of cytomegalovirus (CMV) replication in microglia. With a previously described method (64), murine CMV (MCMV) was cultured in murine microglial cells, and viral replication was assessed by quantifying the cytopathic effect (CPE) of the virus. When compared to control cells, microglial cells treated with interferon gamma (IFN-γ) (100 units/mL) had (A) reduced viral replication and (B)

cultures yield substantial amounts of NO on stimulation with IFN-γ and LPS or TNF-α (58,59), the picture is less clear for human microglial cells. Initial studies of human fetal ameboid microglial cell cultures demonstrated that cytokine-activated human microglia produce little or no NO (60,61). This observation is consistent with the hyporesponsiveness of the human inducible NO synthase (iNOS) gene reported for other populations of human mononuclear phagocytes when stimulated with LPS and IFN-γ.

Recent studies reopened the question of whether human microglia are capable of generating biologically significant amounts of NO. Multiply passaged cultures of human microglia, which select for the *ramified* form, reportedly express iNOS messenger RNA (mRNA) and release substantial amounts of NO (62) following activation of these cells with LPS and TNF-α. Also, in a recent study of hamster microglia, which like human fetal ameboid microglia produce minimal amounts of NO on stimulation with a variety of cytokines, Poly I:C (synthetic double stranded RNA) elicited considerable amounts of NO (63).

Although the functional activities of ROIs remain hypothetical, cytokine-activated murine microglial cells are known to inhibit the intracellular multiplication of *Toxoplasma gondii* by an NO-related mechanism (58). Murine microglia treated with IFN-γ also inhibit the intracellular replication of cytomegalovirus by inducing NO, and this antiviral function is blocked by TGF-β (Fig 3-3) (64). In coculture assay systems, cytokine-activated murine microglia also can mediate the death of neurons (65) and of oligodendrocytes (66) and NO is involved in this cytotoxic activity. Because of their cytotoxic potential, elimination of activated microglia from the brain may be beneficial to neighboring neurons and glial cells. Results of recent studies suggest that one mechanism by which activated microglia could be eliminated from the brain parenchyma is the process of programmed cell death or apoptosis (67). Studies in our laboratory showed that the NO-generating compound sodium nitroprusside induces apoptosis of human microglial cells (Fig 3-4) (68). Thus, NO could play an indirect role in neuroprotection by depleting the brain of activated microglia.

Even though cytokine-activated human microglial cells may be incapable of generating biologically significant amounts of NO, IL-1–stimulated human astrocytes can (60,69). Because microglia are the principal source of IL-1 in the CNS, it has been hypothesized that activated human microglia could play an indirect role in NO-mediated neurotoxicity, as well as in the apoptosis of microglia, by activating astrocyte iNOS (69).

Growth Factors and Proliferation During fetal development, massive numbers of neurons proliferate within the CNS. In addition to their role in removing dead neurons, microglial cells are a potential source of several nerve growth factors (see Table 3-2). Unlike most tissue macrophages, which are considered to be terminally differentiated monocytes, microglial cells themselves also have the capacity to proliferate. Of the

---

increased levels of nitrite, a metabolite of NO, in the culture supernatants. Transforming growth factor-β1 (TGF-β1) (25 pg/mL) added to the microglial cell cultures 24 hours before infection (−24 hours) but not after infection (2 or 24 hours) blocked the antiviral activity of IFN-γ and the IFN-γ–induced production of nitrite. $^{**}p < 0.01$ vs control cells; †† $p < 0.01$ vs IFN-γ–treated cells.

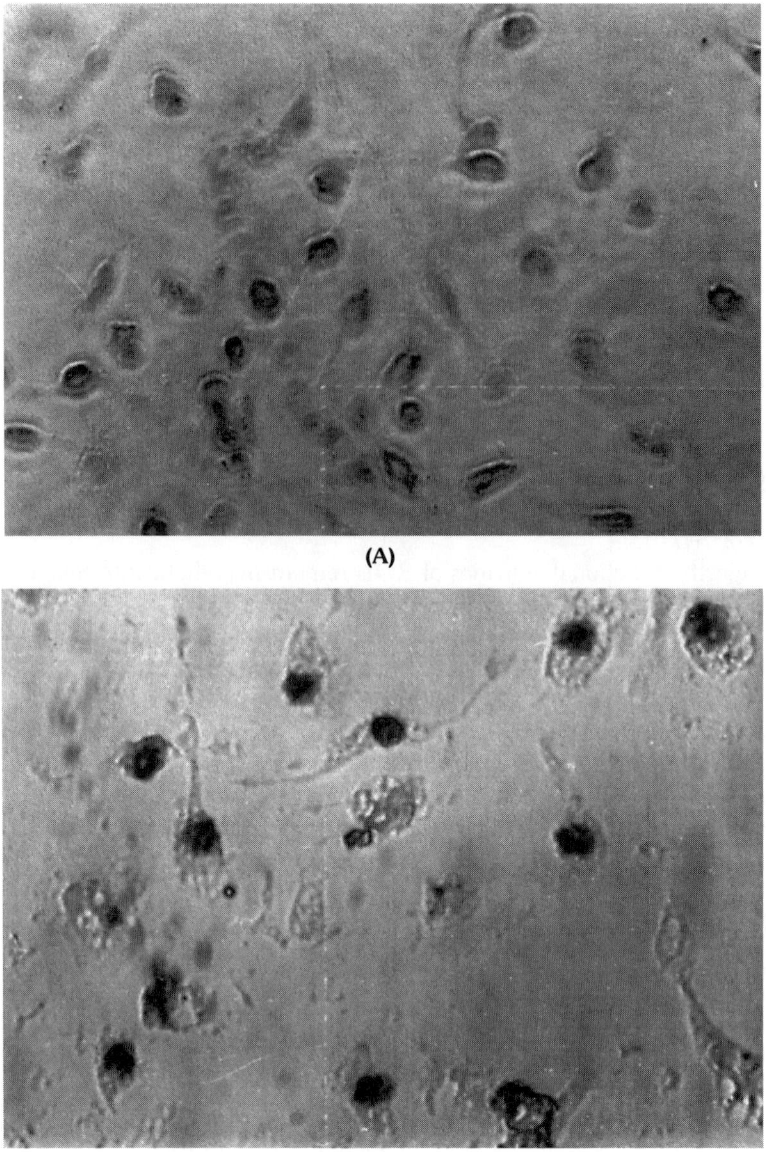

(A)

(B)

Figure 3-4. Programmed cell death (apoptosis) of human fetal microglia induced by nitric oxide (NO). For this experiment, microglial cells were cultured for 24 hours in the (A) absence and (B) presence of the NO-generating chemical sodium nitroprusside (SNP) (2 mM). The cells were then examined by light microscopy (× 400) using the terminal-deoxyneucleotide-transferase mediated dUTP-digoxigenin nick end labeling (TUNEL) technique for detecting apoptosis (68). Only the SNP-exposed cells show the dark-staining nuclei characteristic of apoptotic cells. (C) Gel electrophoresis of DNA extracted from SNP-treated microglia demonstrates low-molecular-weight DNA fragments associated with apoptosis (68). Lane 1: molecular weight markers; lane 2: control (untreated) microglia; lane 3: SNP-exposed microglia. (Reprinted with kind permission from Elsevier Science–NL, Sara Burgerhartstraat 25, 1055 KV Amsterdam, The Netherlands.)

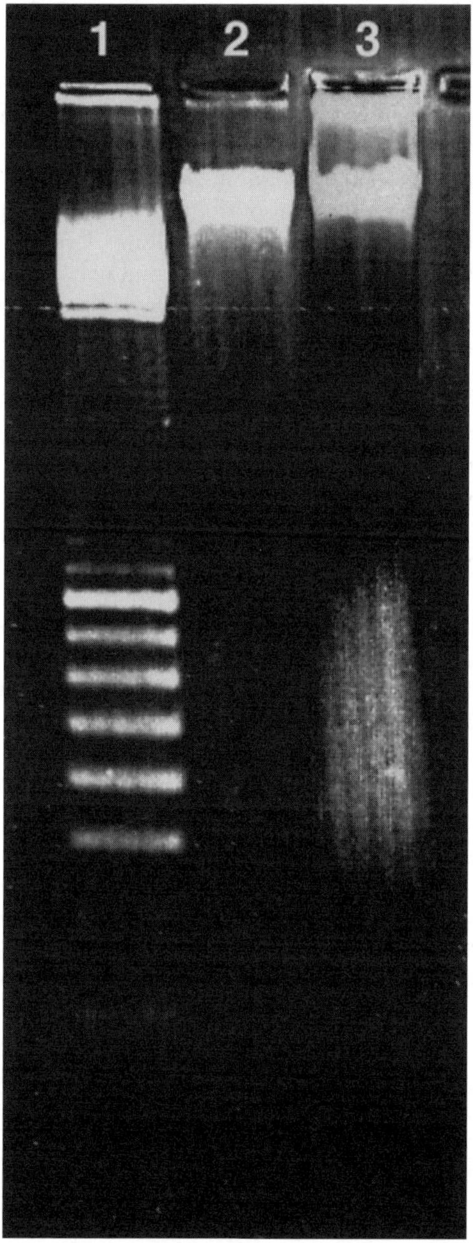

(C)

Figure 3-4. (*continued*)

more than 35 different growth factors that have been recognized for their abilities to influence various steps in neuronal development (70), only a limited number of cytokines have the capacity to induce cell division of microglia. Ameboid rodent microglia proliferate in response to granulocyte-macrophage colony-stimulating factor (GM-CSF), macrophage CSF (M-CSF), IL-3, and IL-5 (71–73). TGF-β, on the other hand, inhibits GM-CSF–induced proliferation of rodent microglia (74).

Human fetal and adult microglia also proliferate in vitro in response to GM-CSF (75). Studies in our laboratory of microglial cell cultures derived from human fetal brain specimens demonstrated that GM-CSF and IL-3, but not TNF-α, IL-1, IL-12, or LPS, stimulate cell proliferation (Table 3-3). In addition to inducing microglial cell proliferation, GM-CSF triggers striking morphologic changes (Fig 3-5B), which are different from the morphologic alterations of microglia in response to TNF-α (Fig 3-5C). In addition to serving as the most potent microglial cell mitogens, GM-CSF and M-CSF appear to retard the process of microglial cell apoptosis (68). Although the cellular source of growth factors that stimulate microglial cell proliferation within the CNS is unknown, astrocytes are a likely candidate.

Complement Factors Microglial cells synthesize several of the early components of the classic complement pathway (see Table 3-2). Activation of complement has been associated with a number of neurologic diseases. Oligodendrocytes and neurons appear to be especially susceptible to complement-mediated injury, and the expression of complement by activated microglia has been implicated in the inflammatory response seen in the brain parenchymal lesions of Alzheimer's disease (76).

Complement production within the CNS may also be important in defense of the brain against invading microorganisms. Normal cerebrospinal fluid is devoid of opsonic activity for the encapsulated bacteria that commonly cause meningitis. However, complement-mediated opsonic activity appears in the cerebrospinal fluid in the early stages of bacterial meningitis, especially in patients who recover from this life-threatening infection (77). Because astrocytes synthesize all of the components of the activation pathways of complement (78) and form the brain's side of the BBB (see Chapter 1), these glial cells are the likely source of cerebrospinal fluid complement.

Table 3-3. Cytokines and Microglial Cell Proliferation[a]

Treatment	*[^{3}H]Thymidine Uptake (cpm/well)*	*PCNA (% positive)*
Control	230.6 ± 10.5	12.0 ± 2.5
IL-3 (20 ng/mL)	1,075.4 ± 67.0[b]	49.7 ± 1.7[b]
GM-CSF (20 ng/mL)	1,742.3 ± 95.8[b]	72.7 ± 4.2[b]

[a]Human fetal microglial cells were cultured for 7 days in medium alone (control) or were treated with cytokines, at indicated concentrations, and cell proliferation was assessed by measuring [^{3}H]thymidine uptake and by proliferating cell nuclear antigen (PCNA) staining (68,75). Values are mean ± standard error of mean of duplicate samples and are representative of three independent experiments.
[b]$p < 0.05$ vs control cells.

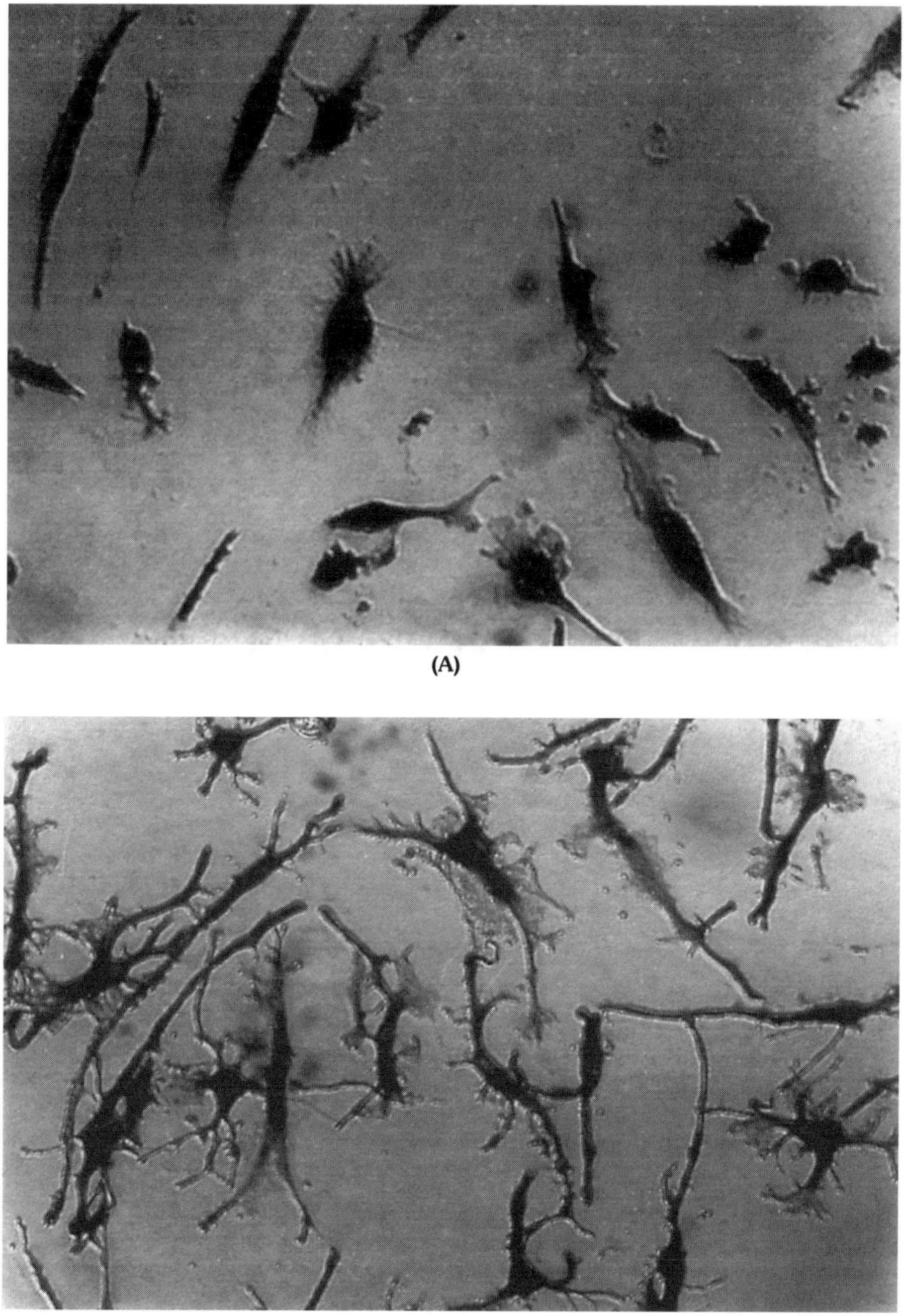

(A)

(B)

Figure 3-5. Effect of granulocyte-macrophage colony-stimulating factor (GM-CSF) and tumor necrosis factor-α (TNF-α) on the morphology of human fetal microglial cells following 7 days in culture. (A) Untreated (control) microglia. (B) GM-CSF (20 ng/mL)–treated microglia. (C) TNF-α (20 ng/mL)–treated microglia. All cell cultures were stained with antibodies specific for human macrophages and examined under light microscopy (× 400).

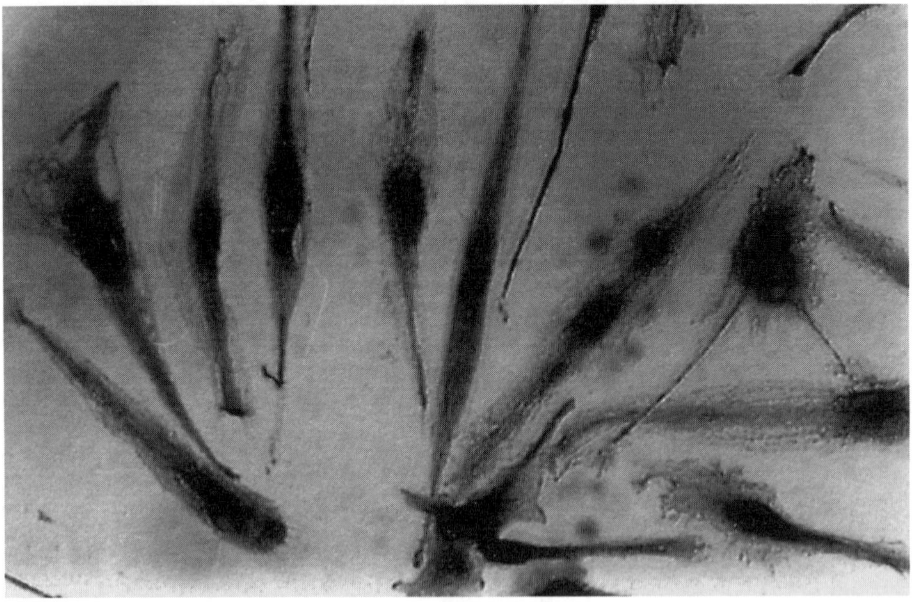

(C)

Figure 3-5. *(continued)*

Antimicrobial Properties The BBB provides a formidable shield for the CNS against microbial invasion. Nevertheless, a number of microorganisms have devised strategies for gaining access to the brain parenchyma, and those that are well adapted for multiplication within the CNS are considered neurotropic (Table 3-4). The idea that microglia may function as the primary defenders of the brain parenchyma dates to del Rio-Hortega (1). However, relatively few studies have examined the antimicrobial activity of microglia, and the results of these studies suggest that microglial cells may be a favored target cell for some neurotropic pathogens.

Bacterial Interactions del Rio-Hortega recognized microglial cells in the CNS lesions of patients with tuberculous meningitis (1). At about the same time, other investigators established that tubercle bacilli gain access to the subarachnoid space via rupture of adjacent tuberculomas within the parenchyma of the brain (79) rather than by hematogenous spread, which occurs in other forms of bacterial meningitis. However, the type of cells involved in infection of the brain parenchyma by *Mycobacterium tuberculosis* is largely unknown.

Studies in our laboratory with human fetal microglial cell cultures demonstrated that nonopsonized *M. tuberculosis* is phagocytized by these microglia via a CD14 receptor–related mechanism (33). When neonatal swine microglial cell cultures are infected with *Mycobacterium bovis*, tubercle bacilli rapidly induce the formation of fused microglia, that is, multinucleated giant cells (MGCs) (80). This phenomenon of MGC formation by microglia depends on a cell surface adhesion molecule, most likely a β_2

Table 3-4. Neurotropic Infectious Agents*

Bacteria	Viruses
Mycobacterium tuberculosis	Herpes group
Treponema pallidum	Herpes simplex virus
Borrelia burgdorferi	Cytomegalovirus
Nocardia asteroides	Epstein-Barr virus
Leptospira	Human herpesvirus 6
Brucella	B virus
Rickettsia	Enteroviruses
Mycoplasma	Polioviruses
	Coxsackieviruses
Fungi	Echoviruses
Cryptococcus neoformans	Retroviruses
Coccidioides immitis	HIV
Histoplasma capsulatum	Human T lymphotropic virus type I
Blastomyces dermatitidis	Rabies virus
Candida	Mumps virus
Zygomycetes	Lymphocytic choriomeningitis virus
Aspergillus	Measles virus
Sporothrix schenckii	Rubella virus
	JC virus
Parasites	Prions
Cysticercus	
Toxoplasma gondii	
Trypanosoma	
Entamoeba histolytica	
Free-living amebas	
Echinococcus	
Schistosoma	
Angiostrongylus cantonensis	
Gnathostoma spinigerum	

*Human pathogens that have the capacity to invade, multiply, and elicit a pathologic response within the brain parenchyma. This list does not include the bacteria that most commonly cause meningitis and brain abscesses, or the parasite *Plasmodium falciparum*, which is the cause of cerebral malaria.

integrin (80,81), and in the case of *M. bovis*–induced MGCs, the proinflammatory cytokine TNF-α (80). Because macrophages are considered the only cell in which tubercle bacilli grow in vivo, it is hypothetically possible that the microglial cell is a favored CNS target for this intracellular pathogen.

In studies of the intracellular opportunist *Nocardia asteroides*, neonatal mouse microglial cells appear to inhibit the intracellular growth of this bacterium, in contrast to astrocytes which support the multiplication of the *Nocardia* organisms (82). In in vivo studies in mice, however, intracellular *Nocardia* bacteria did not appear to be damaged by microglia (83). Thus, the role of microglial cells in the host defense of the CNS against intracellular bacteria (see Table 3-4) remains to be established.

Limited studies have been carried out on the interaction between microglia and *Borrelia burgdorferi*, the etiologic agent of Lyme disease. Studies demonstrated that glioma cells and glial cell cultures release IL-6 and NO in response to intact spirochetes or bacterial sonicates (84,85), suggesting microglia could participate in the pathogenesis of neuroborreliosis.

Because LPS is a potent stimulus of many secretory products of microglia, this bacterial cell wall component could play an important pathogenetic role in brain cell damage associated with gram-negative bacterial meningitis. Interestingly, in vitro studies of the effects of the gram-positive bacterium *Streptococcus pneumoniae* and of pneumococcal cell walls on rat neurons, astrocytes, and microglia demonstrated toxic effects principally in microglia and to a lesser extent in astrocytes but not in neurons, suggesting that microglial cell toxicity may be in part responsible for brain injury during pneumococcal meningitis (86) (see Chapter 8).

Parasite Interactions Probably reflecting the fact that *T. gondii* is the most important infectious cause of CNS mass lesions in AIDS patients (see Chapter 10), this neurotropic parasite has been the best studied in terms of its interaction with microglial cells. In neonatal murine microglial cell cultures, *T. gondii* multiplies readily within nonactivated cells. Treatment of murine microglia with IFN-γ and TNF-α, however, resulted in a marked anti–*T. gondii* effect (87). Other studies of murine microglial cell cultures demonstrated that cells grown in the presence of GM-CSF also had the capacity to restrict the intracellular multiplication of tachyzoites (88). As mentioned earlier, the ability of cytokine-activated microglia to inhibit the intracellular growth of *T. gondii* is related to the production of NO by these cells (58). By way of contrast, IFN-γ– and TNF-α–treated astrocytes are incapable of generating NO, and thereby of limiting the intracellular multiplication of *T. gondii* (89). That IFN-γ, TNF-α, and NO play key mediator roles in microglial cell defense of the brain against *T. gondii* is also supported by in vivo studies of murine cerebral toxoplasmosis (90).

Although a strong case can be made that cytokine-activated microglia contribute to the defense of the murine CNS against *T. gondii*, the role of microglia in human cerebral toxoplasmosis is unclear. In vitro studies showed that IFN-γ– and TNF-α–treated fetal human microglial cells are less readily infected by *T. gondii*. However, once tachyzoites gain entry to human fetal microglia, cytokine treatment has no effect on their intracellular multiplication (91). This animal species difference appears to be explained by the relatively inefficient iNOS in human microglia (60,61). Based on the results of these in vitro studies of human microglia as well as the clinical evidence that development of cerebral toxoplasmosis in HIV-infected patients is associated with a marked reduction in $CD4^+$ T cells, it appears that T lymphocytes may be the primary defenders of the human CNS against *T. gondii* infection (see Chapters 4 and 10).

Fungal Interactions Results of in vivo studies of mice challenged with *Candida albicans* intracerebrally or intravenously strongly suggest that cytokines play a crucial role in defense of the brain against intracerebral infection by this opportunistic fungus (92). Although recent findings suggest that resistance versus susceptibility to CNS *C. albicans* infection cannot be explained simply on the basis of differences in Th1 versus

Th2 cytokine expression (93), IL-1 may be a pivotal cytokine in anti-*Candida* activity within the mouse brain (92).

Few, if any, data have been published regarding the anti-*Candida* activity of microglia. Studies in which *C. albicans* was incubated with enriched microglial cell cultures obtained from healthy human adult brain tissue demonstrated that these cells can serve as APCs to T lymphocytes (94). Also, local (CNS) production of the anti-inflammatory cytokine TGF-β has been implicated in the pathogenesis of a glioblastoma in a patient in whom *C. albicans* meningitis developed (95).

Because of the AIDS epidemic, the incidence of CNS cryptococcosis has increased dramatically (see Chapter 13). Murine models of cryptococcal meningoencephalitis (96–99) have provided evidence that microglial cells and cytokines contribute to resistance of the CNS to infection by *Cryptococcus neoformans*. Human microglia also can inhibit the growth of *C. neoformans* in vitro (100). This fungistatic activity of human microglia is not related to NO production (100), which contrasts sharply with cytokine-treated human astrocytes (101). Pathogenic isolates of *C. neoformans* are encapsulated and require specific anticapsular antibodies for opsonization and efficient phagocytosis via microglial cell Fc receptors (100). Because human microglia appear to have fungistatic but not fungicidal activity against intracellular cryptococci (100), other anticryptococcal defense systems may also be involved in the killing of cryptococci within the brain. Cytotoxic T lymphocytes have direct fungicidal activity against cryptococci (102), and if these cells infiltrate the brain during infection, they could play an important role in eliminating this fungus from the CNS.

Viral Interactions As was pointed out earlier in this review, the recognition of brain macrophages as the principal cell type infected by HIV in patients with AIDS encephalopathy (103) has been an important factor underlying the reawakening of scientific interest in microglia. The complex topic of the neuropathogenesis of HIV is covered in detail elsewhere in this book (see Chapter 18). One controversial issue that relates specifically to the involvement of microglial cells in HIV infection of the brain is whether microglia are actually the mononuclear phagocyte productively infected by the virus. While many studies support the notion that microglia are the only cell type within the CNS that can support a replicating infection by HIV, some data suggest that this dubious distinction belongs to perivascular macrophages or to infected monocytes that have invaded the brain (104). Another point of controversy relates to the role of cytokines in regulating HIV infection in microglia. Cytokines that are known to be produced in abundance by activated microglia (e.g., TNF-α and IL-1) have been strongly implicated in the neuroimmunopathogenesis of HIV (105). These cytokines, when produced by microglia, also upregulate the expression of HIV-1 in chronically infected promonocytes (106,107). Nevertheless, recent findings in our laboratory suggest that IL-1 inhibits HIV-1 replication in acutely infected microglia and that TNF-α has little or no effect (107a).

The potential role of microglia in defense or injury of the CNS has just begun to be considered for other neurotropic viruses, including human T-cell leukemia virus type I (108), herpes simplex virus (see Chapter 16) (109), the swine herpesvirus pseudorabies virus (110), cytomegalovirus (64), measles virus (111), lymphocytic choriomeningitis virus (112), Borna virus (113), rabies virus (113), and Theiler's murine encephalomyelitis virus (114), and for the prion protein associated with Creutzfeldt-Jakob disease (115). While other brain cell types are also likely to be infected by these neurotropic agents, and the most serious clinical consequences are related to neuronal loss or dysfunction, the outcome of the interaction between microorganisms and microglial cells may be an indirect determinant of the survival of neurons.

NEUROTOXICITY

As discussed throughout this chapter, in addition to the role of microglia in restoring homeostasis within the brain following a variety of insults, considerable evidence suggests that microglial cells may also participate in brain pathology. The topic of microglia-induced brain injury has been extensively reviewed by other authors (116,117), and aspects of this topic are also discussed in Chapter 5. While most of the supporting evidence of a pathogenetic role is circumstantial, that is, demonstration of activated microglia within pathologic lesions ("guilt by association"), the main reason why this potential negative side of microglia has captured the attention of many members of the neuroscience community is the diversity of neurologic diseases in which activated microglia have been implicated. These diseases include not only the neurologic sequelae of acute as well as chronic infections, but also neurodegenerative diseases such as Alzheimer's disease (118) and multiple sclerosis (119), and brain injury following hypoxia-ischemia or head trauma (120,121). As more has been learned about the behavioral effects of the secretory products of activated microglia on neurons, these resident defenders of the brain parenchyma have even been considered to play a role in classic psychiatric illnesses such as schizophrenia and depression (122).

CONCLUSIONS

Like many areas of immunology, review of the "old literature" reveals startling insights into virtually all aspects of microglial cell biology, most of which Pio del Rio-Hortega summarized in 1932 (1). Despite an intensive contemporary research effort, the major concepts and controversies raised by del Rio-Hortega about the nature of these resident brain macrophages have not changed. More data have accumulated, of course, regarding the scavenger and defense functions of these cells, and especially about the molecular basis of microglial plasma membrane receptors and the myriad secretory products released from activated cells.

Perhaps as a reflection of increased knowledge, we have gained a better understanding about many important unanswered questions regarding the microglia. What is the origin and the physiologic function of ramified microglia? Are ramified microglia truly quiescent cells or do they normally communicate with other glial cells and with neurons? What are the influences of other brain cells (astrocytes and neurons) and of T lymphocytes on microglial cell function? What is the biologic significance of the animal species differences that have been found in the generation by activated microglia of certain secretory products? Do microglia provide a safe haven for intracellular neurotropic pathogens within the CNS of humans, or are they key defenders of the brain against these pathogens? What role, if any, do reactive microglia play in defense against or the pathogenesis of brain malignancy? Do reactive microglia truly contribute to the process of neuronal degeneration or dysfunction in the wide variety of neurologic and neuropsychiatric diseases in which they have been implicated? Finding definitive answers to these questions promises to keep the neurons of many investigators busy for some time to come.

REFERENCES

1 del Rio-Hortega P. Microglia. In: Penfield W, ed. *Cytology and cellular pathology of the nervous system.* New York: PB Hoeber, 1932: 483–534.

2 Streit WJ. Microglial cells. In: Kentenmann H, Ransom BR, eds. *Neuroglia.* New York: Oxford University Press, 1995:85–96.

3 Gehrmann J, Matsumoto Y, Kreutzberg GW. Microglia: intrinsic immuneffector cell of the brain. *Brain Res Rev* 1995;20:269–287.

4 Perry VH, Lawson LJ. Macrophages in the central nervous system. In: Lewis CE, McGee JO'D, eds. *The macrophage.* Oxford, UK: Oxford University Press, 1992:393–413.

5 Streit WJ, Graeber MB, Kreutzberg GW. Functional plasticity of microglia: a review. *Glia* 1988;1:301–307.

6 Ulvestad E, Williams K, Bjerkvig R, et al. Human microglial cells have phenotypic and functional characteristics in common with both macrophages and dendritic antigen-presenting cells. *J Leukoc Biol* 1994;56:732–740.

7 Kaur C, Ling EA. Study of the transformation of ameboid microglial cells into microglia labeled with the isolectin *Griffonia simplicifolia* in postnatal rats. *Acta Anat* 1991;142:118–125.

8 Lee SC, Liu W, Brosnan CF, Dickson DW. Characterization of primary human fetal dissociated central nervous system cultures with an emphasis on microglia. *Lab Invest* 1992;67:465–476.

9 Schmidtmayer J, Jacobsen C, Miksch G, Sievers J. Blood monocytes and spleen macrophages differentiate into microglia-like cells on monolayers of astrocytes: membrane currents. *Glia* 1994;12:259–267.

10 Lauro GM, Babiloni D, Buttarelli FR, et al. Human microglia cultures: a powerful model to study their origin and immunoreactive capacity. *Int J Dev Neurosci* 1995;13:739–752.

11 Theele DP, Steit WJ. A chronicle of microglial ontogeny. *Glia* 1993;7:5–8.

12 Lawson LJ, Perry VH, Gordon S. Turnover of resident microglia in the normal adult mouse brain. *Neuroscience* 1992;48:405–415.

13 Ling E-A, Wong W-C. The origin and nature of ramified and amoeboid microglia: a historical review and current concepts. *Glia* 1993;7:9–18.

14 Davis EJ, Foster TD, Thomas WE. Cellular forms and functions of brain microglia. *Brain Res Bull* 1994;34:73–78.

15 De Groot CJA, Huppes W, Sminia T, et al. Determination of the origin and nature of brain macrophages and microglial cells in mouse central nervous system, using non-radioactive in situ hybridization and immunoperoxidase techniques. *Glia* 1992;6:301–309.

16 Lassmann H, Hickey WF. Radiation bone marrow chimeras as a tool to study microglia turnover in normal brain and inflammation. *Clin Neuropathol* 1993;12:284–285.

17 Fedoroff S. Development of microglia. In: Kentenmann H, Ransom BR, eds. *Neuroglia.* New York: Oxford University Press, 1995: 162–181.

18 Giulian D, Li J, Bartel S, et al. Cell surface morphology identifies microglia as a distinct class of mononuclear phagocyte. *J Neurosci* 1995;15:7712–7726.

19 Voyvodic JT. Cell death in cortical development: How much? Why? So What? *Neuron* 1996;16:693–696.

20 Brockhaus J, Moller T, Kettenmann H. Phagocytizing ameboid microglial cells studied in a mouse corpus callosum slice preparation. *Glia* 1996;16:81–90.

21 Loughlin AJ, Woodroofe MN, Cuzner ML. Modulation of interferon-γ-induced major histocompatibility complex class II and Fc receptor expression on isolated microglia by transforming growth factor-β1, interleukin-4, noradrenaline and glucocorticoids. *Immunology* 1993;79:125–130.

22 Fabry Z, Raine CS, Hart MN. Nervous tissue

as an immune compartment: the dialect of the immune response in the CNS. *Immunol Today* 1994;15:218–224.

23 Panek RB, Benveniste EN. Class II MHC gene expression in microglia. *J Immunol* 1995;154:2846–2854.

24 Gehrmann J, Banati RB, Kreutzberg GW. Microglia in the immune surveillance of the brain: human microglia constitutively express HLA-DR molecules. *J Neuroimmunol* 1993;48:189–198.

25 Ford AL, Goodsall AL, Hickey WF, Sedgwick JD. Normal adult ramified microglia separated from other central nervous system macrophages by flow cytometric sorting. *J Immunol* 1995;154:4309–4321.

26 Benveniste EN. Cytokine production. In: Kettenmann H, Ransom BR, eds. *Neuroglia*. New York: Oxford University Press, 1995:700–713.

27 Giulian D, Baker TJ, Shih L-C, Lachman LB. Interleukin 1 of the central nervous system is produced by ameboid microglia. *J Exp Med* 1986;164:594–604.

28 Chao CC, Hu S, Close K, et al. Cytokine release from microglia: differential inhibition by pentoxifylline and dexamethasone. *J Infect Dis* 1992;166:847–853.

29 Sébire G, Emilie D, Wallon C, et al. In vitro production of IL-6, IL-1β, and tumor necrosis factor-α by human embryonic microglial and neural cells. *J Immunol* 1993;150:1517–1523.

30 Lee SC, Liu W, Dickson DW, et al. Cytokine production by human fetal microglia and astrocytes. *J Immunol* 1993;150:2659–2667.

31 Ulvestad E, Williams K, Mørk S, et al. Phenotypic differences between human monocytes/macrophages and microglial cells studied in situ and in vitro. *J Neuropathol Exp Neurol* 1994;53:492–501.

32 Galea E, Reis DJ, Fox ES, et al. CD14 mediates endotoxin induction of nitric oxide synthase in cultured brain glial cells. *J Neuroimmunol* 1996;64:19–28.

33 Peterson PK, Gekker G, Hu S, et al. CD14 receptor-mediated uptake of nonopsonized *Mycobacterium tuberculosis* by human microglia. *Infect Immun* 1995;1598–1602.

34 Peterson PK, Hu S, Sheng WS, et al. Thalidomide inhibits tumor necrosis factor-α production by lipopolysaccharide- and lipoarabinomannan-stimulated human microglial cells. *J Infect Dis* 1995;172:1137–1140.

35 Chao CC, Hu S, Sheng WS, Peterson PK. Tumor necrosis factor-alpha production by human fetal microglial cells: regulation by other cytokines. *Dev Neurosci* 1995;17:97–105.

36 Sheng WS, Hu S, Kravitz FH, et al. Tumor necrosis factor alpha upregulates human microglial cell production of interleukin-10 in vitro. *Clin Diagn Lab Immunol* 1995;2:604–608.

37 Chao CC, Hu S, Sheng WS, et al. Tumor necrosis factor-α mediates the release of bioactive transforming growth factor-β in murine microglial cell cultures. *Clin Immunol Immunopathol* 1995;77:358–365.

38 Hetier E, Ayala J, Bousseau A, Prochiantz A. Modulation of interleukin-1 and tumor necrosis factor expression by β-adrenergic agonists in mouse ameboid microglial cells. *Brain Res* 1991;86:407–413.

39 Das KP, McMillan MK, Bing G, Hong J-S. Modulatory effects of [Met^5]-enkephalin on interleukin-1β secretion from microglia in mixed brain cell cultures. *J Neuroimmunol* 1995;62:9–17.

40 Chao CC, Gekker G, Sheng WS, et al. Priming effect of morphine on the production of tumor necrosis factor-α by microglia: implications in respiratory burst activity and human immunodeficiency virus-1 expression. *J Pharmacol Exp Ther* 1994;269:198–203.

41 Otero GC, Merrill JE. Cytokine receptors on glial cells. *Glia* 1994;11:117–128.

42 Chao CC, Gekker G, Hu S, et al. Kappa opioid receptors in human microglia downregulate human immunodeficiency virus-1 expression. *Proc Natl Acad Sci USA* 1996;93:8051–8056.

42a Chao CC, Hu S, Shark KB, et al. Activation of mμ opioid receptors inhibits microglial cell chemotaxis. *J Pharmacol Exp Ther* 1997 (in press).

43 Merrill JE. Tumor necrosis factor alpha, interleukin 1 and related cytokines in brain development: normal and pathological. *Dev Neurosci* 1992;14:1–10.

44 Yong VW. Cytokines, astrogliosis, and neurotropism following CNS trauma. In: Ransohoff RM, Beneviste EN, eds. *Cytokines and the CNS*. Boca Raton, FL: CRC Press, 1996:309–327.

45 Owens T, Renno T, Taupin V, Krakowski M. Inflammatory cytokines in the brain: does the CNS shape immune responses? *Immunol Today* 1994;15:566–571.

46 Dickson DW, Lee SC, Brosnan CF, et al. Neuroimmunology of aging and Alzheimer's disease with emphasis on cytokines. In: Ransohoff RM, Beneviste EN, eds. *Cytokines and the CNS*. Boca Raton. FL: CRC Press, 1996:239–267.

47 Wesselingh SL, Tyor WR, Griffin DE. Cytokines and HIV-associated dementia. In: Ran-

sohoff RM, Beneviste EN, eds. *Cytokines and the CNS*. Boca Raton, FL: CRC Press, 1996:287–307.

48 Sundar SK, Becker KJ, Cierpial MA, et al. Intracerebroventricular infusion of interleukin 1 rapidly decreases peripheral cellular immune responses. *Proc Natl Acad Sci USA* 1989;86:6398–6402.

49 Takao T, Hashimoto K, De Souza EB. Modulation of interleukin-1 receptors in the brain-endocrine-immune axis by stress and infection. *Brain Behav Immun* 1995;9:276–291.

50 van Dam AM, Brouns M, Louisse S, Berkenbosch F. Appearance of interleukin-1 in macrophages and in ramified microglia in the brain of endotoxin-treated rats: a pathway for the induction of non-specific symptoms of sickness? *Brain Res* 1992;588:291–296.

51 Yao J, Harvath L, Gilbert DL, Colton CA. Chemotaxis by a CNS macrophage, the microglia. *J Neurosci Res* 1990;27:36–42.

52 Hayashi M, Luo Y, Laning J, et al. Production and function of monocyte chemoattractant protein-1 and other β-chemokines in murine glial cells. *J Neuroimmunol* 1995;60:143–150.

52a Peterson PK, Hu S, Salak-Johnson J, et al. Differential production of and migratory response to β chemokines by human microglia and astrocytes. *J Infect Dis* 1997;175:478–481.

53 Colton CA, Gilberg DL. Production of superoxide anions by a CNS macrophage, the microglia. *Fed Eur Biochem Soc* 1987;223: 284–288.

54 Suzumura A, Marunouchi T, Yamamoto H. Morphological transformation of microglia in vitro. *Brain Res* 1991;545:301–306.

55 Hu S, Chao CC, Khanna KV, et al. Cytokine and free radical production by porcine microglia. *Clin Immunol Immunopathol* 1996; 78:93–96.

56 Chao CC, Hu S, Peterson PK. Modulation of human microglial cell superoxide production by cytokines. *J Leukoc Biol* 1995;58:65–70.

57 Hu S, Sheng WS, Peterson PK, Chao CC. Cytokine modulation of murine microglial cell superoxide production. *Glia* 1995;13:45–50.

58 Chao CC, Anderson WR, Hu S, et al. Activated microglia inhibit multiplication of *Toxoplasma gondii* via a nitric oxide mechanism. *Clin Immunol Immunopathol* 1993;67:178–183.

59 Bertini G, Savio T, Zaccheo D, et al. NADPH-diaphorase activity in brain macrophages during postnatal development in the rat. *Neuroscience* 1996;70:287–293.

60 Brosnan CF, Battistini L, Raine CS, et al. Reactive nitrogen intermediates in human neuropathology: an overview. *Dev Neurosci* 1994;16:152–161.

61 Peterson PK, Hu S, Anderson RW, Chao CC. Nitric oxide production and neurotoxicity mediated by activated microglia from human versus mouse brain. *J Infect Dis* 1994;170: 457–460.

62 Colasanti M, Persichini T, Di Pucchio T, et al. Human ramified microglial cells produce nitric oxide upon *Escherichia coli* lipopolysaccharide and tumor necrosis factor α stimulation. *Neurosci Lett* 1995;200:144–146.

63 Colton CA. Induction of nitric oxide in cultured microglia: evidence for a cytoprotective role. *Adv Neuroimmunol* 1995;5:491–503.

64 Schut RL, Gekker G, Hu S, et al. Cytomegalovirus replication in murine microglial cell cultures: suppression of permissive infection by interferon-γ. *J Infect Dis* 1994;169:1092–1096.

65 Chao CC, Hu S, Molitor TW, et al. Activated microglia mediate neuronal cell injury via a nitric oxide mechanism. *J Immunol* 1992;149:2736–2741.

66 Merrill JE, Ignarro LJ, Shermann MP, et al. Microglial cell cytotoxicity of oligodendrocytes is mediated through nitric oxide. *J Immunol* 1993;151:2132–2141.

67 Gehrmann J, Banati RB. Microglial turnover in the injured CNS: activated microglia undergo delayed DNA fragmentation following peripheral nerve injury. *J Neuropathol Exp Neurol* 1995;54:680–688.

68 Gehrmann J. Colony-stimulating factors regulate programmed cell death of rat microglia/ brain macrophages in vitro. *J Neuroimmunol* 1995;63:55–61.

69 Chao CC, Hu S, Sheng WS, et al. Cytokine-stimulated astrocytes damage human neurons via a nitric oxide mechanism. *Glia* 1996;16: 276–284.

70 Shepherd GM. Developmental neurobiology. In: Shepherd GM, ed. *Neurobiology*. New York: Oxford University Press, 1994:192–225.

71 Giulian D, Ingeman JE. Colony-stimulating factors as promoters of ameboid microglia. *J Neurosci* 1988;8:4707–4717.

72 Raivich G, Gehrmann J, Moreno-Floros M, Kreutzberg GW. Microglia: growth factor and mitogen receptors. *Clin Neuropathol* 1993;12: 293–295.

73 Ringheim GE. Mitogenic effects of interleukin-5 on microglia. *Neurosci Lett* 1995;210: 131–134.

74 Suzumura A, Sawada M, Yamamoto H, Marunouchi T. Transforming growth factor-β

suppresses activation and proliferation of microglia in vitro. *J Immunol* 1993;151:2150–2158.

75 Lee SC, Lui W, Brosnan CF, Dickson DW. GM-CSF promotes proliferation of human fetal and adult microglia in primary cultures. *Glia* 1994;12:309–318.

76 Walker DG, Kim SU, McGeer PL. Complement and cytokine gene expression in cultured microglia derived from postmortem human brains. *J Neurosci Res* 1995;40:478–493.

77 Zwahlen A, Nydegger UE, Vaudaux P, et al. Complement-mediated opsonic activity in normal and infected human cerebrospinal fluid: early response during bacterial meningitis. *J Infect Dis* 1982;145:635–646.

78 Gasque P, Fontaine M, Morgan BP. Complement expression in human brain. *J Immunol* 1995;154:4726–4733.

79 Rich AR, McCordock HA. Pathogenesis of tuberculous meningitis. *Bull Johns Hopkins Hosp* 1933;52:5–37.

80 Peterson PK, Gekker G, Hu S, et al. Multinucleated giant cell formation of swine microglia induced by *Mycobacterium bovis*. *J Infect Dis* 1996;173:1194–1201.

81 Lee TT, Martin FC, Merrill JE. Lymphokine induction of rat microglia multinucleated giant cell formation. *Glia* 1993;8:51–61.

82 Beaman L, Beaman BL. Interactions of *Nocardia asteroides* with murine glia cells in culture. *Infect Immun* 1993;61:343–347.

83 Beaman BL. Ultrastructural analysis of growth of *Nocardia asteroides* during invasion of the murine brain. *Infect Immun* 1993;61:274–283.

84 Habicht GS, Katona LI, Benach JL. Cytokines and the pathogenesis of neuroborreliosis: *Borrelia burgdorferi* induces glioma cells to secrete interleukin-6. *J Infect Dis* 1991;164:568–574.

85 Tatro JB, Romero LI, Beasley D, et al. *Borrelia burgdorferi* and *Escherichia coli* lipopolysaccharides induce nitric oxide and interleukin-6 production in cultured rat brain cells. *J Infect Dis* 1994;169:1014–1022.

86 Kim YS, Kennedy S, Täuber MG. Toxicity of *Streptococcus pneumoniae* in neurons, astrocytes, and microglia in vitro. *J Infect Dis* 1995;171:1363–1368.

87 Chao CC, Hu S, Gekker G, et al. Effects of cytokines on multiplication of *Toxoplasma gondii* in microglial cells. *J Immunol* 1993;150:3404–3410.

88 Fischer HG, Bielinsky AK, Nitzgen B, et al. Functional dichotomy of mouse microglia developed in vitro: differential effects of macrophage and granulocyte/macrophage colony-stimulating factor on cytokine secretion and antitoxoplasmic activity. *J Neuroimmunol* 1993;45:193–202.

89 Peterson PK, Gekker G, Hu S, Chao CC. Intracellular survival and multiplication of *Toxoplasma gondii* in astrocytes. *J Infect Dis* 1993;168:1472–1478.

90 Gazzinelli RT, Eltoum I, Wynn TA, Sher A. Acute cerebral toxoplasmosis is induced by in vivo neutralization of TNF-α and correlates with the down-regulated expression of inducible nitric oxide synthase and other markers of macrophage activation. *J Immunol* 1993;151:3672–3681.

91 Chao CC, Gekker G, Hu S, Peterson PK. Human microglial cell defense against *Toxoplasma gondii*. *J Immunol* 1994;152:1246–1252.

92 Mazzolla R, Barluzzi R, Puliti M, et al. Biomolecular events involved in the establishment of brain anticandidal resistance. *J Neuroimmunol* 1996;64:9–17.

93 Ashman RB, Bolitho EM, Fulurija A. Cytokine mRNA in brain tissue from mice that show strain-dependent differences in the severity of lesions induced by systemic infection with *Candida albicans* yeast. *J Infect Dis* 1995;172:823–830.

94 Williams K, Bar-Or A, Ulvestad E, et al. Biology of adult human microglia in culture: comparisons with peripheral blood monocytes and astrocytes. *J Neuropathol Exp Neurol* 1992;51:538–549.

95 Peterson PK, Chao CC, Hu S, et al. Glioblastoma, transforming growth factor-β, and *Candida* meningitis: a potential link. *Am J Med* 1992;92:262–264.

96 Blasi E, Barluzzi R, Mazzolla R, et al. Experimental model of intracerebral infection with *Cryptococcus neoformans*: roles of phagocytes and opsonization. *Infect Immun* 1992;60:3682–3688.

97 Blasi E, Barluzzi R, Mazzolla R, et al. Biomolecular events involved in anticryptococcal resistance in the brain. *Infect Immun* 1995;63:1218–1222.

98 Clemons KV, Brummer E, Stevens DA. Cytokine treatment of central nervous system infection: efficacy of interleukin-12 alone and synergy with conventional antifungal therapy in experimental cryptococcosis. *Antimicrob Agents Chemother* 1994;38:460–464.

99 Aguirre K, Havell EA, Gibson GW, Johnson LL. Role of tumor necrosis factor and gamma interferon in acquired resistance to *Cryptococcus neoformans* in the central nervous system of mice. *Infect Immun* 1995;63:1725–1731.

100 Lee SC, Kress Y, Dickson DW, Casadevail A. Human microglia mediate anti-*Cryptococcus*

neoformans activity in the presence of specific antibody. *J Neuroimmunol* 1995;62:43–52.

101 Lee SC, Dickson DW, Brosnan CF, Casadevall A. Human astrocytes inhibit *Cryptococcus neoformans* growth by a nitric oxide-mediated mechanism. *J Exp Med* 1994;180:365–369.

102 Levitz SM, Mathews HL, Murphy JW. Direct antimicrobial activity of T cells. *Immunol Today* 1995;16:387–391.

103 Koenig S, Gendelman HE, Orenstein JM, et al. Detection of AIDS virus in macrophages in brain tissue from AIDS patients with encephalopathy. *Science* 1986;233:1089–1093.

104 Peudenier S, Hery C, Montagnier L, Tardieu M. Human microglial cells: characterization in cerebral tissue and in primary culture, and study of their susceptibility to HIV-1 infection. *Ann Neurol* 1991;29:152–161.

105 Vitkovic L, da Cunha A, Tyor WR. Cytokine expression and pathogenesis in AIDS brain. In: Price RW, Perry SW, eds. *HIV, AIDS, and the brain*. New York: Raven, 1994:203–222.

106 Peterson PK, Gekker G, Hu S, et al. Microglial cell upregulation of HIV-1 expression in the chronically infected promonocytic cell line U1: the role of tumor necrosis factor-α. *J Neuroimmunol* 1992;41:81–88.

107 Peterson PK, Gekker G, Hu S, et al. Morphine amplifies HIV-1 expression in chronically infected promonocytes cocultured with human brain cells. *J Neuroimmunol* 1994;50:167–175.

107a Lokensgard JR, Gekker G, Ehrlich L, et al. Proinflammatory cytokines inhibit HIV-1 SF162 expression in acutely infected human brain cell cultures. *J Immunol* 1997;158: 2449–2455.

108 Hoffman PM, Dhib-Jalbut S, Mikovits JA, et al. Human T-cell leukemia virus type 1 infection of monocytes and microglial cells in primary human cultures. *Proc Natl Acad Sci USA* 1992;89:11784–11788.

109 Esiri MM, Drummond CWE, Morris CS. Macrophages and microglia in HSV-1 infected mouse brain. *J Neuroimmunol* 1995; 201–205.

110 Rinaman L, Card JP, Enquist LW. Spatiotemporal responses of astrocytes, ramified microglia, and brain macrophages to central neuronal infection with pseudorabies virus. *J Neurosci* 1993;13:685–702.

111 Yamabe T, Dhir G, Cowan EP, et al. Cytokine-gene expression in measles-infected adult human glial cells. *J Neuroimmunol* 1994;49:171–179.

112 Frei K, Malipiero UV, Leist TP, et al. On the cellular source and function of interleukin 6 produced in the central nervous system in viral diseases. *Eur J Immunol* 1989; 19:689–694.

113 Akaike T, Weihe E, Schaefer M, et al. Effect of neurotropic virus infection on neuronal and inducible nitric oxide synthase activity in rat brain. *J Neurovirol* 1995;1:118–125.

114 Liuzzi GM, Riccio P, Dal Canto MC. Release of myelin basic protein-degrading proteolytic activity from microglia and macrophages after infection with Theiler's murine encephalomyelitis virus: comparison between susceptible and resistant mice. *J Neuroimmunol* 1995;62:91–102.

115 Mühleisen H, Gehrmann J, Meyermann R. Reactive microglia in Creutzfeldt-Jakob disease. *Neuropathol Appl Neurobiol* 1995;21:505–517.

116 Giulian D. Microglia and neuronal dysfunction. In: Kentenmann H, Ransom BR, eds. *Neuroglia*. New York: Oxford University Press, 1995:671–684.

117 Gehrmann J, Kreutzberg GW. Microglia in experimental neuropathology. In: Kentenmann H, Ransom BR, eds. *Neuroglia*. New York: Oxford University Press, 1995:883–904.

118 McGeer PL, McGeer EG. The inflammatory response system of brain: implications for therapy of Alzheimer and other neurodegenerative diseases. *Brain Res Rev* 1995;21:195–218.

119 Merrill JE. Proinflammatory and antiinflammatory cytokines in multiple sclerosis and central nervous system acquired immunodeficiency syndrome. *J Immunother* 1992;12: 167–170.

120 Giulian D, Corpuz M, Chapman S, et al. Reactive mononuclear phagocytes release neurotoxins after ischemic and traumatic injury to the central nervous system. *J Neurosci Res* 1993;36:681–693.

121 Ivacko JA, Sun R, Silverstein FS. Hypoxic-ischemic brain injury induces an acute microglial reaction in perinatal rats. *Pediatr Res* 1996;39:39–47.

122 Fricchione GL, Bilfinger TV, Stefano GB. The macrophage and neuropsychiatric disorders. *Neuropsychiatr Neuropsychol Behav Neurol* 1996;9:16–29.

4

Cells and Cytokines in Host Defense of the Central Nervous System

YASUHIRO SUZUKI

Although the brain has traditionally been considered an immunologically privileged site, infections in the brain can nevertheless be controlled. Recent studies have shown intensive immunologic infiltration in response to infection and an importance of the immune response in the brain's resistance against infections. It is also true that the immune response can contribute to the development of pathology in the brain (i.e., experimental lymphocytic choriomeningitis virus infection in mice) (see other chapters). However, this chapter does not address this detrimental role of the immune response. The following is an overview of the role of cells and cytokines in resistance against virus- and parasite-induced encephalitis.

THE ROLE OF CELLS AND CYTOKINES IN RESISTANCE AGAINST VIRUS-INDUCED ENCEPHALITIS

Interferon-γ and Tumor Necrosis Factor-α

Development of encephalitis following infection with measles virus (MV) is genetically regulated in mice (1). C3H/He (H-2^k) and C57BL/6 (H-2^b) mice develop a lethal acute encephalitis after intracerebral infection with the neurotropic strain of MV, whereas BALB/c (H-2^d) mice are resistant (1). In BALB/c mice, depletion of $CD8^+$ T cells does not interfere with the clearance of virus from the brain (2). In contrast, following depletion of $CD4^+$ T cells, BALB/c mice become susceptible to MV infection with high mortality rates, indicating that $CD4^+$ T cells are necessary for resistance against the development of encephalitis following MV infection (2). $CD4^+$ T cells obtained from infected BALB/c mice (genetically resistant) produce large amounts of interleukin (IL)-2, interferon (IFN)-γ, and tumor necrosis factor (TNF)-α but no IL-4, IL-6, and IL-10, whereas these T cells from infected C3H/He mice (genetically susceptible) produce little IFN-γ and TNF-α (3). These results suggest that IFN-γ and TNF-α may play an important role in the resistance of BALB/c mice to MV encephalitis. The role of these cytokines in the resistance was examined by treating the mice with monoclonal antibodies (mAbs) against the cytokines to neutralize their activities. Neutralization of IFN-γ activity in BALB/c mice by treatment with anti–IFN-γ mAb results in impairment of viral clearance from their brains and thereby makes them susceptible to MV encephalitis (3). In contrast, neutralization of TNF-α has no effect on survival or virus clearance from the brains of these mice (3). Thus, IFN-γ is a major mediator of the protective activity of $CD4^+$ T cells against the development of MV encephalitis in genetically resistant BALB/c mice.

A similar protective effect of IFN-γ in the brain has been observed in infection with vaccinia virus. In mice immunized with vesicular stomatitis virus (VSV), the growth of wild-type vaccinia virus is inhibited in their brains when the mice are challenged with a mixture of vaccinia recombinant virus expressing the nucleoprotein of VSV and wild-type vaccinia virus. This inhibitory effect of immunized mice on vaccinia virus is partially but significantly abrogated by treatment of the mice with anti–IFN-γ antibody but not by anti–TNF-α antibody (4). Of interest is that replication of wild-type vaccinia virus in the immunized mice is inhibited in their brains but not in their peripheral solid organs (ovaries and testis) (4). This may happen because of accumulation of IFN-γ (locally produced in the brain by infiltrated T cells) in the cerebrospinal fluid (CSF). Because of the blood-brain barrier, which limits exchanges between interstitial fluid and capillaries in the brain (5), cytokines locally produced in the brain can accumulate in the CSF (6–9). IFN-γ but not TNF-α can accumulate in the CSF during acute viral infection in the brain (10,11). These levels of T cell–released IFN-γ may be high enough to exert a significant and biologically relevant nonspecific antiviral effect in protecting choriomeningeal cells, the main targets of vaccinia virus infection (4).

Nitric oxide (NO) appears to play an important role in the protective effect of IFN-γ in resistance against virus infection in the brain. NO is a key component in mediating IFN-γ–induced protection of peripheral macrophages against several virus infections (12). Microglia, the resident macrophages of the brain, and astrocytes, the major numerous glial cell types within the central nervous system, become activated by treatment with IFN-γ plus lipopolysaccharide (LPS) or IFN-γ plus IL-1β, and the activated cells are able to produce NO through activation of inducible NO synthase (iNOS) (13–15) (see Chapters 3 and 5). In addition, NO can inhibit VSV production by infected neurons in vitro (16).

The mechanism of IFN-γ–mediated viral clearance in the brain may also involve an amplification of the ability of microglia and astrocytes to present antigens to T cells in the neighborhood of infected neurons (see Chapter 3). IFN-γ activates these cells to express the major histocompatibility complex (MHC) class II antigens and the other molecules critical for effective antigen presentation (17,18). The molecules induced by IFN-γ include intercellular adhesion molecule-1 (ICAM-1), leukocyte function–associated antigen-3 (LFA-3), and B7. In regard to expression of B7-1 on astrocytes, IFN-γ has been shown to induce expression of this molecule on murine astrocytes (18,19) but not on human astrocytes (20,21). Antigen presentation by these cells most likely contributes to the initiation and maintenance of the protective immune response against infection in the brain.

In addition to the important role of IFN-γ in the inhibition of viral growth and clearance of viruses from the brain just described, this cytokine also has a protective effect against herpes simplex virus (HSV) infection in which viral growth in brains of infected mice is not inhibited (22). Transgenic mice that express IFN-γ restricted to the photoreceptors of the retina survive following intraocular HSV infection, whereas nontransgenic control mice die. Brains of transgenic mice have inflammation and viral titers that are equivalent to those of brains of control mice. However, brains of transgenic mice have markedly lower numbers of central neurons undergoing apoptosis than do those of control mice (22). Upregulation of the proto-oncogene *bcl-2* in neurons occurs only in infected transgenic mice (22). The protein encoded by the *bcl-2* gene is known to be involved in protection from apoptosis of neurons (23). IFN-γ appears to be involved in the protection from death of infected neuron cells in the brain, although the mechanism of the protective effect is unclear.

Interleukin-4 and Interleukin-6

Antiviral antibodies have been shown to be the mechanism by which Sindbis virus (SV) is cleaned from the brain of infected mice (24). In a severe combined immunodeficiency (SCID) mouse model of persistent SV encephalomyelitis, adoptive transfer of hyperimmune serum results in the clearance of infectious virus and viral RNA from the brain, whereas adoptive transfer of sensitized T cells has no effect on viral replication. Treatment of SV-infected primary cultured rat neurons with mAb to the E2 envelope glycoprotein decreases viral protein synthesis, followed by gradual termination of mature infectious virion production (24). Although antibody is responsible for the clearance of virus from the brain, infiltrating T cells and microglia are likely to play an important role in initiating and maintaining the local antiviral antibody response in the brain. Studies using athymic nude mice that lack thymus-dependent T cells showed that the T cells are required for entry of B cells into the brain and for immunoglobulin isotype switching of B cells in the brain (25). In addition, microglia become MHC class II positive soon after infection (26) and may play a role as antigen-presenting cells to activate T cells. Th2-type cytokines (IL-4, IL-5, IL-6) are known to be important for the proliferation and differentiation of B cells for antibody production. Analysis of cytokine messenger RNA (mRNA) expressed in the brain of SV-infected mice revealed predominant Th2-type T-cell responses (27). Thus, the Th2-type cytokines produced by T cells appear to contribute to local antiviral antibody production by B cells in the brains of SV-infected mice, which results in clearance of the virus from the brain.

Interleukin-10

IL-10 significantly inhibits the production of granulocyte-macrophage colony-stimulating factor (GM-CSF), macrophage colony-stimulating factor (M-CSF), and IL-6 by both astrocytes and microglia when the cells are stimulated by components of gram-negative or gram-positive bacteria (LPS, Staphylococcal enterotoxin A, protein A, and purified protein derivative) (28). In contrast, the secretion of these cytokines by the two glial cell populations is not altered by IL-10 when the cells are stimulated by viruses (influenza A and Newcastle disease virus) (28). Thus, the role of IL-10 in the regulation of cytokine production by astrocytes and microglia in the brain may differ between bacterial and viral infections.

Interleukin-12

IL-12 mediates a broad range of effects on both innate and acquired immunity, including augmentation of cytotoxic activity and IFN-γ production of both natural killer (NK) and T cells (29–31) and induction of Th1-type immune responses (32,33). IL-12 gene expression is rapidly induced by viral infections (34). The treatment of mice with IL-12 significantly inhibits VSV infection in their brains (35). Mice treated with IL-12 have significantly decreased VSV titers in their brain homogenates when compared to those in untreated control mice. The inhibition is positively associated with increased expression of iNOS in the brain. Since IL-12 augments the IFN-γ production of both NK and T cells and since IFN-γ activates microglia and astrocytes in collaboration with LPS or IL-1β to produce NO through activation of iNOS (13–15), the protective effect of IL-12 appears to be mediated by IFN-γ. In this regard, administration of IFNs significantly delays the time to death and reduces the mortality rate produced by VSV-induced encephalitis (36).

Treatment with IL-12 also results in enhanced expression of MHC class II antigens and increased T-cell infiltration in the brain as well as diminished VSV-induced apoptosis in the olfactory bulb (35). Since IFN-γ has similar effects in the brain (see Interferon-γ and Tumor Necrosis Factor-α above), IFN-γ may also mediate these effects induced by treatment with IL-12.

Homing of Lymphocytes into the Brain

Expression of ICAM-1 and vascular cell adhesion molecule-1 (VCAM-1) becomes upregulated following infection with SV (37). Studies using a transfer of fluorescent-labeled lymphocytes into infected mice revealed that lymphocyte entry into the brains during maximal inflammation is inhibited by pretreating inoculated cells with antibodies that block LFA-1 (ligand for ICAM-1), but not with those that block very late antigen-4 (VLA-4) (ligand for VCAM-1) (37). These results indicate that LFA-1–ICAM-1 interactions are relevant to lymphocyte entry into the brain during peak inflammation in the infected mice. Of interest is that treatment of the lymphocytes with either anti–LFA-1 or anti–VLA-4 antibodies does not prevent their entry into the brain at the onset of inflammation. This suggests that the earliest recruited cells utilize uncharacterized receptor-ligand interactions during SV infection (37). In contrast to SV infection, VLA-4–VCAM-1 interactions regulate T-cell entry into the brain and influence the development of experimental autoimmune encephalitis (EAE) (38). These differences between SV infection and EAE may happen owing to the paucity of VLA-4 expression on lymphocytes in SV-infected mice (37).

THE ROLE OF CELLS AND CYTOKINES IN RESISTANCE AGAINST PARASITE-INDUCED ENCEPHALITIS

Toxoplasma gondii and *Neospora caninum* cause encephalitis in the hosts. Damage to the central nervous system also occurs in trypanosomiasis and malaria (see Chapters 9 and 11). At this moment, no publications are available regarding the mechanism (or mechanisms) of the protective immunity against development of encephalitis in *N.*

caninum infection. In infection with *T. gondii*, toxoplasmic encephalitis has emerged as a major cause of morbidity and mortality in patients with acquired immunodeficiency syndrome (AIDS) (39,40) (see Chapter 10). Since immunocompetent individuals do not usually have apparent untoward effects, including development of encephalitis (41), it is clear that the immune response is critical for the prevention of the encephalitis. Acute diseases in the setting of *T. gondii* infection are caused by tachyzoites that quickly proliferate within nucleated cells. During the latent chronic stage of infection, the parasite forms cysts in various organs, especially the brain, skeletal muscle, and heart. Toxoplasmic encephalitis in AIDS patients is almost solely caused by recrudescence of a latent chronic infection with *T. gondii* (40,42). Cytokines have been shown to play critical roles in resistance against the development of toxoplasmic encephalitis in animal models.

Interferon-γ

Endogenous IFN-γ is critical in resistance against acute acquired infection with *T. gondii* (43–45) and against recrudescence of the latent chronic infection (toxoplasmic encephalitis) (46,47). Neutralization of the activity of IFN-γ in chronically infected mice by treatment with anti–IFN-γ mAb results in severe acute inflammation and development of large necrosis in their brains (Fig 4-1) (46). In the areas of acute inflam-

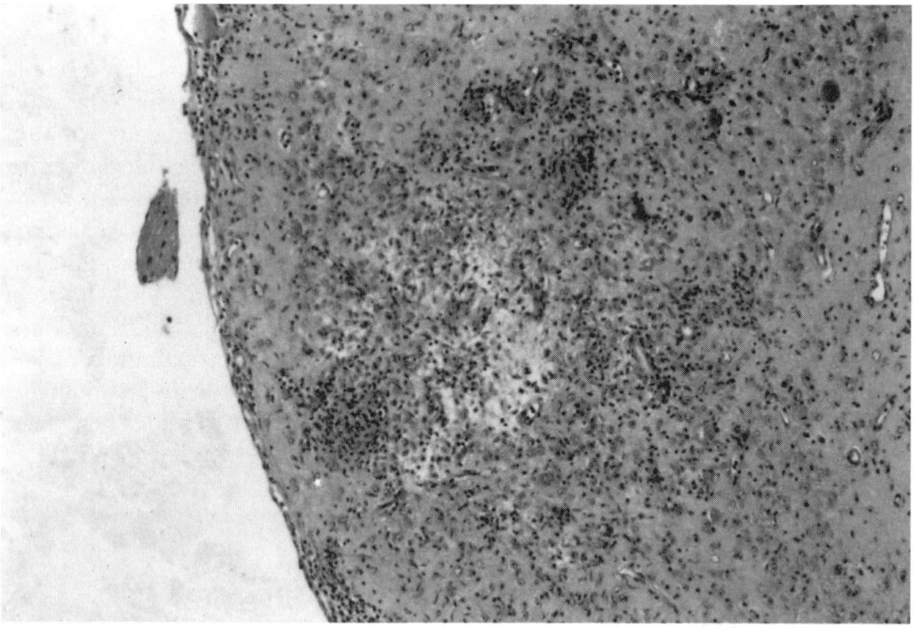

Figure 4-1. Necrosis in the brain of a *Toxoplasma*-infected mouse treated with anti–interferon-γ monoclonal antibody (H & E stain). (From Suzuki Y, Conley FK, Remington JS. Importance of endogenous IFN-γ for prevention of toxoplasmic encephalitis in mice. *J Immunol* Vol. 143, page 2046, September 15, 1989. Copyright 1989, The American Association of Immunologists, with permission.)

mation and necrosis, tachyzoites and *T. gondii* antigens are detected by immunohistology, indicating that such inflammatory responses are caused by a proliferation of tachyzoites. A marked increase in the numbers of tachyzoites in the brains of mice following treatment with anti–IFN-γ mAb is also demonstrated by detecting increased amounts of tachyzoite-specific surface antigen (SAG)-1 and SAG-2 mRNA in their brains (48). Thus, it is clear that IFN-γ plays a critical role in the prevention of toxoplasmic encephalitis by inhibiting the proliferation of tachyzoites in the brains of infected mice.

Both $CD4^+$ and $CD8^+$ T cells obtained from individuals infected with *T. gondii* are able to produce IFN-γ in vitro (44,49–51). However, in vivo, $CD8^+$ T cells appear to be a major source of IFN-γ and the helper function of $CD4^+$ T cells appears to be important to enhance IFN-γ production by $CD8^+$ T cells (44,52). Following infection, both $CD4^+$ and $CD8^+$ T cells infiltrate the brain of mice (53,54). Gazzinelli et al. (47) reported that $CD4^+$ and $CD8^+$ T cells act additively or synergistically to prevent the development of toxoplasmic encephalitis, probably through the production of IFN-γ.

Microglia appear to be major effector cells in the protective immunity mediated by IFN-γ against *T. gondii* in the brain. Both human (55) and murine (15) microglia become activated to inhibit intracellular proliferation of tachyzoites following treatment with IFN-γ plus LPS. TNF-α is involved in the activation of microglia (55,56). NO mediates the inhibitory effect of activated murine microglia on intracellular replication of tachyzoites, as treatment of these cells with N^G-monomethyl-L-arginine (which blocks the generation of NO) ablates their inhibitory activity (15). In contrast, NO is not involved in the inhibitory effect of human microglia (56). The importance of NO in the prevention of toxoplasmic encephalitis was recently reported in a murine model. Hayashi et al. (57) demonstrated that inhibition of NO synthesis by treatment of mice with aminoguanidine following infection results in an increased number of tachyzoites and cysts accompanied by an exacerbated inflammation in their brains.

In addition to the effector role of microglia in resistance against *T. gondii* in the brain, these cells appear to play an important role in antigen presentation to T cells in the brain. Schlüter et al. (58) reported increased expression of MHC class II antigens on microglia during toxoplasmic encephalitis in mice. This activation of microglia is probably through IFN-γ (58). In addition, occasional subependymal and subleptomeningeal astrocytes express MHC class II antigens during acute toxoplasmic encephalitis (59). These astrocytes may also contribute to antigen presentation to T cells. As mentioned previously (see Interferon-γ and Tumor Necrosis Factor-α), IFN-γ activates microglia and astrocytes to induce expression of MHC class II antigens and the other molecules (i.e., ICAM-1, LFA-3, and B7) critical for effective antigen presentation to T cells.

IFN-γ appears to play an important role in the prevention of rupture of cysts in the brain, in addition to its inhibitory effect on the proliferation of tachyzoites. In brains of infected mice treated with anti–IFN-γ mAb, acute inflammation is observed around a certain number of cysts. Tachyzoites and *T. gondii* antigens are detected surrounding the periphery of these cysts, suggesting that cyst disruption occurs in the brains of mAb-treated mice (46). Disrupted cysts in the brain appear to be a significant source of tachyzoites that cause severe toxoplasmic encephalitis (60–63). However, this does not exclude the possibility that cysts ruptured in organs other than the brain are a source of the tachyzoites that appear in the brain, and hence contribute to the development of toxoplasmic encephalitis. The organisms released from the ruptured cysts in such organs can reach the brain through blood (64).

With regard to the effect of IFN-γ on the cyst form of this parasite, Jones et al. (65) reported that treatment with IFN-γ reduces the division of tachyzoites within cultured murine astrocytes, which results in enhanced cyst formation. They also found that cyst rupture occurs after removal of IFN-γ from the culture medium (65). In contrast to these observations, Peterson et al. (66) reported that treatment of murine astrocytes with IFN-γ and LPS has no apparent effect on the survival or growth of tachyzoites. The discrepancy between these observations may be due to the use of different strains of *T. gondii*. The avirulent Pe strain that forms cysts in mice was used in the experiments in the former study (65), whereas the virulent RH strain that appears not to form cysts in mice was used in the experiments in the latter study (66).

As mentioned already, toxoplasmic encephalitis has been the major opportunistic infectious disease in the brains in AIDS patients (39,40,42). Since IFN-γ plays a critical role in resistance against the development of toxoplasmic encephalitis (prevention of cyst rupture and inhibition of proliferation of tachyzoites released from the ruptured cysts in the brain), impairment of IFN-γ production in AIDS patients (67) is likely a major factor in predisposing them to the high incidence of toxoplasmic encephalitis. This strongly suggests that IFN-γ can be an effective treatment of toxoplasmic encephalitis in those patients. We examined the efficiency of recombinant IFN-γ (rIFN-γ) in the treatment of toxoplasmic encephalitis using a murine model (68). Intravenous injection of rIFN-γ markedly reduces the number of areas of acute focal inflammation caused by tachyzoites in the brains of mice with toxoplasmic encephalitis (Fig 4-2) (68). These results indicate that injection of exogenous IFN-γ prevents the proliferation of tachyzoites in the brains of mice with toxoplasmic encephalitis and thereby markedly reduces inflammatory changes.

Tumor Necrosis Factor-α

As mentioned previously, TNF-α plays an important role in the activation of microglia (55,56). Incubation of human (55) and murine (56) microglia with IFN-γ and TNF-α activates these cells to inhibit the intracellular replication of tachyzoites. The importance of TNF-α in the prevention of the proliferation of tachyzoites in the brain has been demonstrated using murine models (48,69). Neutralization of endogenous TNF-α activity by injecting an mAb to this cytokine exacerbates toxoplasmic encephalitis (48,69). The treated mice have significantly higher numbers of areas of acute focal inflammation associated with tachyzoites (Fig 4-3) (69) and larger amounts of tachyzoite-specific SAG-2 mRNA (48) in their brains than do untreated control mice.

The development of toxoplasmic encephalitis in mice is regulated by the gene(s) within the D region of the MHC (H-2) (69–71) (see Chapter 10 in regard to genetic regulation of susceptibility to toxoplasmic encephalitis in mice and AIDS patients). Freund et al. (72) found that polymorphisms in the *TNF-α* gene located in the D region of the H-2 complex correlate with resistance against the development of toxoplasmic encephalitis and with levels of TNF-α mRNA in the brains of infected mice. However, the *L* gene in the D region of the H-2 complex, but not the *TNF-α* gene, was recently identified as important in determining the development of toxoplasmic en-

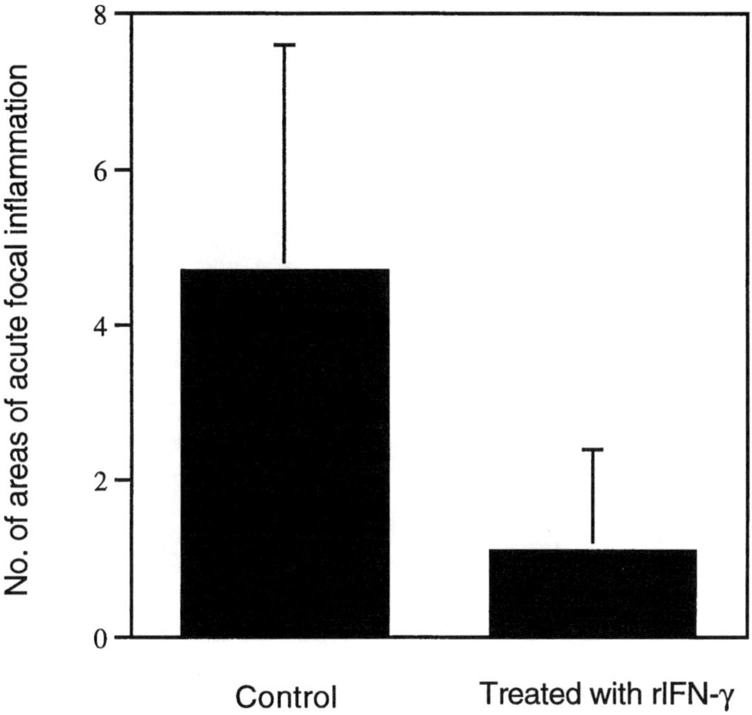

Figure 4-2. Effect of treatment with recombinant interferon-γ (rIFN-γ) on the number of areas of acute focal inflammation in the brains of mice with toxoplasmic encephalitis. Each bar indicates the number per sagittal section of brain. (From Suzuki Y, Conley FK, Remington JS. Treatment of toxoplasmic encephalitis in mice with recombinant gamma interferon. *Infect Immun* Vol. 58, page 3052, September 1990. Copyright 1990, American Society for Microbiology, with permission.)

cephalitis (69,71). When development of toxoplasmic encephalitis was studied in BALB/c and BALB/c-H-2^{dm2} (dm2) mice that have the same *TNF-α* gene, only dm2 mice developed toxoplasmic encephalitis following infection (69,71). Transcripts for TNF-α are detected in the brains of infected dm2 mice but not in BALB/c mice. Injection of neutralizing antibodies against TNF-α results in worsening of the toxoplasmic encephalitis in infected dm2 mice but does not induce toxoplasmic encephalitis in infected BALB/c mice (69). Thus, TNF-α appears to be produced in the brain after toxoplasmic encephalitis has developed and is responsible for preventing the progression of the disease.

Interleukin-4

$CD4^+$ T cells are known to be heterogeneous (Th1 and Th2) with regard to cytokine secretion. Th1 cells preferentially secrete IL-2 and IFN-γ whereas Th2 cells preferen-

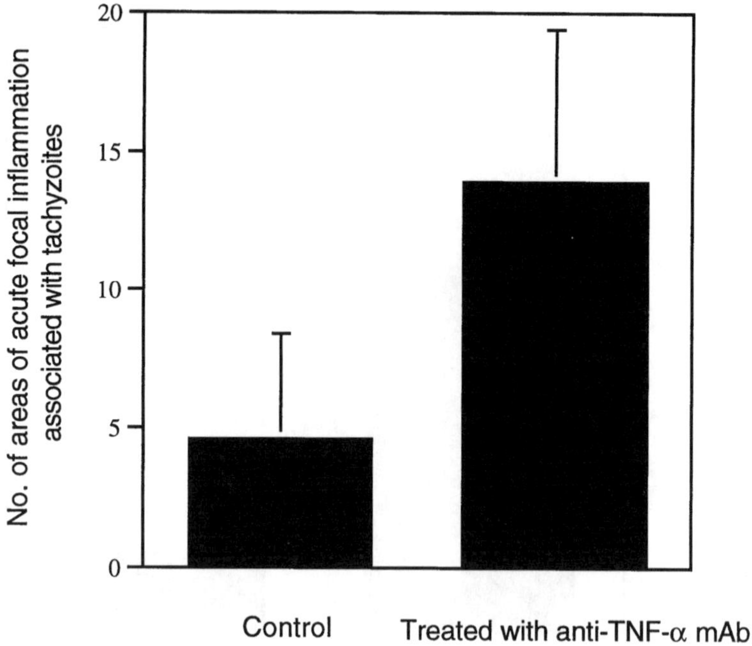

Figure 4-3. Effect of treatment with anti–tumor necrosis factor-α monoclonal antibody (anti-TNF-α mAb) on the number of areas of acute focal inflammation associated with tachyzoites in the brains of BALB/c-H-2^{dm2} mice infected with *T. gondii.* Each bar indicates the number per sagittal section of brain. (From Suzuki Y, Joh K, Kwon OC, et al. MHC class I gene(s) in the D/L region but not TNF-α gene determines development of toxoplasmic encephalitis in mice. *J Immunol* Vol. 153, page 4651, November 15, 1994. Copyright 1994, The American Association of Immunologists, with permission.)

tially produce IL-4, IL-5, IL-6, and IL-10 (73–76). IL-4 has a dominant effect in determining the pattern of cytokines (Th2 type) produced by $CD4^+$ T cells upon subsequent antigen stimulation in vitro (77–80). Since the role of IFN-γ is critical for the prevention of toxoplasmic encephalitis as described in a previous section, colleagues and I examined the role of IL-4 in the pathogenesis of toxoplasmic encephalitis using IL-4 targeted mutant (IL-$4^{-/-}$) mice (81). Surprisingly, IL-4 was protective against the development of toxoplasmic encephalitis. The IL-$4^{-/-}$ mice died during the late stage (from 6 to 20 weeks) of infection, whereas control mice survived. Histologic study revealed significantly higher numbers of cysts and areas of acute focal inflammation associated with tachyzoites in the brains of IL-$4^{-/-}$ mice than control mice at 4 and 8 weeks after infection (81). Significantly larger amounts of tachyzoite-specific SAG-1 mRNA were detected in the brains of the former than in those of the latter mice (Fig 4-4) (81). IL-4 mRNA was detected only in the brains of infected control mice. These results indicate that IL-4 is protective against the development of toxoplasmic encephalitis by preventing the formation of cysts and the proliferation of tachyzoites in the brain.

In addition, in our study, spleen cells of control mice at 8 weeks after infection produced significantly larger amounts of IFN-γ following stimulation in vitro with soluble *T. gondii* antigens than did those of IL-4$^{-/-}$ mice (81). These results indicate that IL-4 plays a role in enhancing IFN-γ production during the late stage of infection. The impaired ability of IL-4$^{-/-}$ mice to produce IFN-γ likely contributes to their susceptibility to the development of severe toxoplasmic encephalitis. Noble and Kemeny (82) recently reported that IL-4 enhances IFN-γ production by T cells that have already been primed (differentiated), whereas it suppresses differentiation of unprimed T cells to IFN-γ–producing cells. During infection with *T. gondii,* IFN-γ production occurs earlier than IL-4 production (83). Thus, it appears that IL-4 does not affect differentiation of unprimed T cells to IFN-γ–producing cells following *T. gondii* infection because of the absence (or very low production) of IL-4 in the early stage of infection,

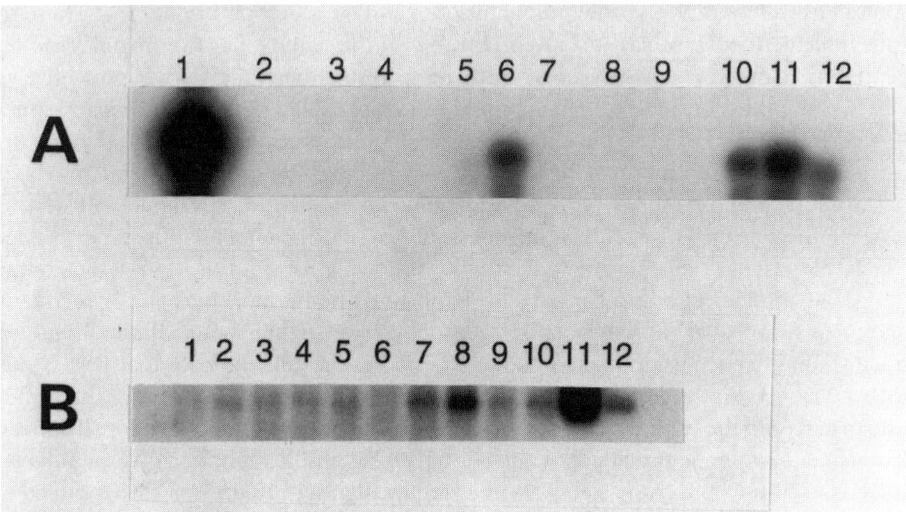

Figure 4-4. Detection of tachyzoite-specific mRNA encoding SAG-1 using polymerase chain reaction–assisted amplification of RNA in the brains of IL-4$^{-/-}$ and control mice infected with *T. gondii*. Mice were killed at 4 (B) and 8 (A) weeks after infection and their brains analyzed for the presence of SAG-1 mRNA. (A) Lane 1, positive control (purified tachyzoites); lane 2, negative control (purified bradyzoites (cysts)); lanes 3 and 4, uninfected control mice; lanes 5 to 7, infected control mice; lanes 8 and 9, uninfected IL-4$^{-/-}$ mice; lanes 10 to 12, infected IL-4$^{-/-}$ mice. (B) Lanes 1 to 6, infected control mice; lanes 7 to 10, infected IL-4$^{-/-}$ mice; lanes 11 and 12, positive control. (From Suzuki Y, Yang Q, Yang S, et al. IL-4 is protective against development of toxoplasmic encephalitis. *J Immunol* Vol. 157, page 2566, September 15, 1996. Copyright 1996, The American Association of Immunologists, with permission.)

whereas it enhances IFN-γ production by differentiated T cells in the late stage of infection.

In contrast to our observation, Roberts et al. (84) recently observed higher numbers of cysts and more severe histologic changes in the brains of control than IL-4$^{-/-}$ mice in the late stage of infection, although the former mice were more resistant against death during the acute stage than were the latter mice. The differences in the genetic backgrounds of the mice and the strain of *T. gondii* used in the two studies (81,84) may have contributed to the different outcomes.

Interleukin-6

IL-6 is a multifunctional cytokine that regulates various aspects of the immune response, acute-phase reaction, and hematopoiesis (85) and acts in the nervous system (86). IL-6 mRNA is expressed in the brains of mice infected with *T. gondii* (47,87,88) and IL-6 is detected in the CSF of infected mice (58). Treatment of toxoplasmic encephalitis in mice with an mAb against IL-6 results in a remarkable decrease in inflammatory responses as well as in the number of tachyzoites and cysts in their brains (89). These results indicate that IL-6 plays an important role in the pathogenesis of toxoplasmic encephalitis. However, it is not clear from these results whether IL-6 is protective or whether it contributes to the development of toxoplasmic encephalitis, because mice treated with anti–IL-6 mAb have paradoxically higher serum levels of IL-6 than do untreated mice (89). Induction of high serum levels of IL-6 by anti–IL-6 mAb has also been observed in endotoxin shock (90) and infection with *Staphylococcus aureus* (91). To determine the role of IL-6 in the pathogenesis of toxoplasmic encephalitis, we examined the development of toxoplasmic encephalitis following infection in IL-6–targeted mutant (IL-6$^{-/-}$) mice. The IL-6$^{-/-}$ mice had significantly higher numbers of *T. gondii* cysts and areas of inflammation associated with tachyzoites in their brains than did control mice (Suzuki et al., unpublished data, 1997). These results indicate that IL-6 is protective against the development of toxoplasmic encephalitis by preventing the formation of cysts and the proliferation of tachyzoites in the brains of infected mice. It appears likely that the therapeutic effect of anti–IL-6 mAb against toxoplasmic encephalitis observed in our previous study (89) was mediated by high serum levels of IL-6 induced by the mAb. In relation to this, Chao et al. (55) reported that treatment of human fetal microglia with IL-6 inhibits intracellular replication of tachyzoites in vitro.

Interleukin-10

IL-10 downregulates IFN-γ synthesis (92,93) and inhibits microbicidal activity for *T. gondii* of macrophages activated by IFN-γ (94). Gazzinelli et al. (48) reported an increase of IL-10 mRNA in the brains of C57BL/6 mice during the late stage of infection (at that time, toxoplasmic encephalitis had developed). Immunohistochemical analysis of the brains of infected mice revealed the presence of IL-10 in mice genetically susceptible to toxoplasmic encephalitis but not in mice genetically resistant against toxoplasmic encephalitis (53). IL-10 may contribute to the development of toxoplasmic encephalitis through its downregulating activity.

Interleukin-12

Recently IL-12 was found to be a critical cytokine in the resistance against *T. gondii* during the early stage of infection (95–97). IL-12 enhances the IFN-γ production that occurs after infection (95). Neutralization of IL-12 by an mAb against this cytokine results in 100% mortality in mice after infection with an avirulent strain of *T. gondii*, whereas control mice survive (95). In contrast to the importance of IL-12 in resistance during the early stage of infection, neutralization of IL-12 during the late stage of infection does not increase mortality in mice with toxoplasmic encephalitis (95). Therefore, IL-12 may not be required for the protective immunity during the late stage of infection.

Transforming Growth Factor-β

Transforming growth factor (TGF)-β mRNA is expressed in the brain of infected mice (88). As mentioned above in the "IFN-γ" section, activation of murine microglia with IFN-γ plus LPS suppresses intracellular growth of tachyzoites in vitro (56). This anti-toxoplasma defense of activated microglia is significantly blocked by neutralizing antibodies against TGF-β, suggesting that TGF-β plays a role in the inhibitory process (56). Consistent with this hypothesis, activation of murine microglia with IFN-γ plus TGF-β inhibited, in a dose-dependent manner, *T. gondii* multiplication (56). In contrast to these findings in the murine model, antitoxoplasma activity of activated human microglia treated with IFN-γ plus LPS is not blocked by neutralizing antibodies to TGF-β (55).

On the other hand, TGF-β is known to have several immunosuppressive activities similar to those of IL-10 (98,99). Hunter et al. (100) reported that TGF-β suppresses the production of IFN-γ by spleen cells from infected SCID mice. Whether TGF-β plays a protective role against the development of toxoplasmic encephalitis or contributes to the development of toxoplasmic encephalitis is unclear.

Macrophage and Granulocyte-Macrophage Colony-Stimulating Factors

The expression of GM-CSF mRNA increases in the brain of mice following infection (48,88). Treatment of murine microglia with GM-CSF results in their activation to inhibit the intracellular replication of tachyzoites (101). The antiparasitic activity of microglia activated by GM-CSF is due to their synthesis of reactive nitrogen intermediates, as their activity is antagonized by N^{G}-monomethyl-L-arginine (101). In contrast to GM-CSF, treatment of murine microglia with M-CSF does not activate them to inhibit the multiplication of tachyzoites (101). GM-CSF may play a protective role in the brains of infected mice to prevent the development of toxoplasmic encephalitis.

Homing of Lymphocytes into the Brain

Deckert-Schlüter et al. (59) demonstrated upregulation of ICAM-1 and VCAM-1 in the endothelia of cerebral blood vessels during toxoplasmic encephalitis. They also reported that most VCAM-1–positive blood vessels are surrounded by inflammatory cells during toxoplasmic encephalitis, whereas only a limited number of ICAM-1–positive blood vessels is surrounded by those cells (59). These observations may suggest that VLA-4–VCAM-1 interactions play an important role in lymphocyte entry into the brain during toxoplasmic encephalitis.

CONCLUSIONS

Table 4-1 summarizes the protective effects of cytokines against the development of encephalitis following virus and parasite infections. T cells are critical for resistance against infection in the brain. Cytokines play important roles in the protective effects of these T cells. IFN-γ is crucial in the activation of microglia and astrocytes. These activated cells can inhibit intracellular proliferation of pathogens through NO-dependent and -independent mechanisms. IFN-γ also induces expression of MHC class II antigens and the other molecules (ICAM-1, LFA-1, and B7) that are critical for effective antigen presentation on microglia and astrocytes. These cells appear to be important as antigen-presenting cells to stimulate T cells in the brain (see Chapter 3). These cells may be able to regulate the activation of T cells. In addition, activated microglia and astrocytes produce the proinflammatory cytokines, that is, TNF-α, IL-1, and IL-6. IFN-γ can upregulate the expression of the adhesion molecules involved in lymphocyte traffic on endothelial cells in vitro, and lymphocytes show much greater adhesion to cere-

Table 4-1. The Protective Cytokines and Their Effects in the Brain Against Development of Encephalitis Induced by Virus and Parasite Infections

Pathogen	***Cytokines***[a]	***Effects Induced by Cytokines***[a]
Measles virus	Interferon-γ[b]	
Vesicular stomatitis virus	Interferon-γ,[b] IL-12	Production of NO, inhibition of apoptosis of neurons
Vaccinia virus	Interferon-γ[b]	
Herpes simplex virus	Interferon-γ	Inhibition of apoptosis of neurons
Sindbis virus	IL-4(?), IL-6(?)	Antiviral antibody production
Toxoplasma gondii	Interferon-γ,[b] tumor, necrosis factor-α IL-4, IL-6, granulocyte-macrophage colony-stimulating factor	Production of NO

[a]Listed only for the cytokines and their effects that have been reported.

[b]Interferon-γ activates microglia and astrocytes to express the MHC class II antigens and the other molecules (i.e., ICAM-1, LFA-3, and B7) that are critical for effective antigen presentation to T cells. Interferon-γ also upregulates the expression of adhesion molecules involved in lymphocyte traffic on cerebrovascular endothelial cells. These activities of this cytokine most likely contribute to its protective effect against the development of encephalitis induced by infections.

IL = interleukin; NO = nitric oxide; MHC = major histocompatibility complex; ICAM-1 = intercellular adhesion molecule-1; LFA-3 = leukocyte function–associated antigen-3.

brovascular endothelial cells in vitro when monolayers are pretreated with IFN-γ, TNF-α, or IL-1 (102,103). Therefore, it is most likely that some of these cytokines induced by infection stimulate the local cerebrovascular endothelium in vivo to induce adhesion and extravasation of lymphocytes (see Chapter 2). Cytokines appear to play crucial roles in each of the critical events in the protective immunity against infection in the brain, such as homing of lymphocytes into the brain, activation of lymphocytes through antigen-presenting cells (microglia and astrocytes), and activation of the effector cells to eliminate pathogens.

REFERENCES

1 Niewiesk S, Brinckmann UG, Bankamp B, et al. Susceptibility to measles virus-induced encephalitis in mice correlates with impaired antigen presentation to cytotoxic T lymphocytes. *Infect Immun* 1993;67:75–81.

2 Finke D, Liebert UG. CD4+ T cells are essential in overcoming experimental murine measles encephalitis. *Immunology* 1994; 83:184–189.

3 Finke D, Brinckmann UG, Meulen VT, Liebert UG. Gamma interferon is a major mediator of antiviral defense in experimental measles virus-induced encephalitis. *J Virol* 1995;69:5469–5474.

4 Kündig TM, Hengartner H, Zinkernagel RM. T cell-dependent IFN-γ exerts an antiviral effect in the central nervous system but not in peripheral solid organs. *J Immunol* 1993; 150:2316–2321.

5 Brightmen MW, Klatzo I, Olsson Y, Reese TS. The blood brain barrier to proteins under normal and pathological conditions. *J Neurol Sci* 1970;10:215–239.

6 Hauser SL, Doolittle TH, Lincoln R, et al. Cytokine accumulations in CSF of multiple sclerosis patients: frequent detection of interleukin-1 and tumor necrosis factor but not interleukin-6. *Neurology* 1990;40:1735–1739.

7 Houssiau FA, Bukasa K, Sindic CJ, et al. Elevated levels of the 26K human hybridoma growth factor (interleukin-6) in cerebrospinal fluid of patients with acute infection of the central nervous system. *Clin Exp Immunol* 1988;71:320–323.

8 Griffin DE, Ward BJ, Jauregui E, et al. Immune activation during measles: interferon-gamma and neopterin in plasma and cerebrospinal fluid in complicated and uncomplicated diseases. *J Infect Dis* 1990;161:449–453.

9 Gallo P, Frei K, Rordorf C, et al. Human immunodeficiency virus type 1 (HIV-1) infection of the central nervous system: an elevation of cytokines in cerebrospinal fluid. *J Neuroimmunol* 1989;23:109–116.

10 Frei K, Leist TP, Meager A, et al. Production of B cell stimulatory factor-2 and interferon gamma in the central nervous system during viral meningitis and encephalitis. *J Exp Med* 1988;168:449–453.

11 Moskophidis D, Frei K, Lohler J, et al. Production of random classes of immunoglobulins in brain tissue during persistent viral infection paralleled by secretion of interleukin-6 (IL-6) but not of IL-4, IL-5, and gamma interferon. *J Virol* 1991;65:1364–1369.

12 Karupiah G, Xie Q, Buller RML, et al. Inhibition of viral replication by interferon-γ-induced nitric oxide synthase. *Science* 1993; 261:1445–1448.

13 Lee SC, Dickson DW, Liu W, Brosnan CF. Induction of nitric oxide synthase activity in human astrocytes by interleukin-1β and interferon-γ. *J Neuroimmunol* 1993;46:19–24.

14 Simmons ML, Murphy S. Roles for protein kinases in the induction of nitric oxide synthase in astrocytes. *Glia* 1994;11:227–234.

15 Chao CC, Anderson WR, Hu S, et al. Activated microglia inhibit *Toxoplasma gondii* via a nitric oxide mechanism. *Clin Immunol Immunopathol* 1993;67:178–183.

16 Bi ZB, Reiss CS. Inhibition of vesicular stomatitis virus infection by nitric oxide. *J Virol* 1995;69:2208–2213.

17 Wong GHW, Bertlett PF, Clark-Lewis I, et al. Interferon-γ induces the expression of H-2 and Ia antigens on brain cells. *J Neuroimmunol* 1985;7:255–278.

18 Shrikant P, Benveniste EN. The central nervous system as an immunocompetent organ: role of glial cells in antigen presentation. *J Immunol* 1996;157:1819–1822.

19 Fierz W, Endler B, Reske K, et al. Astrocytes

as antigen-presenting cells. I. Induction of Ia antigen expression on astrocytes by T cells via immune interferon and its effect on antigen presentation. *J Immunol* 1985;134:3785–3793.

20 Satoh J, Lee YB, Kim SU. T-cell costimulatory molecules B7-1 (CD80) and B7-2 (CD86) are expressed in human microglia but not in astrocytes in culture. *Brain Res* 1995; 704:92–96.

21 Williams K, Ulvestad E, Antel JP. B7/BB-1 antigen expression on adult human microglia studied *in vitro* and *in situ*. *Eur J Immunol* 1994;24:3031–3037.

22 Geiger KD, Gurushanthaih D, Howes EL, et al. Cytokine-mediated survival from lethal herpes simplex virus infection: role of programmed neuronal death. *Proc Natl Acad Sci USA* 1995;92:3411–3415.

23 Dubois-Dauphin M, Frankowski H, Tsujimoto Y, et al. Neonatal motoneurons overexpressing the *bcl-2* protooncogene in transgenic mice are protected from axotomy-induced cell death. *Proc Natl Acad Sci USA* 1994;91:3309–3313.

24 Levine B, Hardwick JM, Trapp BD, et al. Antibody-mediated clearance of alphavirus infection from neurons. *Science* 1991; 254:856–860.

25 Tyor WR, Moench TR, Griffin DE. Characterization of the local and systemic B cell response of normal and athymic nude mice with Sindbis virus encephalitis. *J Neuroimmunol* 1989;24:207–215.

26 Tyor WR, Stoll G, Griffin DE. The characterization of local and systemic Ia expression during Sindbis virus encephalitis in normal and athymic nude mice. *J Neuropathol Exp Neurol* 1990;49:21–30.

27 Wesselingh SL, Levine B, Fox RJ, et al. Intracerebral cytokine mRNA expression during fatal and nonfatal alphavirus encephalitis suggests a predominant type 2 T cell response. *J Immunol* 1994;152:1289–1297.

28 Frei K, Lins H, Schwerdel C, Fontana A. Antigen presentation in the central nervous system. The inhibitory effect of IL-10 on MHC class II expression and production of cytokines depends on the inducing signals and the type of cell analyzed. *J Immunol* 1994;152:2720–2728.

29 Kobayashi M, Fitz L, Ryuan M, et al. Identification and purification of natural killer cell stimulation factor (NKSF), a cytokine with multiple biologic effects on human lymphocytes. *J Exp Med* 1989;170:827–845.

30 Chan SH, Perussia B, Gupta JW, et al. Induction of interferon-γ production by natural killer cell stimulatory factor: characterization of the responder cells and synergy with other inducers. *J Exp Med* 1991;173:869–880.

31 Chehimi A, Valiante N, Andrea AD, et al. Enhancing effect of natural killer stimulatory factor (NKSF/interleukin-12) on cell-mediated cytotoxicity against tumor-derived and virus-derived cells. *Eur J Immunol* 1993;23:1826–1830.

32 Manetti R, Parronchi P, Giudizi MG, et al. Natural killer stimulatory factor (interleukin-12) induces T helper type-1 (Th1)-specific immune responses and inhibits the development of IL-4-producing cells. *J Exp Med* 1993;177:1199–1204.

33 Hsieh CS, Macatonia SE, Tripp CS, et al. Development of Th1 CD4 T cells through IL-12 produced by *Listeria*-induced macrophages. Science 1993;260:547–549.

34 Coutelier JP, Broeck JV, Wolf SF. Interleukin-12 gene expression after viral infection in mice. *J Virol* 1995;69:1955–1958.

35 Bi Z, Quandt P, Komatsu T, et al. IL-12 promotes enhanced recovery from vesicular stomatitis virus infection of the central nervous system. *J Immunol* 1995;155:5684–5689.

36 Gresser L, Tovey MG, Bourali-Maury C. Efficacy of exogenous interferon treatment initiated after onset of multiplication of vesicular stomatitis virus in the brain of mice. *J Gen Virol* 1975;27:395–398.

37 Irani DN, Griffin DE. Regulation of lymphocyte homing into the brain during viral encephalitis at various stages of infection. *J Immunol* 1996;156:3850–3857.

38 Baron JL, Madri JA, Ruddle NH, et al. Surface expression of α-4 integrin by CD4 T cells is required for their entry into brain parenchyma. *J Exp Med* 1993;177:57–68.

39 Levy RM, Bredensen DE, Rosenblum ML. Neurologic manifestations of the acquired immunodeficiency syndrome (AIDS): experience at UCSF and review of the literature. *J Neurosurg* 1985;62:475–495.

40 Luft BJ, Remington JS. AIDS commentary: toxoplasmic encephalitis. *Clin Infect Dis* 1992;15:211–222.

41 Remington JS, McLeod R, Desmonts G. Toxoplasmosis. In: Remington JS, Klein JO, eds. *Infectious diseases of the fetus and newborn infant.* Philadelphia: WB Saunders, 1995:140–267.

42 Wong S-Y, Remington JS. Toxoplasmosis in the setting of AIDS. In: Broder S, Merigan TC Jr, Bolognesi D, eds. *Textbook of AIDS*

medicine. Baltimore: Williams & Wilkins, 1994:223–257.

43 Suzuki Y, Orellana MA, Schreiber RD, Remington JS. Interferon-γ: The major mediator of resistance against *Toxoplasma gondii*. Science 1988;240:516–518.

44 Gazzinelli R, Hakim FT, Hieny S, et al. Synergistic role of $CD4^+$ and $CD8^+$ T lymphocytes in IFN-γ production and protective immunity induced by an attenuated *Toxoplasma gondii* vaccine. *J Immunol* 1991;146:286–292.

45 Johnson LL. A protective role for endogenous tumor necrosis factor in *Toxoplasma gondii* infection. *Infect Immun* 1992;60:1979–1983.

46 Suzuki Y, Conley FK, Remington JS. Importance of endogenous IFN-γ for prevention of toxoplasmic encephalitis in mice. *J Immunol* 1990;143:2045–2050.

47 Gazzinelli RT, Xu Y, Hieny S, et al. Simultaneous depletion of $CD4^+$ and $CD8^+$ T lymphocytes is required to reactivate chronic infection with *Toxoplasma gondii*. *J Immunol* 1992;149:175–180.

48 Gazzinelli RT, Eltoum I, Wynn TA, Sher A. Acute cerebral toxoplasmosis is induced by in vivo neutralization of TNF-α and correlates with the down-regulated expression of inducible nitric oxide synthase and other markers of macrophage activation. *J Immunol* 1993;151:3672–3681.

49 Suzuki Y, Remington JS. The effect of anti-IFN-γ antibody on the protective effect of Lyt-2^+ immune T cells against toxoplasmosis in mice. *J Immunol* 1990;144:1954–1956.

50 Khan IA, Ely KH, Kasper LH. Antigen-specific $CD8^+$ T cell clone protects against acute *Toxoplasma gondii* infection in mice. *J Immunol* 1994;152:1856–1860.

51 Yang TH, Aosai F, Norose K, et al. Enhanced cytotoxicity of IFN-γ-producing $CD4^+$ cytotoxic T lymphocytes specific for *T. gondii*-infected human melanoma cells. *J Immunol* 1995;154:290–298.

52 Suzuki Y, Remington JS. Dual regulation of resistance against *Toxoplasma gondii* infection by Lyt-2^+ and Lyt-1^+, $L3T4^+$ T cells in mice. *J Immunol* 1988;140:3943–3949.

53 Hunter CA, Litton MJ, Remington JS, Abrams JS. Immunochemical detection of cytokines in the lymph nodes and brains of mice resistant or susceptible to toxoplasmic encephalitis. *J Infect Dis* 1994;170:939–945.

54 Schlüter D, Hein A, Dorries R, Deckert-Schlüter M. Different subsets of T cells in conjunction with natural killer cells, macrophages, and activated microglia participate in the intracerebral immune response to *Toxoplasma gondii* in athymic and immunocompetent rats. *Am J Pathol* 1995;146:999–1007.

55 Chao CC, Gekker G, Hu S, Peterson PK. Human microglia cell defense against *Toxoplasma gondii*. *J Immunol* 1994;152:1246–1252.

56 Chao CC, Hu S, Gekker G, et al. Effect of cytokines on multiplication of *Toxoplasma gondii* in microglial cells. *J Immunol* 1993; 150:3404–3410.

57 Hayashi S, Chan CC, Gazzinelli R, Roberge FG. Contribution of nitric oxide to the host parasite equilibrium in toxoplasmosis. *J Immunol* 1996;156:1476–1481.

58 Schlüter D, Deckert-Schlüter M, Schwendemann G, et al. Expression of major histocompatibility complex II antigens and levels of interferon-γ, tumor necrosis factor, and interleukin-6 in cerebrospinal fluid and serum in *Toxoplasma gondii*-infected SCID and immunocompetent CB-17 mice. *Immunology* 1993;78:430–435.

59 Deckert-Schlüter M, Schlüter D, Hof H, et al. Differential expression of ICAM-1, VCAM-1 and their ligands LFA-1, Mac-1, CD43, VLA-4 and MHC class II antigens in murine toxoplasma encephalitis: a light microscopic and ultrastructural immunohistochemical study. *J Neuropathol Exp Neurol* 1994;53:457–468.

60 Zimmerman LE; in discussion of Remington JS. Ocular pathology of toxoplasmosis. *Surv Ophthalmol* 1961;6:832–856.

61 Werner H, Pichl H. Vergleichende Untersuchungen an zystenbildenden Toxoplasmastämmen. II. Mitteilung: Zystenen-swicklung und humorale antikorperbildung. *Zentralbl Bakteriol (Org)* 1959;210:402–416.

62 Huldt G. Studies on experimental toxoplasmosis. *Ann NY Acad Sci* 1971;177:146–155.

63 Frenkel JK. Pathogenesis of toxoplasmosis and of infections with organisms resembling *Toxoplasma*. *Ann NY Acad Sci* 1956;64:215–231.

64 Hofflin JM, Conley FK, Remington JS. Murine model of intracerebral toxoplasmosis. *J Infect Dis* 1987;155:550–557.

65 Jones TC, Bienz KA, Erb P. In vitro cultivation of *Toxoplasma gondii* cysts in astrocytes in the presence of gamma interferon. *Infect Immun* 1986;51:147–150.

66 Peterson PK, Gekker G, Hu S, Chao CC. Intracellular survival and multiplication of *Toxoplasma gondii* in astrocytes. *J Infect Dis* 1993;168:1472–1478.

67 Murray HW, Rubin BY, Masur H, Roberts RB. Impaired production of lymphokines and im-

mune (gamma) interferon in the acquired immunodeficiency syndrome. *N Engl J Med* 1984;310:883–888.

68 Suzuki Y, Conley FK, Remington JS. Treatment of toxoplasmic encephalitis in mice with recombinant gamma interferon. *Infect Immun* 1990;58:3050–3055.

69 Suzuki Y, Joh K, Kwon O-C, et al. MHC class I gene(s) in the D/L region but not the TNF-α gene determines development of toxoplasmic encephalitis in mice. *J Immunol* 1994; 153:4651–4654.

70 Suzuki Y, Joh K, Orellana MA, et al. A gene(s) within H-2D region determines the development of toxoplasmic encephalitis in mice. *Immunology* 1991;74:732–739.

71 Brown CR, Hunter CA, Estes RG, et al. Definitive identification of a gene that confers resistance against *Toxoplasma* cyst burden and encephalitis. *Immunolgy* 1995;85:419–428.

72 Freund YR, Sgarlato G, Jacob CO, et al. Polymorphisms in the tumor necrosis factor α (TNF-α) gene correlate with murine resistance to development of toxoplasmic encephalitis and with levels of TNF-α mRNA in infected brain tissue. *J Exp Med* 1992; 175:683–688.

73 Mosmann TR, Cherwinski H, Bond MW, et al. Two types of murine helper T cell clone. I. Definition according to profiles of lymphokine activities and secreted proteins. *J Immunol* 1986;136:2348–2357.

74 Cherwinski HM, Schumacher JH, Brown KD, Mosmann TR. Two types of mouse helper T cell clone. III. Further differences in lymphokine synthesis between Th1 and Th2 clones revealed by RNA hybridization, functionally monospecific bioassays, and monoclonal antibodies. *J Exp Med* 1987; 166:1229–1244.

75 Mosmann TR, Coffman RL. Th1 and Th2 cells: different patterns of lymphokine secretion lead to different functional properties. *Annu Rev Immunol* 1989;7:145.

76 Fiorentino DF, Bond MW, Mosmann TR. Two types of mouse T helper cells. IV. Th2 clones secrete a factor that inhibits cytokine production by Th1 clones. *J Exp Med* 1989;170:2081–2095.

77 LeGros G, Ben-Sasson SZ, Seder R, et al. Generation of interleukin 4 (IL-4)-producing cells in vivo and in vitro: IL-2 and IL-4 are required for in vitro generation of IL-4-producing cells. *J Exp Med* 1990;172:921–929.

78 Swain SL, Weinberg AD, English M, Huston G. IL-4 directs the development of Th2-like helper effectors. *J Immunol* 1990;145:3796–3806.

79 Betz M, Fox BS. Regulation and development of cytochrome c-specific IL-4-producing T cells. *J Immunol* 1990;145:1046–1052.

80 Seder RA, Paul WE, Davis MM, de St Groth BF. The presence of interleukin 4 during in vitro priming determines the lymphokine-producing potential of $CD4^+$ T cells from T cell receptor transgenic mice. *J Exp Med* 1992;176:1091–1098.

81 Suzuki Y, Yang Q, Yang S, et al. IL-4 is protective against development of toxoplasmic encephalitis. *J Immunol* 1996;157:2564–2569.

82 Noble A, Kemeny DM. Interleukin-4 enhances interferon-γ synthesis but inhibits development of interferon-γ-producing cells. *Immunology* 1995;85:357–363.

83 Beaman MH, Wong SY, Abrams JS, Remington JS. Splenic IL-4 secretion is not associated with the development of toxoplasmic encephalitis. Presented at the second international congress on Biological Response Modifiers, San Diego, 1993. Abstract 81.

84 Roberts CW, Rurguson DPJ, Jebbari H, et al. Different role for interleukin-4 during the course of *Toxoplasma gondii* infection. *Infect Immun* 1996;64:897–904.

85 Akira S, Taga T, Kishimoto T. Interleukin-6 in biology and medicine. *Adv Immunol* 1993;54:1–78.

86 Hirota H, Kiyama H, Kishimoto T, Taga T. Accelerated nerve regeneration in mice by upregulated expression of interleukin (IL)-6 and IL-6 receptor after trauma. *J Exp Med* 1996;183:2627–2634.

87 Deckert-Schlüter M, Albrecht S, Hof H, et al. Dynamics of the intracerebral and splenic cytokine mRNA production in *Toxoplasma gondii*-resistant and -susceptible congenic strains of mice. *Immunology* 1995;85:408–418.

88 Hunter CA, Roberts CW, Alexander J. Kinetics of cytokine mRNA production in the brains of mice with progressive toxoplasmic encephalitis. *Eur J Immunol* 1992; 22:2317–2322.

89 Suzuki Y, Yang Q, Conley FK, et al. Antibody against interleukin 6 reduces inflammation and numbers of cysts in brains of mice with toxoplasmic encephalitis. *Infect Immun* 1994;62:2773–2778.

90 Heremans H, Dillin C, Put W, et al. Protective effect of anti-interleukin (IL)-6 antibody against endotoxin, associated with paradoxically increased IL-6 levels. *Eur J Immunol* 1992;22:2395–2401.

91 Nakane A, Okamoto M, Asano M, et al. Endogenous gamma interferon, tumor necrosis factor, and interleukin-6 in *Staphylococcus aureus* infection in mice. *Infect Immun* 1995;63:1165–1172.

92 Fiorentino DF, Bond MW, Mosmann TR. Two types of mouse T helper cells. IV. Th2 clones secrete a factor that inhibits cytokine production by Th1 clones. *J Exp Med* 1989;170:2081–2095.

93 Firentino DF, Zlotnik A, Vieira P, et al. IL-10 acts on the antigen-presenting cell to inhibit cytokine production by Th1 cells. *J Immunol* 1990;146:3444–3451.

94 Gazzinelli RT, Oswald IP, James S, Sher A. IL-10 inhibits parasite killing and nitrogen oxide production by IFN-γ activated macrophages. *J Immunol* 1992;148:1792–1796.

95 Gazzinelli RT, Wysocka M, Hayashi S, et al. Parasite-induced IL-12 stimulates early IFN-γ synthesis and resistance during acute infection with *Toxoplasma gondii*. *J Immunol* 1994;153:2533–2543.

96 Khan IA, Matsuura T, Kasper LH. Interleukin-12 enhances murine survival against acute toxoplasmosis. *Infect Immun* 1994;62:1639–1642.

97 Hunter CA, Candolfi E, Subauste C, et al. Studies on the role of interleukin-12 in acute murine toxoplasmosis. *Immunology* 1995;84:16–20.

98 Rook AH, Kehrl JH, Wakefield LM, et al. Effects of transforming growth factor-β on the functions of natural killer cells: depressed cytolytic activity and blunting of interferon responsiveness. *J Immunol* 1986;136:3916–3920.

99 McCartney-Francis NL, Wahl SM. Transforming growth factor-β: a matter of life and death. *J Leukoc Biol* 1994;55:401–409.

100 Hunter CA, Bermudez L, Beernink H, et al. Transforming growth factor-β inhibits interleukin-12-induced protection of interferon-γ by natural killer cells: a role for transforming growth factor-β in the regulation of T cell-independent resistance to *Toxoplasma gondii*. *Eur J Immunol* 1995;25:994–1000.

101 Fischer HG, Bielinski AK, Nitzgen B, et al. Functional dichotomy of mouse microglia developed in vitro: differential effects of macrophage and granulocyte/macrophage colony-stimulating factor on cytokine secretion and antitoxoplasmic activity. *J Neuroimmunol* 1993;45:193–202.

102 Hughes CCW, Male DK, Lantos PL. Adhesion of lymphocytes to cerebral microvascular cells: effect of interferon-γ, tumor necrosis factor and interleukin-1. *Immunology* 1988;64:677–681.

103 Elfont RM, Griffin DE, Goldstein GW. Enhanced endothelial cell adhesion of human cerebrospinal fluid lymphocytes. *Ann Neurol* 1995;38:405–413.

5 Glia-Mediated Neurotoxicity

CHUN C. CHAO
SHUXIAN HU
PHILLIP K. PETERSON

The glia (from Greek, meaning *glue*) were known historically for their supportive functions within the central nervous system (CNS). In addition to providing growth factors for neurons, astrocytes play a critical role in the metabolism of neurotransmitters, such as the excitatory amino acid (EAA) glutamate. Results of recent studies suggest that astrocytes also signal neurons directly via this amino acid (1,2). Not so well appreciated by the infectious disease research community, however, is the fact that glial cells greatly outnumber neurons (by about eight to one). Astrocytes are the predominant cell type (comprising approximately 80% of the glia within the cerebral cortex), whereas microglia (15% of the glia) and oligodendrocytes (5% of the glia) are minority cell populations within the brain. Owing to increased research on the neuropathogenesis of CNS disorders, glial cells have become recognized as important immunoregulatory cells of the brain.

Although glia clearly play important supportive roles within the brain, the pathogenetic potential of these cells has received increased attention in recent years. Activated glial cells (microglia and astrocytes) are a hallmark of several neurodegenerative diseases, such as acquired immunodeficiency syndrome (AIDS) dementia and Alzheimer's disease. Microglia are regarded as the ontogenetic and functional equivalents of macrophages in a variety of somatic tissues (for review, see Chapter 3). Histopathologic studies dating to the early part of this century demonstrated that microglial cells differentiate and proliferate at and migrate to sites of inflammation within the CNS (3). In addition to their potential contribution to defense of the CNS (4,5), activated microglia may also be destructive (6). The immunoregulatory activities of microglial cells and astrocytes are apparent following a variety of insults to the CNS, especially during inflammation (7–9). Reactive astrocytes (astrogliosis) are a histopathologic characteristic of several neurodegenerative diseases (10), and impairments of astroglial function by invading microorganisms or their products and by host-derived mediators of inflammation have the potential to contribute to neuropathologic processes as well (11). On the other hand, astrocytes may also have a neuroprotective function under certain pathologic conditions (12,13).

A growing body of evidence supports the hypothesis that activation of glial cells by immune stimuli or cytokines contributes to neuronal cell injury. Although the precise mechanisms underlying glia-mediated neurotoxicity remain to be elucidated, it has been proposed that in addition to cell-to-cell adhesion (14), mediators derived from reactive glial cells are responsible for injury to neighboring neurons. Results of in vitro studies suggest that activated glial cells release a number of neurotoxic factors (Table 5-1), including the proinflammatory cytokines interleukin (IL)-1 and tumor necrosis factor (TNF)-α (15–17), the anti-inflammatory cytokine transforming growth factor (TGF)-β (18), free radicals (i.e., reactive oxygen intermediates (19) and the reactive nitrogen intermediate (RNI) nitric oxide (NO) (20–23)), EAAs (e.g., glutamate (24) and quinolinic acid (25)), platelet-activating factor (26), arachidonic acid (27), and several partially characterized neurotoxins (28,29). The principal aim of this chapter is to review current and emerging concepts about immune activation of glial cells and the subsequent neuronal cell injury that follows in the wake of this process. While numerous neurotoxic factors can be released by activated glial cells under different conditions, we focus on the proinflammatory cytokines and NO, two of the most widely recognized neurotoxic moieties, and discuss the mechanisms underlying their neuropathogenic effects.

THE BRAIN AS AN IMMUNE ORGAN

The concept that the CNS is an immunologically privileged site is supported by evidence that the brain lacks lymphatic drainage (30) and is separated physically from the rest of the organism by the blood-brain barrier (BBB) (31). A growing body of evidence suggests that this concept needs to be modified, because on the brain's side of the BBB are glial cells that respond during inflammation in a manner identical to immunocytes within somatic tissues. Immune stimuli, such as the bacterial cell wall product lipopolysaccharide

Table 5-1. Candidate Neurotoxins Released by Activated Glial Cells

Pro-inflammatory cytokines
Tumor necrosis factor-α
Interleukin-1
Anti-inflammatory cytokines
Transforming growth factor-β
Free radicals
Reactive nitrogen intermediates
Reactive oxygen intermediates
Glutamate/quinolinic acid
Platelet-activating factor
Arachidonic acid
Neurotoxins
Infectious disease agents
Host-derived factors

(LPS), parasites, fungi, viruses, and their constituents, can penetrate the BBB and provoke immune responses within the brain. In addition, pathologic events within the CNS often result in a breakdown of the BBB, which permits cells of the somatic immune system (i.e., T lymphocytes, B cells, monocytes, and neutrophils) to gain access to this protected site (see Chapters 1 and 2). Mediators derived from activated lymphocytes can further potentiate glial cell responses during inflammatory processes. Because of the predominance of glial cells within the CNS and the diverse immunologic properties of these cells, the brain itself can be considered as an immune organ capable of generating immunologic responses during a variety of insults, including an invasion of microorganisms. Inflammation within the CNS may in turn trigger glial cell activation followed by the generation of toxic factors that precipitate neuronal cell death.

Production of Proinflammatory Cytokines

Activated glial cells produce proinflammatory cytokines in response to immune stimulation. Our laboratory and several other research groups showed that LPS is a potent stimulus of microglial cell production of the proinflammatory cytokine TNF-α (32–36). Anti-inflammatory cytokines (i.e., IL-4, IL-6, IL-10, and TGF-β) can inhibit the microglial cell release of TNF-α (36). In contrast to findings with microglial cells, our research group and that of Lee et al. (35) were unable to demonstrate that highly enriched (> 99%) human fetal astrocytes produce detectable amounts of TNF-α in response to LPS, even though others showed that astrocytes derived from rodent species are able to do so (37–39). Whether astrocytes from adult humans will release TNF-α on activation with LPS or other immune stimuli remains to be determined. Nevertheless, the amount of TNF-α released by astrocytes is relatively modest compared to that from microglia.

Activated microglial cells also release another important proinflammatory cytokine, IL-1. Microglial cell release of IL-1, like that of TNF-α, is suppressed by several anti-inflammatory cytokines, such as IL-4, IL-10, and TGF-β (Fig 5-1). Treatment of microglial cells with IL-1 enhances TNF-α production (35,36). Microglial cell membrane–associated IL-1 stimulates astrocyte expression of TNF-α and IL-6 following cell-to-cell contact (35). Since IL-1 and TNF-α may play a critical role in many symptoms of illness associated with infectious and inflammatory diseases (e.g., fever, loss of appetite, sleepiness, and fatigue (40–42)), regulation of the glial cell production of these proinflammatory cytokines may have important implications in the pathogenesis of neurologic disorders in which these symptoms are manifest.

Production of Nitric Oxide

In addition to releasing proinflammatory cytokines, activated glial cells generate NO, which is a highly toxic free radical. This phenomenon is best demonstrated when rodent microglial cells are incubated with immune stimuli, such as interferon (IFN)-γ and LPS (20,21). Whether human microglial cells are capable of generating biologically significant amounts of NO has been a matter of controversy (see Chapter 3). Under certain conditions, however, human astrocytes can release considerable amounts of NO (43–46). In a recent study, cytokine-treated microglial cell cultures of human origin that were multiply passaged in vitro yielded high levels of NO (47). However, this phenomenon was not reproduced in our laboratory in experiments using human fetal

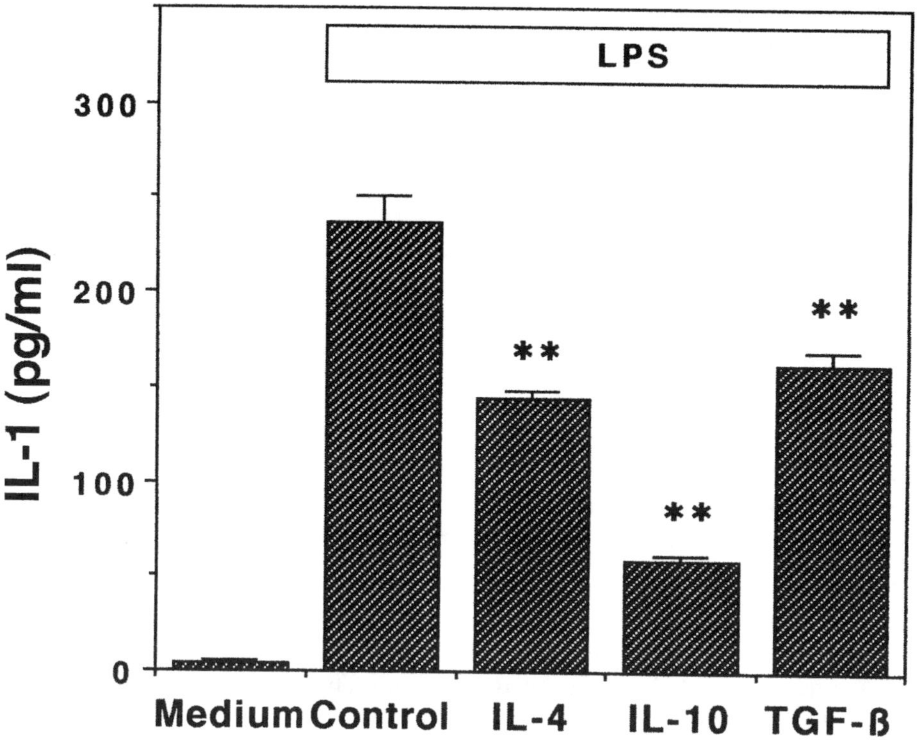

Figure 5-1. Cytokine regulation of microglial cell interleukin (IL)-1 production. Human microglial cell cultures were treated with medium or 1 μg/ml of lipopolysaccharide in the absence (Control) or presence of IL-4 (10 ng/mL), IL-10 (3 ng/mL), and transforming growth factor (TGF)-β (1 ng/mL) for 24 hours. Supernatants were then harvested and assayed for IL-1 as previously described (34). Data are means ± standard error of means of triplicates and are representative of three separate experiments. $^{**}p < 0.01$ versus the control cultures. (Reprinted with permission from University of Chicago Press.)

microglial cell cultures that had been passaged up to 50 times (Hu S, Peterson PK, Chao CC, unpublished data, 1996). The reason for this discrepancy is unknown.

Table 5-2 summarizes the differences in NO production by human versus mouse microglial cell cultures observed in our laboratory. Using probes designed to detect human astrocyte inducible NO synthase (iNOS) messenger RNA (mRNA) expression by reverse transcriptase–polymerase chain reaction (RT-PCR) (23), we were unable to identify any measurable iNOS mRNA in preparations derived from fetal and adult human microglia following stimulation of the cells with IFN-γ plus LPS (Peterson PK, Hu S, Chao CC, unpublished data, 1995). These data suggest that the mRNA transcript for microglial cell iNOS is likely different from that of the astrocyte iNOS message. The biologic consequences of the relatively low levels of NO generated by activated human microglia are unclear at present. Whether the NO produced by human microglia has antimicrobial activity, as reported for rodent microglia (48), has not been clearly defined (5,49,50). Be-

Table 5-2. Species Differences in Microglial Cell Nitric Oxide (NO) Production[a]

Immune Stimuli	*Human*	*Mouse*
Medium	2 ± 1	2 ± 1
Interferon (IFN)-γ (200 U/mL)	1 ± 0	15 ± 2[b]
Lipopolysaccharide (LPS) (1 μg/mL)	2 ± 2	10 ± 2[b]
INF-γ + LPS	9 ± 1[b]	52 ± 4[c]
IFN-γ + LPS + NMMA (500 μM)	4 ± 1[d]	5 ± 2[e]

[a]Human fetal (20-week-old) and mouse neonatal (1-day-old) microglial cell cultures (10^5 cells/well) were treated with medium or indicated immune stimuli for 5 days prior to harvesting supernatants for NO production. N^G-monomethyl-L-arginine (NMMA) is an inducible NO synthase inhibitor. Levels of nitrite, a stable metabolite of NO, were assayed by the Griess reagent as previously described (21). Data are means ± standard error of means of triplicates.
[b]$p < 0.05$.
[c]$p < 0.01$ versus control (medium) cultures.
[d]$p < 0.05$.
[e]$p < 0.01$ versus the IFN-γ 1 LPS group.

cause NO can also function as a neurotransmitter (51), it is possible that the amounts of NO released from human microglia are in a physiologic (nM) rather than a pathologic (μM) range; that is, NO could serve as a communication signal between activated microglia and neurons.

In contrast to microglia, human astrocytes could be a rich source of NO in the CNS. IL-1 plays a pivotal role in the generation of NO by human astrocytes, which is potentiated by either IFN-γ or TNF-α (23,43). IL-1 induces the expression of iNOS mRNA by human astrocytes, which shares identical sequences to that of human hepatocyte iNOS mRNA (23). Treatment of human astrocytes with anti-inflammatory cytokines causes differential inhibition of NO production; that is, IL-4 and IL-10 suppress IFN-γ–enhanced NO production, while TGF-β inhibits TNF-α–potentiated NO production (52). The amount of NO generated by cytokine-activated astrocytes appears to have important biologic effects. For example, production of NO by human astrocytes has been associated with inhibition of the extracellular growth of *Cryptococcus neoformans* (53) as well as the intracellular multiplication of *Toxoplasma gondii* (54). Since activated microglia appear to be a major source of IL-1 within the CNS, it is possible that the role of NO in host defense of the human brain depends on the cooperative interaction between microglial cells and astrocytes.

NEUROTOXICITY

Neurotoxicity in Cultures of Glia and Neurons

Activated microglia or reactive astrocytes have the potential to induce neuronal cell death (55). Even though direct contact of activated glia with neurons may not necessarily be toxic, cytokines or NO released by glia can trigger neuronal cell injury. In cocultures of murine microglia and neurons, cytokine-activated microglia generate considerable amounts of NO, which kills neighboring neurons (20,21). In this coculture model, the anti-inflammatory cytokine IL-4 suppresses microglial cell production of NO and prevents subsequent neuronal cell damage (56). In contrast, human microglia treated with IFN-γ plus LPS produce only a small amount of NO that is insufficient to cause any detectable neuronal cell injury when cocultured with human cerebral cortical neurons (44). Thus, it is unclear at present whether activated human microglia contribute directly to the neuropathogenesis associated with many forms of brain injury. If they do, microglia-mediated neuronal cell damage may involve NO-independent mechanisms, such as production of the proinflammatory cytokines IL-1 and TNF-α (see below).

In striking contrast to findings with human microglia, we recently showed that human astrocytes stimulated with IL-1β plus IFN-γ generate quantities of NO capable of killing neighboring neurons in mixed glial and neuronal cell cultures (23). Even though IL-1β by itself stimulates NO production by astrocytes (23,43), the amount of NO generated (20 μM nitrite, a stable metabolite of NO) is insufficient to cause neuronal cell death. However, IL-1β in combination with potentiating cytokines (e.g., IFN-γ or TNF-α) is capable of initiating the production of neurotoxic amounts of NO by astrocytes (57).

The proposed mechanism of neurotoxicity based on these in vitro studies of mixed glial and neuronal cell cultures may be too simplistic. Many other glial cell factors also must be considered, including the proliferation of astrocytes as well as alterations of certain astrocyte functions, such as glutamine synthetase (GS) activity and glutamate uptake (58). Additionally, other cytokines and mediators of inflammation produced by glia are likely to act in concert in inducing neuronal cell death. Taken together, however, the findings of these studies suggest that activation of astrocytes by cytokines plays a critical role in mediating neurotoxicity in human brain cell cultures.

Cytokine-Induced Neurotoxicity

Cytokines alone may trigger neuronal cell damage under certain conditions. Several studies demonstrated that TNF-α can be neurotoxic (15–17). Experiments in our laboratory found that when cultured for 14 days, fetal murine cerebral cortical cells develop into single neurons and well-differentiated neuronal cell clumps growing atop an astrocyte mat (Fig 5-2A). Treatment of these cell cultures with TNF-α, however, induces marked impairment of neuronal cell development (Fig 5-2B). This effect can be observed as early as day 4 in culture, supporting the notion that TNF-α can hinder the development of neurons in the fetal brain.

One study showed that TNF-α seems to be more lytic to human oligodendrocytes than to neurons (59). A separate study found TNF-α to be neurotoxic in mixed human brain cell cultures indirectly via release of another cytotoxic cytokine, IL-6 (60). Because we did not find IL-6 to be neurotoxic in our human neuronal cell cultures (Hu S, Chao CC, unpublished data, 1996), and some studies actually found it to be neuroprotective in their cell cultures of rodent origin (61–64), caution should be taken when extrapolating data derived from one in vitro model of neurotoxicity to others. While the precise mechanism underlying TNF-α–associated neuronal cell injury is unclear, it may proceed via an indirect pathway involving astrocytes (15). Using human fetal brain cell cultures, we found, for example, that TNF-α potentiates glutamate-mediated neurotoxicity by reducing glutamate uptake and astrocyte GS activity (65).

In addition to its neurotoxic potential, TNF-α exhibits neuroprotective activity in certain in vitro conditions in rodent neuronal cell cultures by a mechanism involving blockade of Ca^{2+} influx (66,67). We observed a similar phenomenon in which either IL-1β or TNF-α protects human cortical neurons against serum deprivation–induced toxicity (Hu S, Peterson PK, Chao CC, unpublished data, 1996). Since serum depriva-

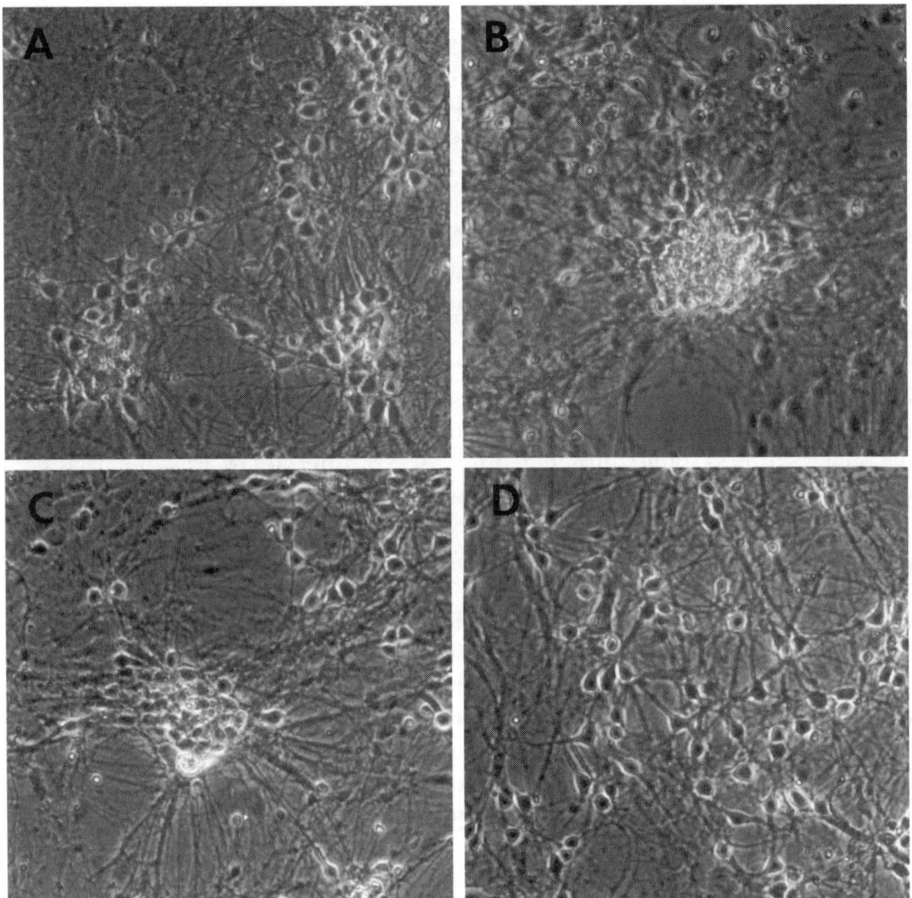

Figure 5-2. Cytokine effects on murine neuronal cell development. Newly dispersed murine fetal cortical cells (containing glia and neurons) were incubated with (A) medium, (B) tumor necrosis factor (TNF)-α (20 ng/mL), (C) interleukin (IL)-1β (1 ng/mL), or (D) IL-4 (20 ng/mL). Neuronal cells were observed for development at 14 days of culture. The TNF-α–treated neurons failed to develop and the neuronal cell clumps that remain are undergoing dissolution, whereas IL-4–treated neurons developed into single cells (× 300).

tion–induced neurotoxicity appears to be mediated via N-methyl-D-aspartate (NMDA) receptors (unpublished data), it is possible that under certain conditions these proinflammatory cytokines may preserve neurons by establishing Ca^{2+} homeostasis. Because IL-1 stimulates astrocyte proliferation (68,69) and astrocytes play a protective role against NMDA-mediated neurotoxicity (70,71), this complex interaction could also account for the neuroprotective effects of IL-1β. However, further studies are warranted to elucidate the mechanism underlying cytokine-mediated neuroprotective effects.

In one study using mixed murine glial and neuronal cell cultures, we found that IL-1β markedly stimulates astrogliosis within the first few days after exposure (Hu S, Chao CC, unpublished data, 1995). However, under our culture conditions, IL-1–treated neuronal cells demonstrated partial impairment of development at 14 days of culture (Fig 5-2C). Interestingly, in the same study the anti-inflammatory cytokine IL-4 appeared to promote murine fetal neuronal cell development in vitro (Fig 5-2D). IL-4–treated neurons developed longer neurites and were more differentiated in culture. The stimulatory activity of IL-4 may be due to its direct effect on astrocyte production of nerve growth factor (NGF) (72). IL-1 also stimulates the release of NGF from rodent astrocytes (73–75), and NGF reportedly promotes neuronal sprouting after injury, especially of cholinergic neurons (76). Whether human astrocytes generate NGF in response to IL-1 stimulation, however, is presently unknown.

Nitric Oxide–Mediated Neuronal Cell Injury

Neurons from rodent brain are highly susceptible to NO-mediated damage, and recent studies demonstrated that fetal human cortical neurons also are vulnerable to NO-mediated toxicity (44). Exposure of human cortical neurons to the NO-generating compound sodium nitroprusside (SNP) induces a dose-dependent toxicity (Fig 5-3A), as reflected by release of lactate dehydrogenase (LDH), a biochemical marker of neuronal cell loss (55). Investigators in our laboratory recently examined the mode of neuronal cell death induced by SNP and found that an apoptotic pathway is involved, as determined by the terminal transferase-mediated uridine triphosphate nick end-labeling (TUNEL) technique (Fig 5-3B). Interestingly, addition of the NMDA receptor antagonist 2-amino-5-phosphonovalerate (2APV) to SNP-treated cultures markedly attenuated NO-mediated apoptosis, suggesting that NO in some way activates NMDA receptors. Whether NO is an important neurotoxin in infectious diseases of the human CNS has yet to be determined. However, NO may contribute to brain injury in patients with the autoimmune brain disease multiple sclerosis (77).

Because cytokines are key mediators in the activation of glial cells, these immune mediators may damage neurons by an indirect mechanism involving glial cell production of NO. Using human mixed glial and neuronal cell cultures, we found that only the combination of IL-1β plus IFN-γ or TNF-α induced amounts of NO (Fig 5-4A) that are capable of killing neurons (Fig 5-4B). Furthermore, the combination of IL-1β and TNF-α elicited NO-mediated neuronal cell injury via a mechanism involving NMDA receptors (57). We also showed that NMDA receptors may be involved in the neurotoxicity mediated by NO following treatment of mixed human glial and neuronal cell cultures with the combination of IL-1β plus IFN-γ (57). In this model, IL-1β plus IFN-γ–mediated neurotoxicity can be attenuated by treatment with NMDA receptor antag-

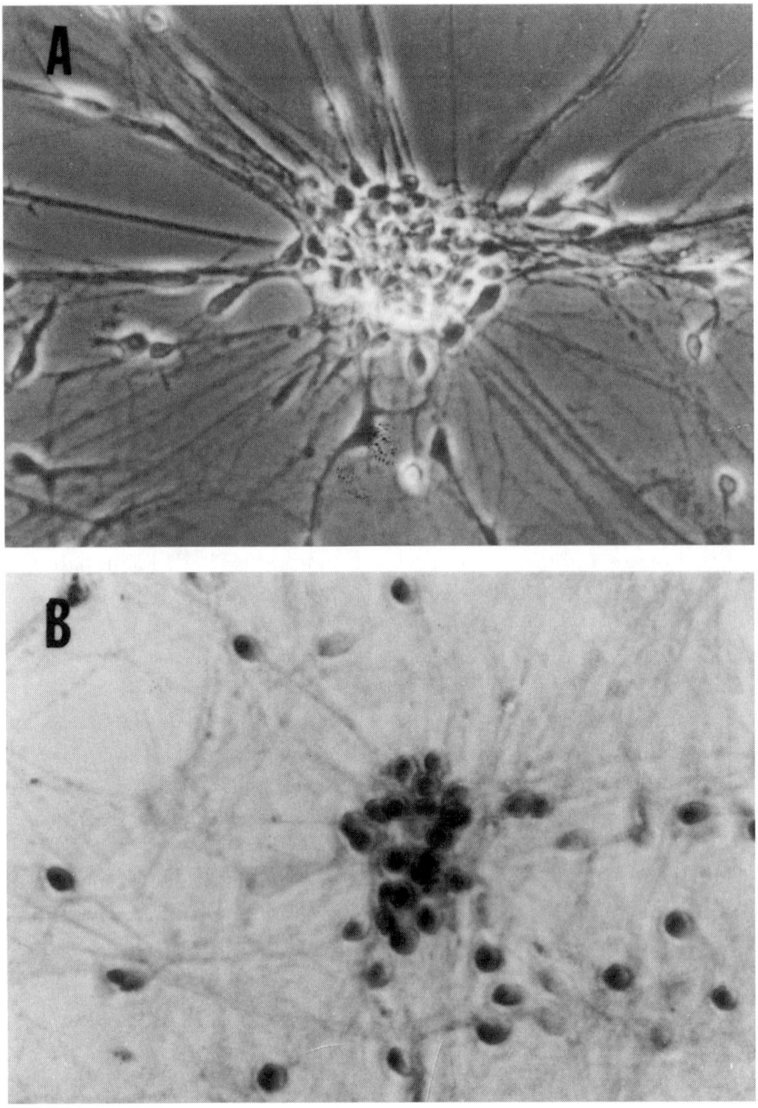

Figure 5-3. Nitric oxide–mediated neuronal cell loss. (A) Highly enriched (> 90%) human fetal neuronal cell cultures were treated with (A) medium or (B) sodium nitroprusside (SNP) (40 μM) for 3 days prior to evaluation by the TUNEL technique under light microscopy (× 200). The SNP-treated cells show the dark-staining nuclei characteristic of apoptotic cells. (C) In a separate experiment, enriched neuronal cell cultures were incubated with medium (Control), 40 μM SNP, or SNP plus 30 μM 2-amino-5-phosphonovalerate (2APV) (an NMDA receptor antagonist) for 3 days prior to harvesting of supernatants for assessment of lactate dehydrogenase (LDH) release (means ± standard error of means of triplicates, n = 3). $^{**}p < 0.01$ versus the control group. $^{\dagger\dagger}p < 0.01$ versus the SNP-treated group.

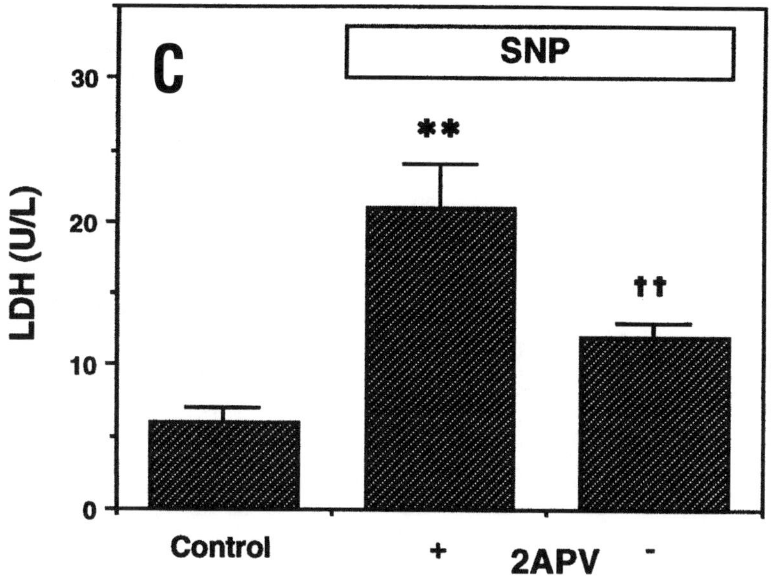

Figure 5-3. *(continued)*

onists without affecting NO production, suggesting that NMDA receptor–mediated neurotoxicity is distal to NO production (23). This finding is in agreement with data showing that NO-mediated neurotoxicity occurs via an NMDA receptor–mediated mechanism (see Fig 5-3). In addition, we also found that IL-1β plus IFN-γ induced apoptotic loss of neurons via an NMDA receptor–mediated mechanism (57).

Although the in vitro studies just cited suggest that high levels of NO are neurotoxic, recent findings in animal studies indicate that different redox states of RNI may have either a neuroprotective or a neurotoxic effect (78). Whether this redox state hypothesis is also true in the human system, however, remains to be elucidated. Thus, the hypothetical contribution of glial cell–derived NO to human neuronal cell damage awaits confirmation under in vivo conditions.

CONCLUSIONS

Activated glial cells appear to play an important pathogenetic role in inflammatory diseases of the brain. Reactive astrocytes and activated microglia are a histopathologic hallmark of several neurodegenerative diseases. Immune mediators, such as proinflammatory cytokines and RNIs, released by activated glial cells, are presently considered to be key candidate neurotoxins. Other mediators, such as reactive oxygen intermediates, EAAs, platelet-activating factors, and arachidonic acid, are also released in inflammatory foci and their contribution to neuronal cell injury has not been clearly defined.

The precise mechanisms underlying inflammation-associated brain injury, however, are still not well understood. Nevertheless, based on studies from our laboratory and the

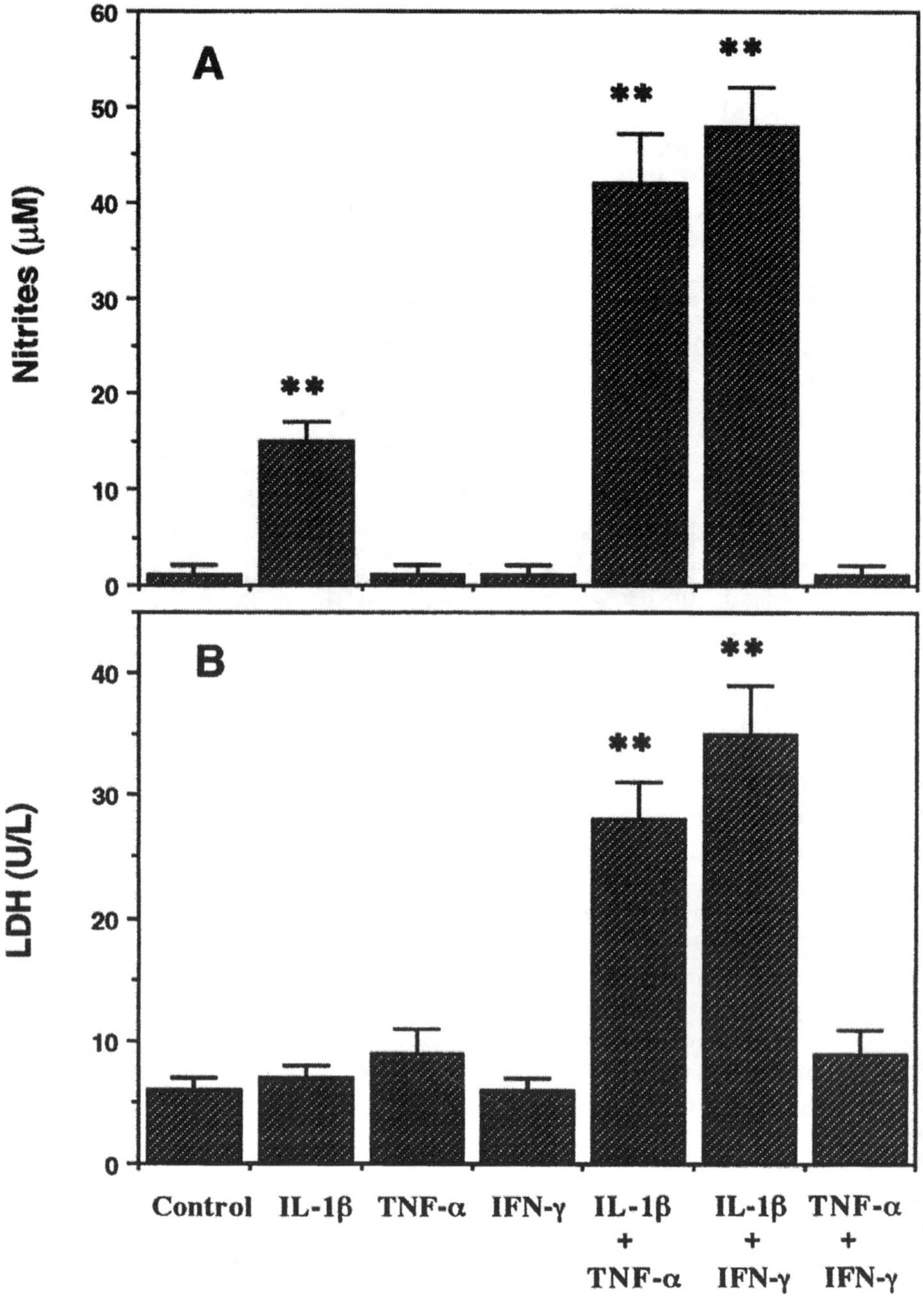

Figure 5-4. Cytokine-mediated neurotoxicity. Mixed human fetal glial and neuronal cell cultures were incubated with medium (Control) or medium containing interleukin (IL)-1β (1 ng/mL), tumor necrosis factor (TNF)-α (20 ng/mL), interferon (IFN)-γ (200 U/mL), or indicated combinations of these cytokines for 10 days prior to harvesting of supernatants for assaying levels of (A) nitrite (a stable metabolite of nitric oxide) or (B) lactate dehydrogenase (LDH). Data are means ± standard error of means of triplicates and are representative of three separate experiments. $^{**}p < 0.01$ versus the control cultures.

work of many other research groups, we propose a unifying model of glia-mediated neurotoxicity (Fig 5-5). In this model, it is suggested that a wide variety of CNS insults can precipitate a cascade of events in which there is a transformation of resting (supporting) glial cells into an activated (destructive) form. Generation of toxic immune mediators (e.g., cytokines and free radicals) by glial cells ensues, ultimately resulting in an excessive activation of NMDA receptors and triggering of an apoptotic intracellular signaling pathway.

During the past 30 years, the development of therapeutic approaches aiming at NMDA receptors has been largely based on both in vivo and in vitro studies derived from animal species. Only recently have in vitro culture models of neurodegeneration using human fetal brain cells been developed (79,80). There is a species difference between human and murine neuronal cell cultures in NMDA receptor-mediated neurotoxicity (Table 5-3). Our in vitro studies of glia-mediated neurotoxicity suggest that an NMDA receptor mechanism could serve as the final pathway leading to neuronal cell death (6,78). Surprisingly little is known, however, about NMDA receptors in the human nervous system. What are the molecular and pharmacologic characteristics of human NMDA receptors? Do these receptors have a direct or indirect interaction with immune mediators, such as cytokines and free radicals? Do human glial cells have NMDA

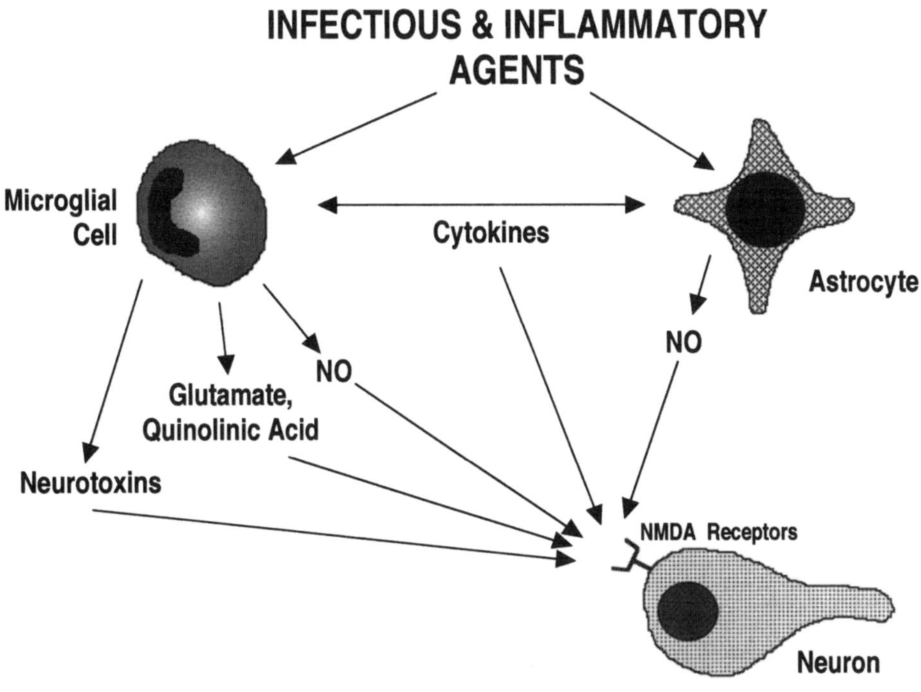

Figure 5-5. Schematic diagram depicting the mediators produced by activated glial cells that induce neurodegeneration by a common final pathway involving NMDA receptor activation. NO = nitric oxide.

Table 5-3. Species Differences in NMDA Receptor–Mediated Neurotoxicity

NMDA Receptor Ligands	*Human*[a]	*Mouse*[b]
Glutamate (300 μM)	15	85
Glutamate (1 mM)	45	100
NMDA (300 μM)	20	95
NMDA (1 mM)	50	100

[a]Fourteen-day-old mixed human glial and neuronal cell cultures derived from 16-week-old fetal abortuses were incubated with the indicated concentrations of NMDA receptor ligands for 5 days prior to microscopic counting of surviving neurons. Data are expressed as percentages of total neuronal cell loss versus control cultures incubated in medium alone.

[b]Fourteen-day-old mixed murine glial and neuronal cell cultures derived from 13-day-old fetuses were incubated with NMDA receptor ligands at the indicated concentrations for 5 minutes and then replaced with culture medium. Surviving neurons were recorded 24 hours later under a light microscope. Data are expressed as percentages of total neuronal cell loss versus control cultures incubated in medium alone.

receptors? If so, what is their role in neurotoxicity or neuroprotection? What processes are involved in deactivation of EAAs in the human brain? What is the source (neuronal or glial cell origin) of excessive EAAs (including glutamate, quinolinic acid, aspartate, glycine)? What specific human neuronal cell types are more susceptible to inflammation-induced neurodegeneration? Finding definitive answers to these questions may lead to development of new therapeutic approaches for a number of neurodegenerative diseases in which activated glial cells have been implicated.

REFERENCES

1 Nedergaard M. Direct signaling from astrocytes to neurons in cultures of mammalian brain cells. *Science* 1994;263:1768–1771.

2 Parpura V, Basarsky TA, Liu F, et al. Glutamate-mediated astrocyte-neuron signaling. *Nature* 1994;369:744–747.

3 del Rio-Hortega P. Microglia. In: Penfield W, ed. *Cytology and cellular pathology of the nervous system*. Vol. 2. New York: Paul P. Hocker, 1932:481–584.

4 Chao CC, Gekker G, Hu S, Peterson PK. Human microglial cell defense against *Toxoplasma gondii*: the role of cytokines. *J Immunol* 1994;152:1246–1252.

5 Lee SC, Kress Y, Dickson DW, Casadevall A. Human microglia mediate anti-*Cryptococcus neoformans* activity in the presence of specific antibody. *J Neuroimmunol* 1995;62:43–52.

6 Chao CC, Hu S, Peterson PK. Glia: the not so innocent bystanders. *J Neurovirol* 1996;2:234–239.

7 Frei K, Fontana A. Immune regulatory functions of astrocytes and microglial cells within the central nervous system. In: Goetzl EJ, Spector VH, eds. *Neuroimmune networks: physiology and diseases*. New York: Alan R. Liss, 1989: 127–136.

8 Giulian D. Ameboid microglia as effectors of inflammation in the central nervous system. *J Neurosci Res* 1987;18:155–171.

9 Hertz L, McFarlin DE, Waksman BH. Astrocytes: auxillary cells for immune responses in the central nervous system. *Immunol Today* 1990;11:265–268.

10 Hatten ME, Liem RKH, Shelanski ML, Mason CA. Astroglia in CNS injury. *Glia* 1991; 4:233–243.

11 Mucke L, Eddleston M. Astrocytes in infectious and immune-mediated diseases of the central nervous system. *FASEB J* 1993;7:1226–1232.

12 Eddleston M, Mucke L. Molecular profile of reactive astrocytes: implications for their role

in neurologic disease. *Neuroscience* 1993; 54:15–36.

13 Nottet HSLM, Jett M, Flanagan CR, et al. A regulatory role for astrocytes in HIV-1 encephalitis: an overexpression of eicosanoids, platelet-activating factor, and tumor necrosis factor-α by activated HIV-1-infected monocytes is attenuated by primary human astrocytes. *J Immunol* 1995;154:3567–3581.

14 Tardieu M, Hery C, Peudenier S, et al. Human immunodeficiency virus type 1-infected monocytic cells can destroy human neural cells after cell-to-cell adhesion. *Ann Neurol* 1992;32:11–17.

15 Bernton EW, Bryant HU, Decoster MA, et al. No direct neurotoxicity by HIV-1 virions or culture fluids from HIV-1 infected T cells or monocytes. *AIDS Res Human Retroviruses* 1992;8:495–503.

16 Gelbard HA, Dzenko KA, DiLoreto D, et al. Neurotoxic effects of tumor necrosis factor alpha in primary human neuronal cultures are mediated by activation of the glutamate AMPA receptor subtype: implications for AIDS neuropathogenesis. *Dev Neurosci* 1993;15:417–422.

17 Talley AK, Dewhurst S, Perry SW, et al. Tumor necrosis factor alpha-induced apoptosis in human neuronal cells: protection by the antioxidant N-acetylcystine and the genes *bcl*-2 and *crm*A. *Mol Cell Biol* 1995;15:2359–2366.

18 Chao CC, Hu S, Tsang M, et al. Effects of transforming growth factor-β on murine astrocyte glutamine synthetase activity: implications in neuronal injury. *J Clin Invest* 1992;90:1786–1793.

19 Tanaka M, Sotomatsu A, Yoshida T, et al. Detection of superoxide production by activated microglia using a sensitive and specific chemiluminescence assay and microglia-mediated PC12 cell death. *J Neurochem* 1994;63:266–270.

20 Boje KM, Arora PK. Microglia-produced nitric oxide and reactive nitrogen oxides mediate neuronal cell death. *Brain Res* 1992;587:250–256.

21 Chao CC, Hu S, Molitor TW, et al. Activated microglia mediate neuronal cell injury via a nitric oxide mechanism. *J Immunol* 1992; 149:2736–2741.

22 Dawson VL, Brahmbhatt HP, Mong JA, Dawson TM. Expression of inducible nitric oxide synthase causes delayed neurotoxicity in primary mixed neuronal-glial cortical cultures. *Neuropharmacology* 1994:33:1425–1430.

23 Chao CC, Hu S, Sheng WS, et al. Cytokine-stimulated astrocytes damage human neurons via a nitric oxide mechanism. *Glia* 1996; 16:276–284.

24 Piani D, Spranger M, Frei K, et al. Macrophage-induced cytotoxicity of N-methyl-D-aspartate receptor positive neurons involves excitatory amino acids rather than reactive oxygen intermediates and cytokines. *Eur J Immunol* 1992;22:2429–2436.

25 Achim CL, Heyes MP, Wiley CA. Quantification of human immunodeficiency virus, immune activation factors, and quinolinic acid in AIDS brains. *J Clin Invest* 1993;91:2769–2775.

26 Gelbard HA, Nottet H, Dzenko KA, et al. Platelet-activating factor: a candidate human immunodeficiency virus type 1-infected neurotoxin. *J Virol* 1994;68:4628–4635.

27 Genis P, Jett M, Bernton EW, et al. Cytokines and arachidonic metabolites produced during human immunodeficiency virus (HIV)-infected macrophage-astroglia interactions: implications for the neuropathogenesis of HIV disease. *J Exp Med* 1992;176:1703–1718.

28 Pulliam L, Herndier BG, Tang NM, McGrath MS. Human immunodeficiency virus-infected macrophages produce soluble factors that cause histological and neurochemical alterations in cultured human brains. *J Clin Invest* 1991;87:503–512.

29 Giulian D, Vaca K, Noonan CA. Secretion of neurotoxins by mononuclear phagocytes infected with HIV-1. *Science* 1991;250:1593–1596.

30 Sabin FR. The origin and development of the lymphatic system. *Johns Hopkins Hosp Rep* 1916;17:347–440.

31 Rapoport SI. *Blood-brain barrier in physiology and medicine*. New York: Raven, 1976.

32 Sawada M, Kondo N, Suzumura A, Marunouchi T. Production of tumor necrosis factor-alpha by microglia and astrocytes in culture. *Brain Res* 1989;491:394–397.

33 Sebire G, Emilie D, Wallon C, et al. In vitro production of IL-6, IL-1β, and tumor necrosis factor-α by human embryonic microglial and neural cells. *J Immunol* 1993;150:1517–1523.

34 Chao CC, Hu S, Close K, et al. Cytokine release from microglia: differential inhibition by pentoxifylline and dexamethasone. *J Infect Dis* 1992;166:847–853.

35 Lee SC, Liu W, Dickson DW, et al. Cytokine production by human fetal microglia and astrocytes: differential induction by lipopolysaccharide and IL-1β. *J Immunol* 1993; 150:2659–2667.

36 Chao CC, Hu S, Sheng WS, Peterson PK. Tumor necrosis factor-alpha production by human fetal microglial cells: regulation by other cytokines. *Dev Neurosci* 1995;17:97–105.

37 Chung IY, Benveniste EN. Tumor necrosis factor-α production by astrocytes: induction by

lipopolysaccharide, IFN-γ, and IL-1β. *J Immunol* 1990;144:2999–3007.

38 Benveniste EN, Tang LP, Law RW. Differential regulation of astrocyte TNF-α expression by the cytokines TGF-β, IL-6 and IL-10. *Int J Dev Neurosci* 1995;13:341–349.

39 Vitkovic L, Chatham JJ, da Cunha A. Distinct expression of three cytokines by IL-1-stimulated astrocytes *in vitro* and in AIDS brain. *Brain Behav Immun* 1995;9:378–388.

40 Hart BL. Biological basis of the behavior of sick animals. *Neurosci Behav Rev* 1988;22:123–137.

41 Obal F Jr, Opp MR, Cady AB, et al. Interleukin 1α and an interleukin 1β fragment are somnogenic. *Am J Physiol* 1990;259:R439–R446.

42 Kapas L, Krueger JM. Tumor necrosis factor-beta induces sleep, fever and anorexia. *Am J Physiol* 1992;263:R703–R707.

43 Lee SC, Dickson DW, Liu W, Brosnan CF. Induction of nitric oxide synthase activity in human astrocytes by interleukin-1β and interferon-gamma. *J Neuroimmunol* 1993;46:19–24.

44 Peterson PK, Hu S, Anderson WR, Chao CC. Nitric oxide production and neurotoxicity mediated by activated microglia from human versus mouse brain. *J Infect Dis* 1994; 170:457–460.

45 Bukrinsky MI, Nottet HSLM, Schmidtmayerova H, et al. Regulation of nitric oxide synthase activity in human immunodeficiency virus type 1 (HIV-1)-infected monocytes: implications for HIV-associated neurologic disease. *J Exp Med* 1995;181:735–745.

46 Koka P, He K, Zack JA, et al. Human immunodeficiency virus 1 envelope proteins induce interleukin 1, tumor necrosis factor alpha, and nitric oxide in glial cultures from fetal, neonatal, and adult human brain. *J Exp Med* 1995;182:941–951.

47 Colasanti M, Persichini T, Di Pucchio T, et al. Human ramified microglial cells produce nitric oxide upon *Escherichia coli* lipopolysaccharide and tumor necrosis factor α stimulation. *Neurosci Lett* 1995;200:144–146.

48 Chao CC, Anderson WR, Hu S, et al. Activated microglia inhibit *Toxoplasma gondii* via a nitric oxide mechanism. *Clin Immunol Immunopathol* 1993;67:178–183.

49 Chao CC, Gekker G, Hu S, Peterson PK. Human microglial cell defense against *Toxoplasma gondii*: the role of cytokines. *J Immunol* 1994;152:1246–1252.

50 Peterson PK, Gekker G, Hu S, et al. CD14 receptor-mediated uptake of nonopsonized *Mycobacterium tuberculosis* by human microglia. *Infect Immun* 1995;63:1598–1602.

51 Dawson TM, Dawson VL, Snyder SH. A novel neuronal messenger molecule in brain: the free radical, nitric oxide. *Ann Neurol* 1992; 32:297–311.

52 Hu S, Sheng WS, Peterson PK, Chao CC. Differential regulation by cytokines of production of nitric oxide by human astrocytes. *Glia* 1995;15:491–494.

53 Lee SC, Dickson DW, Brosnan CF, Casadevall A. Human astrocytes inhibit *Cryptococcus neoformans* growth by a nitric oxide-mediated mechanism. *J Exp Med* 1994;180:365–369.

54 Peterson PK, Gekker G, Hu S, Chao CC. Human astrocytes inhibit intracellular multiplication of *Toxoplasma gondii* by a nitric oxide-mediated mechanism. *J Infect Dis* 1995; 171:516–518.

55 Chao CC, Hu S, Peterson PK. Glia, cytokines and neurotoxicity. *Crit Rev Neurobiol* 1995; 9:189–205.

56 Chao CC, Molitor TW, Hu S. Neuroprotective role of IL-4 against activated microglia. *J Immunol* 1993;151:1473–1481.

57 Chao CC, Hu S, Ehrlich L, Peterson PK. Interleukin-1 and tumor necrosis factor-α synergistically mediate neurotoxicity: involvement of nitric oxide and of N-methyl-D-aspartate receptors. *Brain Behav Immun* 1995;9:355–365.

58 Hu S, Peterson PK, Chao CC. Cytokine-mediated neuronal apoptosis. *Neurochem Int* 1997 (in press).

59 McLaurin J, D'Souza S, Stewart J, et al. Effect of tumor necrosis factor α and β on human oligodendrocytes and neurons in culture. *Int J Dev Neurosci* 1995;13:369–381.

60 Yeung MC, Pulliam L, Lau AS. The HIV envelope protein gp120 is toxic to human brain-cell cultures through the induction of interleukin-6 and tumor necrosis factor-α. *AIDS* 1995;9:137–143.

61 Toulmond S, Vige X, Fage D, Benavides J. Local infusion of interleukin-6 attenuates the neurotoxic effects of NMDA on rat striatal cholinergic neurons. *Neurosci Lett* 1992;144:49–52.

62 Hama T, Miyamoto M, Tsukui H, et al. Interleukin-6 as a neurotrophic factor for promoting the survival of cultured basal forebrain cholinergic neurons from postnatal rats. *Neurosci Lett* 1989;104:340–344.

63 Yamada M, Hatanaka H. Interleukin-6 protects cultured rat hippocampal neurons against glutamate-induced cell death. *Brain Res* 1994; 643:173–180.

64 Rodriguez M, Pavelko KD, McKinney CW, Leibowitz JL. Recombinant human IL-6 suppresses demyelination in a viral model of multiple sclerosis. *J Immunol* 1994;153:3811–3821.

65 Chao CC, Hu S. Tumor necrosis factor-α potentiates glutamate neurotoxicity in human fetal brain cell cultures. *Dev Neurosci* 1994; 16:172–179.

66 Cheng B, Christakos S, Mattson MP. Tumor necrosis factors protect neurons against metabolic-excitotoxic insults and promote maintenance of calcium homeostasis. *Neuron* 1994;12:139–153.

67 Barger SW, Horster D, Furukawa K, et al. Tumor necrosis factors alpha and beta protect neurons against amyloid beta-peptide toxicity: evidence for involvement of a kappa B-binding factor and attenuation of peroxide and Ca^{++} accumulation. *Proc Natl Acad Sci USA* 1995; 92:9328–9332.

68 Giulian D, Lachman LB. Interleukin-1 stimulation of astroglial proliferation after brain injury. *Science* 1985;228:497–500.

69 da Cunha A, Jefferson JJ, Tyor WR, et al. Control of astrogliosis by interleukin-1 and transforming growth factor-β1 in human brain. *Brain Res* 1993;631:39–45.

70 Chao CC, Hu S, Tsang M, et al. Effects of transforming growth factor-β on murine astrocyte glutamine synthetase activity: implications in neuronal injury. *J Clin Invest* 1992; 90:1786–1793.

71 Rosenberg PA, Aizenman E. Hundred-fold increase in neuronal vulnerability to glutamate toxicity in astrocyte-poor cultures of rat cerebral cortex. *Neurosci Lett* 1989;103:162–168.

72 Awatsuji H, Furukawa Y, Hirota M, et al. Interleukin-4 and -5 as modulators of nerve growth factor synthesis/secretion in astrocytes. *J Neurosci Res* 1993;34:539–545.

73 Vige X, Costa E, Wise BC. Mechanism of nerve growth factor mRNA regulation by interleukin-1 and basic fibroblast growth factor in primary cultures of rat astrocytes. *Mol Pharmacol* 1991;40:186–192.

74 Friedman WJ, Altiok N, Fredholm BB, Persson H. Mechanisms of nerve growth factor mRNA regulation by interleukin-1β in hippocampal cultures: role of second messengers. *J Neurosci Res* 1992;33:37–46.

75 Saporito MS, Wilcox HM, Hartpence KC, et al. Pharmacological induction of nerve growth factor mRNA in adult rat brain. *Exp Neurol* 1993;123:295–302.

76 Hefti F. Nerve growth factor promotes survival of septal cholinergic neurons after fimbrial transactions. *J Neurosci* 1986;6:2155–2162.

77 Brosnan CF, Battistini L, Raine CS, et al. Reactive nitrogen intermediates in human neuropathology: an overview. *Dev Neurosci* 1994; 170:457–460.

78 Lipton SA, Choi Y-B, Pan Z-H, et al. A redox-based mechanism for the neuroprotective and neurodestructive effects of nitric oxide and related nitroso-compounds. *Nature* 1993; 364:626–632.

79 Lipton SA, Rosenberg PA. Excitatory amino acids as a final pathway for neurologic disorders. *N Engl J Med* 1994;330:613–622.

80 Lipton SA. HIV-related neuronal injury: potential therapeutic intervention with calcium channel antagonists and NMDA antagonists. *Mol Neurobiol* 1994;8:181–196.

6

Targeting Bacteria to the Central Nervous System

AXEL RING
ELAINE I. TUOMANEN

Bacterial meningitis and encephalitis are caused by a select group of pathogens that gain access to central nervous tissues through the systemic blood circulation or an anatomically adjacent structure such as the paranasal sinuses or the tympanum. Central nervous system (CNS) invasion originating from contiguous tissue is frequently associated with a disruption of tissue continuity as observed with trauma, cholesteatoma, and liquorrhea. In contrast, targeting the CNS from the bloodstream is mechanistically complex and involves disrupting the unique protective screen termed the *blood-brain barrier* (BBB). Current knowledge about the pathogenesis of CNS infection caused by bloodborne organisms is sketchy.

Few bacterial species cause CNS infections and the underlying mechanisms of penetration across the BBB appear to be quite diverse. However, insight into the molecular mechanisms leading to CNS infection promises new avenues for innovative therapeutic approaches to attenuate these devastating infections. This chapter reviews how the major pathogens reach the BBB and the diverse routes used to cross this multilayered barrier. Techniques to further investigate the initial events in meningitis are outlined.

MECHANISMS OF TRAFFICKING TO THE LUMINAL SIDE OF THE BBB

Four major systemic pathogens regularly produce bacterial meningitis: *Escherichia coli* K1 in newborns, and *Streptococcus pneumoniae*, *Neisseria meningitidis*, and *Haemophilus influenzae* in children (1,2). These pathogens share several common attributes:

1 Interaction with the host is initiated by colonization of upper respiratory tract epithelia.

2 Following penetration of the mucosal barrier, the bacteria invade the blood and multiply to high densities despite host defense mechanisms. The chance of BBB traversal increases with the concentration of bacteria in the blood and the duration of bacteremia (3–6).

3 The bacteria attach to the luminal side of the BBB (either endothelial cells or choroid plexus

epithelium) using specific bacterial surface constituents. Binding of bacteria to these cells subsequently leads to either a) transcellular passage or b) paracellular passage. Passing between cells implies disruption of the tight junctions caused either by directly affecting the BBB cell or by indirectly affecting glial cells or basement membrane constituents.

Adhesins for Colonization and Initiation of Bacteremia

Adherence to eukaryotic cells occurs via a wide variety of bacterial surface molecules including fimbriae, pili, and outer membrane proteins in gram-negative bacteria and cell wall components and surface proteins in gram-positive bacteria. These molecules function to allow colonization of the nasopharyngeal epithelial cells, penetration of these cells, traversal of the extracellular matrix of the basement membrane, penetration through the endothelial cells, and establishment of bacteremia.

Neisseria meningitidis Attachment of encapsulated *Neisseria* bacteria to epithelial and endothelial cells largely depends on piliation (7). Pili undergo antigenic variation, being expressed as high- or low-adhesive variants differing in the amino acid composition of the basic pilus component pilin (8). Two pilus-associated proteins, PilC1 and PilC2, regulate pilus assembly (9). The regulation of piliation occurs at the level of DNA expression through a two-component sensor-regulator system, PilA/PilB. Environmental signals are transduced by PilA via phosphorylation of PilB, which in turn binds the promoter of the *pilC1* gene (8).

Although pili affect adherence, they are not involved in cell invasion. In capsule-deficient isolates, the outer membrane proteins Opc, OpaB, and OpaD mediate adherence to, as well as intracellular uptake into, epithelial cell lines. Opc alone plays a similar role in interaction with endothelia in vitro (10,11). Results of a recent study working with primary cultured nasopharyngeal cells suggest that invasiveness is conferred by a 28-kd Opa protein other than Opc (12). However, all findings indicate unanimously that capsular materials as well as the presence of sialylated lipopolysaccharide inhibit adhesive interactions with epithelial and endothelial cells mediated through all outer membrane proteins (10,12).

The complexity of binding capabilities indicates that switching of multiple phase-variable bacterial surface components is essential to the ability of N. *meningitidis* to first adhere to and subsequently invade an epithelial or endothelial barrier. A scenario for the invasive events has been postulated as follows: Carriers harbor both encapsulated and nonencapsulated bacteria. In this stage of infection, expression of high-adhesive pilin and PilC1 acting as an adhesin is advantageous for colonization of the upper respiratory tract. After this initial attachment, as yet unknown factors favor an increased expression of Opc and probably OpaB and OpaD, while the expression of capsule and pili is downregulated. The ability to subsequently cross the epithelial barrier requires the expression of the 28-kd Opa protein and OpaB. The role of Opc during this step may differ between epithelial cell lines and primary human nasopharyngeal cells (10–12). Once inside the cell, a new set of virulence factors must be produced to enable the bacterium to survive in this completely different environment. After the bacterium enters the bloodstream, the production of a capsule is again a vital necessity for the pathogen to evade opsonization and phagocytosis. The expression of low-adhesive pilin may now be an advantage to promote dissemination in the circulation. Sialylation of lipooligosaccharide leads to the generation of an epitope that mimics eukaryotic antigens, thus conferring an immunoresistant phenotype (13).

Haemophilius influenzae *H. influenzae* adheres primarily to nonciliated respiratory epithelial cells via pilus (or fimbrial) and nonpilus adhesins, including surface fibrils and outer membrane proteins (14–17). The presence of a capsule inhibits adherence and entry into epithelial cells (18). *H. influenzae* typically penetrates an epithelial monolayer in vitro by paracellular migration (16). Nevertheless, there is substantial evidence for invasion of epithelial cells by this pathogen, possibly mediated through several outer membrane proteins induced on adherence (16). A 110-kd protein called *Hap*, which shows significant homology to the *H. influenzae* serine-type IgA1 protease, mediates adherence to and invasion of epithelial cells (19). Evidence indicates that the *Haemophilus* bacterium also readily penetrates endothelial cells, an attribute required for completion of invasion from the mucosal surface to the bloodstream. Invasion of human umbilical vein endothelial cells in vitro occurs via a microfilament-dependent pathway. Electron micrographs show that the pathogen eventually passes by transcytosis to the basal plasmalemma within vacuoles (20). However, the contribution of the transcellular pathway to the pathogenesis of bloodstream invasion has yet to be established.

Streptococcus pneumoniae Binding of *S. pneumoniae* to the nasopharynx is affected by two interconvertible colonial phenotypes: opaque and transparent (21–23). Transparent variants effectively colonize the nasopharynx in the infant rat model whereas the opaque phenotype fails to persist on the mucosal surface. While both types of pneumococci can adhere to resting respiratory epithelial cells, the enhanced pathogenicity of the transparent phase variant may be related to its ability to bind additional cell surface determinants on activated human cells (23). At least five distinct adherence interactions between pneumococcal proteins and human glycoconjugates are known (22). Pneumococci do not display fimbriae or other surface adhesive appendages and the precise nature of the adhesins is still to be determined. However, many bacterial surface components that affect pneumococcal adherence have been identified. Cell wall components, particularly phosphorylcholine (24), affect adherence either by directly mediating attachment to human cells or by presenting proteins that are adhesive bridges. Surface proteins that modulate the function of the adhesins include the peptide permeases PlpA, AmiA, and AmiC (25). Binding to fibronectin plays a role in colonization and invasion of a mucosa already injured, thus exposing basement membrane components (26). Such injury can be promoted by several pneumococcal components, including pneumolysin.

The strategy employed by pneumococci to cross the mucosal epithelium into the bloodstream is still unclear. Pneumococci have been detected inside endothelial cells within a vacuolar compartment, suggesting a transcellular migration route leading to exit on the basolateral side. Initial attachments to endothelial and epithelial cells occurs via several glycoconjugate receptors on resting human cells (23,27). However, the triggering of transmigration seems to require activation of the endothelial cell by proinflammatory cytokines, which leads to the appearance of new ligands on the human cell surface. These endogenous molecules upregulated by cellular activation are normally involved in adhesion and recruitment of leukocytes to the site of infection. Pneumococci capitalize on this scenario and specifically target one of these new ligands, the receptor for platelet-activating factor (PAF) (22,28). Binding to the PAF receptor enhances internalization and PAF receptor antagonists block the progression from pneumonia to bacteremia in animal models.

Once the bacteria have entered the vascular system, they encounter an array of different host defense systems that they have to evade on their way to their next target, the BBB. The primary virulence determinant in the bloodstream is the polysaccharide capsule. There are 90 known capsular types, and the current 23-valent polysaccharide vaccine was designed to include the serotypes causing around 90% of the systemic infections in the United States (29).

Bacteria Associated with Infection of Brain Parenchyma

In contrast to bacterial meningitis, which is usually preceded by high-grade bacteremia, multifocal encephalitis is associated with a prolonged, low-grade bacteremia and entry of the pathogen into the CNS at numerous sites along the endothelial BBB. The causative agents include *Staphylococcus aureus, Listeria monocytogenes, Treponema pallidum, Borrelia burgdorferi, Rickettsia prowazekii,* several *Plasmodium* species, fungi, and bacteria causing subacute endocarditis, such as oral streptococci or enterococci. Involvement of the CNS in diseases caused by these pathogens is often a secondary complication occurring during later stages of the infection.

ANATOMY OF THE BBB AS SEEN BY BACTERIA

The BBB consists of the CNS microvessel endothelial cells and pericytes, the basement membrane, and the associated perivascular glia limitans, which in turn is made up by astrocytes and microglia (Fig 6-1) (30–32). In the highly localized area of the blood–cerebrospinal fluid (CSF) barrier, the epithelial cells of the choroid plexus are responsible for the barrier formation. Intercellular tight junctions and scarce pinocytic activity are responsible for the exclusion of large and small blood-borne solutes from the CNS. Thus, penetration of a sealed barrier is significantly different from penetration of the fenestrated endothelia of the peripheral vasculature. It is perhaps mechanistically more related to the events required to trespass an epithelial barrier. Thus, to compare and contrast the capabilities of bacteria to migrate across the BBB, we highlight its anatomy in relation to the major additional capabilities a pathogen must have to enter the CSF after it has penetrated the peripheral epithelial and endothelial barrier already described.

Intercellular Junction Complexes

One critical morphologic correlate of the BBB is the apically located, bipartite, intercellular junction complex that comprises the zonula occludens (tight junction) and the zonula adherens (Fig 6-2). This complex is formed by juxtaposed epithelial cells of the

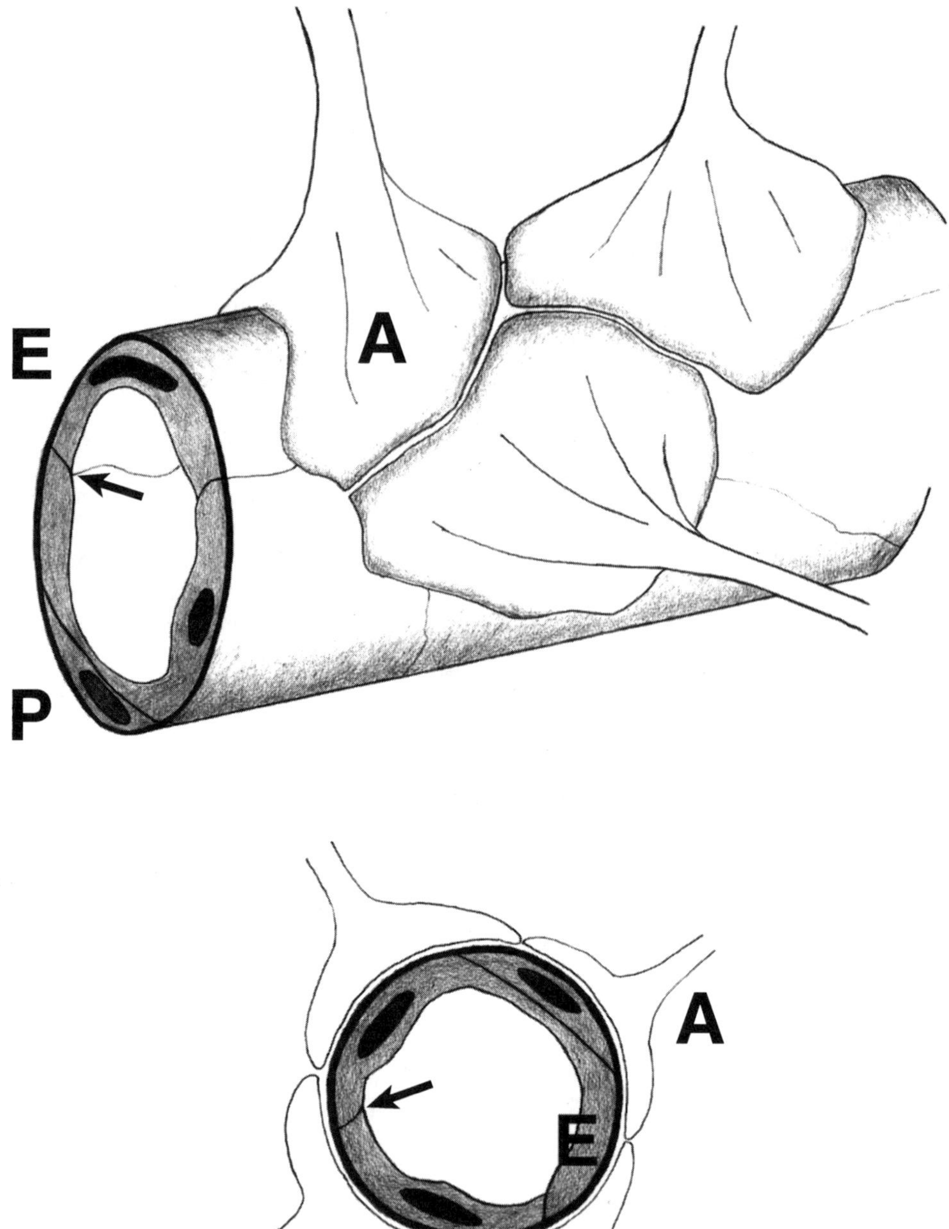

Figure 6-1. Schematic representation of the blood-brain barrier (BBB) anatomy in a three-dimensional and cross-sectional view. A = astrocyte; P = pericyte; E = endothelial cell. The arrows indicate the location of junctional complexes, shown in Figure 6-2.

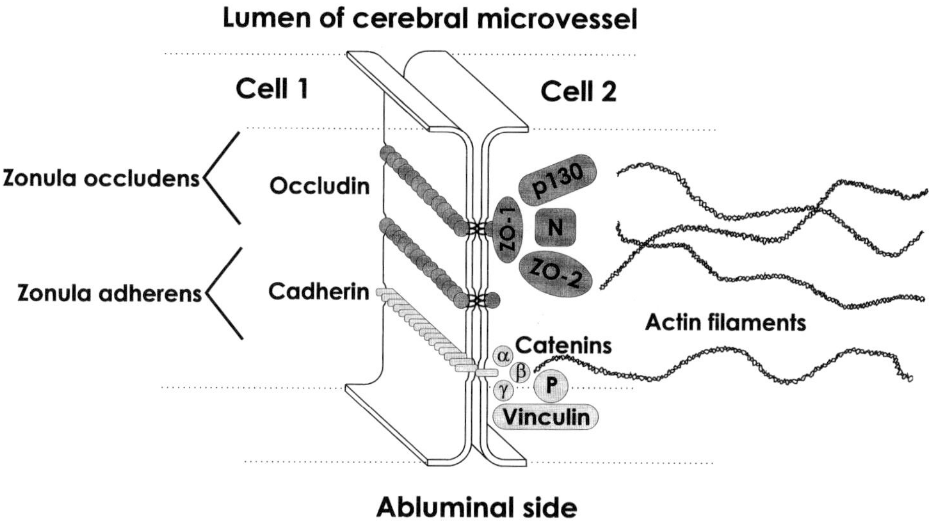

Figure 6-2. The junctional complex composed of the zonula occludens and zonula adherens. N = neurothelin; P = plakoglobin; ZO-1 and ZO-2 = zonula occludens proteins; α, β, and γ = catenins.

choroid plexus at the blood-CSF barrier and by cerebral capillary endothelial cells at the blood-parenchyma barrier (Fig 6-3). Bacteria entering at the blood-CSF interface end up in the ventricles, whereas transit across the more extensive capillary endothelium may lead to infection of the brain parenchyma (as in multifocal encephalitis) as well as the leptomeninx via pial microvessels.

In contrast to peripheral capillaries that by their fenestration act as molecular sieves permitting the passive paracellular passage of hydrophilic substances of a molecular weight lower than 40,000, the continuous seal of the BBB reliably prevents the entry even of small molecules into the CNS (33). Hydrophilic antibiotics such as penicillins and cephalosporins, widely used in the therapy of bacterial meningitis, penetrate into the CSF sufficiently to achieve bactericidal concentrations only after inflammation has disrupted the barrier (34). The electrical resistance that defines in vivo and in vitro the permeability to ions is about 80-fold higher in cerebral microvessels compared to their peripheral counterpart (35,36).

On a molecular level, a critical feature of the BBB tight junctions is that they are circumferential and not interrupted by gap junctions. Compared to the leaky endothelia of peripheral organs and the choroid plexus (37), the zonularity of the tight junction strands, rather than their absolute quantity, represents the unique feature of tight junctions in the brain (33). For this reason, disrupting even a minor portion of the tight junction strands forming the BBB has a large impact on its protective function and would, in principle, suffice to allow bacterial transit.

The molecular organization of tight junctions in the BBB is functionally tripartite, consisting of a transmembrane protein, occludin, that mediates the specific adhesive

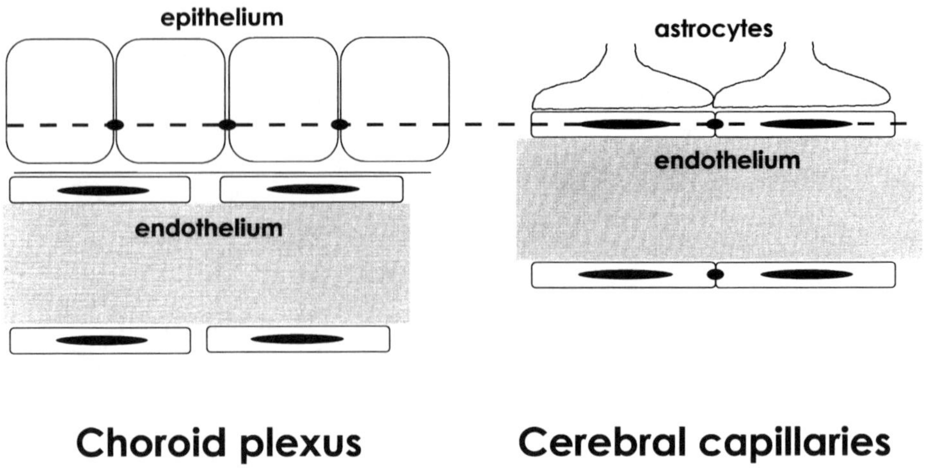

Figure 6-3. Level of the BBB at the blood–cerebrospinal fluid (left) as well as the blood-parenchyma (right) interface. Tight junctions are formed between epithelial cells and endothelial cells of the choroid plexus.

cell-cell contact. With its intracellular domain, it is bound to cytoplasmic plaque proteins including zonula occludens protein 1 (ZO-1) and ZO-2 (38,39), some of which are in turn anchored to cytoskeletal filamentous proteins (40). It has been suggested that dissociation of occludin from ZO-1 might be an early step occurring when the paracellular barrier is disrupted (e.g., induced by bacterial or host-derived molecules during CNS infection) (40). The sealing capacity of tight junctions is also modulated by phosphorylation of junctional components including ZO-1, ZO-2, and cingulin. Targeting of junctional components by bacterial proteins, for example, the interaction of ZO-1 with the elastase of *Pseudomonas* species, can readily alter BBB permeability, providing access from blood to the CNS.

Transcytosis Through the BBB: Pits, Vesicles, and Channels

Another ultrastructural characteristic of the BBB is the low number of pinocytotic vesicles and the high number of mitochondria providing energy to a wide range of specific carrier systems that transport substances like essential nutrients, proteins, metals, vitamins, and ions across the barrier. Macromolecules are assumed to be transported from the luminal (vascular) to the abluminal (brain) side but not vice versa (41). This vectorial carrier function of the BBB is similar to a polarized transporting epithelium (e.g., in the kidney) (41–43). This implies that the mechanisms used by bacteria to target polarized epithelia may be related to those operational while breaching the BBB.

Plasmalemmal pits and vesicles bring solutes into the endothelial cell either in a nonspecific fluid-associated way or in a selective membrane-associated manner. The latter mechanism can be further divided into two types. Adsorptive endocytosis follows electrostatic affiliation of a molecule, with the negatively charged glycocalyx on the surface of cerebral endothelial or plexus epithelial cells. Adsorptive endocytosis, particularly involving binding to sialic acid, N-acetylglucosamine, and other glycoconjugates on the human cell surface through the forces of electrical charge, is the mechanism whereby lectins and cationic ferritin are transported through the cell. Microbial lectins are known to be virulence factors involved in adhesion of a variety of bacteria to eukaryotic cells (44). In these cases, the possible role of adsorptive endocytosis for barrier penetration is yet to be established. Generally, cationization of any protein will enhance its uptake by brain capillaries and delivery through the BBB.

Alternatively, vesicular entry can be more specific when engineered by receptor-mediated endocytosis (33,45,46). Examples of this strategy are the binding of *S. pneumoniae* to the PAF receptor on activated endothelial cells (28) and of *Plasmodium falciparum* to intercellular adhesion molecule 1 (ICAM-1) (47). While fluid-phase macromolecules are eventually directed to endosomes and secondary lysosomes for degradation, molecules endocytosed through membrane-mediated events take transcytotic pathways (45). Insulin, transferrin, low-density lipoprotein (33), the cytokines interleukin (IL)-1α, IL-1β (48), tumor necrosis factor (TNF)-α (49), and IL-6 (50) as well as a broad range of small peptides (51) traverse the BBB via a carrier-mediated pathway following specific receptor binding on the membrane.

These vesicular pathways of transcytosis are physiologic and occur in the absence of BBB disruption. Even the proinflammatory cytokines, though associated with a loss of BBB function, are transported across the barrier without evidence of concomitant increased permeability (48,49). However, the increased BBB permeability engendered by an accumulation of cytokines can play an integral role in microbial passage to the CNS.

Maintenance of the BBB: Astrocytes, Microglia, and Extracellular Matrix Proteins

During the early postnatal phase, astrocytes become instrumental in inducing subsequent maturational changes in the endothelial cells, including further barrier tightening and the installation of specific transport systems (52). Graft experiments have confirmed the requirement of astrocyte participation in BBB induction during embryonic development as well as maintenance in the adult (53). The effect has been attributed to insoluble (54,55) as well as soluble astrocyte-derived factors (56,57). Cyclic adenosine monophosphate increases electrical resistance as well as the expression of BBB marker enzymes, while activators of protein kinase C downregulate tight junction expression (58,59).

Certain extracellular matrix proteins play an essential role in the process of maintaining BBB properties. The effect of contact coculture with astrocytes on the complexity of tight junctions can be mimicked by growth on extracellular matrix protein–coated plastic surfaces and the addition of astrocyte-conditioned medium (60). Growth on fibronectin-coated polycarbonate membranes alone can induce a 13-fold increase (compared to collagen-coated filters) of the transendothelial electrical resistance of bovine brain endothelial cell monolayers (Novak R, Ring A, unpublished data, 1995).

If tight junctions are functionally disturbed by astroglial dysfunction, pathogens could easily translocate into the CNS via a passive route. It has been suggested that *L. monocytogenes* can destroy astrocytes while engineering its passage into the CNS and thus favor BBB disruption (5).

MECHANISMS OF TRAFFICKING THROUGH THE BBB TO THE CNS

Based on the anatomic and physiologic aspects just outlined, there are several possible routes a pathogen can use to cross the BBB once it has made its way to the luminal side of the BBB. One of the major issues in the field of bacterial meningitis that is still unresolved is whether the initial site of entry into the CSF is the choroid plexus or the endothelial BBB. Both routes are conceivable, as the brain extracellular fluid is continuous with the CSF. However, pathologically there is no evidence for brain parenchymal involvement in the earliest stages of meningitis, suggesting a direct route into the CSF space. Several independent findings argue in favor of the choroid plexus as the primary entry site rather than the larger cerebral vessels situated in the subarachnoid space. The choroid plexus is a highly vascularized area equipped with fenestrated endothelial cells, and choroiditis is frequently observed with early meningitis (61). In experimental meningitis the concentration of bacteria in the CSF is the same as that in the ventricles and the lumbar region, even at the beginning of infection (62). Because the CSF flows unidirectionally away from the ventricles down to the lumbar region, the presence of bacteria in the ventricular CSF suggests entry at the level of the choroid plexus. *H. influenzae* is the only bacterium that has been shown to target directly the choroid plexus (63).

In Vitro BBB Models

The recent advances in our knowledge of the interactions of pathogens with the BBB have been made possible partly by the use of in vitro model systems. The availability of in vitro BBB models will play a crucial role in the molecular investigation of bacterial transmigration and the interaction of glial cells, endothelial cells, and bacterial components. These topics have been poorly addressed in the past, in part due to the fact that establishing native cerebral endothelial cell cultures is a time-consuming and complex procedure. Numerous protocols for the preparation of isolated brain microvessels or single endothelial cells from brain homogenates have been developed using human (64–67), porcine (68), bovine (65,69,70), and rat (68,71,72) endothelial cells. The minced tissue is digested with proteolytic enzymes and endothelial cells are purified on density gradients. Though several brain endothelial cell lines have been established (73,74), they do not currently represent an alternative to primary cultures because none of the cell lines express tight junctions with high electrical resistance.

In the two-chamber BBB model, a filter supports a cell monolayer that separates two liquid-filled chambers. The isolated brain microvessel endothelial cells are seeded on filters coated with extracellular matrix proteins (usually fibronectin or collagen) and cocultured with neonatal rat astrocytes or astrocyte-conditioned medium. After several days, the endothelia form monolayers and subsequently develop a high transendothelial electrical resistance characteristic of the BBB and indicative of effective barrier function. The rate of passage of larger macromolecules (e.g., dextran and horseradish peroxidase) can be determined to assess monolayer tightness. The presence of factor VIII and of γ-glutamyl transpeptidase and the uptake of low-density lipoprotein indicate the purity of the preparation.

The purification and cultivation of rat choroid plexus cells and their use in the two-chamber culture system have been described (75,76). An adaptation of this method including astrocyte coculture could prove useful for the investigation of initial bacterial entry into the CSF.

Animal Models

An alternative strategy to investigate microbial interactions with the BBB is to determine molecules of interest using polarized epithelial cells of non-CNS origin that are easily available (e.g., as cell lines) and that have been shown immunohistochemically to share many characteristics with BBB endothelial and plexus epithelial cells (42,77). The relevance for CNS diseases of molecules identified for translocation across epithelia in vitro is then tested in an in vivo animal model. The animal species most widely used for experimental bacterial meningitis models are rabbits and rats. Three types of experimental designs have been used. (1) The infant rat model addresses the transition from bacteremia to CSF infection. (2) The rabbit model uses direct inoculation of microbial products into the cisterna magna with subsequent analysis of CSF cytochemical parameters during the course of disease. (3) The studies of the effects of circulating microbial products on the loss of BBB function have predominantly involved rabbit models. For example, in one study, the intravenous injection of specific glycopeptides derived from the pneumococcal cell wall induced enhanced pinocytotic vesicle trafficking through cerebral endothelial cells (78). In a rat meningitis model, a significant and long-lasting increase of BBB permeability occurred in response to intracerebral bacterial collagenase (79).

Bacterial Molecules Interacting with BBB Constituents

Once at the luminal side of the BBB, the following mechanisms are conceivable for bacterial passage into the subarachnoid space (Fig 6-4):

1 Transcellular passage
   a Through the choroid plexus epithelium leading to the ventricular CSF space
   b Through the cerebral capillary endothelium leading to the brain parenchyma

2 Paracellular transit following disruption of intercellular junctions by
   a Direct effect on the tight junction
   b Compromising glial cell support functions
   c Compromising basal lamina support functions

3 Invasion within human cells during their diapedesis through the BBB

The transcellular route can be further divided into three different mechanisms: a) receptor-mediated uptake and possible release at the abluminal side of the cell (e.g.,

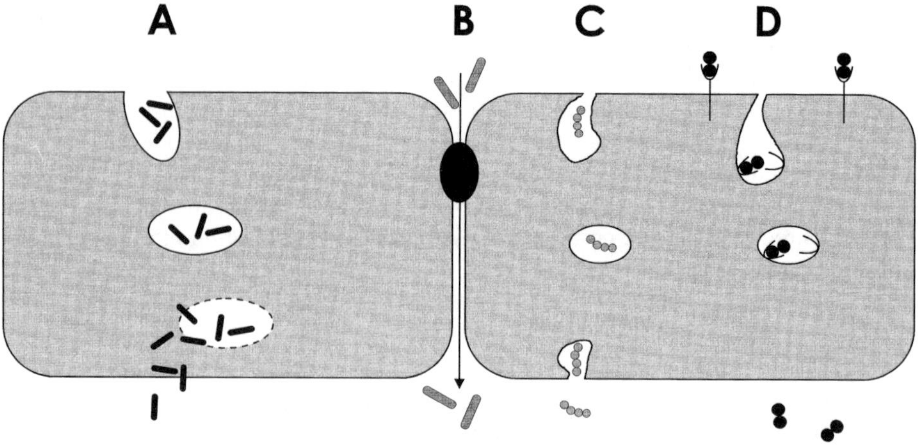

Figure 6-4. Possible routes of transmigration across the BBB. (A) Transcytosis engineered by a pathogen (e.g., *Listeria* species). (B) Paracellular passage (e.g., *Haemophilus influenzae).* (C) Transcellular vesicular transport following adsorptive endocytosis. (D) Receptor-mediated uptake (e.g., pneumococci or *Plasmodium* species).

malarial or pneumococcal organisms), b) enhancement of the normally insignificant pinocytic vesicle transit, and c) invasion engineered by the pathogen by vesicular transport involving endothelial as well as glial cells (e.g., *Listeria* species).

Several lines of evidence favor the choroid plexus as an entry site to the CNS for high-grade pathogens typically causing meningitis, yet the bacterial interactions with these cells remain a mystery. *H. influenzae* binds to ependymal cells and glial cells in a manner dependent on fimbriae (63). The precise molecular ligands remain to be determined.

In contrast to studies with choroid plexus cells, there are considerably more data available concerning the interaction of bacteria with brain endothelial cells. The bacteria that typically cause meningitis can invade peripheral endothelial cells. However, the application of this information to transit across the specialized endothelium of the BBB is still poorly studied. The most comprehensive understanding of the molecular events underlying the targeting of the BBB by bacteria has been gained from studies with *E. coli* capsule type K1 strains causing neonatal meningitis. The importance of the K1 capsule for the ability of *E. coli* to cross the BBB is well established (80). The adherence of *E. coli* to human as well as bovine brain endothelial cells is mediated in part through S-fimbriae (81,82). S-fimbriae display two types of tropism for brain endothelial cells. First, the fimbriae harbor a lectin, SfaS, which binds sialic acid α2-3 galactose on brain cells. In addition, an as yet undefined fimbrial component binds avidly to sulfated glycolipids that are enriched in brain endothelial cells. While S-fimbriae contribute to the tropism of *E. coli* K1 to the brain, binding via S-fimbriae is not accompanied by invasion (83,84). Results of several recent studies indicate that *E. coli* K1 strains capable of invading brain endothelial cells are located intracellularly within vacuoles and probably are then subsequently exocytosed at the basolateral side (83–85). Kim et al. showed that two surface proteins, outer membrane protein A (OmpA) and the 9-kd protein Ibe10, contribute to the invasion potential of *E. coli* K1 causing meningitis (83,84,86). Interestingly, the neurotropism of *E. coli* seems to be conferred partly by the interaction of OmpA with the epitope N-acetylglucosamine β1-4–*N*-acetylglucosamine that is freely accessible on brain endothelial cells but substituted with fucose on systemic endothelial cells (86).

For most other bacterial pathogens that cause meningitis, data on interactions with brain endothelial cells (in contrast to peripheral epithelia and endothelia) are scarce. For pneumococci, in addition to a possible PAF receptor–mediated transcellular pathway, there is evidence that a paracellular route can be opened by separation of tight junctions induced by secreted cell wall subcomponents. Isolated glycopeptides derived from the pneumococcal cell wall induce an enhanced permeability of the BBB in vivo (78). This is consistent with the ability of cell wall components from other bacteria to induce permeability of epithelial tight junctions, for instance, the activity of the cell wall–derived tracheal cytotoxin of *Bordetella pertussis*. In addition to reversible changes in permeability, cell wall components can also cause direct cytotoxicity to endothelial cells (24). Challenge of bovine or rat brain endothelial cells with *H. influenzae* or endotoxin results in a pronounced cytotoxic effect leading to BBB disruption, a phenomenon not seen with invasion of peripheral endothelial cells (20,87,88). The cytopathic effect of the lipid A part of lipopolysaccharide is well known; however, lipopolysaccharide-induced disruption of the brain endothelial monolayer can also occur in the absence of cell death (71). Meningococci adhere to and invade endothelial cells in a manner similar to that for epithelial cells, through their pili and outer membrane proteins as described earlier in this chapter. Pilus-dependent adherence but not Opc-dependent adherence is associated with increased cytotoxicity mediated by lipopolysaccharides. Whereas Opc seems to be directly responsible for endothelial cell invasion, pili act indirectly through binding to the cell surface and synergistically contributing to lipopolysaccharide-induced cell damage (10,11,87).

L. monocytogenes causes meningitis in the newborn period and in patients older than 65 years, suggesting that a compromised T cell–dependent immune status is involved. As a facultative intracellular pathogen, it is able to engineer its direct uptake into endothelial or plexus epithelial cells and subsequently spread to astrocytes, thus undermining the maintenance of the BBB. A second synergistic route involving translocation across the BBB within blood monocytes has been suggested (5).

In summary, all high-grade pathogens discussed here are capable of invading epithelial and endothelial cells, thus suggesting transcellular mechanisms for trafficking across the mucosal and blood-brain barrier. In addition, some of the species discussed can alternatively use a paracellular route mediated through cell injury and barrier disruption. This coordinate interplay of forces eventually favors uptake of a pathogen into the CSF space.

Transmigration Within Human Cells

Several pathogens can arrive at the BBB within human cells. Passage across the BBB within leukocytes has been suggested as a mechanism applied by *Listeria* species (5).

During experimental porcine meningitis, *Streptococcus suis* type 2 was found inside monocytes in the CSF (89). However, the pathophysiologic significance of CSF infection based on leukocyte-borne pathogens is questionable since the initial points of entry for bacteria versus leukocytes seem to be different. Results of histopathologic studies suggest that the earliest entry site for leukocytes is at the dorsal longitudinal sinus along the most superior aspect of the skull (90). Despite equivalent number of bacteria, the leukocyte concentration is significantly lower in the ventricular region than in the lumbar region. This discordance suggests that bacteria entering the CSF in the choroid plexus area translocate independently of leukocytes entering via the dorsal sinuses (62).

Of considerable interest is the ability of malarial parasites to cause cerebral infestation by sequestration of infected erythrocytes in cerebral microvessels. Intracellular parasites modify the surface of the erythrocyte to produce knobs that are highly adhesive for activated endothelial cells (91). The receptors on the BBB that are recognized by the knobs appear on activation of the BBB by cytokines (especially TNF) and include thrombospondin, E-selectin, CD36, ICAM-1, and vascular cell adhesion molecule 1 (VCAM-1). The binding leads to a lining up of maturing parasitized erythrocytes along cerebral capillaries and venules. This may occlude blood flow, particularly if uninfected erythrocytes are recruited into the rosettes. Thus, the parasite never formally invades the endothelial cells of the BBB but induces severe CNS symptoms by specific induction of a unique targeting of a host cell to the brain microvasculature. The nature of the malarial proteins that meditate these changes remains unknown.

CONCLUSIONS AND PROSPECTIVES

The BBB is a complex structure formed by cerebral capillary endothelium and choroid plexus epithelium, as well as associated cell types. As far as its "barrier and carrier" function, the BBB is substantially similar to polarizing transporting epithelia. The analogy to epithelia also appears to be relevant to the obstacles the BBB presents to bacterial transit. Our current knowledge of the molecular processes occurring when bacteria penetrate the barrier is still fragmentary. Recently identified surface components of meningococci, *E. coli*, *H. influenzae*, and pneumococci which promote invasion of host cells will be further evaluated for their relevance to entry into the CSF space, using in vitro and in vivo models of CNS disease. This information will potentially aid in developing new strategies to prevent bacterial access to the brain.

REFERENCES

1 Spellerberg B, Tuomanen EI. The pathophysiology of pneumococcal meningitis. *Ann Med* 1994;26:411–418.

2 Stephens DS, Farley MM. Pathogenic events during infection of the human nasopharynx with *Neisseria meningitidis* and *Haemophilus influenzae*. *Rev Infect Dis* 1991;13:22–33.

3 Tuomanen EI. Entry of pathogens into the central nervous system. *FEMS Microbiol Rev* 1997;18:289–299.

4 Townsend GC, Scheld WM. Microbe-endothelium interactions in blood-brain barrier permeability during bacterial meningitis. *ASM News* 1995;61:294–298.

5 Berche P. Bacteremia is required for invasion of the murine central nervous system by *Listeria monocytogenes*. *Microb Pathog* 1995; 18:323–336.

6 Scolea L, Rosales S, Welliver R, Ogra P. Mechanisms underlying the development of meningitis or epiglottitis in children after *Haemophilus influenzae* type b bacteremia. *J Infect Dis* 1985;151:1162–1165.

7 Virji M, Alexanrescu C, Ferguson DJP, et al. Variations in the expression of pili: the effect on adherence of *Neisseria meningitidis* to human epithelial and endothelial cells. *Mol Microbiol* 1992;6:1271–1279.

8 Nassif X, So M. Interaction of pathogenic *Neisseriae* with nonphagocytic cells. *Clin Microbiol Rev* 1995;8:376–388.

9 Nassif X, Beretti JL, Lowy J, et al. Roles of pilin and PilC in adhesion of *Neisseria meningitidis* to human epithelial and endothelial cells. *Proc Natl Acad Sci USA* 1994;91:3769–3773.

10 Virji M, Makepeace K, Ferguson DJP, et al. Meningococcal Opa and Opc proteins: their role in colonization and invasion of human epithelial and endothelial cells. *Mol Microbiol* 1993;10:499–510.

11 Virji M, Makepeace K, Ferguson DJP, et al. Expression of the Opc protein correlates with invasion of epithelial and endothelial cells by *Neisseria meningitidis*. *Mol Microbiol* 1992; 6:2785–2795.

12 De Vries FP, van der Ende A, van Putten JPM, Dankert J. Invasion of primary nasopharyngeal epithelial cells by *Neisseria meningitidis* is controlled by phase variation of multiple surface antigens. *Infect Immun* 1996;64:2998–3006.

13 Mandrell RE, Griffis JM, Macher BA. Lipooligosaccharides (LOS) of *Neisseria gonorrhoeae* and *Neisseria meningitidis* have components that are immunochemically similar to precursors of human blood group antigens. *J Exp Med* 1988;168:107–126.

14 Farley MM, Stephens DS, Mulks MH, et al. Pathogenesis of IgA1 protease-producing and -nonproducing *Haemophilus influenzae* in human nasopharyngeal organ cultures. *J Infect Dis* 1986;154:752–759.

15 Stephens DS, Hoffman LH, McGee ZA. Interaction of *Neisseria meningitidis* with human nasopharyngeal mucosa: attachment and entry into columnar epithelial cells. *J Infect Dis* 1983;148:369–376.

16 Geme JWS, Falkow S. *Haemophilus influenzae* adheres to and enters cultured human epithelial cells. *Infect Immun* 1990;58:4036–4044.

17 Geme JWS, Cutter D. Evidence that surface fibrils expressed by *Haemophilus influenzae* type b promote attachment to human epithelial cells. *Mol Microbiol* 1995;15:77–85.

18 Geme JWS, Falkow S. Loss of capsule expression by *Haemophilus influenzae* type b results in enhanced adherence to and invasion of human cells. *Infect Immun* 1991;59:1325–1333.

19 Geme JWS, De la Morena ML, Falkow S. A *Haemophilus influenzae* IgA-protease-like protein promotes intimate interaction with human epithelial cells. *Mol Microbiol* 1994; 14:217–233.

20 Virji M, Käyhty H, Ferguson DJP, et al. Interactions of *Haemophilus influenzae* with human endothelial cells in vitro. *J Infect Dis* 1992;165(suppl 1):S115–S116.

21 Tuomanen EI, Austrian R, Masure HR. Pathogenesis of pneumococcal infection. *N Engl J Med* 1995;332:1280–1284.

22 Cundell DR, Masure HR, Tuomanen EI. The molecular basis of pneumococcal infection: a hypothesis. *Clin Infect Dis* 1995;21(suppl 3): S204–S212.

23 Cundell DR, Weiser JN, Shen J, et al. Relationship between colonial morphology and adherence of *Streptococcus pneumoniae*. *Infect Immun* 1995;63:757–761.

24 Geelen S, Battacharyya C, Tuomanen EI. The cell wall mediates pneumococcal attachment and cytopathology to human endothelial cells. *Infect Immun* 1993;61:1538–1543.

25 Cundell DR, Pearce BJ, Sandros J, et al. Peptide permeases from *Streptococcus pneumoniae* affect adherence to eukaryotic cells. *Infect Immun* 1995;63:2493–2498.

26 Van der Flier M, Chhun N, Wizemann TM, et al. Adherence of *Streptococcus pneumoniae* to immobilized fibronectin. *Infect Immun* 1995; 63:4317–4322.

27 Cundell DR, Tuomanen EI. Receptor specificity of adherence of *Streptococcus pneumoniae* to human type-II pneumocytes and vascular endothelial cells in vitro. *Microb Pathog* 1994; 17:361–374.

28 Cundell DR, Gerard NP, Gerard C, et al. *Streptococcus pneumoniae* anchor to activated human cells by the receptor for platelet-activating factor. *Nature* 1995;377:435–438.

29 Shapiro DE, Austrian R. Serotypes responsible for invasive *Streptococcus pneumoniae* infections among children in Connecticut. *J Infect Dis* 1994;169:212–214.

30 Janzer RC. The blood-brain barrier: a cellular basis. *J Inherit Metab Dis* 1993;16:639–647.

31 Pardridge WM. *The blood-brain barrier: cellular and molecular biology*, vol. 1. New York: Raven, 1993.

32 Lassmann H, Zimprich F, Vass K, Hickey WF. Microglial cells are a component of the perivascular glia limitans. *J Neurosci Res* 1991; 28:236–243.

33 Brightman MW. The anatomic basis of the blood-brain barrier. In: Neuwelt EA, ed. *Implications of the blood-brain barrier and its manipulation*, vol. 1. *Basic science aspects.* New York: Plenum Medical Book, 1989:53–83.

34 Strausbaugh LJ. Meningitis, antimicrobial agents and the blood-brain barrier. In: Neuwelt EA, ed. *Implications of the blood-brain barrier and its manipulation,* vol. 2. *Clinical aspects.* New York: Plenum Medical Book, 1989;411–447.

35 Crone C, Olesen SP. Electrical resistance of brain microvascular endothelium. *Brain Res* 1982;241:49–55.

36 Olesen SP, Crone C. Electrical resistance of muscle capillary endothelium. *Biophys J* 1983; 42:31–41.

37 Zeuthen T, Wright EM. Epithelial potassium transport: tracer and electrophysiological studies in choroid plexus. *J Memb Biol* 1981; 60:105–128.

38 Stevenson B, Siliciano J, Mooseker M, Goodenough D. Identification of ZO-1: a high molecular weight polypeptide associated with the tight junction in a variety of epithelia. *J Cell Biol* 1986;103:755–766.

39 Jesaitis L, Da G. Molecular characterization and tissue distribution of ZO-2, a tight junction protein homologous to ZO-1 and the Drosophila discs-large tumor suppressor protein. *J Cell Biol* 1994;124:949–961.

40 Anderson JM, van Itallie CM. Tight junctions and the molecular basis for regulation of paracellular permeability. *Am J Physiol* 1995; 269:G467–G475.

41 Brown D, Stow JL. Protein trafficking and polarity in kidney epithelium: from cell biology to physiology. *Physiol Rev* 1996;76:245–297.

42 Dermietzel R, Krause D. Molecular anatomy of the blood-brain barrier as defined by immunocytochemistry. *Int Rev Cytol* 1991;127:57–109.

43 Broadwell RD. Endothelial cell biology and the enigma of transcytosis through the blood-brain barrier. In: Drewes LR, Betz AL, eds. *Frontiers in cerebral vascular biology: transport and its regulation.* New York: Plenum, 1993:137–141.

44 Patti JM, Allen BL, McGalvin MJ, Höök M. MSCRAMM-mediated adherence of microorganisms to host tissues. *Annu Rev Microbiol* 1994;48:585–617.

45 Broadwell RD. Transcytosis of macromolecules through the blood-brain barrier: a cell biological perspective and critical appraisal. *Acta Neuropathol (Berl)* 1989;79:117–128.

46 Joó F. A new generation of model systems to study the blood-brain barrier: the in vitro approach. *Acta Physiol Hung* 1993;81:207–218.

47 Turner GD, Morrison H, Jones M, et al. An immunohistochemical study of the pathology of fatal malaria. Evidence for widespread endothelial activation and a potential role for intercellular adhesion molecule-1 in cerebral sequestration. *Am J Pathol* 1994;145:1057–1069.

48 Banks WA, Ortiz L, Plotkin SR, Kastin AJ. Human interleukin (IL) 1α, murine IL-1α and murine IL-1β are transported from blood to brain in the mouse by a shared saturable mechanism. *J Pharmacol Exp Ther* 1991;159:988–996.

49 Gutierrez EG, Banks WA, Kastin AJ. Murine tumor necrosis factor alpha is transported from blood to brain in the mouse. *J. Neuroimmunol* 1993;47:169–176.

50 Banks WA, Kastin AJ, Gutierrez EG. Penetration of interleukin-6 across the murine blood-brain barrier. *Neurosci Lett* 1994;179:53–56.

51 Banks WA, Kastin AJ. Saturable transport of peptides across the blood-brain barrier. *Life Sci* 1987;41:1319–1338.

52 Farrel CL, Risau W. Normal and abnormal development of the blood-brain barrier. *Microsc Res Tech* 1994;27:495–506.

53 Abbott NJ, Revest PA, Romero IA. Astrocyte-endothelial interaction: physiology and pathology. *Neuropathol Appl Neurobiol* 1992;18:424–433.

54 Tao-Cheng JH, Nagy Z, Brightman MW. Tight junctions of brain endothelium in vitro are enhanced by astroglia. *J Neurosci* 1987; 7:3293–3299.

55 Bauer HC, Tontsch U, Amberger A, Bauer H. Gamma-glutamyltranspeptidase and Na^+-K^+-ATPase activities in different subpopulations of cloned cerebral epithelial cells: responses to glial stimulation. *Biochem Biophys Res Commun* 1990;168:358–363.

56 Raub TJ, Kuentzel SL, Sawada GA. Permeability of bovine brain microvessel endothelial cells in vitro: barrier tightening by a factor released from astroglioma cells. *Exp Cell Res* 1992; 199:330–340.

57 Dehouck MP, Meresse S, Delorme P, et al. An easier, reproducible and mass-production method to study the blood-brain barrier in vitro. *J Neurochem* 1990;54:1798–1801.

58 Wolburg H, Neuhaus J, Kniesel U, et al. Modulation of tight junction structure in blood-brain barrier endothelial cells. Effects of tissue culture, second messengers and cocultured astrocytes. *J Cell Sci* 1994;107:1347–1357.

59 Beuckmann C, Hellwig S, Galla HJ. Induction of the blood-brain barrier-associated enzyme alkaline phosphatase in endothelial cells from

cerebral capillaries is mediated via cAMP. *Eur J Biochem* 1995;229:641–644.

60 Arthur FE, Shivers RR, Bowman PD. Astrocyte-mediated induction of tight junctions in brain capillary endothelium: an efficient in vitro model. *Dev Brain Res* 1987;36:155–159.

61 Prats N, Briones V, Blanco MM, et al. Choroiditis and meningitis in experimental murine infection with *Listeria monocytogenes*. *Eur J Clin Microbiol Infect Dis* 1992;11:744–747.

62 Daum R, Scheifele D, Syriopoulou V, et al. Ventricular involvement in experimental *Haemophilus influenzae* meningitis. *J. Pediatr* 1978; 93:927–930.

63 Sterk L, van Alphen L, Geelen-van der Broek L, et al. Differential binding of *Haemophilus influenzae* to human tissues by fimbriae. *J Med Microbiol* 1991;35:129–138.

64 Biegel D, Spencer DD, Patcher JS. Isolation and culture of human microvessel endothelial cells for the study of blood-brain barrier properties in vitro. *Brain Res* 1995;692:183–189.

65 Rubin L, Hall D, Porter S, et al. A cell culture model of the blood-brain barrier. *J Cell Biol* 1991;115:1725–1735.

66 Gerhart DZ, Broderius MA, Drewes LR. Cultured human and canine endothelial cells from brain microvessels. *Brain Res Bull* 1988; 21:785–793.

67 Spatz M, Bacic F, McCarron RM, et al. Cholinergic and histaminergic receptors in cultured endothelium derived from human cerebral microvessels. In: Seylaz J, MacKenzie ET, eds. *Neurotransmission and cerebrovascular function I*. New York: Elsevier Science, 1989:105–108.

68 Krause D, Mischek U, Galla HJ, Dermietzel R. Correlation of zonula occludens ZO-1 antigen expression and transendothelial resistance in porcine and rat cultured cerebral endothelial cells. *Neurosci Lett* 1991;128:301–304.

69 Meresse S, Dehouck MP, Delorme P, et al. Bovine brain endothelial cells express tight junctions and monoamine oxidase activity in long-term culture. *J Neurochem* 1989; 53:1363–1371.

70 Van Bree JB, de Boer AG, Danhof M, et al. Characterization of an in vitro blood-brain barrier. Effects of molecular size and lipophilicity on cerebrovascular endothelial transport rates of drugs. *J Pharmacol Exp Ther* 1988; 247:1233–1239.

71 Tunkel AR, Rosser SW, Hansen EJ, Scheld WM. Blood-brain barrier alterations in bacterial meningitis: development of an in vitro model and observations on the effects of lipopolysaccharide. *In Vitro Cell Dev Biol Anim* 1991; 27:113–120.

72 Abbott NJ, Hughes CC, Revest PA, Greenwood J. Development and characterisation of a rat brain capillary endothelial culture: towards an in vitro blood-brain barrier. *J Cell Sci* 1992; 103:23–37.

73 Juillerat-Jeanneret L, Aguzzi A, Wiestler OD, et al. Dexamethasone selectively regulates the activity of enzymatic markers of cerebral endothelial cell lines. *In Vitro Cell Dev Biol Anim* 1992;28:537–543.

74 Lechardeur D, Schwartz B, Paulin D, Scherman D. Induction of blood-brain barrier differentiation in a rat brain-derived endothelial cell line. *Exp Cell Res* 1995;220:161–170.

75 Crook RB, Kasagami H, Prusiner SB. Culture and characterization of epithelial cells from bovine choroid plexus. *J Neurochem* 1981; 37:845–854.

76 Southwell BR, Duan W, Alcorn D, et al. Thyroxine transport to the brain: role of protein synthesis by the choroid plexus. *Endocrinology* 1993;133:2116–2126.

77 Raub TJ, Sawada GA, Kuentzel SL. Expression of a widely distributed, novel sulfated membrane glycoprotein by bovine endothelia and certain transporting epithelia. *J Histochem Cytochem* 1994;42:1237–1250.

78 Spellerberg B, Prasad S, Cabellos C, et al. Penetration of the blood-brain barrier: enhancement of drug delivery and imaging by bacterial glycopeptides. *J Exp Med* 1995;182:1037–1043.

79 Rosenberg GA, Estrada E, Kelley R, Kornfeld M. Bacterial collagenase disrupts extracellular matrix and opens blood-brain barrier in rat. *Neurosci Lett* 1993;160:117–119.

80 Kim KS, Itabashi H, Gemski P, et al. The K1 capsule is the critical determinant in the development of *E. coli* meningitis in the rat. *J Clin Invest* 1992;90:897–905.

81 Stins MF, Prasadarao NV, Ibric L, et al. Binding characteristics of S fimbriated *Escherichia coli* to isolated brain microvascular endothelial cells. *Am J Pathol* 1994;145:1228–1236.

82 Prasadarao NV, Wass CA, Hacker J. Adhesion of S-fimbriated *Escherichia coli* to brain glycolipids mediated by sfaA gene-encoded protein of S-fimbriae. *J Biol Chem* 1993; 268:10356–10363.

83 Prasadarao NV, Wass CA, Weiser JN, et al. Outer membrane protein A of *Escherichia coli* contributes to invasion of brain microvascular endothelial cells. *Infect Immun* 1996;64:146–153.

84 Huang S, Wass CA, Fu Q, et al. *Escherichia coli* invasion of brain microvascular endothelial cells in vitro and in vivo: molecular cloning and characterization of invasion gene ibe10. *Infect Immun* 1995;63:4470–4475.

85 Meier C, Oelschlaeger TA, Merkert H, et al. Ability of *Escherichia coli* isolates that cause meningitis in newborns to invade epithelial and endothelial cells. *Infect Immun* 1996; 64:2391–2399.

86 Prasadarao NV, Wass CA, Kim KS. Endothelial cell GlcNAcb1-4GlcNAc epitopes for outer membrane protein A enhance traversal of *Escherichia coli* across the blood-brain barrier. *Infect Immun* 1996;64:154–160.

87 Dunn KL, Virji M, Moxon ER. Investigations into the molecular basis of meningococcal toxicity for human endothelial and epithelial cells: the synergistic effect of LPS and pili. *Microb Pathog* 1995;18:81–96.

88 Patrick D, Betts J, Frey E, et al. *Haemophilus influenzae* lipopolysaccharide disrupts confluent monolayers of bovine brain endothelial cells via a serum-dependent cytotoxic pathway. *J Infect Dis* 1992;165:865–872.

89 Williams A, Blakemore W. Pathogenesis of meningitis caused by *Streptococcus suis* type 2. *J Infect Dis* 1990;162:474–481.

90 Moxon E, Smith A, Averill D, Smith D. *Haemophilus influenzae* meningitis in infant rats after intranasal inoculation. *J Infect Dis* 1974;129:154–159.

91 Miller LH, Good MF, Milon G. Malaria pathogenesis. *Science* 1994;264:1817–1992.

7

Contribution of Cytokines to Meningeal Inflammation in Bacterial Meningitis

GEORGE H. MCCRACKEN, JR.
XAVIER SÁEZ-LLORENS

Before the advent of antimicrobial therapy, bacterial meningitis was a disease with an almost uniformly fatal outcome. As a result of the introduction of some antibiotics (sulfa agents, penicillin, and chloramphenicol) and of better intensive care techniques, the prognosis of affected patients improved considerably. Subsequently, a worldwide effort was placed on the development of more potent antimicrobial agents and on the sophistication of supportive therapy, with the aim of maximizing successful outcome of this disease. Long-term sequelae and case-fatality rates, however, did not decrease appreciably (1). Thus, in the 1980s it became clear that in addition to promptly eradicating the bacterial pathogen causing meningitis, other therapeutic strategies had to be implemented to achieve significant improvements (2,3). Greater understanding of the basic molecular mechanisms responsible for meningeal inflammation has provided new therapeutic horizons for the treatment of this life-threatening disease.

The inflammatory response has evolved as a means for the host to fight foreign molecules. In infectious processes, inflammation ensues when the immune system recognizes as intruders certain microbial components, such as endotoxins and lipopolysaccharides from gram-negative bacteria and lipoteichoic acids/peptidoglycan fragments from gram-positive organisms. This host reaction is initially mediated by the synthesis of cytokines, which are low-molecular-weight glycoproteins that act systemically (e.g., sepsis) or locally (e.g., meningitis, arthritis, otitis) to produce inflammation (4). At low concentrations, cytokines are believed to play an important protective role in the control of bacterial replication and distant tissue seeding. Concentrations above individual threshold levels, however, can induce overwhelming activation of immune pathways, leading to irreversible cellular damage or death (5).

In this chapter, we describe the molecular pathophysiology of bacterial meningitis based on current concepts, the evidence supporting the participation of several cytokines in the genesis of meningeal inflammation, and the emerging therapeutic implications prompted by an increasing understanding of these molecular mechanisms.

CURRENT CONCEPTS ON PATHOGENESIS AND PATHOPHYSIOLOGY

For a microorganism to cause meningitis, it first has to colonize the host nasopharyngeal mucosa. Beyond the neonatal period, colonization rates vary from 5% to 30% for the most common meningeal pathogens—*Haemophilus influenzae* type b (Hib), *Streptococcus pneumoniae* (pneumococcus), and *Neisseria meningitidis* (meningococcus)—at any given time. To advance successfully beyond this initial pathogenetic step, these bacteria must evade the activity of secretory IgA, avoid the clearance properties of ciliated epithelial cells, adhere to nonciliated epithelium through specific bacterial surface structures and host cell ligands, traverse the epithelium via intracellular or intercellular routes, and invade the submucosa. It is believed that certain respiratory viruses can help bacterial agents to circumvent these host mucosal defenses and facilitate their passage into the intravascular compartment (6,7).

Figure 7-1 presents the putative pathophysiologic steps necessary for a host to develop bacterial meningitis. Once within the bloodstream, bacteria must escape immune surveillance that is mediated initially by the classic and alternative complement pathways. The former requires specific antibodies, which are absent or minimal in some individuals (especially young infants), whereas the effects of the latter can be reduced by the presence of bacterial capsular polysaccharides that inhibit the activity of phagocytes. As microorganisms replicate unchecked and surpass a threshold inoculum, they can seed several distant tissues, including the central nervous system (CNS). The mechanisms by which bacteria gain access to the subarachnoid space are largely unknown. It is believed that the choroid plexus, a site with a rich blood supply and partially devoid of a strict blood-brain barrier (BBB), allows effective penetration of meningeal pathogens into the CNS (8). Whether these organisms utilize specific structures to attach to and traverse cerebral epithelium or enter the choroid plexus inside leukocytes that have been attracted to the site of endothelial injury is still uncertain. Once bacteria reach the cerebrospinal fluid (CSF), they are likely to survive because humoral defenses (immunoglobulin and complement activity) appear to be absent (9). This step heralds the onset of the meningeal host inflammatory response, which eventually manifests as clinical meningitis.

Induction of meningeal inflammation is triggered by the exposure of several cells (i.e., astrocytes, microglia, endothelial cells, leukocytes) to toxic bacterial products released on bacterial replication and death, leading to the synthesis of cytokines and other proinflammatory substances (10). In some instances, initial antimicrobial treatment produces an explosive release of bacterial components, transiently exacerbating this inflammatory response (11). Prominent among these cytokines are tumor necrosis factor (TNF) and interleukin (IL)-1, which are believed to initiate, independently and synergistically, the inflammatory cascade (12). Once these proximal glycopeptides are produced, many secondary mediators such as IL-6, IL-8, platelet-activating factor (PAF), prostaglandins, nitric oxide, and granulocyte-macrophage colony-stimulating factors amplify the pathophysiologic events. The net result is expression of adhesion receptors on endothelial and leukocyte surfaces (receptors of the selectin family required for leukocyte rolling and margination and of the integrin family necessary for firm leukocyte adhesion and transmigration through endothelial barriers), vascular injury, and increased permeability of the BBB (13,14). As a result of the endothelial damage, many

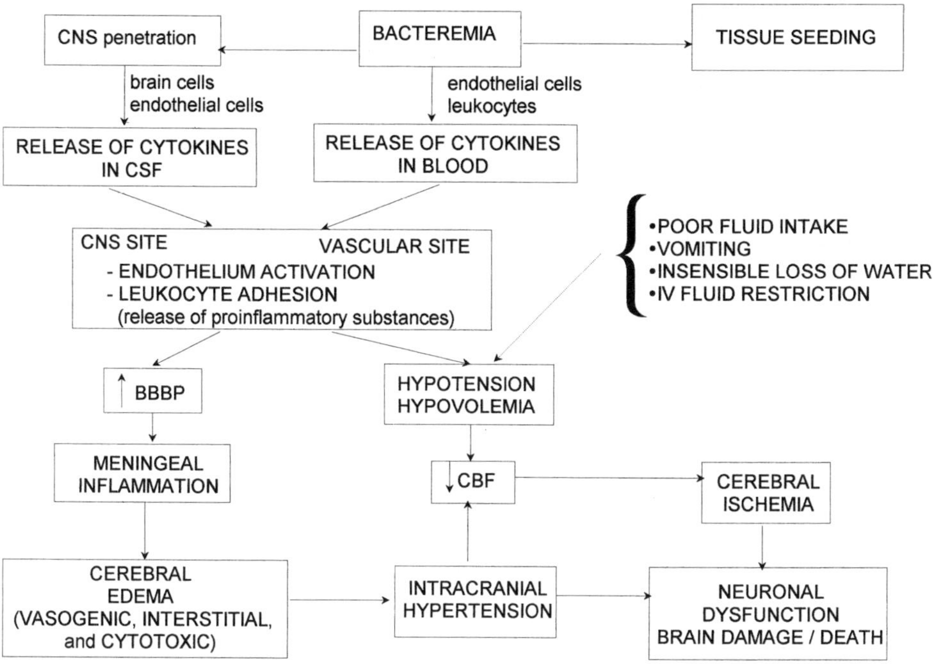

Figure 7-1. Hypothetical pathophysiology of bacterial meningitis. CNS = central nervous system; CSF = cerebrospinal fluid; BBBP = blood-brain barrier permeability; CBF = cerebral blood flow; IV = intravenous.

plasma components traverse freely into the subarachnoid space, contributing to vasogenic edema and to the characteristic pleocytosis and elevated protein concentration detected in the CSF of patients with meningitis. The increased CSF viscosity causes outflow resistance and interstitial edema. Toxicity to cerebral cells induced by several products released by bacteria, neutrophils, and other cellular lineages generates cytotoxic edema. Cerebral edema contributes to the intracranial hypertension seen in most patients with meningitis. The latter causes mechanical obliteration of cerebral vessels that interferes with blood supply. Cerebral blood flow is also reduced by the development of thrombotic phenomena, possibly mediated in part by PAF, and by hypotensive episodes promoted by poor hemodynamic control and restriction of fluids. As a consequence of impaired blood oxygen delivery, anaerobic metabolism ensues and contributes to decreased glucose and increased lactate concentrations in the CSF. Ultimately, if all these events are not modulated promptly and effectively, neuronal dysfunction occurs and can result in transient or permanent brain damage or death.

EVIDENCE SUPPORTING PARTICIPATION OF CYTOKINES

Two preliminary observations supported the hypothesis that common endogenous host inflammatory mediators are instrumental in the development of meningitis. First, diverse stimuli (live microorganisms, cell wall components, and lipopolysaccharide) injected intracisternally in animals elicited a similar pattern of meningeal inflammation. Second, there was a 2- to 3-hour delay from the time of inoculation of bacterial cells or their products into the subarachnoid space to the onset of CSF abnormalities. Two obvious candidates, TNF and IL-1, were initially evaluated for several reasons: the emerging evidence of their seminal participation in sepsis, the ability of bacterial surface components to stimulate their release in vitro, the ability of these peptides to enhance the adherence of neutrophils to endothelium, and the existence of cells within the CNS (astrocytes, microglia, endothelium, meningeal macrophages) capable of cytokine synthesis. Evidence accumulated in recent years, however, incriminated several other secondary mediators, such as IL-6, IL-8, PAF, prostaglandin E_2 (PGE_2), and nitric oxide, in the amplification and perpetuation of the meningeal inflammatory cascade initiated by TNF and IL-1 (15,16).

Tumor Necrosis Factor

This pivotal cytokine is a glycoprotein encoded by a gene located on the short arm of chromosome 6. Although monocyte-macrophage cells seem to be the most important sources of TNF, other activated cellular lineages such as lymphocytes, natural killer cells, Kupffer's cells, synovial phagocytes, and more importantly for the focus of this review, astrocytes and microglial cells of the brain also produce this inflammatory mediator (17).

In experimental meningitis, TNF activity is first detected in the CSF of rabbits 45 minutes after intracisternal inoculation of Hib endotoxin, reaches peak values at 2 hours, and persists for approximately 5 hours, a response almost identical to that seen in humans given endotoxin intravenously (18). The presence of CSF pleocytosis is observed 75 minutes after TNF is detected and peaks 6 to 9 hours after the challenge. Changes in protein, glucose, and lactate concentrations in the CSF are also observed 3 hours after endotoxin administration. Sera obtained simultaneously with CSF samples have no detectable TNF activity, demonstrating exclusive intrathecal synthesis of this cytokine. Importantly, simultaneous intracisternal administration of anti-TNF polyclonal antibody with Hib endotoxin neutralizes CSF TNF activity and is associated with substantial attenuation of the meningeal inflammatory response. Moreover, intracisternal injection of homologous TNF to rabbits induces a more rapid, albeit lesser, inflammatory pattern than that observed after endotoxin challenge; this reaction is prevented by mixing the TNF with its monoclonal antibody before injection.

When live Hib organisms are used to induce meningitis in rabbits, a similar peak TNF concentration is observed at 3 hours after intracisternal challenge, but activity persists for approximately 14 hours (18). This prolonged presence of TNF activity in the CSF is probably best explained by the continuous stimulation of incoming leukocytes, including monocytes, macrophages, and equivalent brain cells, because of persistent endotoxin in the CSF from multiplying and dying bacteria. Interestingly, antimicrobial treatment of Hib-induced meningitis in these rabbits is associated with a brisk release of bacteria-free endotoxin into the CSF from rapidly lysed organisms, resulting in significantly larger concentrations of TNF than those found in untreated animals (19).

Several human studies detected the presence of TNF in the CSF of neonates, infants, children, and adults with bacterial meningitis (20–22). The detection rate at the time of admission varied from 70% to 93%, depending on the timing of the lumbar puncture with respect to the duration of symptoms and to the initiation of antimicrobial treatment. These patients were infected with a variety of meningeal pathogens, including gram-negative enteric bacilli, Hib, *S. pneumoniae, N. meningitidis,* and *Streptococcus agalactiae* (group B). In contrast, bioactive TNF was not found in children with culture-proved viral meningitis or in the CSF of uninfected patients who required lumbar puncture for other reasons (23,24). From a diagnostic perspective, although the absence of detectable TNF in the CSF does not rule out the diagnosis of bacterial meningitis, its presence is highly suggestive of this disease.

Interleukin-1

This cytokine, along with TNF, is thought to be one of the sentinel early mediators of the body's response to microbial invasion and to be responsible for the induction of fever and the acute-phase host reaction that occurs during bacterial infection (25). Formerly called *endogenous pyrogen*, IL-1 is produced and released mainly by mononuclear phagocytes activated by exposure to microorganisms and its products. Besides monocyte-macrophage cells, synovial fibroblasts, epidermal cells, endothelial cells, neutrophils, and astrocytes and microglial cells of the brain also produce this cytokine. IL-1α (the cell-associated form) and IL-1β (the circulating form in body fluids) are coded by a separate gene located on chromosome 2, but both molecules seem to have similar biologic effects (26).

Activity of IL-1 can be detected in the CSF of rats 30 minutes after intracisternal injection of Hib endotoxin, and its concentration is significantly decreased by 2 hours after inoculation (27). Homologous IL-1 inoculated directly into the CSF of rabbits induces meningeal inflammation in a dose-dependent fashion. These inflammatory changes elicited by IL-1, however, are delayed in comparison with those induced by purified Hib endotoxin. Interestingly, TNF activity is not detected in the CSF of these animals, suggesting an independent mechanism of action. Dose-dependent changes in BBB permeability can also be observed when human recombinant IL-1 is inoculated intracisternally in adult rats (28). In all of these experiments, simultaneous inoculation of IL-1 with specific antibodies against this cytokine results in almost complete suppression of meningeal inflammation and BBB functional injury. In several animal meningitis models, intracisternal administration of both proximal cytokines, IL-1 and TNF, is associated with a synergistic increase in the meningeal inflammatory response and in BBB permeability alterations, similar to those changes induced by inoculation of Hib purified endotoxin (29).

Activity of IL-1 is detected in initial CSF samples of almost all neonates, infants, children, and adults with culture-proved bacterial meningitis, and its presence is significantly correlated with CSF inflammatory indices, TNF concentrations, and adverse outcome from the disease (30–32). Neurologic sequelae are associated with IL-1 concentrations higher than 500 pg/mL in CSF obtained at the time of diagnosis. Patients with viral meningitis or with normal CSF have low or nondetectable IL-1 activity.

Other Interleukins

There is accumulating evidence that other interleukins, notably IL-6 and IL-8, may also play an important role in the genesis of meningeal inflammation.

Interleukin-6 The cytokine IL-6, formerly called *hepatocyte-stimulating factor* and *interferon* β2, is a peptide considered the most potent inducer of acute-phase reactants in response to bacterial infection (33). The response to this cytokine is also characterized by fever, leukocytosis, an increase in secretion of corticotropin and glucocorticoids, and activation of the complement and clotting cascades. IL-6 is produced by a variety of cells, including monocytes, endothelial cells, and astrocytes, primarily in response to IL-1 stimulation. Although IL-6 can be detected in the CSF of patients with bacterial meningitis, its presence is not correlated with any of the indices of meningeal inflammation or with severity of disease (34). IL-6 is produced and released shortly afterward but stays detectable for longer periods than do the initial cytokines, TNF and IL-1. Although IL-6 clearly participates during the evolution of the meningeal inflammatory cascade, its exact contribution in the genesis of meningeal inflammation is uncertain. Measurement of IL-6 in CSF can be useful for diagnostic purposes because it constitutes a sensitive marker for the presence of meningitis and, along with detection of TNF, can reliably distinguish viral from bacterial disease (35).

Interleukin-8 This novel cytokine, formerly called *neutrophil-activating peptide-1* and *monocyte-derived neutrophil chemotactic factor*, recently was implicated as a mediator of neutrophil chemoattractant responses induced by TNF and IL-1 (36,37). In addition to these proinflammatory activities, IL-8 regulates neutrophil adhesion to activated receptors on endothelial cells, possibly facilitating the transendothelial migration of polymorphonuclear cells into infected tissues (38). Many cell types, including endothelial cells, monocyte-macrophages, polymorphonuclear leukocytes, astrocytes, microglia, and neuronal cells, produce IL-8 on stimulation by TNF, IL-1, or bacterial endotoxin. Although IL-8 has been detected in the CSF of many patients with bacterial meningitis caused by different pathogens (39–41), experimental studies are needed to precisely define its role in meningeal inflammation.

Other Proinflammatory Substances

In addition to TNF, IL-1, IL-6, and IL-8, other proinflammatory molecules likely participate in the meningeal inflammatory cascade; these substances are also detected in the CSF of patients with bacterial infection of the CNS and include, among others, interferon (IFN)-γ, PAF, PGE_2, and nitric oxide or its degradation products.

IFN-γ is a glycoprotein, mainly secreted by T cells, that enhances macrophage functions and seems to potentiate the immunologic effects induced by TNF. This protein is considered important in the fight against intracellular pathogens (42). It is unknown whether IFN-γ is deleterious when produced in excessive amount.

On induction of phospholipases by TNF and IL-1, membrane phospholipids are enzymatically affected to generate PAF and PGE_2 through different inflammatory pathways. PAF is a potent glycerophosphocholine derivative with a myriad of biologic activities, including aggregation of platelets and leukocytes, and possibly mediation of the formation of thrombi and the activation of clotting factors within vascular compartments (43). Although high amounts of PAF can be detected in the CSF of children with bacterial meningitis, the precise role of this cytokine in meningeal inflammation has not been elucidated (44). PGE_2 is a cyclo-oxygenase product that appears to participate not only in the development of increased permeability of the BBB but also in the down-regulation of TNF and IL-1 synthesis through a negative biofeedback mechanism (45,46). Despite being consistently detected in the CSF of bacterial meningitis patients, the specific effects and interactions of PGE_2 with other inflammatory substances are largely unknown.

Nitric oxide is a recently described free radical molecule that in addition to being a potent vasodilator, an intercellular neuronal messenger, and an inhibitor of the endothelial adhesion of platelets and leukocytes, is considered to induce cytotoxicity when produced in excessive amounts and to possibly mediate the increased permeability of the BBB (47–49). Nitric oxide appears to be induced by TNF and its CSF concentrations are highly correlated with those of TNF and with inflammatory indices (50), and may contribute to anaerobic glycolysis in the CNS. The exact pathophysiologic role of nitric oxide production in bacterial meningitis needs further delineation in experimental studies before it can be determined whether nitric oxide has a salutary or deleterious effect.

Finally, it is important to emphasize that in addition to the participation of molecules with proinflammatory activities, the host also produces several cytokines or substances that exert autoregulatory functions aimed to control excessive inflammation (51). Imbalances in favor of either proinflammatory or anti-inflammatory responses may influence the clinical spectrum of meningitis, varying from uneventful recovery to severe long-term abnormalities or death. Included among these substances are natural receptor inhibitors or antagonists of TNF and IL-1, the recently described anti-inflammatory cytokine IL-10, and endogenous corticosteroids.

THERAPEUTIC IMPLICATIONS OF CYTOKINE PARTICIPATION

Understanding the complex and intricate role of cytokines in the activation of several inflammatory pathways induced during bacterial meningitis is crucial to explain plausibly why the development of more potent antimicrobial agents will not further improve the outcome of the disease and to identify potential targets for adjunctive therapy. Although experimental therapies have been directed against harmful bacterial products (cell wall fragments, endotoxin), we believe that strategies to modulate the production of several proinflammatory cytokines or their activity on endothelium-leukocyte interactions provide greater promise for use in bacterial meningitis (Table 7-1). The timing of these interventions in relation to antibiotic administration and to duration of symptoms is crucial when designing studies in animals or humans.

Table 7-1. Therapeutic Strategies of Potential Clinical Relevance to Modulate Cytokine Effects in Bacterial Meningitis

Mechanism of Action	*Agents*	*Comments*
Regulation of cytokine production	Anticytokine antibodies	Must cross BBB to be effective; many cytokines involved
	Natural cytokine receptor inhibitors	Must cross BBB; not very effective in meningitis induced by live organisms; soluble receptors can render cytokines bioactive substances
	Corticosteroids	Have proved clinical efficacy when administered before the first parenteral antibiotic dose
	Nonsteroidal anti-inflammatory agents	Can interfere with regulatory effects of PG on TNF/IL-1 synthesis; can provoke preferential increase of other inflammatory pathways
	IL-10	Can interfere with CSF eradication of intracellular meningeal pathogens
Regulation of cytokine activity	Anti–endothelium-leukocyte adhesion antibodies	Antibodies against receptors of the integrin family can reduce effective penetration of antibiotics into CSF; agents against receptors of the selectin family are promising
	Anticytotoxic agents	Pentoxifylline can be associated with untoward systemic effects; scavengers of oxygen/nitrogen derivatives and nitric oxide antagonists may interfere with beneficial host responses

BBB = blood-brain barrier; CSF = cerebrospinal fluid; PG = prostaglandins; TNF = tumor necrosis factor; IL = interleukin.

Modulation of Cytokine Production

Several strategies can be utilized to achieve modulation of cytokine activity during bacterial meningitis. These include administering specific antibodies against individual mediators, soluble receptors of these cytokines, and inhibitory agents of cytokine synthesis (corticosteroids, pentoxifylline, nonsteroidal anti-inflammatory drugs, IL-10).

Anti–Cytokine-Specific Antibodies Polyclonal and monoclonal anti-TNF and anti–IL-1 antibodies have been administered to animals with experimental meningitis induced by live organisms or by Hib endotoxin. These investigations demonstrated modulation of the meningeal inflammatory response, especially when homologous anti-TNF and anti–IL-1 antibodies were administered concomitantly (12). To achieve this modulating activity, however, the antibodies have to be administered by the intrathecal route because intravenously injected antibodies are not expected to cross the BBB in adequate amounts, even through inflamed meninges, thus making this therapeutic approach impractical in clinical situations.

Natural Inhibitors of Tumor Necrosis Factor and Interleukin-1 In the past few years, an IL-1 receptor antagonist and a soluble TNF receptor were studied extensively in vitro as well as in animal models of bacterial infections (52,53). The intracisternal inoculation of these inhibitory agents in rabbits with meningitis induced by homologous TNF and IL-1 produced significant modulation of inflammation. In contrast, when live Hib or its purified endotoxin was used to induce meningitis, no significant anti-inflammatory effects of these inhibitory compounds were detected (54). These preliminary data indicate that these natural inhibitors may not be effective in modulating meningeal inflammation induced by a broad inflammatory stimulus such as gram-negative bacteria or their products, and suggest caution in using them to treat bacterial meningitis in humans. In addition, recent data suggest that a soluble TNF receptor type II may have a stabilizing effect on inactive TNF, rendering it a bioactive cytokine in the CSF of patients with meningitis (55).

Corticosteroids To date, corticosteroids are the only anti-inflammatory agents that have successfully passed rigorous assessment in the experimental meningitis model and are widely recommended for use in infants and children with bacterial meningitis (56,57).

Considerable evidence in animal models of meningitis supports the efficacy of dexamethasone, the most studied steroid, in downregulating meningeal inflammation, in reducing cerebral edema and intracranial hypertension, and in attenuating brain damage. Intravenous administration of dexamethasone 1 hour before or simultaneously with Hib endotoxin significantly reduced TNF activity and the meningeal inflammatory indices when compared to delayed or, even more, to no therapy. Additionally, dexamethasone given just before antibiotic therapy in rabbits with live Hib–induced meningitis reduced the inflammatory brisk response resulting from the release into the CSF of bacteria-free endotoxin from dying organisms; this action was also associated with a significant reduction in CSF TNF activity. Treatment with dexamethasone also decreased the CSF pleocytosis induced by intracisternal inoculation of rabbits with TNF or IL-1 or both. Confocal laser scanning microscopy used to investigate the dynamic aspects of rhodamine-labeled leukocytes in the pial microcirculation during the early phase of pneumococcal meningitis demonstrated that early dexamethasone therapy significantly attenuates adherence and subsequent transendothelial passage of leukocytes through the BBB (58).

In vitro studies demonstrated that dexamethasone, when administered to macrophages before endotoxin exposure, inhibits the production of TNF, both by diminishing the quantity of TNF messenger RNA (mRNA) and by preventing its translation (59).

Once endotoxin has induced mRNA for TNF, dexamethasone is incapable of regulating TNF biosynthesis. Dexamethasone also interferes with the production of IL-1 from human monocytes at different levels (60). It markedly decreases IL-1 mRNA by inhibiting the transcription of the IL-1 gene and by selectively decreasing the stability of IL-1 mRNA. In addition, dexamethasone appears to inhibit the translation of the IL-1 precursor and the release of IL-1 into extracellular fluid.

Another mechanism of the anti-inflammatory action of dexamethasone is inhibition of phospholipase activity, thereby decreasing the production of PAF and arachidonic acid metabolites. This action of dexamethasone is probably mediated, at least in part, by stimulation of a group of proteins collectively termed *lipocortins* (61). However, the inhibitory effect of dexamethasone on TNF and IL-1 synthesis by itself can explain its generalized modulatory activity on almost all of the secondary inflammatory mediators presently identified.

Several well-controlled, double-blind, prospective studies of pediatric bacterial meningitis clinically demonstrated the cytokine-modulating activity of dexamethasone (62–68). Most trials associated dexamethasone therapy with an improvement in meningeal inflammatory indices, with a reduction in CSF cytokine concentrations (i.e., TNF, IL-1, PAF, PGE_2), and with fewer audiologic or neurologic sequelae when compared with findings in placebo recipients. A salutary outcome was seen when dexamethasone was given early (i.e., before the first parenteral antibiotic dose) as opposed to late (i.e., after several hours of antimicrobial treatment), thus confirming the critical importance of timing observed in animal models of meningitis to achieve the optimal beneficial effects of steroids (Fig 7-2). Furthermore, a significant reduction in CSF TNF concentrations was evident only when dexamethasone was given before antibiotics, compared with its administration more than 2 hours afterward. Currently, there is concern that routine use of dexamethasone, in virtue of its effect on reducing BBB permeability and penetration of antibiotics into the subarachnoid space, can interfere with CSF eradication of meningeal pathogens, particularly penicillin- and cephalosporin-resistant pneumococcal strains. Although the penetration of certain antibiotics, such as vancomycin, into the CSF of dexamethasone-treated rabbits with pneumococcal meningitis is reduced compared with that in non-steroid-treated animals (69), this does not appear to be the case in children. Vancomycin concentrations in the CSF of dexamethasone-treated children with meningitis were at least twofold to sixfold higher than the MBC_{90} for S. *pneumoniae* (70).

Pentoxifylline Pentoxifylline is a phosphodiesterase inhibitor that affects the functional properties of polymorphonuclear leukocytes once they are activated by endotoxin or cytokines (71). In addition, it increases cyclic adenosine monophosphate, an action that appears to be responsible for more than 50% suppression of endotoxin-induced TNF production by mononuclear cells (72). Results of in vitro studies using mouse macrophages indicate that pentoxifylline blocks TNF mRNA accumulation but has no effect on the efficiency of mRNA translation, whereas dexamethasone has only a modest effect on mRNA accumulation but strongly impedes translational derepression; combined application of both agents causes greater suppression of TNF biosynthesis than that achieved by either agent alone (73).

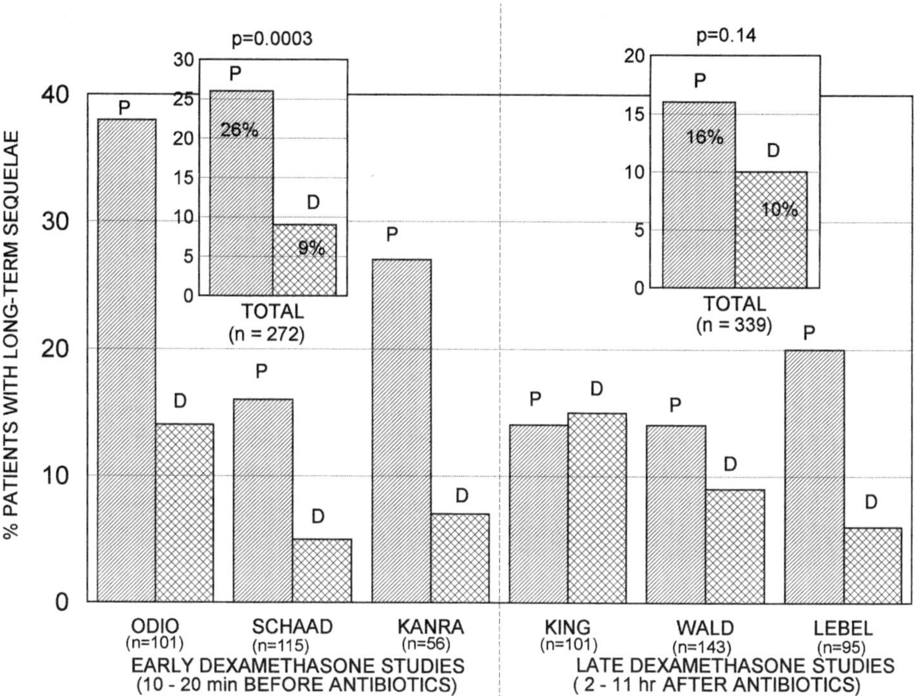

Figure 7-2. Impact of the timing of steroid therapy on the outcome in children with bacterial meningitis (prospective, double-blind, placebo-controlled studies) (62–67). Inset graphs on the left and right represent results of meta-analysis of the data from studies in which dexamethasone was given early or late, respectively. D = dexamethasone; P = placebo.

A continuous intravenous infusion of pentoxifylline in rabbits and rats with meningitis induced by Hib endotoxin ameliorates CSF inflammatory indices and abnormalities in BBB permeability (74,75). In addition, meningeal inflammation induced by intracisternal inoculation of IL-1 in rabbits is markedly attenuated by pentoxifylline treatment. In contrast, pentoxifylline had little effect on rats with meningitis caused by live Hib organisms (76). More experimental studies are needed to delineate the potential modulating effects of this drug on the pathophysiologic cascade of bacterial meningitis.

Nonsteroidal Anti-Inflammatory Agents These drugs block the conversion of arachidonic acid to prostaglandins. Indomethacin reduced CSF PGE_2 concentrations and brain edema in experimental pneumococcal meningitis, but had no effect on inflammation, CSF lactate concentrations, or intracranial pressure (77). Moreover, indomethacin treatment was associated with an increased CSF pleocytosis. Oxindanac is an experimental nonsteroidal agent that has demonstrated broader anti-inflammatory activity in experimental meningitis than that of indomethacin (78). Concern about the use of these agents has been raised because inhibition of the cyclo-oxygenase pathway can preferentially increase lipoxygenase by-products or PAF concentrations and eliminate the regulatory effects of PGE_2 on TNF synthesis.

Interleukin-10 As already mentioned, IL-10 is an anti-inflammatory protein that inhibits the production of proinflammatory cytokines as a means of autoregulatory control of the host's excessive inflammatory response. The potential therapeutic effect of IL-10 was recently studied in a rabbit model of meningitis induced by live Hib and *Listeria* organisms or Hib endotoxin (79). Animals treated with IL-10 showed a significant modulation of meningeal inflammation, although maximal effects were obtained when IL-10 was combined with dexamethasone therapy. Additional experimental studies evaluating other pathophysiologic aspects of meningitis are needed to delineate the specific therapeutic role of this anti-inflammatory cytokine in bacterial meningitis. Of concern is the recent observation that IL-10 in a dose-dependent manner impaired the bactericidal activity of activated mice macrophages against *Listeria monocytogenes*, an intracellular meningeal pathogen (80).

Modulation of Cytokine Activity

Modulation of the activities of several cytokines on endothelium or leukocyte functions is a critical step to limit meningeal inflammation and brain damage during experimental bacterial meningitis. Although agents that reduce cytokine production, as already mentioned, have a nonspecific effect on cytokine activity, selective inhibition of this step can be achieved with drugs that interfere with the adhesion of leukocytes to endothelial cells or with the cytotoxic effects of neutrophil-derived products (see Table 7-1).

Anti–Endothelium-Leukocyte Adhesion Agents

A monoclonal antibody against the CD11/CD18 receptors of the integrin family of leukocyte adhesion molecules that was administered intravenously to rabbits with meningitis induced by live bacteria, endotoxin, or pneumococcal cell walls significantly reduced the severity of meningeal inflammation, brain edema, and impairment of the BBB (81,82). A more profound attenuation of these inflammatory abnormalities was achieved when this antibody was combined with dexamethasone.

Prokaryotic lectin domains of pertussis toxin, similar to those of the selectin family of human receptors, were recently tested in experimental meningitis and associated with decreased CSF pleocytosis and, interestingly, with a dose-dependent reversible increase in BBB permeability that might potentially facilitate delivery of intravenously administered antibiotics to the subarachnoid space (83). Most recently, mice with genetically engineered deficiencies in P- and E-selectins displayed a near-complete inhibition of CSF pleocytosis and BBB permeability in a cytokine (TNF and IL1)-induced meningitis model (84).

Anticytotoxic Agents

Neutrophils contain inside their granules toxic products that are believed to participate actively in the digestion of the BBB, therefore contributing to the increased permeability that occurs during bacterial meningitis. Among these harmful substances are a family of oxidizing chemicals, reactive nitrogen intermediates, and several proteolytic enzymes (85). Some of these toxic products can also be synthesized by other resident CNS cells. Several agents can be potentially useful for decreasing the tissue damage induced by cytotoxic molecules. Pentoxifylline reduces neutrophil degranulation; superoxide dismutase inactivates toxic superoxide radicals, possibly preventing the formation of peroxynitrite (86); catalase scavenges nitric oxide and hydrogen peroxide (87); and competitive inhibitors of L-arginine prevent the synthesis of nitric oxide (88). Investigation of these agents in animals with meningitis is currently ongoing but preliminary results suggest caution with interpretation of some data.

SUMMARY

In the past, meningeal inflammation was believed to ensue after direct toxic effects of invading microorganisms, with subsequent attraction and accumulation of leukocytes within the subarachnoid space induced as a host response to eliminate these foreign intruders. During the last 10 to 15 years, however, this hypothesis was challenged by two reproducible experimental observations: the diversity of infectious agents capable of inducing meningitis and BBB injury in a similar fashion, and the consistent delay of 2 to 3 hours to provoke CSF inflammation after intracisternal inoculation of live bacteria or their cell surface components in rabbits. These findings suggest that common mediators synthesized and released by the host are responsible for the inflammatory response and its pathophysiologic consequences.

Considerable experimental and clinical evidence has implicated a large, and still growing, family of cytokines and other proinflammatory substances that act to initiate and amplify the meningeal inflammatory cascade after being triggered by exposure of brain cells to viable microorganisms or their products. This inflammatory network is initiated by the synthesis of TNF and IL-1, followed by the production of many other secondary mediators. As this proinflammatory cascade evolves, the host also produces several regulatory cytokines and substances that provide a balance between proinflammatory and anti-inflammatory effects. Preference of one or the other pathway ultimately determines the outcome of the disease.

Based on the increasing understanding of the contribution of cytokines to the genesis of meningeal inflammation, abnormal CSF hydrodynamics, cerebral edema, intracranial hypertension, brain ischemia, and neuronal injury, potentially useful therapeutic strategies can be tested in experimental models of meningitis and, if beneficial, progress to clinical investigations. Presently however, only dexamethasone has successfully passed rigorous animal model and clinical scrutiny and is currently widely used in infants and children with bacterial meningitis. In the near future, we expect that other promising therapeutic agents will be successfully tested in patients and improve the outcome of this life-threatening disease.

REFERENCES

1 Sáez-Llorens X, Ramilo O, Mustafa M, et al. Molecular pathophysiology of bacterial meningitis: current concepts and therapeutic implications. *J Pediatr* 1990;116:671–684.

2 Tunkel AR, Wispelwey B, Scheld WM. Bacterial meningitis: recent advances in pathophysiology and treatment. *Ann Intern Med* 1990; 112:610–623.

3 Quagliarello V, Scheld WM. Bacterial meningitis: pathogenesis, pathophysiology, and progress. *N Engl J Med* 1992;327:864–872.

4 Dinarello CA, Mier JW. Lymphokines. *N Engl J Med* 1987;317:940–945.

5 Sáez-Llorens X, McCracken GH Jr. Sepsis syndrome and septic shock in pediatrics: current concepts of terminology, pathophysiology, and management. *J Pediatr* 1993;123:497–508.

6 Tunkel AR, Scheld WM. Pathogenesis and pathophysiology of bacterial meningitis. *Clin Microbiol Rev* 1993;6:118–136.

7 Smith AL. Pathogenesis of *Haemophilus influenzae* meningitis. *Pediatr Infect Dis J* 1987; 6:783–786.

8 Moxon ER, Ostrow PT. Hib meningitis in rats: role of bacteremia in pathogenesis of age-dependent inflammatory responses in CSF. *J Infect Dis* 1977;135:303–308.

9 Simberkoff MS, Moldover NH, Rahal J. Absence of detectable bactericidal and opsonic activities in normal and infected human cerebrospinal fluids: a regional host defense deficiency. *J Lab Clin Med* 1980;95:362–372.

10 Syrogiannopoulos GA, Hansen EJ, Erwin AL, et al. *Haemophilus influenzae* type b endotoxin induces meningeal inflammation. *J Infect Dis* 1988;157:237–244.

11 Mertsola J, Ramilo O, Mustafa M, et al. Release of endotoxin after antibiotic treatment of gram-negative bacterial meningitis. *Pediatr Infect Dis J* 1989;8:904–906.

12 Ramilo O, Sáez-Llorens X, Mertsola J, et al. Tumor necrosis factor and interleukin-1 initiate meningeal inflammation. *J Exp Med* 1990; 172:497–507.

13 Springer TA. Adhesion receptors of the immune system. *Nature* 1990;346:425–434.

14 Moser R, Schleiffenbaum B, Groscurth P, Fehr J. Interleukin-1 and tumor necrosis factor stimulate human vascular endothelial cells to promote transendothelial neutrophil passage. *J Clin Invest* 1989;83:444–455.

15 Pfister HW, Fontana A, Tauber MG, et al. Mechanisms of brain injury in bacterial meningitis: workshop summary. *Clin Infect Dis* 1994;19:463–479.

16 Saukkonen K, Sande S, Cioffe C, et al. The role of cytokines in the generation of inflammation and tissue damage in experimental gram-positive meningitis. *J Exp Med* 1990;171:439–448.

17 Chung IY, Benveniste EN. Tumor necrosis factor production by astrocytes. *J Immunol* 1990; 144:2999–3007.

18 Mustafa M, Ramilo O, Olsen KD, et al. Tumor necrosis factor in mediating experimental *Haemophilus influenzae* type b meningitis. *J Clin Invest* 1989;84:1253–1259.

19 Mustafa M, Ramilo O, Sáez-Llorens X, et al. Role of tumor necrosis factor in experimental and clinical bacterial meningitis. *Pediatr Infect Dis J* 1989;8:907–908.

20 Leist TP, Frei K, Kam-Hansen S, et al. Tumor necrosis factor in cerebrospinal fluid during bacterial but not viral meningitis. *J Exp Med* 1988;167:1743–1748.

21 Waage A, Halstensen A, Shalaby R, et al. Local production of tumor necrosis factor, interleukin-1, and interleukin-6 in meningococcal meningitis. *J Exp Med* 1989;170:1859–1867.

22 McCracken GH, Mustafa M, Ramilo O, et al. Cerebrospinal fluid interleukin-1 beta and tumor necrosis factor concentrations and outcome from neonatal gram-negative enteric bacillary meningitis. *Pediatr Infect Dis J* 1989; 8:155–159.

23 Ramilo O, Mustafa M, Porter J, et al. Detection of interleukin-1 but not tumor necrosis factor in cerebrospinal fluid of children with aseptic meningitis. *Am J Dis Child* 1990;144:349–352.

24 Glimaker M, Kragsbjerg P, Forsgren M, Olcen P. Tumor necrosis factor in cerebrospinal fluid from patients with meningitis of different etiologies: high levels of TNF indicate bacterial meningitis. *J Infect Dis* 1993;167:882–889.

25 Dinarello CA. Interleukin-1 and its biologically related cytokines. *Adv Immunol* 1989; 44:153–205.

26 Dinarello CA. Interleukin-1. *Rev Infect Dis* 1984;6:51–95.

27 Quagliarello VJ, Wispelwey B, Long WJ, Scheld WM. Recombinant human interleukin-1 induces meningitis and blood-brain barrier injury in the rat. *J Clin Invest* 1991; 87:1360–1366.

28 Tunkel AR, Wispelwey B, Scheld WM. Pathogenesis and pathophysiology of meningitis. *Infect Dis Clin North Am* 1990;4:555–581.

29 Sáez-Llorens X, McCracken GH Jr. Mediators of meningitis: therapeutic implications. *Hosp Pract* 1991;26:68–77.

30 Mustafa M, Lebel M, Ranilo O, et al. Correla-

tion of interleukin-1 and cachectin concentrations in cerebrospinal fluid and outcome from bacterial meningitis. *J Pediatr* 1989; 115:208–213.

31 Mustafa M, Ramilo O, Sáez-Llorens X, et al. Prostaglandins, IL-1, and TNF in cerebrospinal fluid of infants and children with bacterial meningitis. *Pediatr Infect Dis J* 1989;8:921–922.

32 Waage A, Halstensen A, Shalaby R, et al. Local production of tumor necrosis factor, interleukin-1, and interleukin-6 in meningococcal meningitis. *J Exp Med* 1989;170:1859–1864.

33 Hirano T, Akira S, Taga T, Kishimoto T. Biological and clinical aspects of interleukin-6. *Immunol Today* 1990;11:443–445.

34 Rusconi F, Parizzi F, Garlaschi L, et al. Interleukin-6 activity in infants and children with bacterial meningitis. *Pediatr Infect Dis J* 1991;10:117–121.

35 Dulkerian SJ, Kilpatrick L, Costarino AT, et al. Cytokine elevations in infants and children with bacterial and aseptic meningitis. *J Pediatr* 1995;126:872–877.

36 Matsushima K, Baldwin ET, Mukaida N. Interleukin-8: novel leukocyte recruitment and activating cytokines. *Chem Immunol* 1992; 51:236–265.

37 Baggiolini M, Walz A, Kunkel SL. Neutrophil-activating peptide-1/interleukin-8, a novel cytokine that activates neutrophils. *J Clin Invest* 1989;84:1045–1050.

38 Huber AR, Kunkel SL, Todd RF, Weiss SJ. Regulation of transendothelial neutrophil migration by endogenous IL-8. *Science* 1991; 254:99–102.

39 Lopez-Cortes LF, Cruz-Ruiz M, Gomez-Mateos J, et al. Interleukin-8 in cerebrospinal fluid from patients with meningitis of different etiologies: its possible role as neutrophil chemotactic factor. *J Infect Dis* 1995;172:581–584.

40 Halstensen A, Ceska M, Brandtzaeg P, et al. Interleukin-8 in serum and cerebrospinal fluid from patients with meningococcal disease. *J Infect Dis* 1993;167:471–475.

41 Seki T, Joh K, Oh-Ishi T. Augmented production of interleukin-8 in cerebrospinal fluid in bacterial meningitis. *Immunology* 1993; 80:333–335.

42 Buchmeier NA, Schreiber RD. Requirement of endogenous interferon-gamma production for resolution of *Listeria monocytogenes* infection. *Proc Natl Acad Sci USA* 1985;82:7404–7408.

43 Pinckard RN, Ludwig JC, McManus LM. Platelet-activating factors. In: Gallin JJ, Goldstein JM, Snyderman R, eds. *Inflammation: basic principles and clinical correlates*. New York: Raven, 1988.

44 Arditi M, Caplan M, Yogev R. Platelet-activating factor levels in CSF of children with Hib meningitis. In: *Program and abstracts from the 29th Interscience Conference on Antimicrobial Agents and Chemotherapy (ICAAC), Houston, Texas, September 1989*:1113. Abstract.

45 Tureen JH, Stella FB, Clyman RI, et al. Effect of indomethacin on brain water content, cerebrospinal fluid pleocytosis, and PGE-2 levels in CSF in experimental pneumococcal meningitis. *Pediatr Infect Dis J* 1987;6:1151–1153.

46 Kunkel SL, Remick DG, Strieter RM, Lanick JW. Mechanisms that regulate the production and effects of tumor necrosis factor. *Crit Rev Immunol* 1989;9:93–117.

47 Haberl RL, Anneser F, Kodel U, Pfister HW. Is nitric oxide involved as a mediator of cerebrovascular changes in the early phase of experimental pneumococcal meningitis? *Neurol Res* 1994;16:108–112.

48 Moncada S, Palmer RNJ, Higgs EA. Nitric oxide: physiology, pathophysiology, and pharmacology. *Pharmacol Rev* 1991;43:109–142.

49 Kubes P, Granger DN. Nitric oxide modulates microvascular permeability. *Am J Physiol* 1992;262:H611–615.

50 Van Furth AM, Seijmonsbergen EM, Groeneveld PHP, et al. Levels of nitric oxide correlate with high levels of tumor necrosis factor in cerebrospinal fluid samples from children with bacterial meningitis. *Clin Infect Dis* 1996; 22: 876–877.

51 Girardin E, Dayer JM. Cytokines and antagonists in septic shock. *J Suisse Med* 1993; 123: 480–491.

52 Ashkenazi A, Marsters SA, Capon DJ, et al. Protection against endotoxic shock by a tumor necrosis factor receptor immunoadhesin. *Proc Natl Acad Sci USA* 1991;88:1535–1539.

53 Fisher E, Marano MA, Van Zee KJ, et al. Interleukin-1 receptor antagonist improves survival and hemodynamic performance in *E. coli* septic shock, but fails to alter host defense to sublethal endotoxemia. *J Clin Invest* 1992; 89:1551–1557.

54 Paris MM, Friedland I, Ehrett S, et al. Effect of interleukin-1 receptor antagonist and soluble tumor necrosis factor receptor in animal models of infection. *J Infect Dis* 1995;171: 161–169.

55 Moller B, Ellerman-Eriksen S, Storgaard M, et al. Soluble tumor necrosis factor receptors conserve TNF bioactivity in meningitis patient spinal fluid. *J Infect Dis* 1996;174:557–563.

56 Tunkel AR, Scheld WM. Acute bacterial meningitis. *Lancet* 1995;346:1675–1680.

57 Schaad UB, Kaplan SL, McCracken GH Jr.

Steroid therapy for bacterial meningitis. *Clin Infect Dis* 1995;20:685–690.

58 Lorenzl S, Koedel U, Dirnagl U, et al. Imaging of leukocyte-endothelium interaction using in vivo confocal laser scanning microscopy during the early phase of experimental pneumococcal meningitis. *J Infect Dis* 1993;168:927–933.

59 Beutler B, Krochin N, Milsark IW, et al. Control of tumor necrosis factor synthesis: mechanisms of endotoxin resistance. *Science* 1986; 232:977–980.

60 Kern JA, Lamb RJ, Reed JC, et al. Dexamethasone inhibition of interleukin-1 beta production by human monocytes. *J Clin Invest* 1988; 81:237–244.

61 Northup JK, Braun KA, Johnson LK, et al. Evaluation of the anti-inflammatory and phospholipase-inhibitory activity of calpactin/lipocortin. *J Clin Invest* 1988;82:1437–1452.

62 Lebel MH, Freij BJ, Syrogiannopoulos GA, et al. Dexamethasone therapy for bacterial meningitis. *N Engl J Med* 1988;319:964–971.

63 Odio CM, Faingezicht I, Paris MM, et al. The beneficial effects of early dexamethasone administration in infants and children with bacterial meningitis. *N Engl J Med* 1991; 324:1525–1531.

64 Schaad UB, Lips U, Gnehm HE, et al. Dexamethasone therapy for bacterial meningitis in children. *Lancet* 1993;342:1525–1531.

65 King SM, Law B, Langley JM, et al. Dexamethasone therapy for bacterial meningitis: better never than late? *Can J Infect Dis* 1994; 5:219–225.

66 Wald ER, Kaplan SL, Mason EO, et al. Dexamethasone therapy for children with bacterial meningitis. *Pediatrics* 1995;95:21–28.

67 Kanra GY, Ozen H, Secmeer G, et al. Beneficial effects of dexamethasone in children with pneumococcal meningitis. *Pediatr Infect Dis J* 1995;14:490–494.

68 Kennedy WA, Hoyt MJ, McCracken GH Jr. The role of corticosteroid therapy in children with pneumococcal meningitis. *Am J Dis Child* 1991;145:1374–1378.

69 Paris MM, Hickey SM, Uscher MI, et al. Effect of dexamethasone on therapy of experimental penicillin and cephalosporin-resistant pneumococcal meningitis. *Antimicrob Agents Chemother* 1994;38:1320–1324.

70 Klugman KP, Friedland IR, Bradley JS. Bactericidal activity against cephalosporin-resistant *Streptococcus pneumoniae* in cerebrospinal fluid of children with acute bacterial meningitis. *Antimicrob Agents Chemother* 1995; 39:1988–1992.

71 Sullivan GW, Carper HT, Novick WJ, Mandell GL. Inhibition of the anti-inflammatory action of interleukin-1 and tumor necrosis factor on neutrophil function by pentoxifylline. *Infect Immun* 1988;56:1722–1729.

72 Strieter RM, Resnick DG, Ward PA, et al. Cellular and molecular regulation of tumor necrosis factor production by pentoxifylline. *Biochem Biophys Res Commun* 1988;155:1230–1236.

73 Han J, Thompson P, Beutler B. Dexamethasone and pentoxifylline inhibit endotoxin-induced tumor necrosis factor synthesis at separate points in the signaling pathway. *J Exp Med* 1990;172:391–394.

74 Sáez-Llorens X, Ramilo O, Mustafa MM, et al. Pentoxifylline modulates meningeal inflammation in experimental bacterial meningitis. *Antimicrob Agents Chemother* 1990;34:837–843.

75 Sáez-Llorens X, Ramilo O, Mustafa M, et al. Modulation of meningeal inflammation by treatment with pentoxifylline. *Pediatr Infect Dis J* 1989;8:922–923.

76 Sable CA, Aubin MA, Scheld WM. Pentoxifylline effect on Hib-induced alteration in blood-brain barrier permeability in experimental meningitis. In: *Program and abstracts of the 31st ICAAC, Chicago, September 29-October 2, 1991*:252. Abstract.

77 Kadurugamura JL, Hengstler B, Bray MA, Zak O. Inhibition of C5-induced inflammatory reaction by PGE-2 in experimental meningitis. *J Infect Dis* 1989;160:715–719.

78 Kadurugamura JL, Hengstler B, Zak O. Effects of anti-inflammatory drugs on arachidonic acid metabolites and cerebrospinal fluid proteins during pneumococcal meningitis in rabbits. *Pediatr Infect Dis J* 1987;6:1153–1154.

79 Paris MM, Hickey S, Trujillo M, et al. Effect of interleukin-10 in experimental bacterial meningitis. In: *Program and abstracts of the 35th Interscience Conference on Antimicrobial Agents and Chemotherapy (ICAAC), San Franscisco, September 17-20, 1995*:B22. Abstract.

80 Frei K, Nadal D, Pfister HW, Fontana A. Listeria meningitis: identification of a cerebrospinal fluid inhibitor of macrophage listericidal function as interleukin-10. *J Exp Med* 1993; 178:1255–1261.

81 Tuomanen EI, Saukkonen K, Sande S, et al. Reduction of inflammation, tissue damage, and mortality in bacterial meningitis in rabbits treated with monoclonal antibodies against adhesion-promoting receptors of leukocytes. *J Exp Med* 1989;170:959–969.

82 Sáez-Llorens X, Jafari HS, Severien C, et al. Enhanced attenuation of meningeal inflammation and brain edema by concomitant administration of anti-CD18 antibodies and dexamethasone in experimental meningitis. *J Clin Invest* 1991;88:2003–2011.

83 Rozdzinski E, Spellerberg B, Van der Flier M, et al. Peptide from a prokaryotic adhesin blocks leukocyte migration in vitro and in vivo. *J Infect Dis* 1995;172:785.

84 Tang T, Frenette PS, Hynes RO, et al. Cytokine-induced meningitis is dramatically attenuated in mice deficient in endothelial selectins. *J Clin Invest* 1996;97:2485–2490.

85 Ganz T, Selsed ME, Babior BM, Curnutte JT. Neutrophils and host defense. *Ann Intern Med* 1988;109:127–142.

86 Beckman JS, Beckman TW, Chen J, et al. Apparent hydroxyl radical production by peroxynitrite: implications for endothelial injury from nitric oxide and superoxide. *Proc Natl Acad Sci USA* 1990;87:1620–1624.

87 Pfister HW, Koedel U, Lorenzl S, Tomasz A. Antioxidants attenuate microvascular changes in the early phase of experimental pneumococcal meningitis in rats. *Stroke* 1992; 23:1798–1804.

88 Koshland DE Jr. The molecule of the year. *Science* 1992;258:1861. Editorial.

8 Neuronal Injury in Meningitis

MARTIN G. TÄUBER
YOUNG S. KIM
STEPHEN L. LEIB

Approximately 15,000 cases of bacterial meningitis occur each year in the United States, while other parts of the world have a substantially higher incidence. Even when treated with highly effective antibiotics, the disease is fatal in 5% to 40% of the patients and causes neurologic sequelae in as many as 30% of the survivors (1,2). Neurologic sequelae can be grouped into three categories: 1) hearing impairment, which is most commonly the result of direct inflammatory invasion of the inner ear via the cochlear aqueduct (3–5); 2) obstructive hydrocephalus; and 3) brain parenchymal damage, reflected by sensory-motor syndromes, cerebral palsy, mental retardation, learning deficits, cortical blindness, and seizure disorders. The neuropathologic corollary of these sequelae has been characterized by histopathologic studies in patients dying of meningitis. These studies show areas of acute neuronal injury (swelling, followed by shrinkage and pyknosis) in patients dying within the first days after the onset of symptoms, and widespread complete loss of neurons in more chronic stages (6–9). Loss of neurons can be associated with areas of focal ischemic necrosis or with hemorrhagic cerebrocortical infarction (6–8), supporting a role of vascular involvement in brain injury. The loss of neurons is typically accompanied by evidence of activation of astrocytes, by a marked increase in microglial cells, and in more chronic cases, by vascular proliferation in the damaged parenchyma (6,7,9). These neuropathologic findings in humans unequivocally document neuronal loss and glial reaction during meningitis.

The molecular mediators involved in the parenchymal processes leading to neuronal injury during meningitis have not been conclusively identified (10). It is likely that a better understanding of these mechanisms will lead to new therapeutic approaches to complement antibiotic therapy. Studies with dexamethasone are testimony to the potential value of adjunctive therapies for bacterial meningitis. Hearing impairment, overall neurologic outcome, and mortality were improved in patients treated with dexamethasone plus antibiotics compared to those treated with antibiotics alone (11–13). Nevertheless, dexamethasone is probably not the ideal adjunctive drug for meningitis. The benefits of dexamethasone are likely mediated by a broad, nonselective anti-inflammatory effect. Also, some evidence suggests that the drug may have some adverse effects on neuronal survival in the hippocampus (14), even though the relevance of these findings with regard to the human disease is not known. It appears that therapies which target harmful processes more selectively than corticosteroids may be more effective or remain effective during more advanced stages of the disease, when the effectiveness of anti-inflammatory drugs is limited.

In addition to delay of treatment, two factors seem to affect the incidence of neuronal injury during bacterial meningitis: the age of the patient and the infecting organism. The disease that consistently causes the most severe neuronal injury is neonatal meningitis. In most newborns, meningitis is caused by group B streptococci (GBS) or *Escherichia coli*, and mortality rates can be as high as 35% (15–17). Only 50% of survivors of GBS meningitis are neurologically intact, while 21% have severe neurologic sequelae (18). Given the extremely serious nature of neonatal meningitis, we have developed a model of neonatal meningitis in infant rats infected with GBS, to learn more about the mechanisms that lead to brain injury in this disease (19). The new model is characterized by the development of extensive neuronal injury and has proved very useful to start elucidating the mechanisms that lead to neuronal injury during meningitis. In this chapter, we review the lessons learned from this model and from parallel studies in primary cell cultures of rat brain cells.

IN VITRO STUDIES IN PRIMARY CULTURES OF BRAIN CELLS

Toxicity of Bacterial Products in Cultures of Neurons, Astrocytes, and Microglia

An important element of our strategy to identify neurotoxic mediators in bacterial meningitis is the use of cultures of brain cells, specifically neurons, astrocytes, and microglia. In initial studies, we explored whether bacterial products of meningeal pathogens can directly induce cellular injury in these cells. This work was based on the assumption that bacterial products released from the meningeal pathogen in the cerebrospinal fluid (CSF) space can diffuse at significant concentrations into the brain parenchyma and interact there with various brain cells. We exposed cultures of primary neurons, of primary and transformed astrocytes, and of primary and transformed microglia to bacterial products (heat-killed organisms, cell wall from pneumococci or GBS, endotoxin) and found that primary neurons were remarkably resistant to any toxic effects of bacterial products (20). In contrast, pneumococcal products produced dose-dependent toxicity in astrocytes and microglia, with maximal toxicity reached at concentrations of approximately 100 μg/mL of bacterial cell wall (20). Cell wall from GBS was also toxic to glial cells, albeit slightly less than pneumococcal cell wall (21). Endotoxin added in a serum-free culture system was not toxic to any cell type, but when 10% fetal calf serum was added with endotoxin, toxicity similar to that of pneumococcal products was observed in astrocytes and microglia, indicating the need for endotoxin-binding serum factors in this system (22). These results show that astrocytes and microglia, but not neurons, are sensitive to the direct effects of bacterial products.

Neuronal Toxicity of Proinflammatory Cytokines

Since bacterial products were not directly toxic to neurons, we examined whether tumor necrosis factor (TNF)-α or interleukin (IL)-1, the two most prominent proinflammatory cytokines identified in the CSF during meningitis, were neurotoxic. Control experiments confirmed that the neurons were sensitive to the excitatory amino acid glutamate, as expected, with approximately 40% toxicity induced by 1 mM glutamate exposure over 24 hours. At concentrations of the cytokines found during bacterial meningitis (23,24), neither TNF-α nor IL-1 induced significant toxicity in the primary neuronal cultures. The combination of the two cytokines was also not toxic. Only at very high, supraphysiologic concentrations (5×10^{-6} M for TNF-α and 1×10^{-8} M for IL-1) did we find significant toxicity (Kim YS, Täuber MG, unpublished observations, 1994). The relevance of these findings is currently unclear and it is important to note that we tested only for acute toxicity in this system and did not exclude that physiologic concentrations of the cytokines induced delayed apoptotic cell death, a possibility that was recently raised (25).

Neuronal Toxicity of Bacterial Products in Mixed Neuronal-Glial Cocultures

Since bacterial products did not appear to cause direct neurotoxicity but showed activity in glial cells, we explored whether the effects of bacterial products on glial cells had adverse effects on neurons in cocultures. Experiments were performed either with neuronal cultures plated on astrocyte feeder layers, or with microglial cells added to neurons directly cultured on polylysine-coated dishes (at 1:5 ratio). In both cases, addition of a crude preparation of pneumococcal cell wall to the cocultures produced toxicity in neurons in a dose-dependent way (21). To identify the nature of the neurotoxic factor, we examined the effects of an excitatory amino acid antagonist (MK-801, 10 μg/mL) and of nitric oxide (NO) inhibition L-N$^{\omega}$-amino-L-arginine methyl ester (L-NAME, 10 μM). In both coculture systems, MK-801 did not protect neurons, but L-NAME was protective (21). These results indicate that NO production contributed to neuronal injury in cocultures with astrocytes or microglia stimulated with bacterial products. NO production in this system was further confirmed by increased concentrations of nitrite in the supernatants of glial cultures stimulated with bacterial products (21). These findings are similar to published studies, in which gram-negative bacterial products and cytokines induced NO-mediated neuronal injury by glial cells (26–28).

We further explored whether reactive oxygen intermediates (ROIs), in addition to NO, contributed to neuronal injury in cocultures of neurons on an astrocyte feeder layer. The addition of α-phenyl-*tert*-butyl-nitrone (PBN, 100 μM), a spin-trapping agent that can biologically neutralize various ROIs, partially reversed the neurotoxicity induced by bacterial products in these cocultures, suggesting that in addition to NO, ROIs may also contribute to neuronal injury in this system (Kim YS, Täuber MG, unpublished observations). This combined effect of NO and ROIs could be mediated by the formation of the cytotoxic molecule peroxynitrite from NO and superoxide, a possibility that needs to be explored further.

Combined Effects of Excitatory Amino Acids and Glial Cell–Derived Neurotoxicity

In light of the role of excitatory amino acids (EAAs) in causing neuronal injury in animal models of bacterial meningitis (see below), we also explored whether EAAs influenced the neuronal injury caused by bacteria-stimulated glial cultures in vitro. We exposed neurons cultured on an astrocyte feeder layer to low, mildly toxic concentrations of glutamate, pneumococcal cell wall, GBS cell wall, or the combination of either bacterial product with glutamate. The combination of the bacterial product and glutamate was significantly more toxic than either stimulus alone (synergism) (21). Treatment with PBN (100 μM) completely prevented the neurotoxicity induced by glutamate alone, glutamate plus pneumococcal cell wall, or glutamate plus GBS cell wall (Kim YS, Täuber MG, unpublished observations, 1996). These results suggest that the mediator(s) of glia-induced neuronal injury after stimulation with bacterial products and EAAs interacts in their neurotoxic potential, and that the generation of ROIs, in addition to NO, is a critical contributor to the neuronal injury in this setting.

Summary of In Vitro Findings

Our in vitro studies (Table 8-1) identified several molecular mediators that could play a role in causing neuronal injury during meningitis. These include NO and ROIs, both of which can be derived from glial cells stimulated by bacterial products, and excitatory amino acids. The three classes of neurotoxic mediators not only can contribute to neuronal injury individually, but also may potentiate each other in their neurotoxic effects. Our experiments did not conclusively address whether cytokines are directly neurotoxic because we did not test for delayed apoptotic neuronal injury. The in

Table 8-1. Summary of Neurotoxic Mediators Identified in Primary Cultures of Neurons and Cocultures of Neurons with Glia

	Neurotoxicity in	
Experimental Stimulus	*Pure Neuronal Cultures*	*Mixed Neuron/ Glia Cultures*
Pneumococcal cell wall (≤ 200 μg/mL)	±	++
Group B streptococcus (≤ 200 μg/mL)	±	++
LPS, no serum (≤ 5 μg/mL)	–	–
LPS (≤ 5 μg/mL) plus 10% serum	–	++
Bacterial products + L-NAME	ND	–
Bacterial products + PBN	ND	–
Bacterial products + MK-801	ND	++
Glutamate (1 mM)	++	++
Glutamate (15 μM) + cell wall (10 μg/mL)	ND	+++
Glutamate (15 μM) + cell wall (10 μg/mL) + PBN	ND	–

– = no toxicity in neurons; ± = minimal toxicity; + to +++ = increasing toxicity; ND = not done; LPS = lipopolysaccharide. L-NAME = L-N$^{\omega}$-amino-L-arginine methyl ester; PBN = α-phenyl-*tert*-butyl-nitrone.

vitro studies just summarized provided valuable guides for the studies described below, in which we evaluated the role of these same mediators in causing brain injury in vivo.

IN VIVO STUDIES IN A MODEL OF NEONATAL MENINGITIS IN INFANT RATS

Description of the Model

We initially attempted to develop a model of neonatal meningitis, in which meningitis resulted from systemic infection, as described by others (29,30). However, positive CSF cultures developed in less than 50% of bacteremic animals, and histopathologic examination of the brains of animals with meningitis showed only minimal CSF inflammation and no structural abnormalities. We therefore developed a new model using intracisternal injection of the infecting pathogen to reliably produce a more severe form of meningitis.

The methods used to produce meningitis and to examine animals have been published (19,31). Briefly, infant rats (10–12 days old) were infected by direct intracisternal inoculation of 10 μL of a suspension of an encapsulated GBS type III (gift of Dr. Rubens, Seattle). The inoculum was varied over several orders of magnitude and its size positively correlated with several clinical and histologic aspects of the severity of the disease (19).

Eighteen hours after infection, animals underwent a standardized assessment that included a clinical scoring (19) and sampling of CSF (10–20 μL). At this time, animals showed clinical signs of disease (lethargy, obtundation, seizures) and had high CSF bacterial titers (19). Blood cultures were also consistently positive. Following sampling of CSF and blood, animals were started on antibiotic therapy (ceftriaxone, 100 mg/kg subcutaneously every 24 hours). Depending on the inoculum size used to infect the animals, between 50% and 100% of the animals treated with antibiotics survived the acute infection. Untreated, the disease was uniformly fatal.

Neuronal Injury

Histopathologically, the disease in this model showed features remarkably similar to those described in neonates and infants dying of neonatal meningitis (19). An intense granulocytic inflammation involved the entire subarachnoid space as well as the ventricular space. Granulocytes were first seen in the subarachnoid space 4 hours after intracisternal inoculation, and CSF inflammation was fully developed by 18 hours and remained visible for at least 5 days after initiation of antibiotic therapy. Eighteen to 20 hours after the animals were infected, subarachnoid and intraparenchymal vessels showed marked dilatation and were engorged with erythrocytes. The transient vasculopathy, which disappeared uniformly within hours after institution of antibiotic therapy, was seen despite careful perfusion of the brains at the time of death, suggesting that some vessels were not actively perfused at the height of the untreated infection.

Nissl staining with cresyl violet revealed two distinct forms of neuronal injury: extensive cortical injury and selective injury to the dentate gyrus of the hippocampus (19). In the cortex, the injury pattern consisted of areas of reduced neuronal density, which were first seen approximately 18 hours after the time of infection and were fully developed by 24 hours. Foci of neuronal injury appeared throughout the cortex, often in areas that also showed the vasculopathy described above, and tended to be wedge shaped and thus suggestive of ischemic damage (Figs 8-1 and 8-2). Neurons in these cortical areas showed morphologic signs compatible with necrosis, such as marked swelling of the cell body and loss of cellular demarcation and cytoarchitecture. During therapy with antibiotics, the border between injured areas and areas with preserved neurons became sharply demarcated (19). By the third day, larger areas of injury showed the histologic appearance of a cortical pannecrosis, and became infiltrated with a population of mononuclear cells not present earlier (19). Extensive cortical lesions developed into cystic areas 2 weeks after the start of infection (19).

The pattern of injury in the hippocampus showed features that were distinctly different from those described in the cortex. Neurons in the granule cell layers of the dentate gyrus, predominantly in the lower blade (31), became markedly condensed, rounded, and shrunken (suggestive of apoptosis), beginning approximately 20 hours after infection (Fig 8-3). The apoptotic nature of this form of neuronal injury was further supported by positive terminal-deoxynucleotide-transferase mediated dUTP-digoxigenin nick end-labelling (TUNEL) staining in the dentate gyrus, but not the cortex.

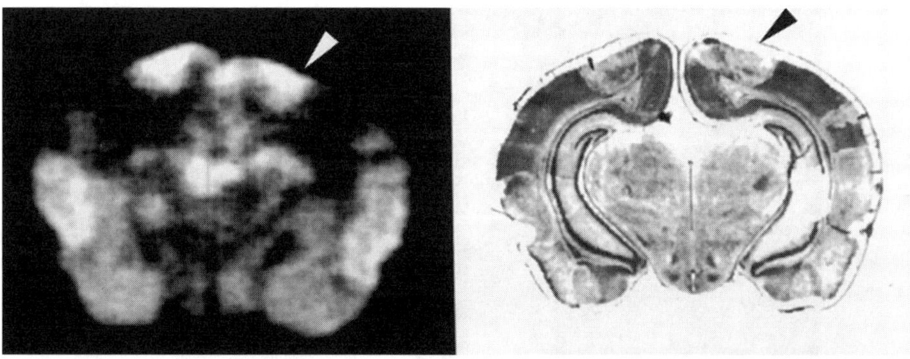

Figure 8-1. Infant rat with group B streptococcal (GBS) meningitis 24 hours after the time of infection. The T2-weighted magnetic resonance image (MRI) (left) shows patchy pathology with increased signal, suggestive of edema, throughout the brain with prominent involvement of the cortex (white arrow). The corresponding pathology section (cresyl violet) shows areas of decreased neuronal density in wedge-shaped distribution in the same location as the MRI abnormalities (black arrow). (MRI performed by Zina Vexler, PhD, USCF)

Approximately 10% of the condensed, rounded cells in the dentate gyrus were positive for the TUNEL staining, while less than 1% were positive in other areas of the brain, including the cortex and the CA1 to CA3 areas of the hippocampus (the most ischemia-sensitive areas of the hippocampus) (32). During the next 2 to 3 days, the neurons disappeared from the injured dentate gyrus, which became instead infiltrated by mononuclear cells (19). As with the cortical injury, the frequency of hippocampal injury depended on the inoculum size, and the extent of cortical and hippocampal injury correlated significantly ($r = 0.72$, $p < 0.001$).

Control animals injected with saline solution rather than bacterial suspension showed none of the changes in the subarachnoid space, cortex, or hippocampus described for infected animals. Also, animals infected with an isogenic, capsule-deficient mutant of the GBS (courtesy of Dr. Rubens, Seattle) developed a mild meningitis that was self-limited without antibiotic therapy and did not lead to brain injury as shown by histopathologic examination. This is compatible with previous studies using pneumococci and *Haemophilus influenzae* type b which found that the absence of a capsule prevents the development of a productive infection in the CSF (33–35), a finding attributable to the documented antiphagocytic properties of the bacterial polysaccharide capsule (34).

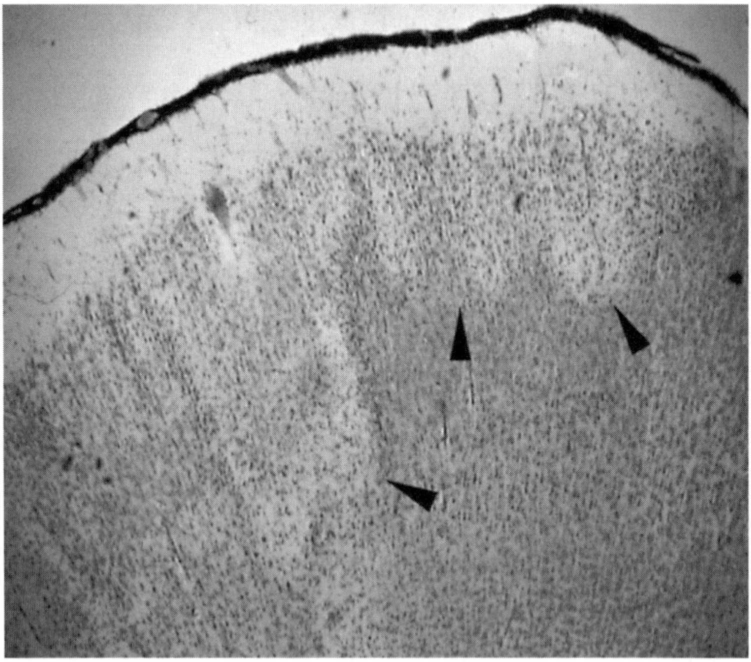

Figure 8-2. Higher-magnification view of an injured cortex in an animal with GBS meningitis 24 hours after the time of infection (cresyl violet). There are distinct areas of neuronal loss in a vascular distribution (arrows).

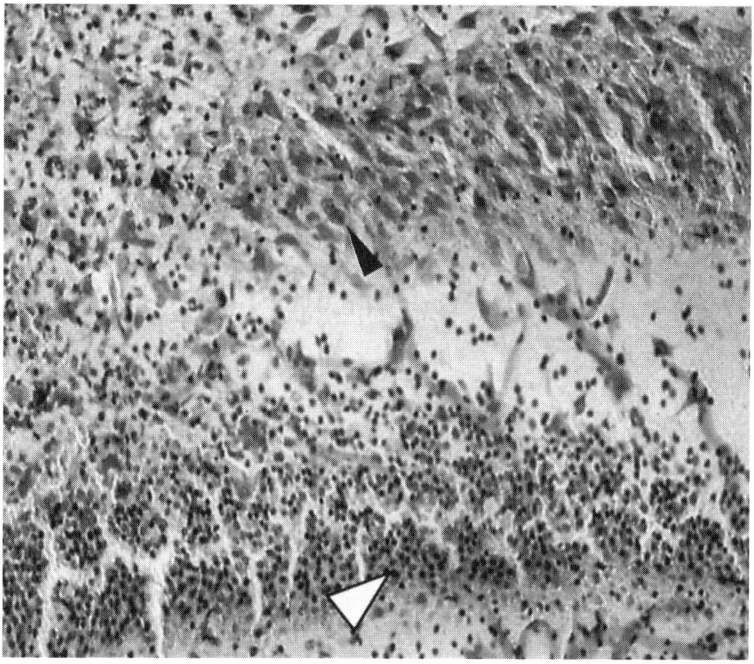

Figure 8-3. High-magnification view of the dentate gyrus of the hippocampus in a rat with GBS meningitis, 24 hours after the time of infection (cresyl violet). Most cells of the dentate gyrus are highly abnormal, with condensed, shrunken nuclei suggestive of apoptosis (white arrow). For comparison, see the normal neurons in the hilus (black arrow).

Glial Reaction

Based on immunocytochemical studies with antibodies that detect microglia (Ox-42), these cells reacted early and profoundly to the meningitic process in the infant rat model (Fig 8-4). In uninfected animals, microglia formed a homogeneous, continuous network of multiple, thin processes that contact each other. In contrast, microglial processes during meningitis became thicker and shorter and contacts between individual microglial cells were lost. Some areas of the cortex became devoid of staining almost completely in animals with severe meningitis. As the injury process progressed, Ox-42–positive cells with more rounded, larger cell bodies and only very few, short processes ("ameboid microglia") appeared. These ameboid cells were seen particularly in areas of severe injury (Leib SL, Täuber MA, unpublished observations, 1995). These changes of microglia are very reminiscent of similar changes seen with other forms of CNS injury, including ischemia in the neonatal rat (36–38).

Changes in astrocytes, as determined by immunocytochemistry for the glial fibrillary acidic protein (GFAP) specific for astrocytes, were delayed compared to those seen in

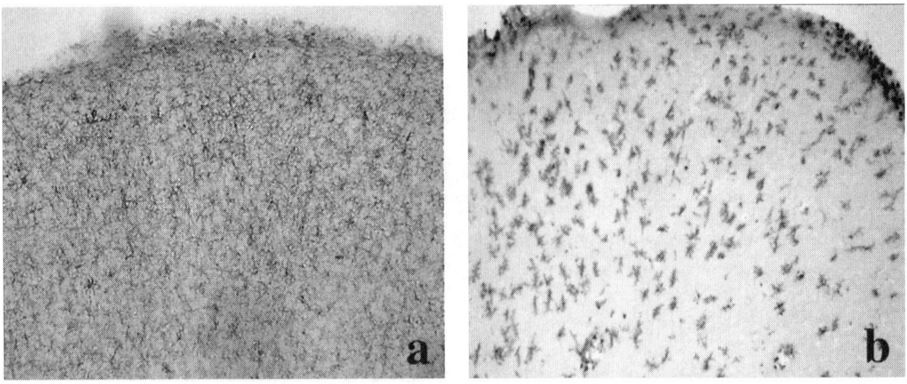

Figure 8-4. Immunocytochemistry for microglia with Ox-42 antibodies. (a) In an uninfected animal, the pattern is normal, with fine reticular, homogeneous staining throughout the brain with microglia with very small cell bodies. (b) In an animal with GBS meningitis at 20 hours after infection, the staining pattern is markedly altered, with reduced cellular processes, swollen cell bodies, and an apparent loss of microglial cells.

microglia. In normal animals, astrocyte staining for GFAP was weak throughout the brain, with few positive cells in the cortex and more positive cells in white matter tracts and the hippocampus. An intense reaction of the astrocytes to meningitis became apparent approximately 3 days after infection developed, and peaked at approximately 10 days. Positive cells often showed morphologic signs of activation with enlarged cell bodies and processes, and were seen along the surface of the cortex in the vicinity of the CSF inflammation, and along the border of areas of cortical injury. Within severely injured areas, GFAP staining was absent (19). Similar changes in astrocyte morphology were observed in humans with fatal bacterial meningitis (7).

Effect of Anti-Inflammatory Therapy in the Infant Rat Model of GBS Meningitis

To assess the role of inflammation in our model, we examined the effect of dexamethasone (1 mg/kg subcutaneously twice per day) started at the time of infection. Twenty hours after infection was induced, dexamethasone-treated animals had significantly lower clinical illness scores in spite of CSF bacterial titers that were approximately 1 $\log_{10}$/mL higher than those in untreated control animals ($p < 0.01$) (19). All animals were then treated with ceftriaxone, 100 mg/kg every 12 hours. Brains examined 2 to 3 days after the time of infection showed a marked reduction in subarachnoid and ventricular inflammation. This reduction was associated with a significant improvement of neuronal injury in the cortex in animals treated with dexamethasone plus antibiotics compared to infected control animals treated with antibiotics alone (19). The injury score for the hippocampus was not significantly different between the treated and untreated animals. Importantly in light of a recent report that dexamethasone may increase hippocampal injury (14), we failed to detect a harmful effect of dexamethasone. However, there was not much hippocampal injury in these experiments, thus limiting the power of our study to detect a difference.

We also examined the effect of a monoclonal antibody directed against TNF-α (courtesy of Dr. E. Huguenel, Bayer Corporation). Animals received saline solution or 20 mg/kg of the antibody intraperitoneally at the time of infection, CSF samples were examined 18 hours later, and the extent of neuropathologic changes was assessed 24 hours after the time of infection. Treatment with the antibody significantly reduced mortality ($p < 0.05$) and apoptotic neuronal injury in the dentate gyrus of the hippocampus ($p < 0.01$), but had no significant effect on CSF inflammation and cortical, ischemic neuronal injury (38a). To test whether the lack of effect on inflammation and cortical injury was a reflection of inadequate CSF concentrations of the antibody, we performed a second experiment in which the antibody was directly administered into the cisterna magna, resulting in estimated concentrations 10-to-100-fold higher than those after systemic administration. Again the antibody significantly improved apoptotic hippocampal injury without a measurable effect on cortical injury. These results suggest that TNF is only one of several cytokines contributing to the meningeal inflammation, but plays an essential role in inducing hippocampal apoptosis in this model.

Role of Cerebral Ischemia in Experimental GBS Meningitis

Bacterial meningitis is associated with marked changes in cerebral blood flow. In the early phase of meningitis, an increase in blood flow is observed in experimental models (39,40). This hyperemia appears to be mediated by NO (19) and oxidative radicals (41–43). In advanced meningitis, cerebral blood flow is reduced both in patients (44–47) and in experimental models, including our rabbit models of pneumococcal meningitis (48,49). Several clinical studies found an association between severe cerebral blood flow reduction and adverse outcomes in both children and adults with meningitis, suggesting that ischemia is an important mediator of brain damage in meningitis in humans (12,44,46,50).

Cerebral blood flow reduction during meningitis can be global or focal, the latter most likely resulting from vascular involvement of the cerebral arteries and veins by the subarachnoid space inflammation. Focal vascular involvement is apparent both by histologic examination (7,9) and by angiography, and may lead to temporary vasospasm or to more permanent thrombosis and vascular occlusion (45,47,51). In fatal neonatal meningitis, inflammatory vasculitis is uniformly present (8), possibly indicating that the cerebral vasculature of the neonate is particularly susceptible to inflammatory damage (17). This may explain in part the high frequency of severe sequelae in neonatal meningitis. The global hypoperfusion of the brain in advanced meningitis appears to result at least in part from pathophysiologic alterations. Brain edema, a common complication of bacterial meningitis, can lead to intracranial hypertension (52,53). This, in conjunction with systemic hypotension, leads to a reduction in cerebral perfusion pressure, which in turn can result in global cerebral hypoperfusion, because the autoregulation of cerebral blood flow is impaired during meningitis (40,54).

To explore the role of ischemia in causing neuronal injury in our model of GBS neo-

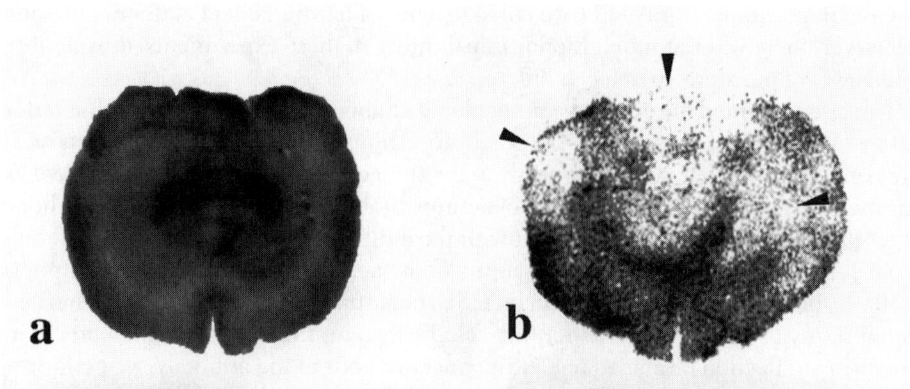

Figure 8-5. Measurement of cerebral blood flow by the iodo-[^{14}C]-antipyrine method. (a) In an uninfected control animal, there is intense, homogeneous signal by autoradiography. (b) In contrast, an animal with severe meningitis 22 hours after the time of infection shows global decreases of signal with superimposed areas of severe hypoperfusion (arrows).

natal meningitis in rats, we performed studies of cerebral blood flow by using the iodo-[^{14}C]-antipyrine method described by Lyons et al. (55). These studies showed that meningitis led to a global decrease in blood flow, on which focal deficits, primarily in the cortex, were superimposed (Fig 8-5). The focal deficits showed a pattern very similar to the pattern of neuronal injury documented by histopathology. These studies thus documented that the changes in cerebral blood flow expected to occur during meningitis do occur in our infant rat model and support the hypothesis that cerebral ischemia, particularly in the cortex, is an important factor in the development of neuronal injury. A critical role of cerebral blood flow for the development of brain injury is further documented by the results obtained with blockers of nitric oxide synthase (NOS) and ROIs, summarized below.

Nitric Oxide and Nitric Oxide Synthase in Experimental GBS Meningitis

Several recent reports indicated that NO may play a harmful role in meningitis, including in modulating cerebral blood flow (56–58). We therefore explored its role in our infant rat model of GBS meningitis. First, we documented the production of NO during meningitis by measuring CSF nitrite concentrations. Confirming reports by others in humans and animal models (57,58), we found CSF nitrite concentrations increased approximately 50-fold during meningitis compared to concentrations in uninfected control animals (58a). We then explored whether the increase of NO production was associated with an increased expression of the inducible NOS (iNOS) in the brain. Western blots of brain homogenates from animals with meningitis and control animals showed that the disease led to the expression of iNOS, which was undetectable in uninfected animals, while the constitutive neuronal NOS (nNOS) was present in similar quantities in normal and infected animals. Next, we measured enzyme activity of the two isoforms in brain homogenates and confirmed that iNOS activity was dramatically induced during meningitis, while the constitutive nNOS activity did not differ between infected and control animals. However, removal of the subarachnoid and ventricular space prior to homogenizing the brain reduced iNOS activity to levels close to those of uninfected control animals. Further studies using immunocytochemistry and in situ hybridization confirmed that iNOS was confined to the inflammatory cells in the subarachnoid and ventricular space and to the vessel wall of the subarachnoid vasculature (Fig 8-6). Importantly, there was no significant expression of iNOS in the brain parenchyma up to 48 hours after the time of infection (58a). This indicates that NO

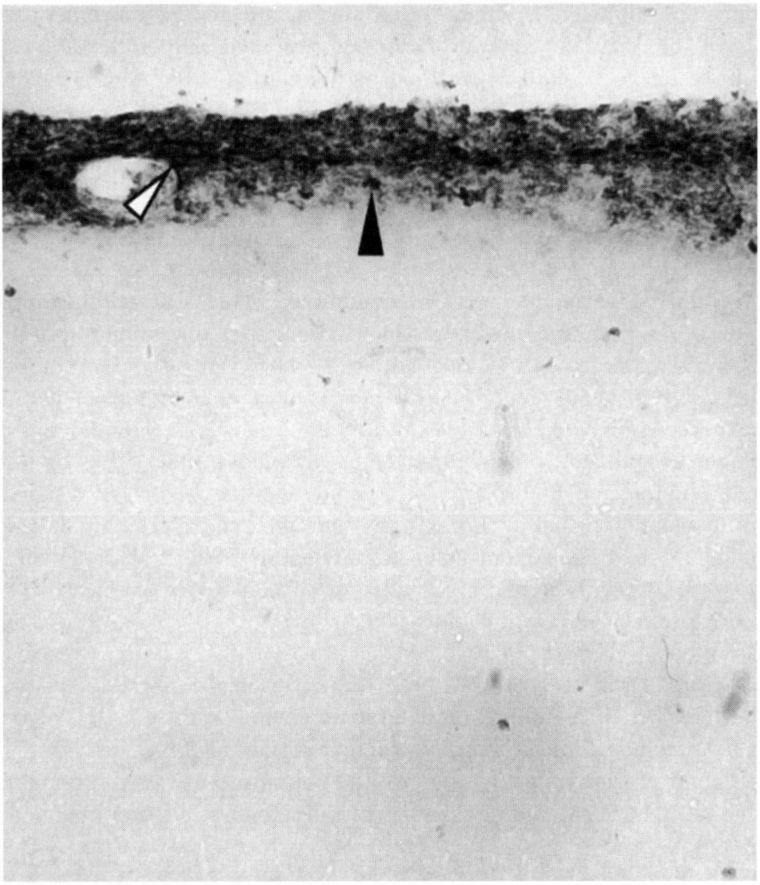

Figure 8-6. Immunocytochemistry for inducible nitric oxide synthase in an animal with GBS meningitis 24 hours after the time of infection. There is marked signal colocalizing with the inflammatory cells in the subarachnoid space (black arrow). Higher magnification (not shown) suggests that the signal is mostly localized to granulocytes. In addition, there is positive signal in the vessel wall of the subarachnoid vasculature (white arrow).

production by iNOS, in contrast to its role in our in vitro experiments (see above), is not a likely mechanism of neuronal injury within the brain parenchyma. NO from other sources within the brain parenchyma, notably from nNOS, may contribute to neuronal injury, as postulated for cerebral ischemia (59,60).

Effect of the Nitric Oxide Synthase Inhibitor Aminoguanidine in Experimental GBS Meningitis

Given the profound upregulation of iNOS and NO production by meningitis in our model, we evaluated the effect of inhibiting iNOS by administration of aminoguanidine (130 mg/kg subcutaneously every 8 hours), an NOS inhibitor with activity primarily against iNOS. When animals were treated with aminoguanidine beginning at the time of infection, CSF nitrite concentrations were significantly reduced as evidence for NOS inhibition by the drug (58a). However, aminoguanidine treatment led to a significant increase in brain injury, both when the drug was started at the time of infection and when it was started 1 hour after institution of antibiotic therapy, 19 hours after the time of infection (58a). Thus, while iNOS was upregulated in our model, its inhibition with aminoguanidine was detrimental for the neuropathologic outcome. Given the absence of iNOS upregulation in the brain parenchyma, it is not surprising that inhibition of iNOS with aminoguanidine did not reduce neuronal injury, but its detrimental effect still needed to be explained.

In light of the recognized role of NO in regulating vascular tone and the upregulation of iNOS in the vessel wall of the subarachnoid vasculature, it was an obvious step to examine whether treatment with aminoguanidine had a negative effect on cerebral blood flow as a possible explanation for its harmful effect on neuropathologic outcome. To indirectly assess cerebral blood flow, we determined the extent of cerebral perfusion at the time of death by perfusing animals with the highly water-soluble dye neutral red (61). Compared to uninfected control animals, animals with meningitis had a significant reduction in cerebral perfusion 20 hours after infection, in a pattern of both a global decrease and focal areas of marked hypoperfusion. Treatment with aminoguanidine further exacerbated the extent of cerebral hypoperfusion, particularly the extent of areas with severe hypoperfusion (58a). Thus, it appears likely that the harmful effect of aminoguanidine in this model is the result of increased cerebral ischemia in animals treated with this drug. These findings indicate that the NO produced in the cerebral vasculature during meningitis has a beneficial function by counteracting the processes that lead to cerebral ischemia. Importantly, these findings suggest that inhibition of NOS as a strategy for adjunctive therapy of bacterial meningitis has the potential for severe undesirable effects on cerebral blood flow and cannot, at least at the present time, be recommended for clinical studies (62).

Role of Oxidative Injury in Experimental GBS Meningitis

Many aspects of the meningitic process may involve oxidative radical generation and subsequent oxidative tissue injury (63). We therefore performed experiments to obtain evidence for the production of ROIs in the brain during meningitis and explored the effect of the potent oxidative radical scavenger PBN. Using a method to directly visualize the production of superoxide (perfusion of the brain with a manganese-containing buffer, followed by incubation with diaminobenzidine (DAB) (64)), we were able to document superoxide production in all animals with meningitis, primarily in two areas, colocalized with the inflammatory cells in the subarachnoid and ventricular space, and along penetrating cortical vessels (32) (Fig 8-7). Further evidence for the occurrence of oxidative injury was obtained by measuring end products of lipid peroxidation, an indicator of oxidative injury, in the brains of control animals and animals with meningitis (65,66). Meningitis led to a marked increase of lipid peroxidation, as measured by the concentration of maleonate and 4-hydroxyalkenals ($p < 0.001$) (32). Pretreatment

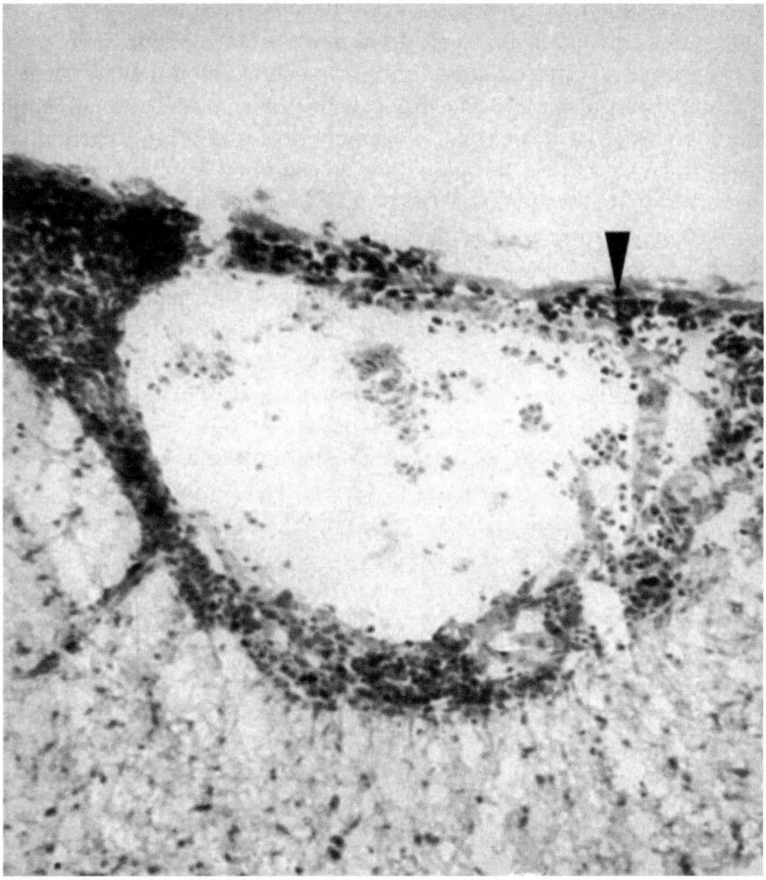

Figure 8-7. Manganese and diaminobenzidine staining in an animal with GBS meningitis 20 hours after the time of infection. Black crystals, as evidence for local superoxide production, are clearly seen in the subarachnoid space in association with inflammatory cells (black arrow). The positive signals are in close vicinity to a large vessel traversing the subarachnoid space.

with PBN (100 mg/kg subcutaneously every 8 hours) completely prevented the increase in brain lipid peroxidation and superoxide production. In parallel, pretreatment also completely prevented the development of brain injury, both in the cortex and in the hippocampus (32). These findings lend strong support to the hypothesis that meningitis leads to ROI production in the brain, which is associated with the development of neuronal injury, and that scavengers of ROIs are beneficial in this disease.

Based on these results, we then studied the effect of treatment with PBN (100 mg/kg intraperitoneally every 4 to every 8 hours, starting 18 hours after the time of infection, concomitant with antibiotics. We chose this time point because it represents the earliest time when neuronal injury becomes histologically apparent, while the full extent of injury is not yet established. Treatment at this later time was also highly effective in that injury was significantly reduced in the cortex ($p < 0.005$) and even more profoundly in the dentate gyrus of the hippocampus ($p < 0.001$) (32). Taken together, these data thus strongly point to a critical role of oxidative injury in bacterial meningitis.

Given the previously stressed importance of cerebral blood flow in our model, we assessed whether part of the beneficial effects of PBN on brain oxidative injury and neuropathology could be linked to a beneficial effect of PBN on cerebral perfusion. Animals with meningitis were treated with saline solution or PBN (100 mg/kg subcutaneously every 8 hours) beginning at the time of infection, and cerebral perfusion was assessed 20 hours later by the neutral red method (61). As in previous experiments, meningitis led to a significant reduction in cerebral perfusion. In animals pretreated with PBN, blood flow reduction was significantly less severe than that in untreated infected animals ($p < 0.05$) (32). Thus, one of the effects of scavenging of ROIs with PBN in the present model is amelioration of cerebral ischemia. These findings indicate that the production of ROIs in association with the cerebral vasculature contributes to the development of cerebral hypoperfusion and that prevention of cerebral ischemia is an important mechanism by which PBN exerts its neuroprotective effects, at least when given early in the disease.

Excitatory Amino Acids as Mediators of Neuronal Injury

The mediators most clearly identified as causing direct neuronal injury during meningitis are the EAAs (glutamate, aspartate). EAAs mediate neuronal injury in a variety of brain disorders (reviewed in (67)). In ischemia, the best-studied example of EAA-mediated injury, increased concentrations of EAAs in brain interstitial fluid result from increased release and reduced uptake from ischemic neurons and glial cells (68,69). EAAs act through binding to receptor-gated ion channels on neurons, among which the N-methyl-D-aspartate (NMDA) subtype may be the most critical for the induction of neuronal injury, at least in the developing central nervous system (70,71). NMDA-mediated neuronal injury results from an increase in intracellular calcium and appears to depend on the production of both ROIs and NO, the latter by neurons containing nNOS (59,60).

A role for EAAs in mediating neuronal injury in meningitis is supported by the following evidence. In a rabbit model, we showed that glutamate concentrations in brain interstitial fluid, as measured by microdialysis probes, are significantly increased in pneumococcal meningitis (72). Similar results were also found in experimental *E. coli* meningitis (73). We obtained more direct evidence for a causative role of EAAs in neuronal injury in our infant rat model of neonatal meningitis, in which we examined kynurenic acid, a nonselective inhibitor of the neurotoxic effect of EAAs (74). Animals randomly received 300 mg/kg of kynurenic acid or saline solution (controls) subcutaneously every 24 hours, and brain injury was examined 1 to 3 days later (antibiotics were given to all animals 20 hours after the time of infection). Kynurenic acid–treated animals had significantly less injury, both in the cortex and in the hippocampus at the end of the experiments. These results suggest that EAAs do play a role in mediating both cortical and hippocampal neuronal injury observed in our model.

SUMMARY

The development of a new model of neonatal meningitis in infant rats that is characterized by extensive neuronal injury of both necrotic and apoptotic characteristics has allowed us to start elucidating the pathways that lead to neuronal injury in meningitis (Fig 8-8). Guided by experiments in brain cell cultures, our in vivo work focused on the role of NO, ROIs, and EAAs. With regard to the necrotic injury in the cortex, cerebral ischemia has emerged as a critical mechanism of injury, and NO and ROIs seem to have opposing effects, with NO ameliorating ischemia and ROIs contributing to the vascular changes that lead to ischemia. In keeping with the ischemic nature of the cortical injury, EAAs have emerged as one important class of mediators of cortical neuronal injury. Whether NO and ROIs, in addition to their effect on cerebral vasculature, also act as neurotoxic molecules within the brain parenchyma needs to be explored in future studies.

Our results also suggest that the mechanisms of hippocampal injury may be different from those of cortical injury. First, the nature of injury in the hippocampus is apoptotic, rather than necrotic. Second, the affected hippocampal structure, the dentate gyrus, is not particularly sensitive to ischemic damage, whereas the ischemia-sensitive areas of the hippocampus, the CA1 to CA3 regions, were uniformly preserved in the present model. Third, a TNF-α antibody was significantly protective against hippocampal injury, while it had no measurable effect on the ischemic injury in the cortex. These findings suggest that ischemia is not the primary mechanism of apoptotic neuronal injury in the hippocampus. Rather, TNF and glutamate may act more directly on this structure, possibly as a result of the close physical proximity of the dentate gyrus to the ventricular inflammation. Both TNF and EAAs might induce, as their common toxic mediator, the production of ROIs, which play an essential role in the development of the hippocampal injury.

Further studies are needed to more clearly identify the molecular mediators of both the necrotic and the apoptotic injury present in the model of GBS meningitis in infant rats. The data presented suggest that this will be possible, and that the resulting knowledge will lead to a much more refined understanding of the molecular mechanisms of brain injury in meningitis. It is our hope that this refined understanding will help to develop potent new strategies for the adjunctive therapy of bacterial meningitis that will significantly improve the neurologic outcome of this disease.

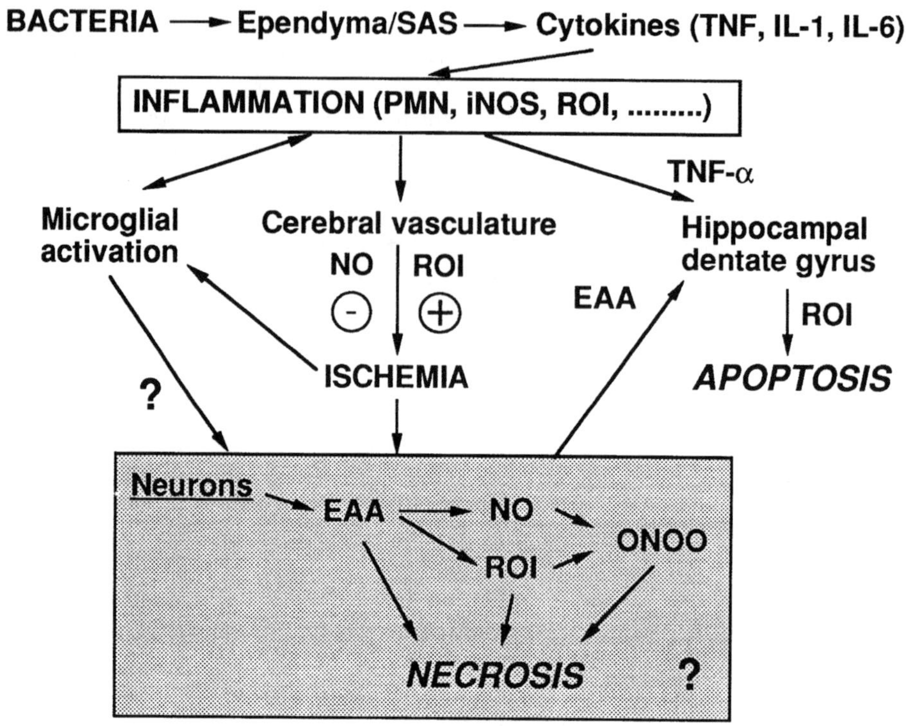

Figure 8-8. Schematic summary of the pathogenesis of brain injury in the infant rat model of neonatal meningitis caused by GBS. For details, see text. SAS = subarachnoid space; TNF = tumor necrosis factor; IL = interleukin; PMN = polymorphonuclear granulocytes; iNOS = inducible nitric oxide synthase; ROI = reactive oxygen intermediates; NO = nitric oxide; EAA = excitatory amino acids; ONOO = peroxynitrite.

REFERENCES

1 Klein JO, Feigin RD, McCracken GH Jr. Report of the task force on diagnosis and management of meningitis. *Pediatrics* 1986; 78:959–982.

2 Wenger JD, Hightower AW, Facklam RR, et al. Bacterial Meningitis Study Group. Bacterial meningitis in the United States, 1986: report of a multistate surveillance study. *J Infect Dis* 1990;162:1316–1323.

3 Kaplan SL, Hawkins EP, Kline MW, et al. Invasion of the inner ear by *Haemophilus influenzae* type b in experimental meningitis. *J Infect Dis* 1989;159:923–930.

4 Kay R. The site of the lesion causing hearing loss in bacterial meningitis: a study of experimental streptococcal meningitis in guinea-pigs. *Neuropathol Appl Neurobiol* 1991; 17:485–493.

5 Bhatt SM, Lauretano A, Cabellos C, et al. Progression of hearing loss in experimental pneumococcal meningitis: correlation with cerebrospinal fluid cytochemistry. *J Infect Dis* 1993;167:675–683.

6 Cairns H, Russell DS. Cerebral arteritis and phlebitis in pneumococcal meningitis. *J Pathol Bacteriol* 1946;58:649–665.

7 Adams RD, Kubic CS, Bonner FJ. The clinical and pathological aspects of influenzal meningitis. *Arch Pediatr* 1948;65:354–376, 408–441.

8 Berman PH, Banker BQ. Neonatal meningitis.

A clinical and pathological study of 29 cases. *Pediatrics* 1966;38:6–24.

9 Smith JF, Landing BH. Mechanisms of brain damage in *H. influenzae* meningitis. *J Neuropathol Exp Neurol* 1960;19:248–265.

10 Pfister HW, Fontana A, Täuber MG, et al. Mechanisms of brain injury in bacterial meningitis: workshop summary. *Clin Infect Dis* 1994;19:463–479.

11 Lebel MH, Freij BJ, Syrogiannopoulos GA, et al. Dexamethasone therapy for bacterial meningitis. Results of two double-blind, placebo-controlled trials. *N Engl J Med* 1988; 319:364–371.

12 Odio CM, Faingezicht I, Paris M, et al. The beneficial effects of early dexamethasone administration in infants and children with bacterial meningitis. *N Engl J Med* 1991; 324:1525–1531.

13 Girgis NI, Farid Z, Mikhail IA, et al. Dexamethasone treatment for bacterial meningitis in children and adults. *Pediatr Infect Dis J* 1989; 8:848–851.

14 Zysk G, Brück W, Gerber J, et al. Anti-inflammatory treatment influences neuronal apoptotic cell death in the denate gyrus in experimental pneumococcal meningitis. *J Exp Neurol Neuropathol* 1996;55:722–728.

15 Francis BM, Gilbert GL. Survey of neonatal meningitis in Australia: 1987–1989. *Med J Aust* 1992;156:240–243.

16 Anderson SG, Giulbert GL. Neonatal gram negative meningitis: a 10-year review, with reference to outcome and relapse of infection. *J Paediatr Child Health* 1990;1990:212–216.

17 Smith AL, Haas J. Neonatal bacterial meningitis. In: Scheld WM, Whitley RJ, Durack DT, eds. *Infections of the central nervous system.* New York: Raven, 1991:313–333.

18 Edwards MS, Rench MA, Haffar AAM, et al. Long-term sequelae of group B streptococcal meningitis in infants. *J Pediatr* 1985; 106:717–722.

19 Kim YS, Sheldon RA, Elliot BR, et al. Brain damage in neonatal meningitis caused by group B streptococci in rats. *J Neuropathol Exp Neurol* 1995;54:531–539.

20 Kim YS, Kennedy S, Täuber MG. Toxicity of *Streptococcus pneumoniae* in neurons, astrocytes, and microglia in vitro. *J Infect Dis* 1995;171:1363–1369.

21 Kim YS, Täuber MG. Neurotoxicity of glia activated by gram-positive bacterial products depends on nitric oxide production. *Infect Immun* 1996;68:3148–3153.

22 Ulevitch RJ. Recognition of bacterial endotoxins by receptor-dependent mechanisms. *Adv Immunol* 1993;53:267–289.

23 Ramilio O, Sáez-Llorens X, Mertsola J, et al. Tumor necrosis factor α/cachectin and interleukin 1β initiate meningeal inflammation. *J Exp Med* 1990;172:497–507.

24 Waage A, Halstensen A, Shalaby R, et al. Local production of tumor necrosis factor α, interleukin 1, and interleukin 6 in meningococcal meningitis. *J Exp Med* 1989; 170:1859–1867.

25 Talley AK, Dewhurst S, Perry SW, et al. Tumor necrosis factor alpha-induced apoptosis in human neuronal cells: protection by the antioxidant N-acetylcysteine and the genes bcl-2 and crmA. *Mol Cell Biol* 1995;15:2359–2366.

26 Chao CC, Hu S, Sheng WS, et al. Cytokine-stimulated astrocytes damage human neurons via a nitric oxide mechanism. *Glia* 1996; 16:276–284.

27 Chao CC, Hu S, Molitor TW, et al. Activated microglia mediate neuronal cell injury via a nitric oxide mechanism. *J Immunol* 1992;149:2736–2741.

28 Skaper SD, Facci L, Leon A. Inflammatory mediator stimulation of astrocytes and meningeal fibroblasts induces neuronal degeneration via nitridergic pathway. *J Neurochem* 1995; 64:266–276.

29 Ferrieri P, Burke B, Nelson J. Production of bacteremia and meningitis in infant rats with group B streptococcal serotypes. *Infect Immun* 1980; 27:1023–1032.

30 Kim KS, Bayer AS. Efficacy of BMY-28142 in experimental bacteremia and meningitis caused by *Escherichia coli* and group B streptococci. *Antimicrob Agents Chemother* 1985; 28:51–54.

31 Leib SL, Kim SY, Ferriero DM, Täuber MG. Neuroprotective effect of excitatory amino acid antagonist kynurenic acid in experimental bacterial meningitis. *J Infect Dis* 1996; 173:166–171.

32 Leib SL, Kim YS, Chow LL, et al. Reactive oxygen intermediates contribute to necrotic and apoptotic neuronal injury in an infant rat model of bacterial meningitis due to group B streptococci. *J Clin Invest* 1996;98:2632–2639.

33 Tomasz A, Saukkonen K. The nature of cell wall derived inflammatory components of pneumococci. *Pediatr Infect Dis J* 1989; 8:902–903.

34 Tuomanen E, Tomasz A, Hengstler B, Zak O. The relative role of bacterial cell wall and capsule in the induction of inflammation in pneumococcal meningitis. *J Infect Dis* 1985; 151:535–540.

35 Quagliarello VJ, Long WJ, Scheld WM. Morphologic alterations of the blood-brain barrier with experimental meningitis in the rat. *J Clin Invest* 1986;77:1085–1095.

36 McRae A, Gilland E, Bona E, Hagberg H. Microglial activation after neonatal hypoxia-ischemia. *Dev Brain Res* 1995;84:245–252.

37 Gehrmann J, Kreuzberg GW. Monoclonal antibodies against macrophage/microglial immunocytochemical studies of early microglial activation in experimental pathology. *Clin Neuropathol* 1993;12:301–306.

38 Andersson BP, Perry VH, Gordon S. The acute inflammatory response to lipopolysaccharide in CNS parenchyma differs from that in other body tissue. *Neuroscience* 1992;48:169–186.

38a Bogdan I, Leib SL, Chow L, Täuber MG. Tumor necrosis factor-α contributes to apoptosis in hippocampal neurons during experimental group B streptococcal meningitis. *J Infect Dis* (in revision).

39 Pfister HW, Koedel U, Haberl RL, et al. Microvascular changes during the early phase of experimental bacterial meningitis. *J Cereb Blood Flow Metab* 1990;10:914–922.

40 Tureen JH, Dworkin RJ, Kennedy SL, et al. Loss of cerebrovascular autoregulation in experimental meningitis in rabbits. *J Clin Invest* 1990;85:577–581.

41 McKnight A, Keyes W, Hudak M, Jones M. Oxygen free radicals and the cerebral arteriolar response to group B streptococci. *Pediatr Res* 1992;31:640–644.

42 Pfister HW, Ködel U, Dirnagl U, et al. Effect of catalase on regional cerebral blood flow and brain edema during the early phase of experimental pneumococcal meningitis. *J Infect Dis* 1992;166:1442–1445.

43 Pfister HW, Koedel U, Lorenzl S, Tomasz A. Antioxidants attenuate microvascular changes in the early phase of experimental pneumococcal meningitis in rats. *Stroke* 1992; 32:1798–1804.

44 Paulson OB, Brodersen P, Hansen EL, Kristensen HS. Regional cerebral blood flow, cerebral metabolic rate of oxygen, and cerebrospinal fluid acid-base variables in patients with acute meningitis and with acute encephalitis. *Acta Med Scand* 1974;196:191–198.

45 Förderreuther S, Tatsch K, Einhäupl KM, Pfister HW. Abnormalities of cerebral blood flow in the acute phase of bacterial meningitis in adults. *J Neurol* 1992;239:431–436.

46 Ashwal S, Stringer W, Tomasi L, et al. Cerebral blood flow and carbon dioxide reactivity in children with bacterial meningitis. *J Pediatr* 1990; 117:523–530.

47 Pfister HW, Borasio GD, Dirnagl U, et al. Cerebrovascular complications of bacterial meningitis in adults. *Neurology* 1992;42:1497–1504.

48 Täuber MG, Burroughs M, Niemöller UM, et al. Differences of pathophysiology in experimental meningitis caused by three strains of *Streptococcus pneumoniae*. *J Infect Dis* 1991;163:806–811.

49 Tureen JH, Täuber MG, Sande MA. Effect of hydration status on cerebral blood flow and cerebrospinal fluid lactic acidosis in rabbits with experimental meningitis. *J Clin Invest* 1992;89:947–953.

50 Goitein KJ, Tamir I. Cerebral perfusion pressure in central nervous system infections of infancy and childhood. *J Pediatr* 1983;103:40–43.

51 Thomas VH, Hopkins IJ. Arteriographic demonstration of vascular lesions in the study of neurologic deficit in advanced *Haemophilus influenzae* meningitis. *Dev Med Child Neurol* 1972;14:783–787.

52 Quagliarello V, Scheld WM. Bacterial meningitis: pathogenesis, pathophysiology, and progress. *N Engl J Med* 1992;327:864–872.

53 Fishman RA. Brain edema. *N Engl J Med* 1975;293:706–711.

54 McMenamin JB, Volpe JJ. Bacterial meningitis in infancy: effects on intracranial pressure and cerebral blood flow velocity. *Neurology* 1984; 34:500–504.

55 Lyons DT, Vasta F, Vannucci RC. Autographic determination of regional cerebral blood flow in the immature rat. *Pediatr Res* 1987; 21:471–476.

56 Tureen J. Effect of recombinant human tumor necrosis factor-alpha on cerebral oxygen uptake, cerebrospinal fluid lactate, and cerebral blood flow in the rabbit: role of nitric oxide. *J Clin Invest* 1995;95:1086–1091.

57 Koedel U, Bernatowicz A, Paul R, et al. Experimental pneumococcal meningitis: cerebrovascular alterations, brain edema, and meningeal inflammation are linked to the production of nitric oxide. *Ann Neurol* 1995;37:313–323.

58 Buster BL, Weintrob AC, Townsend GC, Scheld WM. Potential role of nitric oxide in the pathophysiology of experimental bacterial meningitis in rats. *Infect Immun* 1995; 63:3835–3839.

58a Leib SL, Kim YS, Black SM, Tureen JH, Täuber MG. Inducible nitric oxide synthase activity attenuates brain injury in rats. *Ann Neurol* (submitted).

59 Ferriero DM, Sheldon RA, Black SM, Jing C. Selective destruction of nitric oxide synthase neurons with quisqualate reduces damage after

hypoxia-ischemia in the neonatal rat. *Pediatr Res* 1995;38:912–918.

60 Huang Z, Huang PL, Panahia N, et al. Effects of cerebral ischemia in mice deficient in neuronal nitric oxide synthase. *Science* 1994; 265:1883–1885.

61 Selman WR, VanDerVeer C, Whittingham TS, et al. Visually defined zones of focal ischemia in the rat brain. *Neurosurgery* 1987;21:825–830.

62 Leib SL, Kim YS, Black SM, et al. Detrimental effect of nitric oxide inhibition in experimental bacterial meningitis. *Ann Neurol* 1996;39:555. Letter.

63 Carney JM, Floyd RA. Protection against oxidative damage to CNS by α-pheyl-*tert*-butyl nitrone (PBN) and other spin-trapping agents: a novel series of nonlipid free radical scavengers. *J Mol Neurosci* 1991;3:47–57.

64 Kontos CD, Wei EP, Williams JI, et al. Cytochemical detection of superoxide in cerebral inflammation and ischemia. *Am J Physiol* 1992; 263:H1234–H1242.

65 Esterbauer H, Cheeseman KH. Determination of aldehydic lipid peroxidation products: malonaldehyde and 4-hydroxynonenal. *Methods Enzymol* 1990;186:407–421.

66 Melchiorri D, Reiter RJ, Sewerynek E, et al. Melatonin reduces kainate-induced lipid peroxidation in homogenates of different brain regions. *FASEB* 1995;9:1205–1210.

67 Choi DW. Glutamate neurotoxicity and disease of the nervous system. *Neuron* 1988;1:623–634.

68 Koh J-Y, Gwang BJ, Lobner D, Choi DW. Potentiated necrosis of cultured cortical neurons by neurotrophins. *Science* 1995;268:573–575.

69 Sugiyama K, Brunori A, Mayer ML. Glial uptake of excitatory amino acids influences neuronal survival in cultures of mouse hippocampus. *Neuroscience* 1989;32:779–791.

70 Choi DW. Excitotoxic cell death. *J Neurobiol* 1992;23:1261–1276.

71 McDonald JW, Johnston MV. Physiological and pathophysiological roles of excitatory amino acids during central nervous system development. *Brain Res Rev* 1990;15:41–70.

72 Guerra-Romero L, Tureen JH, Founrier MA, et al. Amino acids in cerebrospinal and brain interstitial fluid during experimental pneumococcal meningitis. *Pediatr Res* 1993; 33:510–513.

73 Perry V, Young RSK, Aquilla WJ, During MJ. Effect of experimental *Escherichia coli* meningitis on concentrations of excitatory and inhibitory amino acids in the rabbit brain: in vivo microdialysis study. *Pediatr Res* 1993; 34:187–191.

74 Simon RP, Young RSK, Stout S, Cheng J. Inhibition of excitatory neurotransmission with kynurinate reduces brain edema in neonatal anoxia. *Neurosci Lett* 1986;71:361–364.

9 Mechanisms of Cerebral Malaria

DOMINIC KWIATKOWSKI

THE CLINICAL PROBLEM

Cerebral malaria is responsible for many more deaths than any other form of infectious encephalopathy. It makes its greatest impact in sub-Saharan Africa, where cerebral malaria and severe malarial anemia are estimated to kill a million children each year (1). In parts of the tropics and subtropics where transmission of malaria is more patchily distributed, it is often seen in adults and particularly migrant workers. In this era of global travel, it is an essential part of the differential diagnosis of coma anywhere in the world.

The central feature of cerebral malaria is coma due to *Plasmodium falciparum* infection. Many malaria patients become drowsy or disoriented but this is generally not called cerebral malaria, although the condition may be due to the same underlying cause. The criterion used by most research studies is failure to localize pain, which in children amounts to a Blantyre coma score of 2 or less (2). There are frequently convulsions, which can be protracted and are often subclinical. There may be additional neurologic abnormalities, including opisthotonus and other bizarre posturings, as well as hemiparesis and more subtle localizing features. But a significant proportion of patients simply have coma, without any clinical evidence of convulsions or other neurologic signs.

The case fatality rate varies geographically, and is typically in the range of 10% to 30% (2–4). Neurologic sequelae are relatively uncommon in adults but in African children they affect about 10% of survivors (2,5). Such sequelae often resolve with time and a recent study found that by 6 months only 4% of patients were still affected (6). There is a question of whether cerebral malaria leaves a substantial number of children with subtle forms of cognitive or motor impairment. The available psychometric data indicate that this is not the case (7), although it is a difficult question to evaluate in developing countries.

The clinical spectrum of cerebral malaria can be illustrated by three brief case histories. The first is a Vietnamese adult with high parasitemia who has jaundice and renal failure before falling into coma, and dies 3 days later of pulmonary edema. The second is a Gambian child with moderate parasitemia who, while playing with friends, suddenly starts to convulse and dies in coma a few hours later. The third is another Gambian child with exactly the same presenting symptoms who is profoundly comatose for 24 hours before waking up abruptly and returning to full activity within 4 days. The first scenario, which is common in Southeast Asia and in Western travelers who contract malaria, shows that cerebral malaria can be simply one component of a multisystem illness (8). But this scenario is extremely rare in African children with cerebral malaria in whom the function of other vital organs is generally not impaired. What the second and third examples illustrate is the remarkable polarity of clinical outcome in African children with cerebral malaria. Around 15% die within 48 hours, while most others walk out of the hospital within 4 or 5 days. This capacity for cerebral malaria patients to recovery rapidly from profound coma is in striking contrast to other forms of infectious encephalopathy, and suggests a transient toxic effect or metabolic derangement.

There have been numerous attempts to explain the coma in terms of a systemic biochemical disturbance. Although no satisfactory explanation has been identified, there are some important contributory factors. The most obvious is hypoglycemia, which occurs in about 20% of children with cerebral malaria (9). This is sometimes secondary to quinine-induced hyperinsulinemia (10), but in African children it is a primary complication with complex underlying mechanisms, and is associated with a poor prognosis (11,12). Occasionally a comatose child with falciparum malaria will wake up immediately after receiving a glucose infusion, but unfortunately this happens in only a very small proportion of children, and generally the child remains comatose despite correction of the hypoglycemia (9). Thus, hypoglycemia is important to the clinician, both as a complication to be treated urgently and as a prognostic marker, but it is not the main mechanism of coma. Lactic acidosis is another important complicating factor that signals a poor prognosis (10,12,13), but it is not a constant feature, nor is it usually of such severity as to explain the coma. Plasma electrolyte concentrations are generally normal, although hyponatremia can occur (14).

The diverse presentation of cerebral malaria can make it difficult to focus on the primary problem. For example, roughly a third of African children with cerebral malaria also have profound anemia or respiratory distress due to lactic acidosis (15). In Southeast Asia, as mentioned already, cerebral malaria commonly occurs in combination with multiorgan failure (8). But it is possible to dissect away from these complications a large number of instances where *P. falciparum* infection causes fatal coma without other organ failure or any obvious biochemical explanation. The crucial issues are the mechanism of the fatal coma, and why survivors are able to make such a speedy recovery. Research into these key questions is hampered by the lack of any comparable animal model.

Another question is why cerebral malaria and other life-threatening complications occur in some infected individuals but not others. In many tropical communities, the average child is reinfected several times each year, and severe complications arise with only a small minority of infections. The proportion has been estimated at 1% in The Gambia (16), but in populations exposed to a very large number of infective bites (e.g., 300 bites per person per year in parts of Tanzania (17)) the figure is clearly much lower than this. As will be described, recently there have been some significant discoveries concerning parasite and host factors that determine whether an infected individual is likely to develop cerebral malaria.

The following sections discuss our present understanding of the molecular and cellular processes that underlie the coma of cerebral malaria. The first point to emphasize is that in cerebral malaria, the parasites do not actually invade the brain. After a short sojourn in the liver in the initial phase of infection, *P. falciparum* resides exclusively within erythrocytes and is thus confined to the circulation. Whatever causes cerebral malaria must be secondary to pathologic events that are initiated from within the vascular compartment. There are two major hypotheses as to the primary mechanism, namely, parasite sequestration and the host inflammatory response. Readers who seek a comprehensive account of the debate up to 1992 are referred to the article by White and Ho (18). Over the years there have been vigorous arguments between champions of the different theories (19–22), but it is increasingly recognized that both processes may be involved.

PARASITE SEQUESTRATION

One of the things that distinguishes *P. falciparum* from other human malarial parasites is that in the later stages of parasite development, infected erythrocytes adhere to vascular endothelium and sequester in the tissues. Patients who die of cerebral malaria are usually found at autopsy to have parasitized erythrocytes congregating within small blood vessels of the brain (22,23). An example of this phenomenon is shown in Figure 9-1a. Although the total cerebral blood flow is not significantly impaired, there is evidence of cerebral anaerobic glycolysis associated with reduced oxygen consumption, consistent with microvascular obstruction causing a local metabolic disturbance (24).

The difficulty with sequestration as the sole explanation for cerebral malaria is that all *P. falciparum* infections sequester; that is, sequestration occurs with mild malaria as well as severe malaria. It also occurs at many sites other than the brain, including the heart, liver, kidneys, and skeletal muscles. Therefore, the question is whether cerebral malaria is caused by parasites preferentially sequestering in the brain. What is the evidence that patients with cerebral malaria have more parasites sequestered in cerebral blood vessels than do infected individuals who do *not* develop cerebral malaria? Or do they have denser sequestration in crucial locations such as the brainstem? A handful of pathologic studies tried to address this issue (23,25–29) but case definitions have tended to be lax and the literature remains controversial (21,22). The main deficit is truly quantitative data, and carefully controlled autopsy studies are urgently needed. It is an extremely tough problem for two reasons: Quantitating regional sequestration in a complex structure such as the brain is technically difficult, and the control subjects should strictly be individuals who are undergoing an uncomplicated episode of malaria fever, but who by definition rarely come to autopsy. Despite our ignorance concerning this key question, there is a wide consensus that sequestration plays an important role in the pathogenesis of cerebral malaria, though opinions differ as to whether it is the primary cause (22) or simply a contributory factor (21).

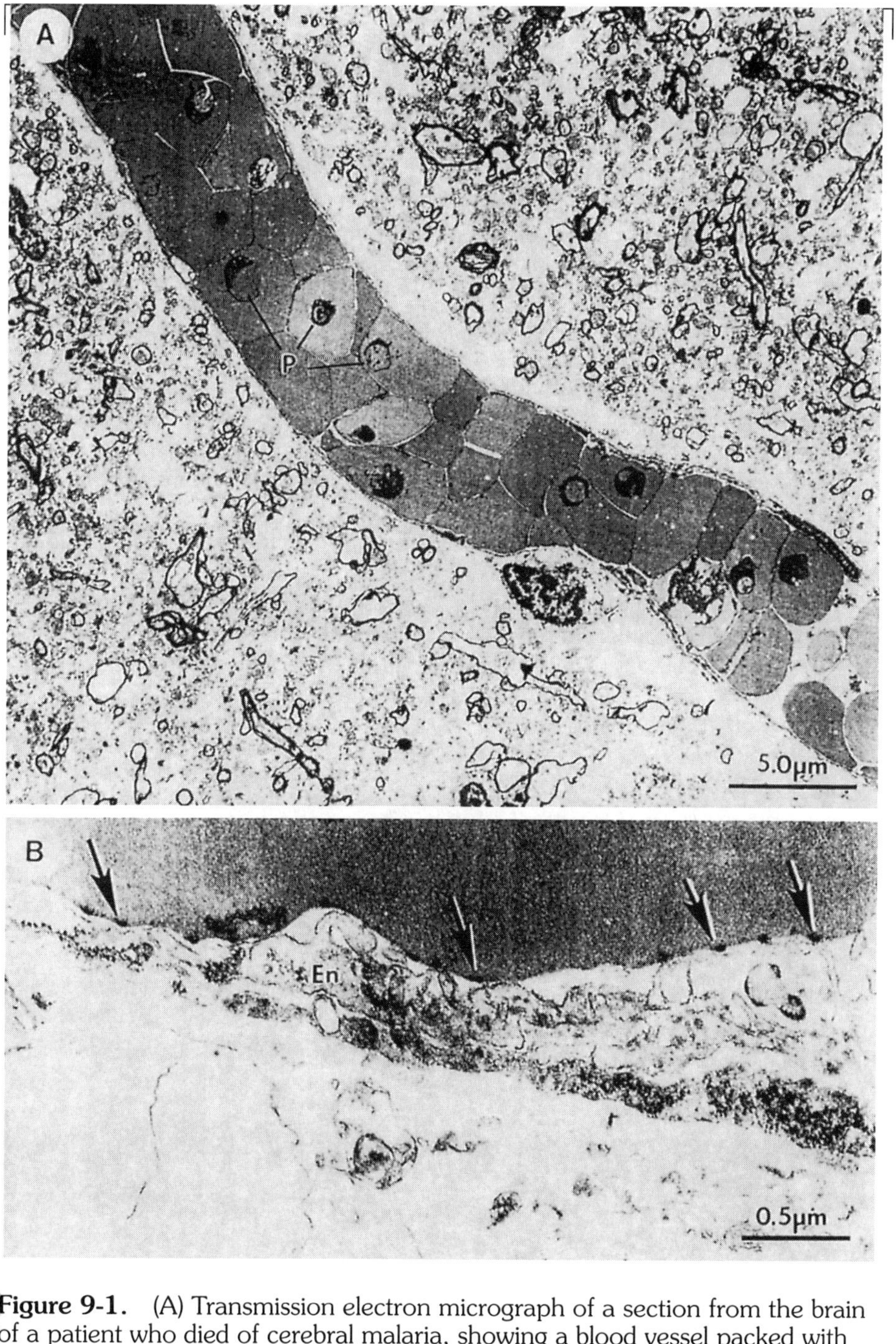

Figure 9-1. (A) Transmission electron micrograph of a section from the brain of a patient who died of cerebral malaria, showing a blood vessel packed with erythrocytes, most of which are infected. (Reproduced by permission from Berendt AR, Ferguson DJ, Gardner J et al. Molecular mechanisms of sequestration in malaria *Parasitology* 1994;108:S19–S28.) (B) Detail from the periphery of the blood vessel showing the characteristic knobs (arrows) at the surface of an infected blood cell in close apposition to the plasma membrane of the endothelial cell (En). (Courtesy of D.J.P. Ferguson, N. Day, and N.J. White.)

Molecular Basis of Cytoadherence

The last couple of years have seen huge advances in our understanding of the molecular basis of sequestration. For some time it has been recognized that parasite sequestration within small blood vessels is mediated by an interaction between molecules that the mature trophozoite causes to be expressed on the surface of the host erythrocyte, and receptors that are expressed on vascular endothelium (reviewed elsewhere (30,31)). This process can be reproduced in vitro, as shown in Figure 9-2. The endothelial receptors include a number of well-known adhesion molecules, and the outstanding issue has been the nature of the binding ligand on the surface of the parasitized erythrocyte. Until recently there was doubt in some quarters as to whether this constituted a single molecular entity, and whether it was truly synthesized by the parasite or, alternatively, formed from host membrane components. Most of these doubts were dispelled by an outstanding series of papers describing an extremely diverse multigene family that determines the major binding ligand and thereby explains the parasite's capacity to vary its cytoadherence phenotype (32–34).

The endothelial receptor utilized by the greatest variety of parasite strains is CD36 (35,36). Some but not all strains of parasite bind to intercellular adhesion molecule-1 (ICAM-1) (37,38) and this specific phenotypic property may be of considerable pathologic significance, as will be discussed later. One intriguing question was whether the parasite binds to ICAM-1 at the same site used by its natural ligand, leukocyte function

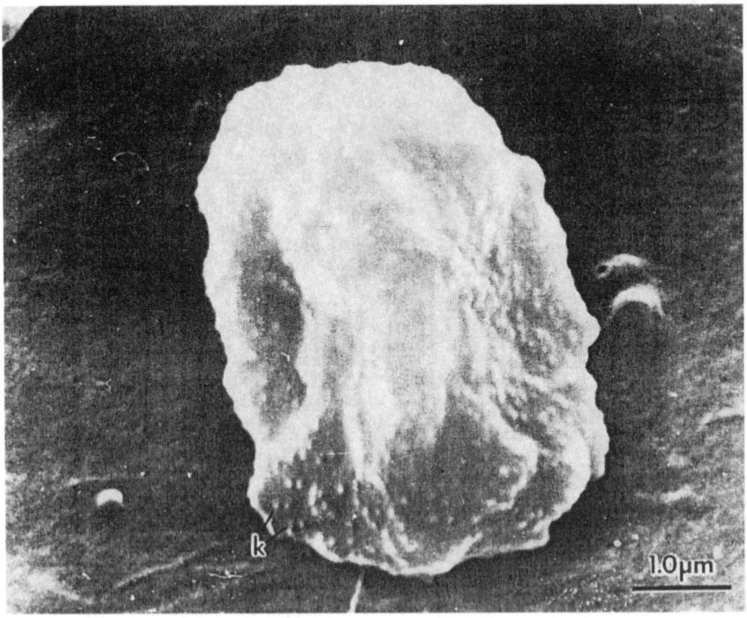

Figure 9-2. Scanning electron micrograph of an infected red blood cell, characterized by the presence of knobs (k) at its surface, cytoadhering to the smooth surface of a human umbilical vein endothelial cell monolayer. (Courtesy of D.J.P. Ferguson and A.R. Berendt.)

antigen-1 (LFA-1), and peptide mapping studies showed that it utilizes a distinct binding site (39,40). Studies under artificial flow conditions indicated that ICAM-1 mediates a rolling attachment that is relatively resistant to shear stress, whereas CD36 causes a high-efficiency static attachment (41). On this basis it has been proposed that parasites initially engage endothelium at high wall shear stress by means of a rolling interaction mediated by ICAM-1, followed by immobilization and stabilization via CD36 and other receptors. Other endothelial receptors to which parasitized erythrocytes bind are thrombospondin (42), E-selectin (43), vascular cell adhesion molecule-1 (VCAM-1) (43), and chondroitin sulfate (44). It is quite possible that other endothelial receptors for parasite binding have yet to be discovered.

The quest for the binding ligand on the surface of the parasitized erythrocyte has been, for malariologists, something of a holy grail. Its biologic interest has arisen from a set of fundamental observations made over the past 15 years or so. Firstly, cytoadherence phenotype varies greatly, not just between strains but also within a given strain over time. Secondly, infected individuals develop specific antibody responses to a neoantigen that is expressed on the surface of the erythrocyte, and several features indicate that this neoantigen is also the determinant of cytoadherence phenotype. Both antigenic type and cytoadherence phenotype become apparent at roughly the midpoint of the asexual growth cycle, both are highly trypsin sensitive, and both can be made to vary by successive passages through splenectomized and spleen-intact animals. There is evidence from rodent and simian models that antibodies to the neoantigen can suppress infection, which would be good news for vaccine developers if it were not so antigenically variable between strains. Finally, both cytoadherence properties and surface antigen expression are capable of true phenotypic variation; that is, parasites with widely different phenotypes can arise within a population derived from a single parasite. One experiment showed a parasite isolate from a single patient to contain some clones that bound to CD36, some that bound to ICAM-1, and some that bound to both (45). Single cells taken from one clone gave rise to a series of new cytoadherence and antigenic phenotypes, and the rate of appearance of these new phenotypes indicated an extraordinarily high switching rate, approximately 2% per generation.

The antigenic determinant and putative binding ligand on the surface of the infected erythrocyte is termed *P. falciparum* erythrocyte membrane protein-1 (PfEMP-1). The first clues as to its nature came from experiments on the simian parasite *Plasmodium knowlesi* (46) and subsequently *P. falciparum* (47), which revealed a family of large ($\geq$ 200 kd) trypsin-sensitive surface proteins, identified by radioiodination, that could be immunoprecipitated by homologous (but not heterologous) strain-specific antibodies. The evidence linking this protein family to cytoadherence was initially circumstantial, in that the strain-specific antisera used to immunoprecipitate PfEMP-1 also blocked cytoadherence in a strain-specific manner. It was not easy to proceed from these observations to a biochemical characterization of PfEMP-1, partly due to its low abundance but also because of its rapid phenotypic variation and the consequent heterogeneity of large-scale parasite cultures. The latter difficulty was recently circumvented by the observation that binding phenotypes differ in their sensitivity to sequence-specific proteases, which has allowed highly specific parasite subpopulations to be selected by a combination of protease treatment and receptor panning (48). One important conclusion of this analysis is that a single infected erythrocyte is capable of binding to at least three different types of endothelial receptors (in this case ICAM-1, CD36, and thrombospondin).

The molecular structure of PfEMP-1 began to be unravelled in 1994 with a remarkable convergence of results from independent laboratories. Russell Howard's group in Santa Clara, California, described the cloning of two related PfEMP1 genes from a single parasite isolate, and showed that antibodies generated against recombinant protein fragments reacted with the surface of parasitized erythrocytes and blocked cytoadherence to CD36, both in a strain-specific manner (32). At around the same time, while attempting to locate the chloroquine resistance gene, Tom Wellem's group at the National Institutes of Health (NIH), Bethesda, Maryland, discovered an extremely diverse family of *P. falciparum* genes encoding proteins whose size of 200 to 350 kd corresponded to that of PfEMP-1 (33). The sequence agreed with that found by the California group. These are now termed *var* genes, and each parasite has been estimated to contain 50 to 150 copies on multiple chromosomes. The predicted protein structure includes a variable extracellular segment, and this contains several regions of homology to a binding ligand that the parasite utilizes at a different stage of the life cycle, during erythrocyte invasion. The story was rounded off by the groups of Lou Miller in Bethesda and Chris Newbold in Oxford, who utilized a parasite clone tree to show that expression of variant antigenic determinants is correlated with expression of individual *var* genes (34). The members of the clone tree that were able to bind to ICAM-1 all expressed the same *var* gene, which was absent in lines that did not bind to ICAM-1.

This is clearly just the beginning of the story and it raises some fascinating questions. How is *var* gene expression regulated? How frequently can it switch within the lifetime of a single parasite? Is the switching process preprogrammed, or can it respond to extracellular signals? Is the genomic organization of *var* genes subject to continual rearrangements, and are individual *var* genes hypervariable? How is PfEMP-1 transported to the erythrocyte surface—does it have to cross the membranes of the parasite and parasitophorous vacuole, or is there an alternative route? How many potential binding domains does it contain, and when two different parasite strains bind to the same endothelial adhesion molecule, do they utilize the same binding domain? Is a significant part of the extracellular segment of PfEMP-1 conserved and, if so, why is the antibody response directed to the variable regions? Might it be possible to engineer a vaccine against relatively conserved regions of the molecule?

Although PfEMP-1 and the *var* genes explain a great deal of the cytoadherence phenomenon, they may not be the whole story. There is evidence that the presence of the parasite can alter the surface of the host cell by modification of the erythrocyte membrane protein band 3 (49). It is possible that these modifications play a role in sequestration, as synthetic peptides derived from band 3 (or antibodies generated against such peptides) can inhibit cytoadherence in vitro (50,51).

At the ultrastructural level, attachment to endothelial cells tends to be localized at small < 0.1 μm) bumps on the surface of the parasitized erythrocyte called *knobs* (23). These are illustrated in Figures 1B and 2. They are associated with submembranous aggregates of electron-dense material, which includes a histidine- and lysine-rich protein known as PfHRP-1 (52). It has been proposed that the basic residues on PfHRP-1 form salt bridges with the acidic terminal segment of PfEMP-1, thereby anchoring the binding ligand at the knobs (33). Initially it was thought that knobs were essential for binding, until it was discovered that cultured parasites can generate knobless forms which retain the ability to adhere to endothelial cells. The shift to a knobless phenotype is commonly associated with subtelomeric deletions of chromosome 2, where the PfHRP-1 gene is sited (53). Although knobs are not a prerequisite for binding in vitro, it is conceivable that their morphology favors sequestration in vivo. Another ultrastructural feature that was recently noted is the presence of immunoglobulin-containing fibrillar strands on the surface of infected erythrocytes, and it has been suggested that these may also play a role in parasite sequestration (54).

Clinical Correlates of Cytoadherence Phenotype

As noted at the beginning of this section, most malariologists believe cerebral sequestration to be a crucial step in the development of cerebral malaria, but quantitative data to support this relationship have proved difficult to obtain. Now that more is known about the molecular basis of sequestration, the question can be rephrased. Is there any evidence that cerebral malaria is associated with parasite types that bind to endothelial receptors preferentially expressed in cerebral blood vessels?

To address this question, investigators studied the in vitro binding properties of fresh parasite isolates taken from the peripheral blood of patients with cerebral or other severe complications of malaria, and compared them to isolates from patients with uncomplicated malaria fever. The earlier studies, which involved a relatively small sample size, measured binding to C32 melanoma cells (which serve as an artificial model of CD36-dependent binding) or to purified CD36 or ICAM-1 (38,55,56). These investigations revealed no significant relationship between cerebral malaria and parasite binding phenotype. Recently a much larger case-control study conducted in Kenyan children assessed binding against a panel of putative endothelial receptors including CD36, ICAM-1, thrombospondin, E-selectin, and VCAM-1 (56a). As expected, the strongest binding was observed to CD36, but there was no evidence that this was increased in cerebral malaria. The ICAM-1 data were a little more interesting in that binding to this receptor was significantly higher in patients with malaria fever than in those with asymptomatic parasitemia, and slightly higher still in those with cerebral malaria (although the latter difference was not statistically significant).

From these data, the clinical evidence in favor of cerebral malaria being determined by cytoadherence phenotype looks unimpressive. However, these studies should be interpreted in light of what we now know about the huge amount of phenotypic variation that is going on in a population of 10^{10} parasites, which is roughly the number present in a symptomatic individual. By sampling peripheral blood, we get a snapshot of the "average" phenotype of a mixed population of young parasites. This may be unrepresentative of the mature parasites that sequester within a specific tissue, because the local pattern of endothelial receptor expression will cause selective enrichment of certain parasite phenotypes at that site. Thus, it could be argued that if cerebral malaria is indeed caused by a specific cytoadherence phenotype, it might not be evident from the studies mentioned here.

Because of the limited information that can be gleaned from analysis of peripheral blood, there is growing interest in obtaining autopsy samples to explore the relationship between parasite phenotype and endothelial receptor expression in different parts of the body. As discussed already, case-control autopsy studies are fraught with practical difficulties, but a number of researchers are now addressing the problem. The best available data are from a study in Thai adults, which showed that fatal malaria was associated with an upregulation of ICAM-1 and E-selectin expression in the cerebral microvasculature (29). In contrast, CD36 and thrombospondin were weakly expressed in the brain. Quantitative analysis revealed highly significant colocalization of parasite sequestration with ICAM-1 expression in cerebral vessels and a lesser degree of colocalization with CD36 and E-selectin. The mechanisms of ICAM-1 upregulation in malaria are discussed in the later section on host responses.

Rosettes

Adherence to endothelium is not the only mechanism by which parasitized erythrocytes interfere with microcirculatory flow. Some strains of *P. falciparum* cause the parasitized erythrocyte to bind to uninfected erythrocytes, forming cellular aggregates known as *rosettes* (Fig 9-3). In contrast to endothelial cytoadherence, rosetting has been correlat-

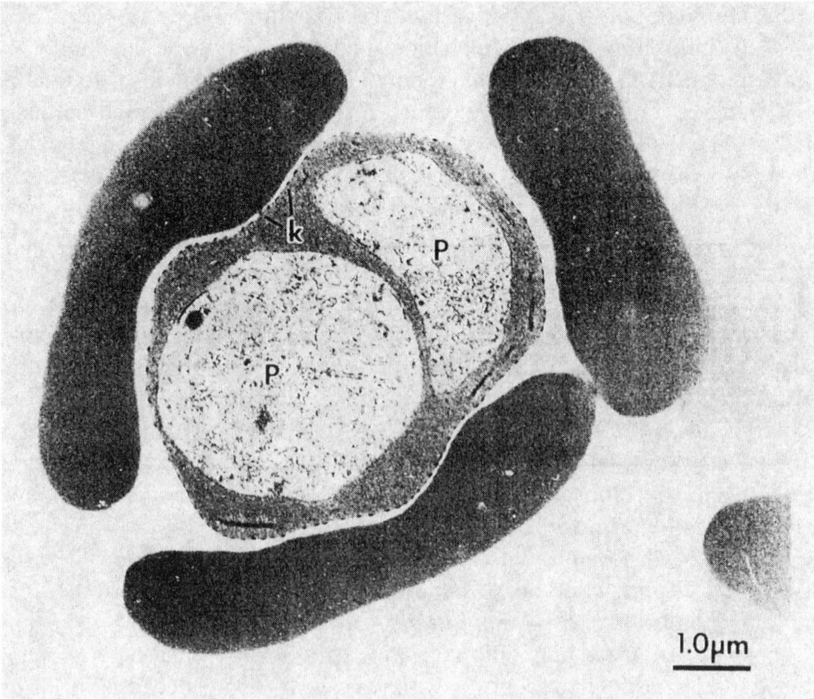

Figure 9-3. Transmission electron micrograph of a rosette. Note the close apposition of the uninfected erythrocytes to the central erythrocyte, which is infected with two parasites (P) and has surface knobs (k). (Courtesy of D.J.P. Ferguson and A.R. Berendt.)

ed with disease severity (57–59). An elegant rheologic study showed that rosettes can withstand arterial levels of flow stress, and that it requires five times more force to remove a cell from a rosette than is typically needed to disrupt endothelial cytoadherence (60).

Rosetting has also been studied under flow conditions using video microscopy of perfused rat mesocecal vessels (61). In the latter study, rosettes were disrupted in arterioles but they appeared to re-form in venules, resulting in increased resistance to flow. It has been pointed out (18) that if rosettes simply obstruct flow, they should lead to a tailback of both parasitized and unparasitized erythrocytes, and this would not explain the dense accumulations of parasitized erythrocytes typically observed at sites of sequestration (see Fig 9-1). But by slowing flow, rosettes may act to reduce wall shear stress and thereby create favorable conditions for parasitized erythrocytes to adhere to endothelium.

Like cytoadherence, rosetting is subject to phenotypic variation (45), raising the question of whether PfEMP-1 might be involved. However, the available evidence suggests that rosetting is associated with much smaller (22 and 28 kd) surface proteins termed *rosettins* (62). The putative rosetting ligand forms lectin-like attachments to various carbohydrate moieties on the uninfected erythrocyte, which might explain why erythrocytes of blood group O form smaller rosettes than do those of blood group A or B (63). Rosettes can be disrupted by various sulfated glycoconjugates including dextran sulfate, fucoidan, and sulfatide, suggesting intriguing possibilities for therapeutic intervention (64,65).

THE HOST RESPONSE

The role of host mediators in the pathogenesis of cerebral malaria has attracted much controversy in the past. Now it is widely accepted that the course of infection is influenced by host inflammatory mediators and adhesion molecules, and the challenge is to unravel the complex relationships that exist between parasite sequestration, the host response, and cerebral pathology.

Early attempts to incriminate host mediators in the pathogenesis of cerebral malaria involved experimental studies of rhesus monkeys dying of *P. knowlesi* infection (19). These data suggested that the central problem was the generation of kinins and other vasoactive inflammatory mediators that caused leakiness of the blood-brain barrier and consequently cerebral edema. This led to the belief that steroids were a valuable form of treatment. Subsequent clinical studies proved that these arguments did not apply to human cerebral malaria. Careful investigations in Thai adults with cerebral malaria revealed that the blood–cerebrospinal fluid barrier is essentially intact (66) and that cerebral edema may occur as a terminal event but is otherwise uncommon (67). Clinical trials showed that dexamethasone treatment does not improve recovery from cerebral malaria and can cause potentially dangerous side effects (68a). With the benefit of hindsight, these erroneous theories stemmed from an inappropriate experimental model. The rhesus monkey (*Macaca mulatta*) is not a natural host for *P. knowlesi* (69). Almost 100% of erythrocytes become parasitized and the infected monkey usually dies within a week of infection, retaining consciousness till just before death. In contrast, humans with fewer than 1% of erythrocytes infected with *P. falciparum* can develop coma, and complete recovery is possible. The lack of a suitable animal model has been one of the major obstacles to progress in this field of research.

In view of the devastating clinical effects of cerebral malaria, it is remarkable that autopsy reveals so few inflammatory changes in the brain (23). As described earlier, the most conspicuous feature is the accumulation of mature parasitized erythrocytes within capillaries and venules (see Fig 9-1). Focal hemorrhages may be observed, usually around small subcortical vessels, and these are commonly associated with a local inflammatory infiltrate, but the gross histology is otherwise relatively benign (70). Clinical measurements of intracranial pressure are broadly consistent with this pathologic picture. Most Thai adults with cerebral malaria have a normal intracranial pressure (66). When lumbar puncture is performed in African children with cerebral malaria, cerebrospinal fluid opening pressures tend to be modestly elevated (71–73). It has been suggested that this is secondary to increased cerebral blood volume (71), although some children have diffuse brain swelling of uncertain cause (74).

Thus, cerebral malaria research has followed a different path from that of most other infectious encephalopathies, in that it is difficult to identify inflammatory processes within the brain itself. Attention has focused instead on the generation of cytokines and other mediators within the vascular compartment. These are thought to cause pathology in two ways: 1) by affecting parasite sequestration, and 2) by interfering with cerebral function, either by their direct action on neurotransmission or by promoting metabolic disturbances such as hypoglycemia.

Tumor Necrosis Factor

Whereas cerebral malaria occurs with a small minority of infections, malaria in nonimmune individuals is invariably associated with fever. This occurs when billions of schizonts rupture out of host erythrocytes to release their progeny. Several lines of evidence have implicated tumor necrosis factor (TNF) as a critical mediator of malaria fever. Notably, malaria fever paroxysms are associated with a sharp rise in circulating TNF levels (75); the ability of TNF to induce fever has been well characterized (76); and monoclonal antibodies against TNF are capable of inhibiting the fever (77). Other endogenous pyrogens are generated during malarial infection and may contribute to the fever: They include interleukin (IL)-1β (78), IL-1α (79), IL-6 (80,81), and lymphotoxin (LT)-α (82). It is likely that the production of these mediators is modulated by interferon (IFN)-γ (79,83) and IL-10 (83), which are also present in malaria patients. This review uses TNF as an illustrative paradigm for cytokine-induced symptomatology, because it has been studied the most extensively, but clearly this is only part of the story.

A number of clinical studies showed that high TNF levels are associated with cerebral malaria (79,80,84). Several mechanisms have been proposed to explain this association (Fig. 9-4). One arose initially from investigations of the neurologic complications that occur during *Plasmodium berghei* anka infection in CBA-Ca mice (85,86). Although the pathology differs in several respects from that of human cerebral malaria, these data were the first to indicate that TNF released during malarial infection might

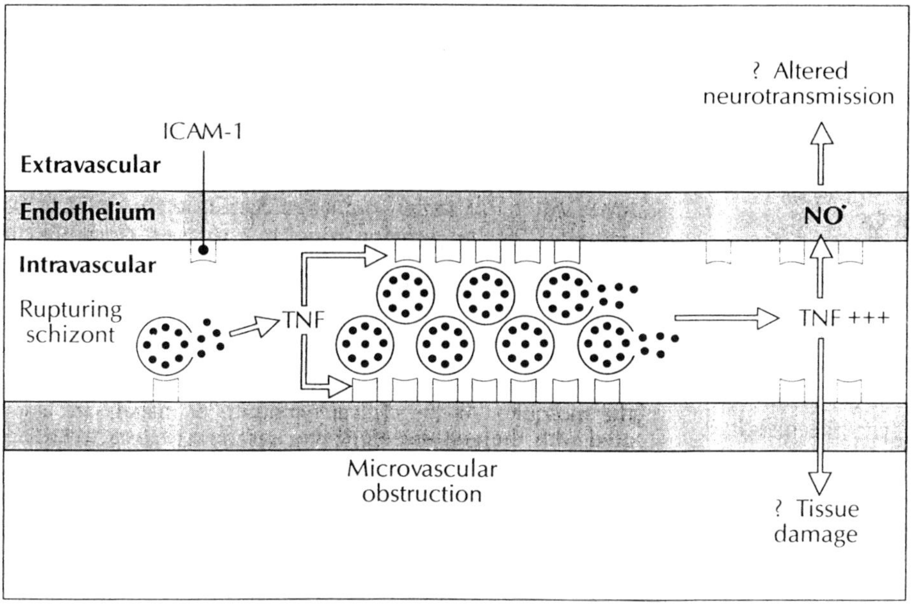

Figure 9-4. Putative interaction between host cytokine response and parasite cytoadherence in the pathogenesis of cerebral malaria. After binding to endothelium by various receptors, schizonts rupture to release toxins that stimulate circulating leukocytes to produce tumor necrosis factor (TNF). This leads to upregulation of intercellular adhesion molecule-1 (ICAM-1) expression and thereby enhances sequestration. The pathology results both from microvascular obstruction and from the local release of inflammatory mediators, which may promote ring hemorrhages or may directly interfere with neurotransmission. NO = nitric oxide. (Reproduced from Kwiatkowski D. Malaria: becoming more specific about non-specific immunity *Curr Opin Immunol* 1992;4:425–431.)

enhance endothelial adhesiveness and thereby promote sequestration in cerebral vessels. This was supported by the observation that some strains of *P. falciparum* bind to endothelium via ICAM-1, which is upregulated by TNF (37). E-selectin, another cytoadherence receptor, is also potentially inducible by TNF (43). In addition to promoting sequestration, a high level of TNF is likely to be one of the explanations why some cerebral malaria patients have hypoglycemia and lactic acidosis, which are associated with a poor prognosis (12,79,87).

From these observations, it was thought that monoclonal anti-TNF antibodies might be valuable in the treatment of cerebral malaria. However, a recent large study in Gambian children showed no effect on mortality, and a possible deleterious effect on neurological sequelae (87a). It is presently unclear whether this result disproves the general principle of anti-cytokine treatment for cerebral malaria, or whether it reflects on the specific properties of the antibody used.

Nitric Oxide

There is presently much debate about the role of nitric oxide (NO) in malarial pathogenesis. It is probably generated through several routes. Cytokines produced during malaria, such as IFN-γ plus TNF, can stimulate murine macrophages to produce NO. There is also evidence that substances released by rupturing schizonts can directly stimulate NO release by murine macrophages, independently of TNF (88). Although there has been doubt concerning the ability of human macrophages to produce inducible NO synthase (iNOS), there is growing evidence that this can happen in certain circumstances, and it was recently reported that iNOS is expressed in leukocytes of African children with *P. falciparum* infection (89). It also appears that the malaria parasite makes its own form of NO synthase (90).

There have been many reports that NO can inhibit the growth of malaria parasites at various stages of their life cycle within the human host (reviewed by Clark and Rockett (91)). But Clark and colleagues argue that when NO is generated from vascular endothelium, it can cross the blood-brain barrier and inhibit glutamate-induced calcium entry in postsynaptic neurons. This would lead to a reduction of neuronal NO synthase activity, thereby suppressing excitatory neurotransmission and effectively anesthetizing the individual (92). This would be a most elegant explanation of why the deep coma of cerebral malaria does not preclude a rapid and full recovery. The problem is how to test it in a clinical setting. Since NO has a short half-life, its production has to be assessed indirectly. This is conventionally done by measuring nitrite and nitrate levels in urine and plasma, but it is extremely difficult to exclude the confounding effect of dietary intake. Moreover, circulating nitrite/nitrate levels may be a poor indicator of NO generation within the brain, where the critical pathologic events are postulated to occur. Some attempts have been made to address the problem by comparing circulating or urinary nitrite/nitrate levels in children with different degrees of malaria severity: The results of two studies tend to support the theory (93,94) and those of one go against it (89).

Protection Versus Pathology

It is likely that the true biologic role of TNF and other inflammatory mediators produced in malaria is to protect the host. Some years before TNF was formally identified, there was evidence that unknown serum factor(s) elicited by endotoxin injection could attenuate the growth of malarial parasites in mice (95,96,96a). TNF may not be the only factor responsible but it appears to play a major role. Parasite growth is suppressed when mice are injected with recombinant TNF, or made to overexpress TNF by transgenic methods (97,98,99). In vitro studies indicate that TNF is not directly parasiticidal (98,100) and a variety of experimental evidence, summarised elsewhere (87,101) , indicates that TNF acts to kill parasites by promoting such responses as temperature elevation, phagocytosis by both neutrophils and macrophages, and the release of NO and reactive oxygen intermediates.

Thus the question arises of what distinguishes a TNF response that is protective from one that leads to cerebral malaria. Pathology is probably a consequence of deviation from appropriate levels of TNF production, and not the result of TNF production per se. The pathology induced by a given amount of TNF depends on the parasite's tendency to sequester, and probably other factors such as parasite density. TNF production is likely to be determined by a number of variables: strain variation in toxin expression by the parasite (102), the propensity of the host to produce TNF (103), the population dynamics of the parasite within the host (104), and the acquisition of antibodies against the parasite components that induce TNF (105–107) and other immune adaptations of the host.

As mentioned at the beginning of the chapter, one of the most puzzling and central questions about cerebral malaria is why it affects only a small proportion of infected individuals. What causes one child in an African village to become comatose when her siblings and friends suffer only fever, or may even be asymptomatic, with just the same levels of parasitemia? Part of the answer may be that cerebral malaria is a chance event, occurring when an unusually large proportion of the sequestered parasite population happens to congregate in a critical region of the brain. However in recent years it has become evident that genetic factors, involving both parasite and host, may be of critical importance.

An obvious area of interplay between parasite and host genetic factors is the relationship between the many different forms of PfEMP-1 and the variable patterns of endothelial receptor expression that are manifest by the host. Although many researchers see this as the likely root cause of the 'chance event' of cerebral malaria, it is an extraordinarily complex issue to resolve at the clinical level. Efforts are now underway to develop molecular techniques that might be used to explore this question in autopsy samples from fatal cases of cerebral malaria.

An equally important factor may be that both parasite and host appear to be genetically polymorphic with respect to TNF induction. Different strains of *P. falciparum* vary in their ability to induce TNF production by human monocytes, and wide differences in TNF-inducing activity have been observed among parasite clones derived from a single wild isolate (102). The genetic and structural basis of this polymorphism is unknown, but the available evidence suggests that like cytoadherence phenotype and surface antigen expression (45), the TNF-inducing phenotype can undergo variation within a population of clonal origin (102). A recent clinical study found that wild isolates from patients with cerebral malaria had, on average, somewhat higher TNF-inducing activity than did parasites from patients with mild malaria, but there was considerable overlap between the two groups (108). Thus, it is too early to draw any conclusions about how phenotypic variation in TNF induction affects disease severity, but it is remarkable that wild isolates appear to differ by up to 100-fold in the amount of TNF they induce in vitro, given the importance of this cytokine in both protection and pathology.

Genetic differences in the regulation of TNF by the host may also be important. At −308 nucleotides relative to the transcription start site of TNF is a biallelic polymorphism, the variant being a G to A transition (109). A large case-control study in Gambian children found that homozygotes for the $-308_{g \rightarrow a}$ allele had a relative risk of 4 for cerebral malaria, and of 7 for death or severe neurologic sequelae due to cerebral malaria (103). Importantly, the association with cerebral malaria was independent of variation in neighboring HLA alleles. This finding would fit with previous data on circulating TNF levels, which are abnormally elevated in cerebral malaria and highest in children who die or have neurologic sequelae (79). The implication of these findings is that the $-308_{g \rightarrow a}$ allele tends to upregulate TNF transcription and thereby determines susceptibility to cerebral malaria. Analysis of this hypothesis at the cellular level is limited by the difficulty of conducting receptor gene studies in human macrophages, and there are data both for (110) and against (111) a functional role for this particular polymorphism. Thus, it is conceivable that the association may have arisen through linkage of the $-308_{g\rightarrow a}$ allele to a functional polymorphism in a neighboring region of the genome. This question is currently being addressed in my laboratory by fine genetic mapping of the disease association in different populations, coupled with a functional analysis of the promoter elements that govern the TNF response to malaria in human macrophages.

The above findings provide some initial glimpses into mechanisms by which the malaria parasite and its host may have co-evoloved to their mutual advantage. Although the TNF response might seem disadvantageous for the host, causing fever and sometimes more serious complications, in evolutionay terms this may be an acceptable price to pay for a rapidly-elicited host defense mechanism against rapid parasite growth. The parasite may have little to lose by eliciting TNF since the process is density-dependent and is this unlikly to eradicate the infection (104). The problem is that humans have to cope with many different infections where similar 'negotiations' between parasite and host are involved—meningococcal disease and tuberculosis to name but two examples—and the appropriate level of TNF response for one type of infection may be inappropriate for another. The need for human populations to cope with a succession of different infectious epidemics suggests that there is no such thing as a single 'optimal' level of cytokine response. Such evolutionary pressures may underlie the variability that is found in the cytokine response to infection, and cerebral malaria may be partly a consequence of this natural diversity.

ACKNOWLEDGEMENTS

I thank David Ferguson, Tony Berendt, Nick Day and Nick White for the electronmicrographs in this chapter.

REFERENCES

1 Gilles HM, Warrell DA. *Bruce-Chwatt's essential marlariology.* London: Arnold, 1993.

2 Molyneux ME, Taylor TE, Wirima JJ, Borgstein A. Clinical features and prognostic indicators in paediatric cerebral malaria: a study of 131 comatose Malawian children. *Q J Med* 1989;71:441–459.

3 Boele van Hensbroek M, Onyiorah E, Jaffar S, et al. A trial of artemether or quinine in children with cerebral malaria. *N Engl J Med* 1996;335:69–75.

4 Hien TT, Day NPJ, Phu NH, et al. A controlled trial of artemether or quinine in Vietnamese adults with severe falciparum malaria. *N Engl J Med* 1996;335:76–83.

5 Brewster DR, Kwiatkowski D, White NJ. Neurological sequelae of cerebral malaria in children. *Lancet* 1990;336:1039–1043.

6 Boele van Hensbroek M, Palmer A, Jaffar S, et al. Residual neurological sequelae following childhood cerebral malaria. *J Pediatr* 1997 (in press).

7 Muntendam AH, Jaffar S, Bleichrodt N, Boele van Hensbroek M. Absence of neuropsychological sequelae following cerebral malaria in Gambian children. *Trans R Soc Trop Med Hyg* 1996;90:391–394.

8 Warrell DA, Molyneux ME, Beales P. Severe and complicated malaria. 2nd ed. *Trans R Soc Trop Med Hyg* 1990;84(suppl 2):1–65.

9 White NJ, Marsh K, Turner RC, et al. Hypo-

glycaemia in African children with severe malaria. *Lancet* 1987;1:708–711.

10 White NJ, Warrell DA, Chanthavanich P, et al. Severe hypoglycemia and hyperinsulinemia in falciparum malaria. *N Engl J Med* 1983;309:61–66.

11 Taylor TE, Molyneux ME, Wirima JJ, et al. Blood glucose levels in Malawian children before and during the administration of intravenous quinine for severe falciparum malaria. *N Engl J Med* 1988;319:1040–1046.

12 Krishna S, Waller DW, ter Kuile F, et al. Lactic acidosis and hypoglycaemia in children with severe malaria: pathophysiological and prognostic significance. *Trans R Soc Trop Med Hyg* 1994;88:67–73.

13 Taylor TE, Borgstein A, Molyneux ME. Acid-base status in paediatric *Plasmodium falciparum* malaria. *Q J Med* 1993;86:99–109.

14 English MC, Waruiru C, Lightowler C, et al. Hyponatraemia and dehydration in severe malaria. *Arch Dis Child* 1996;74:201–205.

15 Marsh K, Forster D, Waruiru C, et al. Indicators of life-threatening malaria in African children. *N Engl J Med* 1995;332:1399–1404.

16 Greenwood BM, Bradley AK, Greenwood AM, et al. Mortality and morbidity from malaria among children in a rural area of The Gambia, West Africa. *Trans R Soc Trop Med Hyg* 1987;81:478–486.

17 Smith T, Charlwood JD, Kihonda J, et al. Absence of seasonal variation in malaria parasitaemia in an area of intense seasonal transmission. *Acta Trop* 1993;54:55–72.

18 White NJ, Ho M. The pathophysiology of malaria. *Adv Parasitol* 1992;31:83–173.

19 Maegraith BG. Aspects of the pathogenesis of malaria. *Southeast Asian Trop Med Public Health* 1981;12:251–261.

20 Phillips RE, Warrell DA. The pathophysiology of severe falciparum malaria. *Parasitol Today* 1986;2:271–282.

21 Clark IA, Rockett KA. How important is mechanical blockage of blood vessels in human cerebral malaria? *Parasitol Today* 1994;10:409–411.

22 Berendt AR, Turner G, Newbold CI. Cerebral malaria: the sequestration hypothesis. *Parasitol Today* 1994;10:412–414.

23 MacPherson GG, Warrell MJ, White NJ, et al. Human cerebral malaria: a quantitative ultrastructural analysis of parasitized erythrocyte sequestration. *Am J Pathol* 1985;119:385–401.

24 Warrell DA, Veall N, Chanthavanich P, et al. Cerebral anaerobic glycolysis and reduced cerebral oxygen transport in human cerebral malaria. *Lancet* 1988;2:534–537.

25 Dudgeon LS, Clarke C. An investigation on fatal cases of pernicious malaria caused by *Plasmodium falciparum* in Macedonia. *Q J Med* 1918;12:372–390.

26 Kean BH, Smith JA. Death due to aestvo-autumnal malaria. A resume of one hundred autopsy cases 1925–42. *Am J Trop Med Hyg* 1944;24:317–322.

27 Spitz S. Pathology of acute falciparum malaria. *Mil Med* 1946;99:555–572.

28 Pongponratn E, Riganti M, Punpoowong B, Aikawa M. Microvascular sequestration of parasitized erythrocytes in human falciparum malaria: a pathological study. *Am J Trop Med Hyg* 1991;44:168–175.

29 Turner GD, Morrison H, Jones M, et al. An immunohistochemical study of the pathology of fatal malaria. Evidence for widespread endothelial activation and a potential role for intercellular adhesion molecule-1 in cerebral sequestration. *Am J Pathol* 1994;145:1057–1069.

30 Berendt AR, Ferguson DJP, Newbold CI. Sequestration in *Plasmodium falciparum* malaria: sticky cells and sticky problems. *Parasitol Today* 1990;6:247–254.

31 Pasloske BL, Howard RJ. Malaria, the red cell, and the endothelium. *Annu Rev Med* 1994;45:283–295.

32 Baruch DI, Pasloske BL, Singh HB, et al. Cloning the *P. falciparum* gene encoding PfEMP1, a malarial variant antigen and adherence receptor on the surface of parasitized human erythrocytes. *Cell* 1995;82:77–87.

33 Su XZ, Heatwole VM, Wertheimer SP, et al. The large diverse gene family var encodes proteins involved in cytoadherence and antigenic variation of *Plasmodium falciparum*-infected erythrocytes. *Cell* 1995;82:89–100.

34 Smith JD, Chitnis CE, Craig AG, et al. Switches in expression of *Plasmodium falciparum* var genes correlate with changes in antigenic and cytoadherent phenotypes of infected erythrocytes. *Cell* 1995;82:101–110.

35 Barnwell JW, Ockenhouse CF, Knowles DM. Monoclonal antibody OKM5 inhibits the in vitro binding of *Plasmodium falciparum*-infected erythrocytes to monocytes, endothelial, and C32 melanoma cells. *J Immunol* 1985;135:3494–3497.

36 Oquendo P, Hundt E, Lawler J, Seed B. CD36 directly mediates cytoadherence of *Plasmodium falciparum* parasitized erythrocytes. *Cell* 1989;58:95–101.

37 Berendt AR, Simmons DL, Tansey J, et al. Intercellular adhesion molecule-1 is an endothelial cell adhesion receptor for *Plasmodium falciparum*. *Nature* 1989;341:57–59.

38 Ockenhouse CF, Ho M, Tandon NN, et al. Molecular basis of sequestration in severe and uncomplicated *Plasmodium falciparum* malaria: differential adhesion of infected erythrocytes to CD36 and ICAM-1. *J Infect Dis* 1991;164:163–169.

39 Berendt AR, McDowall A, Craig AG, et al. The binding site of ICAM-1 for *Plasmodium falciparum*-infected erythrocytes overlaps, but is distinct from, the LFA-1 binding site. *Cell* 1992;68:71–81.

40 Ockenhouse CF, Betageri R, Springer TA, Staunton DE. *Plasmodium falciparum*-infected erythrocytes bind ICAM-1 at a site distinct from LFA-1, Mac-1, and human rhinovirus. *Cell* 1992;68:63–69.

41 Cooke BM, Berendt AR, Craig AG, et al. Rolling and stationary cytoadhesion of red blood cells parasitized by *Plasmodium falciparum:* separate roles for ICAM-1, CD36 and thrombospondin. *Br J. Haematol* 1994; 87:162–170.

42 Roberts DD, Sherwood JA, Spitalnik SL, et al. Thrombospondin binds falciparum malaria parasitized erythrocytes and may mediate cytoadherence. *Nature* 1985;318:64–66.

43 Ockenhouse CF, Tegoshi T, Maeno Y, et al. Human vascular endothelial cell adhesion receptors for *Plasmodium falciparum*-infected erythrocytes: roles for endothelial leukocyte adhesion molecule 1 and vascular cell adhesion molecule 1. *J Exp Med* 1992;176:1183–1189.

44 Rogerson SJ, Chaiyaroj SC, Ng K, et al. Chondroitin sulfate A is a cell surface receptor for *Plasmodium falciparum*-infected erythrocytes. *J Exp Med* 1995;182:15–20.

45 Roberts DJ, Craig AG, Berendt AR, et al. Rapid switching to multiple antigenic and adhesive phenotypes in malaria. *Nature* 1992; 357:689–692.

46 Howard RJ, Barnwell JW, Kao V. Antigenic variation of *Plasmodium knowlesi* malaria: identification of the variant antigen on infected erythrocytes. *Proc Natl Acad Sci USA* 1983; 80:4129–4133.

47 Leech JH, Barnwell JW, Miller LH, Howard RJ. Identification of a strain-specific malarial antigen exposed on the surface of *Plasmodium falciparum*-infected erythrocytes. *J Exp Med* 1984;159:1567–1575.

48 Gardner JP, Pinches RA, Roberts DJ, Newbold CI. Variant antigens and endothelial receptor expression in *Plasmodium falciparum. Proc Natl Acad Sci USA* 1996;93:3503–3508.

49 Crandall I, Sherman IW. *Plasmodium falciparum* (human-malaria)-induced modifications in human erythrocyte band 3 protein. *Parasitology* 1991;102(pt 3):335–340.

50 Crandall I, Collins WE, Gysin J, Sherman IW. Synthetic peptides based on motifs present in human band 3 protein inhibit cytoadherence/sequestration of the malaria parasite *Plasmodium falciparum. Proc Natl Acad Sci USA* 1993;90:4703–4707.

51 Crandall I, Sherman IW. Antibodies to synthetic peptides based on band 3 motifs react specifically with *Plasmodium falciparum* (human malaria)-infected erythrocytes and block cytoadherence. *Parasitology* 1994; 108:389–396.

52 Kilejian A, Sharma YD, Karoui H, Naslund L. Histidine-rich domain of the knob protein of the human malaria parasite *Plasmodium falciparum. Proc Natl Acad Sci USA* 1986; 83:7938–7941.

53 Pologe LG, Ravetch JV. A chromosomal rearrangement in a *P. falciparum* histidine-rich protein gene is associated with the knobless phenotype. *Nature* 1986;322:474–477.

54 Scholander C, Treutiger CJ, Hultenby K, Wahlgren M. Novel fibrillar structure confers adhesive property to malaria-infected erythrocytes. *Nat Med* 1996;2:204–208.

55 Marsh K, Marsh VM, Brown J, et al. *Plasmodium falciparum:* the behaviour of clinical isolates in an *in vitro* model of infected red blood cell sequestration. *Exp Parasitol* 1988; 65:202–208.

56 Ho M, Singh B, Looareesuwan S, et al. Clinical correlates of *in vitro Plasmodium falciparum* cytoadherence. *Infect Immun* 1991; 59:873–878.

56a Newbold C, Black G, et al. Receptor specific adhesion and clinical disease in *Plasmodium falciparum. Am J Trop Med Hyg* 1997, in press.

57 Carlson J, Helmby H, Hill AVS, et al. Human cerebral malaria: association with erythrocyte rosetting and lack of anti-rosetting antibodies. *Lancet* 1990;336:1457–1460.

58 Treutiger C-J, Hedlund I, Helmby H, et al. Rosette formation in *Plasmodium falciparum* isolates and anti-rosette activity of sera from Gambians with cerebral or uncomplicated malaria. *Am J Trop Med Hyg* 1992; 46:503–510.

59 Rowe A, Obeiro J, Newbold CI, Marsh K. *Plasmodium falciparum* rosetting is associated with malaria severity in Kenya. *Infect Immun* 1995;63:2323–2326.

60 Nash GB, Cooke BM, Carlson J, Wahlgren M. Rheological properties of rosettes formed by red blood cells parasitized by *Plasmodium falciparum. Br J Haematol* 1992;82:757–763.

61 Kaul DK, Roth EF Jr, Nagel RL, et al. Rosetting of *Plasmodium falciparum*-infected red blood cells with uninfected red blood cells en-

hances microvascular obstruction under flow conditions. *Blood* 1991;78:812–819.

62 Helmby H, Cavelier L, Pettersson U, Wahlgren M. Rosetting *Plasmodium falciparum*-infected erythrocytes express unique strain-specific antigens on their surface. *Infect Immun* 1993;61:284–288.

63 Carlson J, Wahlgren M. *Plasmodium falciparum* erythrocyte rosetting is mediated by promiscuous lectin-like interactions. *J Exp Med* 1992;176:1311–1317.

64 Rogerson SJ, Reeder JC, al Yaman F, Brown GV. Sulfated glycoconjugates as disrupters of *Plasmodium falciparum* erythrocyte rosettes. *Am J Trop Med Hyg* 1994;51:198–203.

65 Rowe A, Berendt AR, Marsh K, Newbold CI. *Plasmodium falciparum:* a family of sulphated glycoconjugates disrupts erythrocyte rosettes. *Exp Parasitol* 1994;79:506–516.

66 Warrell DA, Looareesuwan S, Phillips RE, et al. Function of the blood-cerebrospinal fluid barrier in human cerebral malaria: rejection of the permeability hypothesis. *Am J Trop Med Hyg* 1986;35:882–889.

67 Looareesuwan S, Warrell DA, White NJ, et al. Do patients with cerebral malaria have cerebral oedema? A computed tomography study. *Lancet* 1983;1:434–437.

68 Warrell DA, Looareesuwan S, Warrell MJ, et al. Dexamethasone proves deleterious in cerebral malaria. A double-blind trial in 100 comatose patients. *N Engl J Med* 1982; 306:313–319.

68a Hoffman SL, Rustama D, Punjabi NH, et al. Hig-dose dexamethasone in quinine-treated patients with cerebral malaria: a double-blind placebo-controlled trial. *J Infect Dis* 1988; 158:325–331.

69 Butcher GA. Models for malaria: nature knows best. *Parasitol Today* 1996;12:378–382.

70 Francis N, Warrell DA. Pathology and pathophysiology of human malaria. In: Gilles HM, Warrell DA, eds. *Bruce-Chwatt's essential malariology*. London: Arnold, 1993:50–59.

71 Newton CRJC, Kirkham FJ, Winstanley PA, et al. Intracranial pressure in African children with cerebral malaria. *Lancet* 1991; 337:573–576.

72 Kwiatkowski D, Molyneux M, Taylor T, et al. Cerebral malaria. *Lancet* 1991;337:1281–1282.

73 Waller D, Crawley J, Nosten F, et al. Intracranial pressure in childhood cerebral malaria. *Trans R Soc Trop Med Hyg* 1991; 85:362–364.

74 Newton CRJC, Peshu N, Kendall B, et al. Brain swelling and ischaemia in Kenyans with cerebral malaria. *Arch Dis Child* 1994; 70:281–287.

75 Karunaweera ND, Grau GE, Gamage P, et al. Dynamics of fever and serum levels of tumor necrosis factor are closely associated during clinical paroxysms in *Plasmodium vivax* malaria. *Proc Natl Acad Sci USA* 1992; 89:3200–3203.

76 Dinarello CA, Cannon JG, Wolff SM, et al. Tumor necrosis factor (cachectin) is an endogenous pyrogen and induces production of interleukin-1. *J Exp Med* 1986; 163:1433–1450.

77 Kwiatkowski D, Molyneux ME, Stephens S, et al. Anti-TNF therapy inhibits fever in cerebral malaria. *Q J Med* 1993;86:91–98.

78 Cannon JG, van der Meer JWM, Kwiatkowski D, et al. Interleukin-1 beta in human plasma: optimization of blood collection, plasma extraction and radioimmunoassay methods. *Lymphokine Res* 1988;7:457–467.

79 Kwiatkowski D, Hill AVS, Sambou I, et al. TNF concentration in fatal cerebral, non-fatal cerebral, and uncomplicated *Plasmodium falciparum* malaria. *Lancet* 1990; 336:1201–1204.

80 Kern P, Hemmer CJ, van Damme J, et al. Elevated tumor necrosis factor alpha and interleukin-6 serum levels as markers for complicated *Plasmodium falciparum* malaria. *Am J Med* 1989;57:139–143.

81 Molyneux ME, Taylor TE, Wirima JJ, Grau GE. Tumour necrosis factor, interleukin-6, and malaria. *Lancet* 1991;337:1098.

82 Clark IA, Gray KM, Rockett EJ, et al. Increased lymphotoxin in human malarial serum, and the ability of this cytokine to increase plasma interleukin-6 and cause hypoglycaemia in mice: implications for malarial pathology. *Trans R Soc Trop Med Hyg* 1992;86:602–607.

83 Wenisch C, Parschalk B, Narzt E, et al. Elevated serum levels of IL-10 and IFN-gamma in patients with acute *Plasmodium falciparum* malaria. *Clin Immunol Immunopathol* 1995; 74:115–117.

84 Grau GE, Taylor TE, Molyneux ME, et al. Tumor necrosis factor and disease severity in children with falciparum malaria. *N Engl J Med* 1989;320:1586–1591.

85 Grau GE, Fajardo LF, Piguet P-F, et al. Tumor necrosis factor (cachectin) as an essential mediator in murine cerebral malaria. *Science* 1987;237:1210–1212.

86 Grau GE, Pointaire P, Piguet P-F, et al. Late administration of monoclonal antibody to leucocyte function-antigen 1 abrogates incipient murine cerebral malaria. *Eur J Immunol* 1991;21:2265–2267.

87 Clark IA, Rockett KA, Cowden WB. TNF in

malaria. In: Beutler B, ed. *Tumor necrosis factors. The molecules and their emerging role in medicine.* New York: Raven, 1992:303–328.

87a Boele van Hensbroek M, Palmer A, Onyiorah E, et al. The effect of a monoclonal antibody to tumour necrosis factor on survival from childhood cerebral malaria. *J Infect Dis* 1996; 174:1091–1097.

88 Rockett KA, Kwiatkowski D, Bate CAW, et al. *In vitro* induction of nitric oxide by an extract of *Plasmodium falciparum. J Infect* 1996; 32:187–196.

89 Anstey NM, Weinberg JB, Hassanali MY, et al. Nitric oxide in Tanzanian children with malaria: inverse relationship between malaria severity and nitric oxide production/nitric oxide synthase type 2 expression. *J Exp Med* 1996;184:557–567.

90 Ghigo D, Todde R, Ginsburg H, et al. Erythrocyte stages of *Plasmodium falciparum* exhibit a high nitric oxide synthase (NOS) activity and release an NOS-inducing soluble factor. *J Exp Med* 1995;182:677–688.

91 Clark IA, Rockett KA. Nitric oxide and parasitic disease. *Adv Parasitol* 1996;37:1–56.

92 Clark IA, Rockett KA, Cowden WB. Proposed central role of nitric oxide in conditions clinically similar to cerebral malaria. *Lancet* 1992; 340:894–895.

93 Kremsner P, Winkler S, Wilding E, et al. High plasma levels of nitrogen oxides are associated with severe disease and correlate with rapid parasitological and clinical cure in *Plasmodium falciparum* malaria. *Trans R Soc Trop Med Hyg* 1996;90:44–47.

94 Al Yaman FM, Mokela D, Genton B, et al. Association between serum levels of reactive nitrogen intermediates and coma in children with cerebral malaria in Papua New Guinea. *Trans R Soc Trop Med Hyg* 1996;90:270–273.

95 Martin LK, Einheber A, Sadun EH, Wren RE. Effect of bacterial endotoxin on the course of *Plasmodium berghei* infection. *Exp Parasitol* 1967;20:186–199.

96 Clark IA. Does endotoxin cause both the disease and parasite death in acute malaria and babesiosis? *Lancet* 1978; ii:75–78.

96a Taverne J, Dockrell HM, Playfair JHL. Endotoxin-induced serum factor kills malarial parasites in vitro. *Infect Immun* 1981; 33:83–89.

97 Clark IA, Hunt NH, Butcher GA, Cowden WB. Inhibition of murine malaria (*Plasmodium chabaudi*) in vivo by recombinant interferon-gamma or tumor necrosis factor, and its enhancement by butylated hydroxyanisole. *J Immunol* 1987;139:3493–3496.

98 Taverne J, Tavernier J, Fiers W, Playfair JHL. Recombinant tumour necrosis factor inhibits malaria parasites *in vivo* but not *in vitro. Clin Exp Immunol* 1987;67:1–4.

99 Taverne J, Sheikh N, de Souza JB, et al. Anaemia and resistance to malaria in transgenic mice expressing human tumour necrosis factor. *Immunology* 1994;82:397–403.

100 Jensen JB, Vande Waa JA, Karadsheh AJ. Tumor necrosis factor does not induce *Plasmodium falciparum* crisis forms. *Infect Immun* 1987;55:1722–1724.

101 Kwiatkowski D. Malarial toxins and the regulation of parasite density. *Parasitol Today* 1995;11:206–212.

102 Allan RJ, Rowe A, Kwiatkowski D. *Plasmodium falciparum* varies in its ability to induce tumor necrosis factor. *Infect Immun* 1993;61:4772–4776.

103 McGuire W, Hill AVS, Allsopp CEM, et al. Variation in the TNF-α promoter region is associated with susceptibility to cerebral malaria. *Nature* 1994;371:508–511.

104 Kwiatkowski D, Nowak M. Periodic and chaotic host-parasite interactions in human malaria. *Proc Natl Acad Sci USA* 1991; 88: 5111–5113.

105 Bate CAW, Taverne J, Davé A, Playfair JHL. Malaria exoantigens induce T-independent antibody that blocks their ability to induce TNF. *Immunology* 1990;70:315–320.

106 Playfair JHL, Taverne J, Bate CAW, de Souza JB. The malaria vaccine: anti-parasite or anti-disease? *Immunol Today* 1990;11:25–27.

107 Bate CAW, Kwiatkowski D. Inhibitory immunoglobulin M antibodies to tumor necrosis factor-inducing toxins in patients with malaria. *Infect Immun* 1994;62:3086–3091.

108 Allan RJ, Beattie P, Bate CAW, et al. Strain variation in TNF induction by parasites from children with falciparum malaria. *Infect Immun* 1995;63:1173–1175.

109 Wilson AG, di Giovine FS, Blakemore AIF, Duff GW. Single base polymorphism in the human tumour necrosis factor alpha gene detectable by *Nco*I restriction of PCR product. *Hum Mol Genet* 1992; 1:353.

110 Wilson AG, Symons JA, McDowell TA, et al. Effects of a polymorphism in the human TNF-alpha promoter on transcriptional activation. *Proc Natl Acad Sci USA* 1997; in press.

111 Stuber F, Udalova IA, Book M, et al. -308 TNF polymorphism is not associated with survival in severe sepsis and is unrelated to lipopolysaccharide inducibility of the human TNF promoter. *J Inflammation* 1996;46:42–50.

10

Toxoplasmosis of the Central Nervous System

JOSE G. MONTOYA
JACK S. REMINGTON

TOXOPLASMOSIS OF THE CENTRAL NERVOUS SYSTEM

Toxoplasmosis of the central nervous system (CNS) in congenitally infected newborns was first reported in 1939 (1). Although brain involvement in adults was rarely reported in the ensuing years, the remarkable report by Vietzke and his colleagues in 1968 highlighted *Toxoplasma gondii* as a cause of life-threatening infection of the brain in patients with malignancy (2). Thereafter, numerous reports expanded on *T. gondii* as a cause of CNS disease in the immunocompromised host (3–5). The most recent development in the saga of the parasite as a cause of serious disease of the brain was the advent of acquired immunodeficiency syndrome (AIDS). Prior to routine use of prophylaxis for toxoplasmosis, as many as 25% to 50% of AIDS patients with pre-existing *T. gondii* antibodies developed toxoplasmic encephalitis (6,7).

T. gondii is transmitted primarily via the oral route and the definitive hosts are members of the cat family (8). The primary encounter between this intracellular pathogen and its incidental human host most often goes unrecognized. This primary event leads to a chronic (latent) infection that can reactivate in a setting of impaired host immunity. In approximately 10% of immunocompetent adults and children, acute infection results in a self-limited and nonspecific illness that rarely requires treatment. The most frequently observed clinical manifestation is lymphadenopathy and fatigue without fever (8,9). Immunity in the immunocompetent host is lifelong. Reinfection occurs but does not appear to result in clinically apparent disease.

In contrast to the usually benign course of the initial infection in immunologically intact hosts, reactivation of the chronic infection can occur in severely immunocompromised individuals and result in widespread dissemination of the parasite, often with a devastating outcome. The CNS is almost always the most seriously affected site.

Wolf, Cowen, and Paige (1) first reported toxoplasmic encephalitis in humans. In 1939, these investigators described a newborn who presented with seizures on the third day of life, intracranial calcifications, hydrocephalus, and chorioretinitis. Autopsy revealed widespread encephalomyelitis characterized by multiple focal areas of inflammation and necrosis. Some of the lesions in the cerebral cortex showed a distinct tendency to become calcified. In the right eye there was a localized zone of chorioretinitis. *T. gondii* was observed in lesions of both the brain and the eye (1).

Before 1968, there were only sporadic reports of life-threatening infection with *Toxoplasma* in patients with cancer. In that year, Vietzke et al. (2) reported the first series of patients with malignancy in whom *T. gondii* was the cause of encephalitis. The major pathologic lesion in their six patients was a necrotizing encephalitis of the gray matter. The authors noted the remarkable predilection of the organism for the CNS, its misdiagnosis premortem, and the mortality associated with this disease in the brain.

In 1979, McLeod et al. (10) first reported *Toxoplasma* species as a cause of brain abscess. This occurred in a heart transplant recipient who was seronegative before transplantation and who had received a heart from a seropositive donor. With the onset of the AIDS epidemic, toxoplasmosis was recognized as a cause of both diffuse lesions and abscesses in the brain and spinal cord of these patients (6,7,11,12).

THE ORGANISM

T. gondii is an obligate intracellular protozoan that exists in nature in three forms: the oocyst (which releases sporozoites), the tissue cyst (which contains and may release bradyzoites), and the tachyzoite (8). Strains isolated from a variety of hosts on five continents revealed a perfect correlation between virulence for mice and a single clonal lineage that was geographically widespread and found in both domestic animals and humans (13). Clear differences were observed in the frequency of parasite genotypes when *T. gondii* isolates from animals versus humans were compared. Type III strains were common in animals but were observed significantly less often in human toxoplasmosis. Most human cases were caused by type II strains. Type II strains were significantly more often associated with reactivation of chronic infections and accounted for 65% of cases in AIDS patients. Type I strains were significantly more often associated with human congenital toxoplasmosis (14). For a more complete discussion of the organism itself, including its cell biology, molecular biology, antigenic structure, and immunobiology, the reader is referred to recent reviews (15–18).

Oocyst

Oocysts are formed in the gastrointestinal tract only in members of the cat family (19) and are excreted in the feces for periods varying from 7 to 20 days. As many as 10 million oocysts can be shed in the feces in a single day (8) and will become infectious (by sporulation) in 1 to 21 days, depending on temperature and availability of oxygen.

Tachyzoite

Tachyzoites are crescentic in shape, measure 2 to 4 μm wide and 4 to 8 μm long, and require an intracellular habitat to survive and multiply. They reside and multiply within vacuoles in their host's cells (20), can infect most phagocytic and nonphagocytic cell types (21,22), and multiply approximately every 4 to 6 hours to form rosettes. Continuous multiplication leads to cell disruption and the release of organisms that go on to invade contiguous cells (23–25) or are phagocytosed and transported to other areas of the body by blood and lymph (26). They are propagated in the laboratory in the peritoneum of mice (27) and in tissue cultures of mammalian cells (28). Tachyzoites are seen in the primary or reactivating infection; their presence is the hallmark of acute infection.

Cyst

The tissue cyst is formed within a host cell and can vary in size from cysts that contain only a few organisms (bradyzoites) to those at least 200 μm in size that contain several thousand bradyzoites (29). Cysts stain well with periodic acid–Schiff (PAS), Wright-Giemsa, Gomori methenamine silver, and immunoperoxidase stains. They appear spherical in the brain and conform to the shape of muscle fibers in heart and skeletal muscles. The CNS, eye, and skeletal, smooth, and heart muscles appear to be the most common sites of latent infection (30). Because of this persistence in tissues, demonstration of cysts in histologic sections does not necessarily mean that the infection was recently acquired or that it is clinically relevant.

Cysts develop within a host cell vacuole following stage differentiation from tachyzoite to bradyzoite and may retain a relatively large size while still within the host cell cytoplasm. It has been suggested that in brain tissue, while the tachyzoite form appears to be indiscriminate in the type of host cell parasitized, cyst formation occurs predominantly within neurons (31,32). Cysts also can be formed in astrocytes cultured in vitro, but not in cultured microglial cells (33). In an electron microscopy study of the pathologic changes in brains of infected mice, Ferguson et al. (34) observed the cysts to be intracellular throughout the period of study (22 months). However, the observation that cysts persist only within cells is controversial (35). It has been proposed that growth of the tissue cysts results in degeneration and death of the host cell (33,36) and thus, that the majority of cysts in the brain are located extracellularly.

Stage Conversion

Tachyzoites and bradyzoites reveal a different phenotype within the intracellular habitat of their host (22). Tachyzoites multiply rapidly and synchronously, forming rosettes and lysing the cell, whereas the more slowly replicating bradyzoites form tissue cysts (37,38). Molecules are expressed in a stage-specific manner and are responsible for certain phenotypic differences between tachyzoites and bradyzoites (22,39). There are major differences in the total protein profiles and in the antigenic structure of tachyzoites and cysts, suggesting the existence of cyst-specific and bradyzoite-specific molecules (40–44). Interferon (IFN)-γ and nitric oxide are triggers of conversion of tachyzoites to bradyzoites in vitro and perhaps also in vivo (45–47).

LIFE CYCLE

T. gondii has a complex life cycle (48). The parasite undergoes two cycles in separate biotypes, an enteroepithelial sexual cycle in the small bowel of members of the cat family and an extraintestinal asexual cycle in cats as well as in all other infected animals including humans. The two most common routes of infection in humans are oral ingestion of the parasite and the transplacental route (congenital transmission to the fetus). The principal forms of the parasite that transmit the infection are the tissue cyst and oocyst. Ingestion of undercooked or raw meat that contains cysts or of water or food contaminated with oocysts leads to the acute infection. Following ingestion, the outer walls of the cysts or oocysts are disrupted by enzymatic degradation and the parasites are liberated into the intestinal lumen. They become tachyzoites and spread to invade virtually all cells and tissues of the body. In the cat, the definitive host, the sexual cycle occurs in the small intestine.

EPIDEMIOLOGY

Toxoplasmosis is a zoonosis; the definitive host is the cat, and all other hosts are incidental. In humans, the prevalence of positive *Toxoplasma* serologic test titers increases with age and there are considerable geographic differences in prevalence rates. Differences in the epidemiology of *T. gondii* infection in various geographic locales and between population groups within the same locale can be explained by differences in exposure to sources of the infection.

Congenital Infection

The incidence of congenital toxoplasmosis in newborns directly correlates with two factors, the prevalence of newly acquired infection among women who are at risk and the public health programs instituted for prevention, detection, and treatment of the infection during pregnancy. Toxoplasmic encephalitis in newborns is a preventable disease. In countries with a high prevalence of infection such as France and Austria, a significant decline in the incidence of congenital toxoplasmosis was observed after the introduction of national programs that required examination of every pregnant woman for *Toxoplasma* infection (8,49). Although screening for *Toxoplasma* infection is mandatory during pregnancy in some Western European countries such as Austria and France, in the United States routine serologic screening is not conducted. It has been estimated that as many as 4100 of the 4.1 million infants born annually in recent years in the United States are congenitally infected with this parasite. The majority of infected infants do not have clinical signs at birth but untoward sequelae frequently develop later in life (8). These sequelae primarily are the result of damage to the brain and eye.

AIDS

The incidence of toxoplasmic encephalitis in human immunodeficiency virus (HIV)–infected individuals directly correlates with three factors: the prevalence of *Toxoplasma* antibodies among the general HIV-infected population, the degree of immunosuppression in HIV-infected individuals, and the institution of effective prophylactic treatment regimens against the development of toxoplasmic encephalitis. The *T. gondii* seropositivity rate among HIV-infected patients varies from 10% to 45% in the United States and from 50% to 80% in certain areas of Western Europe and Africa (50). It is from this background of dually infected individuals that toxoplasmic encephalitis develops. Thirty percent to 50% of HIV and *Toxoplasma* seropositive individuals ultimately develop toxoplasmic encephalitis if prophylaxis is not used. The risk of toxoplasmosis in HIV-infected, *T. gondii* seropositive individuals can be stratified by their $CD4^+$ T-cell count. Approximately 90% of patients who develop toxoplasmic encephalitis do so when their $CD4^+$ T-cell count is less than 200 cells/μL. Leport et al. (51) reported the incidence of toxoplasmic encephalitis to be 13% at 1 year in HIV-infected individuals who were not taking prophylactic regimens; in their study, patients with AIDS and a $CD4^+$ count less than 50 cells/μL had a 1-year incidence of toxoplasmic encephalitis of 33%. Several prophylactic drug regimens are effective for the primary or secondary prevention of toxoplasmic encephalitis in AIDS patients (52–55).

Hodgkin's Disease and Organ Transplant

Even before the emergence of AIDS, toxoplasmic encephalitis had been recognized as a cause of incapacitating disease and death among immunosuppressed patients (2,3,5,56), especially in those whose underlying disease or therapy caused a deficiency in cell-mediated immunity. Patients with hematologic malignancies, especially those with Hodgkin's disease, are at a particularly high risk to develop relapse of toxoplasmosis (3,5). Among organ transplant patients, those with heart, lung, kidney, and bone marrow transplants develop toxoplasmosis at a higher rate (3,5,56).

PATHOGENESIS

Primary Infection

In all mammalian species, *Toxoplasma* organisms multiply intracellularly at the site of invasion (the gastrointestinal tract appears to be the major route for and the initial site of infection in nature); after host cell disruption, parasites invade adjacent cells from which they spread throughout the body via lymphatics and the bloodstream (57). With the appearance of humoral and cellular immunity, only the parasites protected by an intracellular habitat or within cysts survive. An effective immune response significantly reduces the number of *T. gondii* in all tissues. Thereafter, tachyzoites are rarely demonstrable histologically in tissues of infected humans, including brain tissue (57). In contrast, in laboratory mice, depending on the strain of mice and of *T. gondii*, numerous cysts may be present in the brains. Despite the ability to isolate cysts from normal brains of chronically infected humans, the cyst form is rarely observed in histologic preparations.

Chronic (Latent) Infection and Target Organs

The tissue cyst form is responsible for residual infection and persists primarily in the brain, skeletal and heart muscle, and eye (30,58,59). It appears that predilection of this parasite for some body sites is host dependent (60). In mice, rats, and humans, the brain is considered the most common site of residual infection. One study isolated the cyst form of *T. gondii* from autopsy samples of brain or skeletal muscle (or both) from 5 (9.6%) of 52 seropositive patients (none had clinical or pathologic evidence of active infection); both brain and skeletal muscle were sites of residual infection (30).

In mice and rats, studies on the localization and persistence of *T. gondii* in tissues revealed that the parasite may survive in brain tissue indefinitely (59,61). This apparent predilection for the brain has been used to maintain *T. gondii* in "animal banks"; the parasite is obtained from brains of such mice or rats and is passed to other laboratory animals by intraperitoneal inoculation. *T. gondii* is uniformly present for a period of at least 2 years in rats and for the life of the infected mice.

It appears that initially in some mammals, the parasite localizes preferentially in certain organs such as the reticuloendothelial system and lungs. There is a significant initial delay between the time of infection and the time of invasion of the CNS. It is unclear whether the reason for this delay resides in the unique features of the endothelial cells lining the vasculature of the brain. It is possible that these cells or other components of the blood-brain barrier establish an effective obstacle to initial invasion into the CNS. However, once *T. gondii* has reached the brain, it is able to persist in a residual form for the life of the host (30,59).

In marked contrast to mice and humans, studies in sheep, goats, pigs, horses, and cattle revealed that latent *T. gondii* infection is more frequently found in skeletal muscles than in neural tissues (60,62,63). This apparent predilection for muscle tissue agrees with results from other studies in livestock that suggest that *T. gondii* establishes more residual infection in the brains of mice and rats than in livestock.

Although residual infection is higher in the brains of laboratory mice and rats than in other tissues, experimental data do not support the concept that *T. gondii* is a neurotropic organism. It is unclear whether *T. gondii* penetrates the brain more easily than other organs of some animals or whether it is more difficult for the brain, as an immunologically privileged site, to eradicate the organism during the initial acute infection and once residual infection has been established.

Extension of *T. gondii* to the Brain via the Bloodstream

In infants with congenital toxoplasmosis, the location of necrotic foci and lesions in general suggests that *T. gondii* reaches the brain via the bloodstream (8). There is a remarkable variability in the distribution of lesions and parasites among different reported cases.

In AIDS patients, the simultaneous development of multifocal brain lesions suggests that although toxoplasmic encephalitis arises from reactivation of a latent infection, the multiple areas of the brain that are affected are likely the result of hematogenous spread of the parasite (64,65).

Invasion of the Brain

To invade the brain, *T. gondii* must first encounter a unique collection of anatomic, biochemical, and transport specializations expressed by vascular endothelial cells within the CNS (the blood-brain barrier) (66). The impermeability of brain capillaries of this barrier in adult brain depends on the junctions linking the endothelial cells that line them. A first step in the invasion of *T. gondii* into the brain most likely involves penetration of the endothelial cells of the CNS microvasculature. The ability of the parasite to replicate within human endothelial cells of other body sites has been reported (67).

Entry of *T. gondii* into mammalian cells has been studied in detail in a variety of experimental models (21,22). Entry into cells is an active, parasite-directed event. Invasion by *T. gondii,* as seen in HeLa cell cultures by cinematographic and electron microscopic investigations, is a rapid event taking 15 to 40 seconds (25,68,69). It is likely that the parasite penetrates the cells of the brain microvasculature localized in the blood-brain barrier by an active process similar to that observed with HeLa cells. The mechanical events that occur have been reported in detail (70–75).

Localization Within the Brain

It appears that *T. gondii* has greater affinity for some areas of the brain than others. For instance, in most autopsy series of AIDS patients with toxoplasmic encephalitis, there is almost universal involvement of the cerebral hemispheres and a remarkable predilection for the basal ganglia (76,77). In a consecutive autopsy study of 204 patients who died with AIDS, 46 (23%) had morphologic evidence of cerebral toxoplasmosis. In 38 (83%) of the 46, toxoplasmosis was restricted to the CNS. Of all the CNS lesions, the cerebral hemispheres were affected in 91% and the rostral basal ganglia in 78% (76). In congenital toxoplasmosis, necrosis of the brain is most intense in the cortex and basal ganglia and at times in the periventricular areas (1,78). Studies of the localization of *T. gondii* cysts within brains of otherwise normal mice also indicated comparatively greater numbers in the cerebral hemispheres and olfactory bulbs than in the cerebellum, medulla, and pons (79).

It is not clear why the parasite has a predilection for the cerebral hemispheres and basal ganglia of newborns with congenital toxoplasmosis, AIDS patients with toxoplasmic encephalitis, and laboratory mice with toxoplasmic encephalitis. There are quantitative and possibly qualitative differences in the function of the blood-brain barrier in different regions of the brain and spinal cord (80). The uptake of radioisotope-tagged urea into various regions of the CNS of cats revealed a predilection for the cerebral cortex and basal ganglia (81). This phenomenon may relate to differences in blood supply between the particular areas. Whether a predilection of the blood supply for certain areas of the brain such as the cerebral hemispheres and basal ganglia explains the propensity of *T. gondii* for these areas is unknown.

Encephalitis

In immunocompetent individuals, the primary infection is most often undetected clinically. In almost all cases, this primary event and the resultant seeding of different organs lead to a chronic or latent infection without clinical significance. This chronic stage of infection corresponds to the symptomatic persistence of the cyst form in multiple tissues. It is believed that periodically the quiescent cyst form spontaneously "ruptures" in immunocompetent individuals; cyst disruption in this setting is a clinically silent process effectively contained by the immune system. Cyst rupture in these individuals likely results in small inflammatory nodules, with a limited degree of neuronal cell death and architectural damage (37).

In severely immunocompromised individuals, *T. gondii* can cause severe and life-threatening encephalitis. Encephalitis in these individuals can be caused by primary infection, but most often is a result of reactivation of the latent infection. It is believed that reactivation of chronic infection is the result of disruption of the cyst form followed by the uncontrolled proliferation of organisms and tissue destruction in a setting of impaired host immunity. In individuals with deficient cell-mediated immunity, rapid, uncontrolled proliferation of *T. gondii* results in progressively enlarging necrotic lesions (77,82). It has been postulated that toxoplasmic encephalitis can result directly from cyst disruption in the brain parenchyma or from cyst disruption at extraneural body sites followed by subsequent spread to the brain (64).

Evidence for the occurrence of cyst disruption in vivo has been published (37,83–85). In the brains of chronically infected mice, it is not unusual to find small and large cysts in close proximity, suggesting that cyst disruption results in the formation of satellite ("daughter") cysts (83). However, it is not known whether such satellite cysts result from disruption of larger cysts or whether they develop at the same time as the larger cysts in the same area (8). A study of a Panamanian night monkey infected with *T. gondii* demonstrated the histologic sequence of apparently intact cysts surrounded by a microglial reaction, and the transition from intact cyst to disintegrating cyst, and thereafter to glial nodule formation with *T. gondii* antigen (85). Tissue cyst disruption was observed in immunocompetent mice chronically infected with *T. gondii* (37,47). The early stages following disruption were associated with a marked influx of inflammatory cells, giving rise to microglial nodules. In the study of Ferguson et al. (37), most of the cysts within the host cells did not elicit an inflammatory reaction. A number of inflammatory cells were also noted around an apparently intact cyst (37). The presence of inflammatory cells associated with an apparently intact cyst and the rapid development of an inflammatory nodule around the disrupted cysts observed in immunocompetent mice are similar to those seen in the night monkey (85). Cyst disruption followed by recrudescence of active proliferation of tachyzoites and progressive encephalitis has also been observed in immunosuppressed hosts (82).

HISTOPATHOLOGY

Damage to the CNS by *T. gondii* is characterized by multiple foci of enlarging necrosis and microglial nodules. Necrosis is the most prominent feature of the disease because of vascular involvement by the lesions (Fig 10-1).

Congenital Infection

In infants who die in the newborn period there are extensive diffuse and focal alterations of the parenchymal architecture (1,78,86,87). Lesions consist of numerous glial nodules similar to those observed in some viral encephalitides (88). The lesions are most

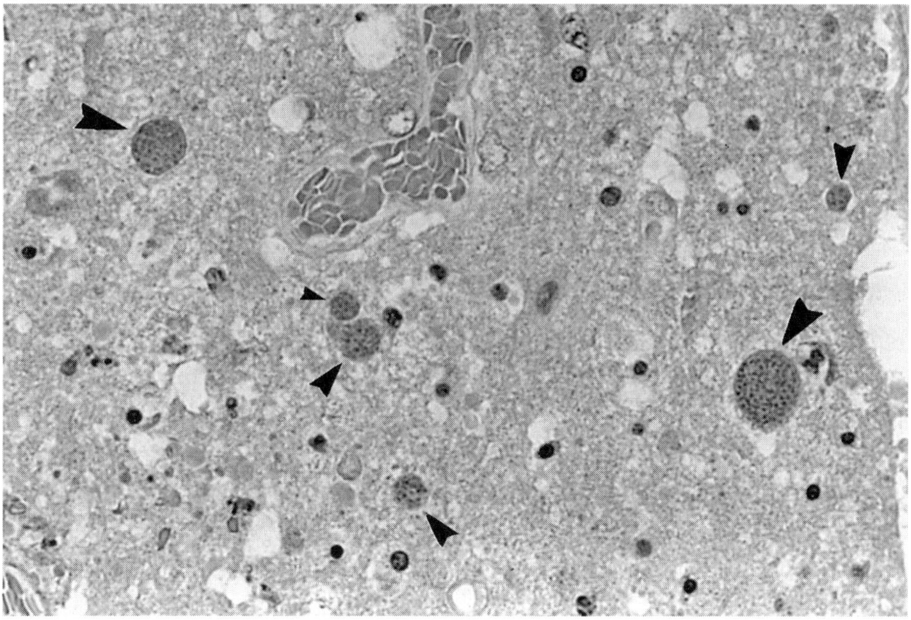

Figure 10-1. Toxoplasmic encephalitis. Cross section of brain showing multiple *T. gondii* cysts (arrowheads) of different sizes in a background of necrotic brain. (Courtesy of Dr. J. M. Seitz, Bonn, Germany.)

intense in the cortex and basal ganglia and at times in the periventricular areas; they distinctively reveal the formation of prominent glial nodules so much so that Wolf et al. (1) termed these nodules *miliary granulomas*.

Necrosis may progress to an actual formation of cysts, which have eosinophilic material at the center of the cyst cavity. At the periphery of the cystic areas, focal calcification of necrotic individual nerve cells may be evident. Calcification within zones of necrosis may be extensive, forming broad bands of calcific material involving most of the cortical layers, or it may be scattered diffusely throughout the foci of necrosis. The calcium salts are deposited in coarse granules or in finely divided particles, which gives the appearance of "calcium dust." Many cells become completely calcified, whereas others contain only a few, finely divided particles of finely divided calcium. The extent of calcification appears to depend on the severity of the reaction and duration of infection (89). *Toxoplasma* tachyzoites and cysts are seen in and adjacent to necrotic foci near or in the glial nodules, in perivascular regions, and in cerebral tissue uninvolved by inflammatory change (87).

Periaqueductal and periventricular vasculitis with necrosis can be pathognomonic of toxoplasmosis (78,88). The necrotic brain tissue autolyzes and is gradually shed into the ventricles. The protein content of such ventricular fluid may be in the range of grams per deciliter and may contain significant amounts of *Toxoplasma* antigens (88). If the cerebral aqueduct of Sylvius is blocked by the ependymitis, the lateral and third ventricles begin to resemble an abscess cavity that contains accretions of *Toxoplasma* and inflammatory cells (90). Hydrocephalus develops in these children, and the necrotic brain tissue may calcify and become visible on neuroimaging studies. Destruction of brain tissue, especially intense periventricular necrosis, rather than obstruction of ventricular passages, appears to account for the development of hydrocephalus in some patients (1,86).

Immunocompromised Patients

The presence of multiple brain abscesses is the most characteristic feature of toxoplasmic encephalitis in severely immunocompromised patients and is particularly characteristic in patients with AIDS. These abscesses usually have three distinctive zones without capsule formation (7):

1 A central avascular zone that contains very few organisms and a solid and coagulated necrotic center filled with amorphous eosinophilic debris (7,91); vessels, if present, are occluded by fibrin thrombi and necrotic material.

2 An intermediate zone, congested with blood vessels, only spotty areas of necrosis, and numerous free extracellular and intracellular tachyzoites. This zone rarely exhibits cysts. An inflammatory reaction surrounds the necrotic areas; the intensity of this cellular infiltrate is variable and consists of acute and chronic inflammatory cells, reactive astrocytes, and macrophages (7,76,77,91). Perivascular cuffing by lymphocytes, plasma cells, and macrophages is also present (7,91). Endothelial cell swelling and proliferation are observed.

3 An outer zone in which necrosis is rare and vascular lesions are minimal; more *T. gondii* cysts with fewer tachyzoites are observed. Leptomeningitis, which is infrequent, is usually seen only in direct association with areas of encephalitis. Arteritis of large vessels is absent (7).

Organizing and chronic abscesses are occasionally seen in AIDS patients with toxoplasmic encephalitis, particularly in those who have received a lengthy course of anti-*Toxoplasma* therapy (77,91).

Diffuse "encephalitic" cerebral toxoplasmosis in AIDS patients has been reported (11). Gross postmortem findings in the brain may be normal. Microscopic examination of the basal ganglia reveals small necrotic lesions with central coagulation necrosis characteristic of toxoplasmosis, surrounded by an inflammatory reaction containing numerous cysts (11). Examination of the cerebral hemispheres, brainstem, and cerebellum reveals numerous widespread microglial nodules in the brain parenchyma, most of which contain *Toxoplasma* cysts or free tachyzoites (11).

RESISTANCE AGAINST *T. GONDII*

For a more in-depth discussion of the role of $CD4^+$ and $CD8^+$ T lymphocytes, lymphokine-activated killer (LAK), natural killer (NK), and $\gamma\delta$ T cells and cytokines, the reader is referred to Chapter 4.

Systemic Immune Response

Infection with *T. gondii* induces both humoral and cell-mediated immune responses. A well-orchestrated and effective systemic immune response is responsible for the early disappearance of *T. gondii* from peripheral blood during the acute infection and limits the parasite burden in the CNS. Although cellular immunity appears to be the most important in the defense of the brain, it is likely that this arm of the immune response acts in concert with antibodies in extraneural sites and perhaps also in the inflamed brain.

Innate Resistance

Experiments performed with activated human and murine macrophages suggest that these cells play an important role in resistance to *Toxoplasma* infection (92–97). *T. gondii* or *Toxoplasma* antigen can activate macrophages to produce tumor necrosis factor (TNF), interleukin (IL)-12, IL-1, and IL-15. IL-12 acts in concert with IL-1 and IL-15 to stimulate NK cells to produce significant amounts of IFN-γ. IFN-γ activates macrophages to produce reactive nitrogen intermediates and oxygen free radicals, which inhibit *T. gondii* replication (Fig 10-2).

NK and LAK cells from mice and humans have been implicated in the host immune response against *T. gondii* (98–102). Human LAK cells of both the NK- and T-cell phenotype from seronegative donors are cytotoxic for cells infected with the parasite (100). Infection with *T. gondii* triggers murine NK spleen cells to produce large amounts of IFN-γ (103,104). Since resistance against *T. gondii* infection does not develop in nude mice (105,106), nude rats (107), or severe combined immunodeficient (SCID) mice (108,109), it appears that nonspecific immunity alone is inadequate to control this infection.

Humoral Immunity

Passive transfer of immune sera or of monoclonal antibody to uninfected animals confers some protection against challenge with *T. gondii* (110–113). Although humoral immunity alone does not provide significant protection against virulent strains of the parasite, some studies demonstrated protection against challenge with less virulent strains. It is likely that humoral immunity in concert with cellular immunity plays a role in the host defense against *T. gondii*.

Genetic Susceptibility

Several experimental studies in mice and observational studies in humans raised the possibility that host genetic factors may contribute to the development and severity of the clinical entity of toxoplasmic encephalitis (114–119).

In mice, development of toxoplasmic encephalitis is regulated by a gene or genes located within the H-2D region (115,118,119). Suzuki et al. (115) reported that mice with the b or k allele at the H-2D region developed severe encephalitis during the chronic

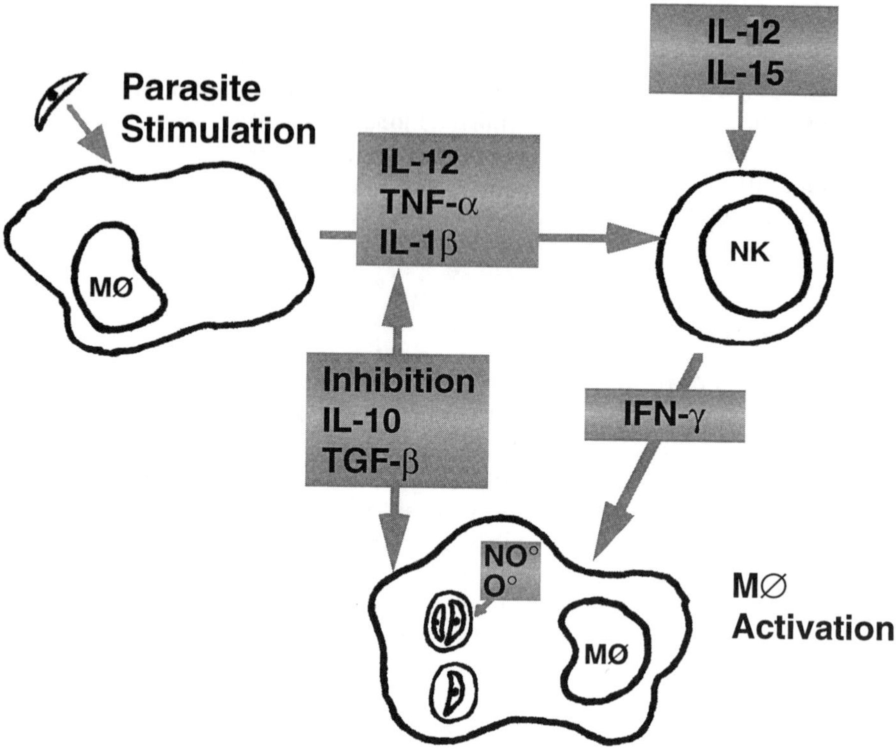

Figure 10-2. T cell–independent mechanism of resistance to *T. gondii*. *T. gondii* organisms or antigens stimulate macrophages to produce interleukin (IL)-12, IL-1, tumor necrosis factor (TNF)-α, and IL-15. IL-1β and IL-15 act in concert with IL-12 to induce production of interferon (IFN)-γ by natural killer (NK) cells. IFN-γ activates macrophages to produce reactive nitrogen intermediates and oxygen free radicals that can inhibit parasite replication. IL-10 and transforming growth factor (TGF)-β act as inhibitors of this T cell–independent mechanism of resistance. MØ = macrophages; NO = nitric oxide; O = oxygen. (Adapted from Hunter C, Remington J. Immunopathogenesis of toxoplasmic encephalitis. *J Infect Dis* 1994;170:1057–1067.)

stage of infection, whereas those with the d allele at the region of the H-2 complex did not. Brown and McLeod (120) reported the importance of class I major histocompatibility complex (MHC) genes at the H-2L region in regulating the formation of *T. gondii* cysts in the brains of mice. Further work by Suzuki et al. (116) and others (119) demonstrated that in mice, within the H-2 region, a MHC class I gene(s) in the D/L region, the L^d gene, determines the parasite burden in the brain and whether toxoplasmic encephalitis will occur.

The fact that not all AIDS patients with positive serology for *T. gondii* develop toxoplasmic encephalitis suggests the possibility that genetic factors may also play a role in the predisposition of AIDS patients to this disease. In a recent study, Suzuki et al. (114) found that HLA-DQ3 was significantly more frequent in white North American AIDS patients with toxoplasmic encephalitis (85%) than in the general white population (51.8%; $p = 0.007$, corrected $p = 0.028$) or randomly selected control AIDS patients who had not developed toxoplasmic encephalitis (40%, $p = 0.016$). In contrast, the frequency of HLA-DQ1 was lower in toxoplasmic encephalitis patients than in healthy control subjects (40% versus 66.5%, $p = 0.027$); this difference, however, did not reach statistical significance when corrected for the number of variables tested. Thus, HLA-DQ3 appears to be a genetic marker of susceptibility to the development of toxoplasmic encephalitis in AIDS patients, and DQ1 may be a resistance marker. These HLA associations with disease suggest that the development of toxoplasmic encephalitis in HIV-infected patients is regulated by genes in or near the HLA complex. Studies will be required to determine whether genetic control of susceptibility to toxoplasmic encephalitis is similar in white individuals from countries outside North America and in patients in other ethnic groups.

T Cells

The major mechanism of resistance against *T. gondii* in murine models of the infection is mediated by T cells (121,122). The association between toxoplasmosis and conditions that affect T cell–mediated immunity (e.g., patients with lymphomas or AIDS) provides indirect evidence for the role of these cells in resistance against this parasite in humans (2,6,50,123). Adoptive transfer experiments of immune T cells confer resistance against *T. gondii* in nude rats (107), SCID mice (108,109), and immunocompetent mice (121,122). Studies in the latter indicated that $CD8^+$ T cells are primarily responsible for resistance, although significant protection is also conferred by $CD4^+$ T lymphocytes (121,122). In addition to their production of cytokines, it has been proposed that T cells confer protection against *T. gondii* through lysis of parasite-infected cells (124–126). $CD8^+$ T cells from *T. gondii*–infected mice can lyse *T. gondii*–infected cells (124) and $CD4^+$ and $CD8^+$ T cells from humans infected with *T. gondii* are cytotoxic against *T. gondii*–infected cells (126–128). The role of MHC class II and I molecules in the cytotoxic activity of $CD4^+$ and $CD8^+$ T cells is unresolved. Whereas some investigators provided evidence of MHC restriction mediating this cytotoxic activity (126), others suggested that such activity might be MHC nonrestricted (129).

Rapid induction of a remarkable primary $\gamma\delta$ T-cell response may be an important component of the early immune response to *T. gondii* in humans (130–133). The percentage of $\gamma\delta$ T cells in peripheral blood is increased in patients with acute toxoplasmic lymphadenitis compared with control subjects (131,132). Preferential expansion and activation of human $\gamma\delta$ T cells, in particular $V\gamma9^+$ $V\delta2^+$ $\gamma\delta$ T cells, occur when peripheral blood T cells from either *T. gondii* seronegative or seropositive individuals are incubated with autologous peripheral blood mononuclear cells infected with the parasite (130). $\gamma\delta$ T cells are cytotoxic for *T. gondii*–infected cells in an MHC unrestricted manner, and produce IFN-γ, IL-2, and TNF-α, but not IL-4 when incubated with cells infected with the parasite (130). More recently, analysis of $\gamma\delta$ T cells in patients with congenital toxoplasmosis revealed evidence for anergy of these cells with or without clonal Vδ2$^+$ $\gamma\delta$ T-cell expansion in the acute phase of *T. gondii* infection. The Vδ2$^+$ $\gamma\delta$ T-cell tolerance was lost in these infected infants earlier than was $\alpha\beta$ T-cell tolerance (133).

Cytokines

Cytokines are important in the pathogenesis of toxoplasmosis and toxoplasmic encephalitis (134,135). For a more complete discussion of the role of cytokines in *T. gondii* infection, see Chapter 4.

IFN-γ appears to be the major mediator of host resistance against *T. gondii* (136). Administration of murine recombinant IFN-γ to mice infected with *T. gondii* prevents their death or prolongs their survival (137). Protective immunity conferred by adoptive transfer of immune T cells in mice can be ablated by coadministration of IFN-γ antibodies (138).

IFN-γ plays a significant role in the prevention or development of toxoplasmic encephalitis in mice. Monoclonal antibody against IFN-γ appears to predispose to disruption of *Toxoplasma* cysts in chronically infected mice (47). Treatment with IFN-γ significantly reduces the inflammatory response and numbers of tachyzoites in mice with toxoplasmic encephalitis (139).

Studies of the role of TNF-α in murine toxoplasmosis revealed conflicting results. Administration of TNF-α in one study protected mice against lethal challenge with *T. gondii* (140) whereas in another study, administration of TNF-α resulted in increased mortality (141). Administration of TNF-α neutralizing antibody in infected mice resulted in the death of mice and an increase in the number of *T. gondii* cysts in the brains of the survivors (142,143).

IL-6 serum levels in mice rise during the course of lethal *T. gondii* infection and appear to correlate with clinical status (16). Administration of anti–IL-6 monoclonal antibody remarkably reduces the frequency of tachyzoites and *T. gondii* cysts in the brains of mice with toxoplasmic encephalitis (144).

IL-10 plays an important role in vivo in downregulating monokine and IFN-γ responses to acute *T. gondii* infection (145). IL-12 appears to be important in the early immune response against *T. gondii*. *T. gondii* can directly stimulate macrophages to produce IL-12 and TNF-α, which act in concert to induce NK-cell production of IFN-γ (146). This event appears to be a first line of defense before development of T-cell responses (147). Both IL-1 and IL-15 are important in the IL-12–mediated resistance to *T. gondii* in vivo (148). Endogenous production of IL-15 is important for optimal production of IFN-γ by NK cells in vitro (149). Administration of exogenous recombinant IL-15 with soluble *Toxoplasma* lysate antigen (TLA) provides complete protection against lethal parasite challenge, whereas treatment with either recombinant IL-15 or TLA alone is not protective (150). Adoptive transfer of CD8$^+$ T cells, but not CD4$^+$ T cells, from TLA/recombinant IL-15–vaccinated mice protects naive mice from lethal infection (150).

Immune Response Mechanisms Within the Brain

Remarkable numbers of $CD4^+$ and $CD8^+$ T cells have been observed in the CNS of mice with toxoplasmic encephalitis (151). Infiltration of T cells into the CNS correlates with the appearance of parasites and early signs of astrocyte activation (152).

Levels of cytokine messenger RNA (mRNA) transcripts have been studied during toxoplasmic encephalitis in the CNS of susceptible mice (152–155). IL-4 transcripts were detected early in the development of toxoplasmic encephalitis while IL-2 transcripts appeared later. These data suggest that different Th1- and Th2-type responses may be present at different times during toxoplasmic encephalitis (152).

Elevated levels of mRNA transcripts for IFN-γ and TNF-α have also been demonstrated in the CNS of mice susceptible to toxoplasmic encephalitis (152–155). Administration of anti–IFN-γ (47) or anti–TNF-α (154) results in a remarkable increase in the degree of inflammation in the brains of infected mice. Levels of IL-10 transcripts are elevated in the brains of mice susceptible to toxoplasmic encephalitis (154) but not in the brains of mice resistant to toxoplasmic encephalitis (151).

Astrocytes and microglia may play an important role in the immune response against *T. gondii* within the CNS. In the early stages of toxoplasmic encephalitis in both humans and mice, there is a remarkable and widespread astrocytosis restricted to areas in which the parasite is detected (135). *T. gondii* can invade, survive, and multiply in astrocytes (156) (also, see chapter by Peterson in this book). Uptake of *T. gondii* into neonatal murine astrocytes is parasite driven and its survival within these cells does not appear to be affected by treatment with IFN-γ and lipopolysaccharide (LPS) (156). Thus, it has been postulated that on entry into the CNS, *T. gondii* would find astrocytes to be a safe harbor (156).

In contrast to astrocytes, microglia appear to be equipped with at least two strategies to defend the brain against infection with *T. gondii* (156–158): an intrinsic mechanism for killing tachyzoites internalized by a phagocytic process and a nitric oxide–independent mechanism that is upregulated by murine IFN-γ (mIFN-γ) and LPS (156,158). Also, see Chapter by Chao in this book. IFN-γ/LPS–treated microglia limit *T. gondii* growth (158). More than 90% of this anti-*Toxoplasma* activity of activated microglia is blocked by neutralizing antibodies to TNF-α or IL-6 (158). Whether microglia are major effector cells in the CNS against *T. gondii* remains uncertain (135). Increased expression of MHC class II antigens has been demonstrated in microglia, but not astrocytes of *T. gondii*–infected SCID and immunocompetent C.B-17 mice that develop toxoplasmic encephalitis (159), suggesting that microglia may play a role in the presentation of *T. gondii* antigens.

A prominent upregulation of intercellular cell adhesion molecule-1 (ICAM-1) and of Ia on cerebral endothelia, microglia, ependyma, and choroid plexus epithelium during acute and chronic murine toxoplasmic encephalitis has been reported (160). Microglia also express Mac-1 and leukocyte function–associated antigen-1 (LFA-1), which are both ligands of ICAM-1, as well as CD45. The vascular cell adhesion molecule-1 (VCAM-1) is restricted to endothelia of cerebral blood vessels, which frequently show perivascular cuffing of inflammatory cells. In this model, upregulation of Ia, the cellular adhesion molecules, and their ligands correlates with disease activity (160).

CLINICAL MANIFESTATIONS

For a more complete description of the clinical manifestations of CNS toxoplasmosis, the reader is referred to recent published reviews on this subject (8,50).

Congenital Toxoplasmosis in the Infant

Congenital *Toxoplasma* infection in the newborn is most frequently a subclinical or inapparent infection (161,162). Less common are the severe signs of the disease that occur when the fetus is infected very early in gestation. These include hydrocephalus, chorioretinitis, jaundice, and cerebral calcifications. None of these signs are pathognomonic for toxoplasmosis and they can be mimicked by congenital infection with other pathogens including cytomegalovirus, herpes simplex virus, *Treponema pallidum*, and rubella virus.

It is important to recognize that in newborns, it is not possible to rely on clinical manifestations alone to raise the possibility of congenital toxoplasmosis. For instance, an asymptomatic newborn of a mother who acquired the infection during pregnancy can develop an incapacitating visual impairment in the second or third decade of life whether or not toxoplasmic chorioretinitis goes unrecognized early in life (8).

When the infection is clinically apparent in the newborn, the manifestations of the disease are usually severe and signs referable to the CNS are always present. These patients rarely recover without sequelae, even when treatment is instituted (8). Other infants present with convulsions, bulging fontanel, nystagmus, or an abnormal increase in head circumference. These patients may respond to treatment and their development may be normal thereafter (8).

Toxoplasmosis in Patients with AIDS

The clinical syndrome of toxoplasmic encephalitis is variable and nonspecific in patients with AIDS (50,65,163). The clinical presentation varies from a subacute, insidious process evolving over weeks, to an acute confusional state with or without focal neurologic deficits evolving over days. Clinical findings include alteration in mental status, seizures, motor weakness, cranial nerve disturbances, sensory abnormalities, cerebellar signs, meningismus, movement disorders, and neuropsychiatric manifestations. Constitutional symptoms and signs such as fever and malaise are variable.

The tragedy of this disease in AIDS patients rests with the fact that it impairs cognitive and motor functions. The most common focal neurologic manifestations are hemiparesis and abnormalities of speech. Secondary to brainstem involvement, cranial nerve lesions occur. Because *T. gondii* causes predominantly encephalitis with little or no meningeal involvement, signs of meningeal irritation are rare (50). Seizures, cerebral hemorrhage, and diffuse toxoplasmic encephalitis may present acutely and progress rapidly to death (11,164–166).

Spinal cord toxoplasmosis in AIDS patients can present with motor or sensory disturbances of single or multiple extremities, bladder, or bowel (50). Cervical and thoracic myelopathy and conus medullaris syndromes have also been reported (167–170).

DIAGNOSIS

For a more comprehensive discussion of the methods used for the diagnosis of CNS toxoplasmosis in the congenitally acquired disease and in the immunocompromised host, the reader is referred to excellent reviews elsewhere (8,50).

Laboratory tests currently available for the diagnosis of toxoplasmic encephalitis include serologic studies, histologic studies (hematoxylin and eosin, immunoperoxidase (Fig 10-3), Wright-Giemsa, and PAS stains), isolation of the parasite by mouse or tissue culture inoculation, polymerase chain reaction (PCR), and radiographic studies (Figs 10-4 and 10-5).

Congenital Toxoplasmosis

Once the occurrence of acute maternal infection acquired during pregnancy has been established, the diagnosis of whether fetal infection has occurred is best accomplished by PCR on amniotic fluid (171,172). Diagnosis of infection in the newborn can be established by demonstration of IgM, IgA, or IgE antibodies in cord serum not contaminated with maternal blood and in peripheral blood and cerebrospinal fluid (8). In their absence, follow-up testing is the only means of making a serologic diagnosis of subclinical congenital toxoplasmosis. The diagnosis can also be established by isolation of the

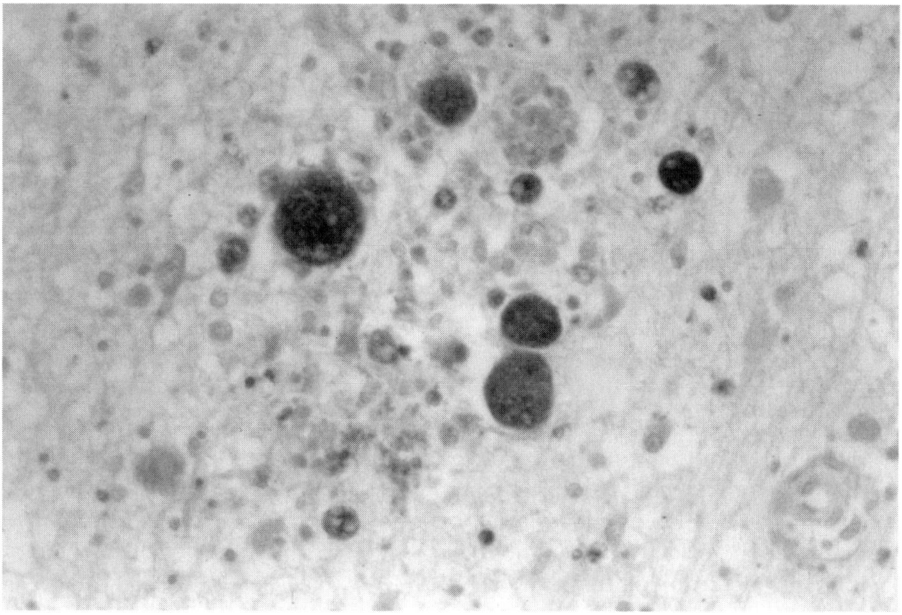

Figure 10-3. Toxoplasmic encephalitis. Cross section of the brain demonstrating intracellular and extracellular *Toxoplasma* antigens by immunoperoxidase stain.

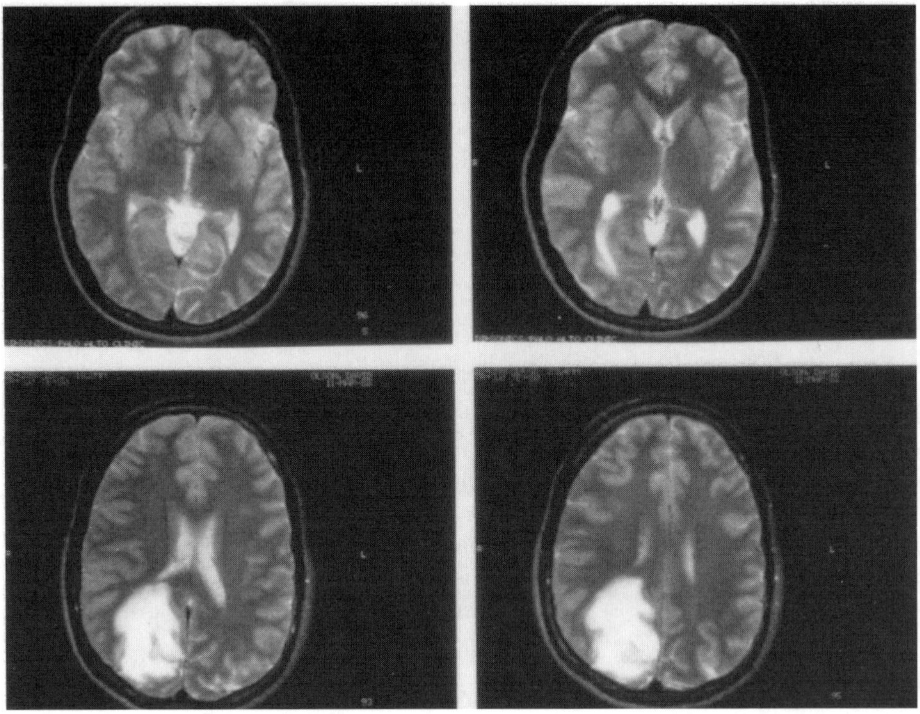

Figure 10-4. Magnetic resonance images of a brain with toxoplasmic encephalitis, obtained after administration of a contrast agent (gadolinium diethylenetriamine penta-acetic acid), demonstrate abnormalities in the blood-brain barrier. Accumulation of the contrast agent is seen as high signal intensity.

parasite from amniotic fluid, placenta, or both (8). Cerebral calcifications on x-ray films, computed tomography scans, or magnetic resonance images, and the presence of chorioretinitis should heighten suspicion of *T. gondii* as the cause of the disease.

AIDS Patients

Serologic tests are usually only helpful to establish that the HIV-positive individual has been exposed to *T. gondii* and that such individuals are at risk to develop toxoplasmic encephalitis once AIDS develops. Isolation of the parasite and staining, including the use of immunoperoxidase and Wright-Giemsa stains, can be attempted on preparations of almost any body fluid or tissue suspected of being infected with *T. gondii*. PCR can detect *T. gondii* DNA in the cerebrospinal fluid of approximately 70% of patients with toxoplasmic encephalitis (173,174) and has also been successful in demonstrating the parasite DNA in peripheral blood, bronchoalveolar lavage material, and vitreal fluid of these patients (175,176).

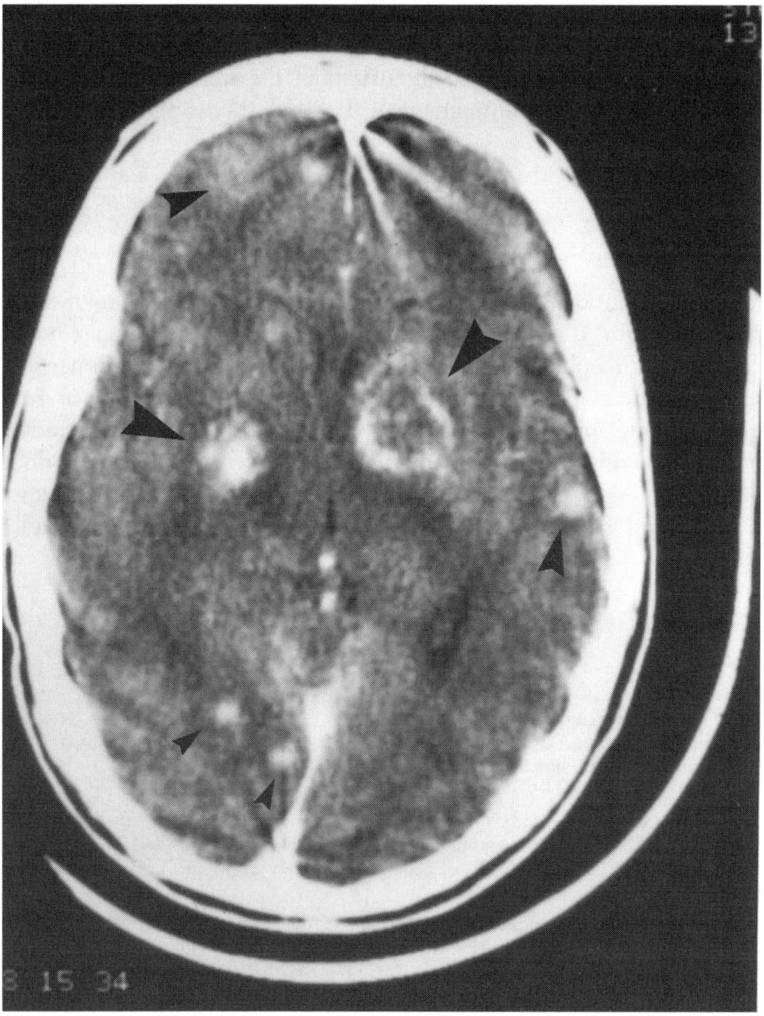

Figure 10-5. Computed tomography scan of a brain with toxoplasmic encephalitis reveals multiple round, ring-enhancing, nodular lesions in both hemispheres (arrows). The distribution and multiplicity of these lesions are typical of toxoplasmic encephalitis.

TREATMENT

Pyrimethamine, a dihydrofolate reductase inhibitor, has remarkable activity against *T. gondii* and is considered to be the most effective anti-*Toxoplasma* agent. Folinic acid should always be administered concomitantly to avoid dose-related bone marrow suppression. At present there is no role for monotherapy in the treatment of CNS toxoplasmosis. A second drug such as sulfadiazine or clindamycin should always be added.

The role of other agents, including azithromycin, clarithromycin, atovaquone, dapsone, and trimethoprim-sulfamethoxazole, is less clear; they should only be used as alternative regimens. For a more detailed discussion of the treatment of toxoplasmic encephalitis in the newborn and in patients with AIDS, the reader is referred elsewhere (8,50).

CONCLUSIONS

In regard to the immunopathogenesis of toxoplasmosis in the CNS, many questions remain unanswered (this is not unique to toxoplasmosis). Among them are the following: Does toxoplasmic encephalitis result from cyst disruption in the brain per se (e.g., can cyst disruption alone at multiple intracerebral sites account for as many as 4 to 12 brain abscesses during one episode of toxoplasmic encephalitis in a particular patient) or is it due to parasitemia following cyst disruption at an extraneural site, or is it due to both? Why is there a predilection of pathology for the basal ganglia? What is the role of the cytokines produced within the human brain in the development of toxoplasmic encephalitis?

REFERENCES

1 Wolf A, Cowen D, Paige BH. Toxoplasmic encephalomyelitis III. A new case of granulomatous encephalomyelitis due to a protozoan. *Am J Pathol* 1939;15:657–694.

2 Vietzke WM, Gelderman AH, Grimley PM, Valsamis MP. Toxoplasmosis complicating malignancy. Experience at the National Cancer Institute. *Cancer* 1968;21:816–827.

3 Ruskin J, Remington JS. Toxoplasmosis in the compromised host. *Ann Intern Med* 1976; 84:193–199.

4 Carey RM, Kimball AC, Armstrong D, Lieberman PH. Toxoplasmosis. Clinical experiences in a cancer hospital. *Am J Med* 1973;54:30–38.

5 Israelski D, Remington J. Toxoplasmosis in the non-AIDS immunocompromised host. *Curr Clin Top Infect Dis* 1993;13:322–356.

6 Luft BJ, Conley F, Remington JS, et al. Outbreak of central-nervous-system toxoplasmosis in western Europe and North America. *Lancet* 1983;1:781–784.

7 Post MJ, Chan JC, Hensley GT, et al. Toxoplasmosis encephalitis in Haitian adults with acquired immunodeficiency syndrome: a clinical-pathologic-CT correlation. *Am J Neuroradiol* 1983;4:155–162.

8 Remington JS, McLeod R, Desmonts G. Toxoplasmosis. In: Remington JS, Klein JO, eds. *Infectious diseases of the fetus and newborn infant*. 4th ed. Philadelphia: WB Saunders, 1995:140–267.

9 Remington JS, Gentry LO. Acquired toxoplasmosis: infection versus disease. *Ann NY Acad Sci* 1970;174:1006–1017.

10 McLeod R, Berry PF, Marshall WHJ, et al. Toxoplasmosis presenting as brain abscesses. Diagnosis by computerized tomography and cytology of aspirated purulent material. *Am J Med* 1979;67:711–714.

11 Gray F, Gherardi R, Wingate E, et al. Diffuse "encephalitic" cerebral toxoplasmosis in AIDS. *J Neurol* 1989;236:273–277.

12 Luft BJ, Brooks RG, Conley FK, et al. Toxoplasmic encephalitis in patients with acquired immune deficiency syndrome. *JAMA* 1984; 252:913–917.

13 Sibley LD, Boothroyd JC. Virulent strains of *Toxoplasma gondii* comprise a single clonal lineage. *Nature* 1992;359:82–85.

14 Howe DK, Sibley LD. *Toxoplasma gondii* comprises three clonal lineages: correlation of parasite genotype with human disease. *J Infect Dis* 1995;172:1561–1566.

15 Wong SY, Remington JS. Biology of *Toxoplasma gondii*. AIDS 1993;7:299–316.

16 Beaman M, Remington J. Cytokines and

resistance against *Toxoplasma gondii*: evidence from in vivo and in vitro studies. In: Sonnenfeld G, Czarniecki C, Nacy C, et al, eds. *Cytokines and resistance to nonviral pathogenic infections*. New York: Biomedical, 1992:111–119.

17 McLeod R, Mack D, Brown C. *Toxoplasma gondii*. New advances in cellular and molecular biology. *Exp Parasitol* 1991;72:109–121.

18 Cesbron M-F, Dubremetz J-F, Sher A. The immunobiology of toxoplasmosis. *Res Immunol* 1993;144:7–8.

19 Freyre A, Dubey JP, Smith DD, Frenkel JK. Oocyst-induced *Toxoplasma gondii* infections in cats. *J Parasitol* 1989;75:750–755.

20 Gustafson PV, Agar HD, Cramer DI. An electron microscope study of toxoplasma. *Am J Trop Med Hyg* 1954;3:1008–1021.

21 Werk R. How does *Toxoplasma gondii* enter host cells? *Rev Infect Dis* 1985;7:449–457.

22 Smith J. An ubiquitous intracellular parasite: the cellular biology of *Toxoplasma gondii*. *Int J Parasitol* 1995;25:1301–1309.

23 Bommer W, Hofling KH, Heunert HH. Multiplication of *Toxoplasma* in cell cultures. *Dtsch Med Wochenschr* 1969;94:1000–1002.

24 Lund E, Lycke E, Sourander P. A cinematographic study of *Toxoplasma gondii* in cell cultures. *Br J Exp Pathol* 1961;42:357–362.

25 Hirai K, Hirato K, Yanagwa R. A cinematographic study of the penetration of cultured cells by *Toxoplasma gondii*. *Jpn J Vet Res* 1966;14:83–90.

26 Jones TC, Yeh S, Hirsch JG. The interaction between *Toxoplasma gondii* and mammalian cells. I. Mechanism of entry and intracellular fate of the parasite. *J Exp Med* 1972;136:1157–1172.

27 Jacobs L. The biology of toxoplasma. *Am J Trop Med Hyg* 1953;2:365–389.

28 Cook MK, Jacobs L. Cultivation of *Toxoplasma gondii* in tissue cultures of various derivations. *J Parasitol* 1958;44:172–182.

29 Remington JS. Experiments on the transmission of toxoplasmosis. *Surv Ophthalmol* 1961;6:856–876.

30 Remington JS, Cavanaugh EN. Isolation of the encysted form of *Toxoplasma gondii* from human skeletal muscle and brain. *N Engl J Med* 1965;273:1308–1310.

31 Sims TA, Hay J, Talbot IC. An electron microscope and immunohistochemical study of the intracellular location of *Toxoplasma* tissue cysts within the brains of mice with congenital toxoplasmosis. *Br J Exp Pathol* 1989;70:317–325.

32 Ferguson DJ, Hutchison WM. The host-parasite relationship of *Toxoplasma gondii* in the brains of chronically infected mice. *Virchows Arch* 1987;411:39–43.

33 Jones TC, Bienz KA, Erb P. In vitro cultivation of *Toxoplasma gondii* cysts in astrocytes in the presence of gamma interferon. *Infect Immun* 1986;51:147–156.

34 Ferguson DJP, Graham DI, Hutchinson WM. Pathological changes in the brains of mice infected with *Toxoplasma gondii*: a histological immunocytochemical and ultrastructural study. *Int J Exp Pathol* 1991;72:463–474.

35 Ferguson DJ, Hutchison WM. An ultrastructural study of the early development and tissue cyst formation of *Toxoplasma gondii* in the brains of mice. *Parasitol Res* 1987;73:483–491.

36 Van Der Zypen E. Light and electron microscopic studies on the development of toxoplasma cysts in the brain of the white mouse. *Z F Parasitenkunde* 1966;28:31–44.

37 Ferguson DJ, Hutchison WM, Pettersen E. Tissue cyst rupture in mice chronically infected with *Toxoplasma gondii*. *Parasitol Res* 1989;75:599–603.

38 Pavesio C, Chiappino M, Setzer P, Nichols B. *Toxoplasma gondii*: differentiation and death of bradyzoites. *Parasitol Res* 1992;78:1–9.

39 Gross U, Bohne W. *Toxoplasma gondii*: strain- and host cell-dependent induction of stage differentiation. *J Eukaryot Microbiol* 1994; 41:10S.

40 Parmley SF, Yang S, Harth G, et al. Molecular characterization of a 65 kilodalton *Toxoplasma gondii* antigen expressed abundantly in the matrix of tissue cysts. *Mol Biochem Parasitol* 1994;66:283–296.

41 Zhang YW, Smith JE. *Toxoplasma gondii*: identification and characterization of a cyst molecule. *Exp Parasitol* 1995;80:228–233.

42 Kasper LH. Identification of stage-specific antigens of *Toxoplasma gondii*. *Infect Immun* 1989;57:668–672.

43 Woodison G, Smith JE. Identification of the dominant cyst antigens of *Toxoplasma gondii*. *Parasitology* 1990;100:389–392.

44 Tomavo S, Fortier B, Soete M, et al. Characterization of bradyzoite-specific antigens of *Toxoplasma gondii*. *Infect Immun* 1991; 59:3750–3753.

45 Bonhe W, Heesemann J, Gross U. Reduced replication of *Toxoplasma gondii* is necessary for induction of bradyzoite-specific antigens: a possible role for nitric oxide in triggering stage conversion. *Infect Immun* 1994;62:1761–1767.

46 Bonhe W, Heesemann J, Gross U. Induction of bradyzoite specific *Toxoplasma gondii* antigens in γ-interferon-treated mouse macrophages. *Infect Immun* 1993;61:1141–1145.

47 Suzuki Y, Conley FK, Remington JS. Importance of endogenous IFN-γ for prevention of toxoplasmic encephalitis in mice. *J Immunol* 1989;143:2045–2050.

48 Frenkel JK. Toxoplasmosis: parasite life cycle pathology and immunology. In: Hammond DM, Long PL, eds. *The coccidia*. Baltimore: University Park Press, 1973:343–410.

49 Aspock H, Flamm H, Picher O. Toxoplasmosis surveillance during pregnancy—10 years of experience in Austria. *Mitt Osterr Ges Tropenmed Parasitol* 1986;8:105–113.

50 Wong S, Remington J. Toxoplasmosis in the setting of AIDS. In: Broder S, Merigan T Jr, Bolognesi D, eds. *Textbook of AIDS medicine*. Baltimore: Williams & Wilkins, 1994:223–257.

51 Leport C, Chene G, Morlat P, et al. Pyrimethamine for primary prophylaxis of toxoplasmic encephalitis in patients with human immunodeficiency virus infection: a double-blind, randomized trial. *J Infect Dis* 1996;17:91–97.

52 Kovacs J. Toxoplasmosis in AIDS: keeping the lid on. *Ann Intern Med* 1995;123:230–231.

53 Beaman M, Luft B, Remington J. Prophylaxis for toxoplasmosis in AIDS. *Ann Intern Med* 1992;117:163–164.

54 Podzamczer D, Miró J, Bolao F, et al. Twice-weekly maintenance therapy with sulfadiazine-pyrimethamine to prevent recurrent toxoplasmic encephalitis in patients with AIDS. *Ann Intern Med* 1995;123:175–180.

55 Podzamczer D, Salazar A, Jiménez J, et al. Intermittent trimethoprim-sulfamethoxazole compared with dapsone-pyrimethamine for the simultaneous primary prophylaxis of pneumocystis pneumonia and toxoplasmosis in patients infected with HIV. *Ann Intern Med* 1995;122:755–761.

56 Slavin M, Meyers J, Remington J, Hackman R. *Toxoplasma gondii* infection in marrow transplant. In: *33rd International Conference on Antimicrobial Agents and Chemotherapy*. New Orleans: American Society Microbiology, 1993:124.

57 Krahenbuhl JL, Remington JS. The immunology of toxoplasma and toxoplasmosis. In: Cohen S, Warren KS, eds. *Immunology of parasitic infections*. 2nd ed. London: Blackwell Scientific, 1982:356–421.

58 Remington JS, Jacobs L, Kaufman HE. Studies on chronic toxoplasmosis: the relation of infective dose to residual infection and to the possibility of congenital transmission. *Am J Ophthalmol* 1958;46:261–267.

59 Ruchman I, Fowler JC. Localization and persistence of toxoplasma on tissues of experimentally infected white rats. *Proc Soc Exp Biol Med* 1951;76:793–796.

60 Dubey JP, Lunney JK, Shen SK, et al. Infectivity of low numbers of *Toxoplasma gondii* oocysts to pigs. *J Parasitol* 1996;82:438–443.

61 Disko R, Braveny I, Greutelaers MT. Affinity of *Toxoplasma gondii*. *Zentralbl Bakteriol* 1978;242:565–571.

62 Dubey JP. Long-term persistence of *Toxoplasma gondii* in tissues of pigs inoculated with *T. gondii* oocysts and effect of freezing on viability of tissue cysts in pork. *Am J Vet Res* 1988;49:910–913.

63 Jacobs L, Moyle G, Ris RR. The prevalence of toxoplasmosis in New Zealand sheep and cattle. *Am J Vet Res* 1963;24:673–675.

64 Hofflin JM, Conley FK, Remington JS. Murine model of intracerebral toxoplasmosis. *J Infect Dis* 1987;155:550–557.

65 Luft BJ, Remington JS. Toxoplasmic encephalitis in AIDS. CID 1992;15:211–222.

66 Laterra J, Goldstein GW. Brain microvessels and microvascular cells in vitro. In: Pardridge WM, ed. *The blood-brain barrier. Cellular and molecular biology*. New York: Raven, 1993:1–24.

67 Woodman JP, Dimier IH, Bout DT. Human endothelial cells are activated by IFN-γ to inhibit *Toxoplasma gondii* replication. *J Immunol* 1991;147:2019–2023.

68 Bommer W. The life cycle of virulent toxoplasma in cell cultures. *Aust J Exp Biol Med Sci* 1969;47:505–512.

69 Nguyen BT, Stadtsbaeder S. Modes of entry of *Toxoplasma gondii* trophozoites into normal mouse peritoneal macrophage and HeLa cell monolayers. A phase-contrast microcinematographic study. *Z Parasitenkd* 1979;60:135–146.

70 Nichols BA, Chiappino ML, O'Connor GR. Secretion from the rhoptries of *Toxoplasma gondii* during host-cell invasion. *J Ultrastruct Res* 1983;83:85–98.

71 Leriche MA, Dubremetz JF. Exocytosis of *Toxoplasma gondii* dense granules into the parasitophorous vacuole after host cell invasion. *Parasitol Res* 1990;76:559–562.

72 Michel R, Schupp K, Raether W, Bierther FW. Formation of a close junction during invasion of erythrocytes by *Toxoplasma gondii* in vitro. *Int J Parasitol* 1980;10:309–313.

73 Dubremetz JF, Rodriguez C, Ferreira E. *Toxoplasma gondii*: redistribution of monoclonal antibodies on tachyzoites during host cell invasion. *Exp Parasitol* 1985;59:24–32.

74 Jones TC, Hirsch JG. The interaction between *Toxoplasma gondii* and mammalian cells. II. The absence of lysosomal fusion with phagocytic vacuoles containing living parasites. *J Exp Med* 1972;136:1173–1194.

75 Aikawa M, Komata Y, Asai T, Midorikawa O. Transmission and scanning electron microscopy of host cell entry by *Toxoplasma gondii*. *Am J Pathol* 1977;87:285–296.

76 Strittmatter C, Lang W, Wiestler OD, Klleihues P. The changing pattern of human immunodeficiency virus associated cerebral toxoplasmosis: a study of 46 postmortem cases. *Acta Neuropathol (Berl)* 1992;83:475–481.

77 Navia BA, Petito CK, Gold JW, et al. Cerebral toxoplasmosis complicating the acquired immune deficiency syndrome: clinical and neuropathological findings in 27 patients. *Ann Neurol* 1986;19:224–238.

78 Frenkel JK, Friedlander S. Toxoplasmosis. *Pathology of neonatal disease. Pathogenesis, diagnosis and treatment.* Public Health Service publication no. 141. Washington, DC: US Government Printing Office, 1951:1–107.

79 Verma MP, Bowles L. Concentration of *Toxoplasma gondii* in the brain tissue of animals: a histological study confirmed by biological isolations. *J Parasitol* 1967;53:254–257.

80 Bradbury M. *The concept of a blood-brain barrier.* Chichester: Wiley-Interscience, 1979.

81 Schoolar JC, Barlow CF, Roth LJ. The penetration of carbon-14 urea into cerebrospinal fluid and various areas of the cat brain. *J Neuropathol* 1960;19:216–227.

82 Frenkel JK, Nelson BM, Arias SJ. Immunosuppression and toxoplasmic encephalitis: clinical and experimental aspects. *Hum Pathol* 1975;6:97–111.

83 Lainson R. Observations on the development and nature of pseudocysts and cysts of *Toxoplasma gondii*. *Trans R Soc Trop Med Hyg* 1958;52:396–407.

84 Van der Waaij D. Formation, growth and multiplication of *Toxoplasma gondii* cysts in mouse brains. *Trop Geogr Med* 1959; 11:345–370.

85 Frenkel JK, Escajadillo A. Cyst rupture as a pathogenic mechanism of toxoplasmic encephalitis. *Am J Trop Med Hyg* 1987; 36:517–522.

86 Zuelzer WW. Infantile toxoplasmosis, with a report of three cases, including two in which the patients were identical twins. *Arch Pathol* 1944;38:1–19.

87 Rodney MB, Mitchell N, Redner B, Turin R. Infantile toxoplasmosis: report of a case with autopsy. *Pediatrics* 1950;5:649–663.

88 Frenkel JK. Pathology and pathogenesis of congenital toxoplasmosis. *Bull NY Acad Med* 1974;50:182–191.

89 Callahan WP Jr, Russell WO, Smith MG. Human toxoplasmosis. A clinicopathologic study with presentation of five cases and review of the literature. *Medicine* 1946;25:343–397.

90 Frenkel JK. Toxoplasmosis. Mechanisms of infection, laboratory diagnosis and management. *Curr Top Pathol* 1971;54:27–75.

91 Carrazana EJ, Rossitch EJ, Samuels MA. Cerebral toxoplasmosis in the acquired immune deficiency syndrome. *Clin Neurol Neurosurg* 1989;91:291–301.

92 Vischer WA, Suter E. Intracellular multiplication of *Toxoplasma gondii* in adult mammalian macrophages cultivated in vitro. *Proc Soc Exp Bio Med* 1954;86:413–419.

93 Nakayama I. Effects of immunization procedures in experimental toxoplasmosis. *Keio J Med* 1965;14:63–72.

94 Stadtsbaeder S, Nguyen BT, Calvin-Preval MC. Respective role of antibodies and immune macrophages during acquired immunity against toxoplasmosis in mice. *Ann Immunol (Paris)* 1975;126c:461–474.

95 Remington JS, Krahenbuhl JL, Mendenhall JW. A role for activated macrophages in resistance to infection with *Toxoplasma*. *Infect Immun* 1972;6:829–834.

96 Jones TC, Len L, Hirsch JG. Assessment in vitro of immunity against *Toxoplasma gondii*. *J Exp Med* 1975;141:466–482.

97 Anderson SEJ, Remington JS. Effect of normal and activated human macrophages on *Toxoplasma gondii*. *J Exp Med* 1974; 139:1154–1174.

98 Dannemann BR, Morris VA, Araujo FG, Remington JS. Assessment of human natural killer and lymphokine-activated killer cell cytotoxicity against *Toxoplasma gondii* trophozoites and brain cysts. *J Immunol* 1989; 143:2684–2691.

99 Sharma SD, Hofflin JM, Remington JS. In vivo recombinant interleukin 2 administration enhances survival against a lethal challenge with *Toxoplasma gondii*. *J Immunol* 1985; 135:4160–4163.

100 Subauste CS, Dawson L, Remington JS. Human lymphokine-activated killer cells are cytotoxic against cells infected with *Toxoplasma gondii*. *J Exp Med* 1992;176:1511–1519.

101 Hauser WE Jr, Tsai V. Acute toxoplasma infection of mice induces spleen NK cells that are cytotoxic for *Toxoplasma gondii* in vitro. *J Immunol* 1986;136:313–319.

102 Goyal M, Ganguly NK, Mahajan RC. Natural killer cell cytotoxicity against *Toxoplasma gondii* in acute and chronic murine toxoplasmosis. *Med Sci Res* 1988;16:375–377.

103 Hunter CA, Subauste C, Cleave V, Remington JS. Production of IFN-γ by NK cells from *Toxoplasma gondii* infected SCID mice: regulation by IL-10, IL-12, and TNF-α. *Infect Immun* 1994;62:2818–2824.

104 Sher A, Oswald I, Hieny S, Gazzinelli R. *Toxoplasma gondii* induces a T-independent IFN-γ response in natural killer cells that requires both adherent accessory cells and tumor necrosis factor-α. *J Immunol* 1993; 150:3982–3989.

105 Lindberg RE, Frenkel JK. Toxoplasmosis in nude mice. *J Parasitol* 1977;63:219–221.

106 Frenkel JK, Taylor DW. Toxoplasmosis in immunoglobulin M-suppressed mice. *Infect Immun* 1982;38:360–367.

107 Duquesne V, Auriault C, Darcy F, et al. Protection of nude rats against *Toxoplasma* infection by excreted-secreted antigen-specific helper T cells. *Infect Immun* 1990;58:2120–2126.

108 Beaman MH, Araujo F, Remington JS. Protective reconstitution of the SCID mouse against reactivation of toxoplasmic encephalitis. *J Infect Dis* 1994;169:375–383.

109 Johnson LL. SCID mouse models on acute and relapsing chronic *Toxoplasma gondii* infections. *Infect Immun* 1992;60:3719–3724.

110 Foster BG, McCulloch WF. Studies of active and passive immunity in animals inoculated with *Toxoplasma gondii*. *Can J Microbiol* 1968;14:103–110.

111 Pavia CS. Protection against experimental toxoplasmosis by adoptive immunotherapy. *J Immunol* 1986;137:2985–2990.

112 Johnson AM, McDonald PJ, Neoh SH. Monoclonal antibodies to *Toxoplasma* cell membrane surface antigens protect mice from toxoplasmosis. *J Protozool* 1983;30:351–356.

113 Sharma SD, Araujo FG, Remington JS. *Toxoplasma* antigen isolated by affinity chromatography with monoclonal antibody protects mice against lethal infection with *Toxoplasma gondii*. *J Immunol* 1984;133:2818–2820.

114 Suzuki Y, Wong SY, Grumet FC, et al. Evidence for genetic regulation of susceptibility to toxoplasmic encephalitis in AIDS patients. *J Infect Dis* 1996;173:265–268.

115 Suzuki Y, Joh K, Orellna MA, et al. A gene(s) within the H-2D region determines the development of toxoplasmic encephalitis in mice. *Immunology* 1991;74:732–739.

116 Suzuki Y, Joh K, Kwon O-C, et al. MHC class I gene(s) in the D/L region but not the TNF-α gene determines development of toxoplasmic encephalitis in mice. *J Immunol* 1994; 153:4649–4654.

117 Brinkmann V, Remington JS, Sharma SD. Protective immunity in toxoplasmosis: correlation between antibody response, brain cyst formation, T-cell activation, and survival in normal and B-cell-deficient mice bearing the H-2^k haplotype. *Infect Immun* 1987; 55:990–994.

118 Deckert-Schülter M, Schülter D, Schmidt D, et al. *Toxoplasma* encephalitis in congenic B10 and BALB mice: impact of genetic factors in the immune response. *Infect Immun* 1994; 62:221–228.

119 Brown C, Hunter C, Estes R, et al. Definitive identification of a gene that confers resistance against *Toxoplasma* cyst burden and encephalitis. *Immunology* 1995;85:419–428.

120 Brown CR, McLeod R. Class I MHC genes and $CD8^+$ T cells determine cyst number in *Toxoplasma gondii* infection. *J Immunol* 1990; 145:3438–3441.

121 Gazzinelli RT, Hakim FT, Hieny S, et al. Synergistic role of CD4+ and CD8+ T lymphocytes in IFN-γ production and protective immunity induced by an attenuated *Toxoplasma gondii* vaccine. *J Immunol* 1991;146:286–292.

122 Suzuki Y, Remington JS. Dual regulation of resistance against *Toxoplasma gondii* infection by Lyt-2+ and Lyt-1+, L3T4+ T cells in mice. *J Immunol* 1988;140:3943–3946.

123 Israelski DM, Remington JS. Toxoplasmosis in patients with cancer. *Clin Infect Dis* 1993; 17(suppl):S423–S435.

124 Subauste CS, Koniaris AH, Remington JS. Murine CD8+ cytotoxic T lymphocytes lyse *Toxoplasma gondii*-infected cells. *J Immunol* 1991;147:3955–3959.

125 Hakim FT, Gazzinelli RT, Denkers E, et al. CD8+ T cells from mice vaccinated against *Toxoplasma gondii* are cytotoxic for parasite-infected or antigen-pulsed host cells. *J Immunol* 1991;147:2310–2316.

126 Yano A, Aosai F, Ohta M, et al. Antigen presentation by *Toxoplasma gondii*-infected cells to CD4+ proliferative T cells and CD8+ cytotoxic cells. *J Parasitol* 1989;75:411–416.

127 Montoya JG, Lowe KE, Clayberger C, et al. Both human $CD4^+$ and $CD8^+$ T lymphocytes are cytotoxic against *Toxoplasma gondii* infected cells. *Infect Immun* 1996;64:176–181.

128 Curiel T, Krug E, Purner M, et al. Cloned human CD4+ cytotoxic T lymphocytes specific for *Toxoplasma gondii* lyse tachyzoite-infected target cells. *J Immunol* 1993; 151:2024–2031.

129 Khan IA, Smith KA, Kasper LH. Induction of antigen-specific human cytotoxic T cells by *Toxoplasma gondii. J Clin Invest* 1990; 85:1879–1886.

130 Subauste C, Chung J, Do D, et al. Preferential activation and expansion of human peripheral blood γδ T cells in response to *Toxoplasma gondii* in-vitro and their cytokine production and cytotoxic activity against *T. gondii*-infected cells. *J Clin Invest* 1995; 96:610–619.

131 de Paoli P, Basaglia G, Gennari D, et al. Phenotypic profile and functional characteristics of human gamma and delta T cells during acute toxoplasmosis. *J Clin Microbiol* 1992; 30:729–731.

132 Scalise F, Gerli R, Castellucci G, et al. Lymphocytes bearing of γδ T-cell receptor in acute toxoplasmosis. *Immunology* 1992;76:668–670.

133 Hara T, Ohashi S, Yamashita Y, et al. Human Vδ2+ γδ T-cell tolerance to foreign antigens of *Toxoplasma gondii. Proc Natl Acad Sci USA* 1996;93:5136–5140.

134 Beaman MH, Wong SY, Remington JS. Cytokines, toxoplasma and intracellular parasitism. *Immunol Rev* 1992;127:97–117.

135 Hunter C, Remington J. Immunopathogenesis of toxoplasmic encephalitis. *J Infect Dis* 1994;170:1057–1067.

136 Suzuki Y, Orellana MA, Schreiber RD, Remington JS. Interferon-γ: the major mediator of resistance against *Toxoplasma gondii. Science* 1988;240:516–518.

137 McCabe RE, Luft BJ, Remington JS. Effect of murine interferon gamma on murine toxoplasmosis. *J Infect Dis* 1984;150:961–962.

138 Suzuki Y, Remington JS. The effect of anti-IFN-γ antibody on the protective effect of LYT-2+ immune T cells against toxoplasmosis in mice. *J Immunol* 1990;144:1954–1956.

139 Suzuki Y, Conley FK, Remington JS. Treatment of toxoplasmic encephalitis in mice with recombinant gamma interferon. *Infect Immun* 1990;58:3050–3055.

140 Chang HR, Grau GE, Pechere JC. Role of TNF and IL-1 in infections with *Toxoplasma gondii. Immunology* 1990;69:33–37.

141 Black CM, Israelski DM, Suzuki Y, Remington JS. Effect of recombinant tumour necrosis factor on acute infection in mice with *Toxoplasma gondii* or *Trypanosoma cruzi. Immunology* 1989;68:570–574.

142 Johnson L. A protective role for endogenous tumor necrosis factor in *Toxoplasma gondii* infection. *Infect Immun* 1992;60:1979–1983.

143 Chang H, Pechere J, Piguet P. Role of tumour necrosis factor in chronic murine *Toxoplasma gondii* encephalitis. *Immunol Infect Dis* 1992; 2:61–68.

144 Suzuki Y, Yang Q, Conley F, et al. Antibody against interleukin-6 reduces inflammation and numbers of cysts in brains of mice with toxoplasmic encephalitis. *Infect Immun* 1994; 62:2773–2778.

145 Gazinelli RT, Wysocka M, Hieny S, et al. In the absence of endogenous IL-10, mice acutely infected with *Toxoplasma gondii* succumb to a lethal immune response dependent on CD4+ T cells and accompanied by overproduction of IL-12, IFN-γ, and TNF-α. *J Immunol* 1996;157:798–805.

146 Gazzinelli R, Hieny S, Wynn T, et al. Interleukin 12 is required for the T-lymphocyte-independent induction of interferon γ by an intracellular parasite and induces resistance in T-cell-deficient hosts. *Proc Natl Acad Sci USA* 1993;90:6115–6119.

147 Bancroft GJ, Schreiber RD, Bosma GC, et al. A T cell-independent mechanism of macrophage activation by interferon-gamma. *J Immunol* 1987;139:1104–1107.

148 Hunter CA, Chizzonite R, Remington JS. IL-1β is required for IL-12 to induce production of IFN-γ by NK cells. *J Immunol* 1995; 155:4347–4354.

149 Carson W, Ross M, Baiocchi R, et al. Endogenous production of interleukin 15 by activated human monocytes is critical for optimal production of interferon-gamma by natural killer cells in vitro. *J Clin Invest* 1995; 96:25–78.

150 Khan I, Kasper L. IL-15 augments CD8+ T cell-mediated immunity against *Toxoplasma gondii* infection in mice. *J Immunol* 1996; 157:2103–2108.

151 Hunter CA, Litton MJ, Remington JS, Abrams JS. Immunocytochemical detection of cytokines in the lymph nodes and brains of mice resistant or susceptible to toxoplasmic encephalitis. *J Infect Dis* 1994;170:939–945.

152 Hunter CA, Roberts CW, Alexander J. Kinetics of cytokine mRNA production in the brains of mice with progressive toxoplasmic encephalitis. *Eur J Immunol* 1992;22:2317–2322.

153 Hunter C, Abrams J, Beaman M, Remington J. Detection of cytokine mRNA in the central nervous system of SCID mice infected with *Toxoplasma gondii*: importance of TNF-α, IFN-γ, IL-6, and IL-10 in T-cell-independent

regulation of resistance to *T. gondii*. *Infect Immun* 1993;61:4038–4044.

154 Gazzinelli R, Eltoum I, Wynn T, Sher A. Acute cerebral toxoplasmosis is induced by in vivo neutralization of TNF-α and correlates with the down-regulated expression of inducible nitric oxide synthase and other markers of macrophage activation. *J Immunol* 1993;151:3672–3680.

155 Hunter CA, Roberts CW, Murry M, Alexander J. Detection of cytokine mRNA in the brains of mice with toxoplasmic encephalitis. *Parasite Immunol* 1992;14:405–413.

156 Peterson P, Gekker G, Hu S, Chao C. Intracellular survival multiplication of *Toxoplasma gondii* in astrocytes. *J Infect Dis* 1993; 168:1472–1478.

157 Chao CC, Hu S, Gekker G, et al. Effects of cytokines on multiplication of *Toxoplasma gondii* in microglial cells. *J Immunol* 1993; 150:3404–3410.

158 Chao C, Gekker G, Hu S, Peterson P. Human microglial cell defense against *Toxoplasma gondii*. *J Immunol* 1994;152:1246–1252.

159 Schluter D, Deckert-Schluter M, Schwendemann G, et al. Expression of major histocompatibility complex class II antigens and levels of interferon-γ, tumour necrosis factor, and interleukin-6 in cerebrospinal fluid and serum in *Toxoplasma gondii*-infected SCID and immunocompetent C.B-17 mice. *Immunology* 1993;78:430–435.

160 Deckert-Schüter M, Schlüter D, Hof H, et al. Differential expression of ICAM-1, VCAM-1 and their ligands LFA-1, Mac-1, CD43, VLA-4, and MHC class II antigens in murine *Toxoplasma* encephalitis: a light microscopic and ultrastructural immunohistochemical study. *J Neuropathol Exp Neurol* 1994;53:457–468.

161 Lelong M, Alison F, Desmonts G, et al. Thoughts on 7 cases of congenital toxoplasmosis. Different clinical aspects of this infirmity. *Arch Fr Pediatr* 1959;15:433–448.

162 Alford C, Foft J, Blankenship W, et al. Subclinical central nervous system disease of neonates: a prospective study of infants born with increased levels of IgM. *J Pediatr* 1969;75:1167–1178.

163 Subauste C, Wong S-Y, Remington JS. AIDS-associated toxoplasmosis. In: Sande M, Volberding P, eds. *The medical management of AIDS*. 5th ed. Philadelphia: WB Saunders, 1996:343–362.

164 Casado-Naranjo I, Lopez-Trigo J, Ferrandiz A, et al. Hemorrhagic abscess in a patient with the acquired immunodeficiency syndrome. *Neuroradiology* 1988;31:289.

165 Chaudhari AB, Singh A, Jindal S, Poon TP. Hemorrhage in cerebral toxoplasmosis. A report on a patient with the acquired immunodeficiency syndrome. *S Afr Med J* 1989; 76:272–274.

166 Khuong MA, Matheron S, Marche C, et al. Diffuse toxoplasmic encephalitis without abscess in AIDS patients. In: *30th Interscience Conference on Antimicrobial Agents and Chemotherapy*. Atlanta: 1990: Abstract 1157.

167 Mehren M, Burns PJ, Mamani F, et al. Toxoplasmic myelitis mimicking intramedullary spinal cord tumor. *Neurology* 1988; 38:1648–1650.

168 Herskovitz S, Siegel SE, Schneider AT, et al. Spinal cord toxoplasmosis in AIDS. *Neurology* 1989;39:1552–1553.

169 Harris TM, Smith RR, Bognanno JR, Edwards MK. Toxoplasmic myelitis in AIDS: gadolinium-enhanced MRI. *J Comput Assist Tomogr* 1990;14:809–811.

170 Kayser C, Campbell R, Sartorious C, Barlett M. Toxoplasmosis of the conus medullaris in a patient with hemophilia A-associated AIDS. *J Neurosurg* 1990;73:951–953.

171 Wong S-Y, Remington J. Toxoplasmosis in pregnancy. *Clin Infect Dis* 1994;18:853–862.

172 Hohlfeld P, Daffos F, Costa J-M, et al. Prenatal diagnosis of acongenital toxoplasmosis with polymerase-chain-reaction test on amniotic fluid. *N Engl J Med* 1994;331:695–699.

173 Parmley S, Goebel F, Remington J. Detection of *Toxoplasma gondii* in cerebrospinal fluid from AIDS patients by polymerase chain reaction. *J Clin Microbiol* 1992;30:3000–3002.

174 Schoondermark-van de Van E, Galama J, Kraaijeveld C, et al. Value of the polymerase chain reaction for the detection of *Toxoplasma gondii* in cerebrospinal fluid from patients with AIDS. *Clin Infect Dis* 1993;16:661–666.

175 Dupouy-Camet J, Lavareda de Souza L, Maslo C, et al. Detection of *Toxoplasma gondii* in venous blood from AIDS patients by polymerase chain reaction. *J Clin Microbiol* 1993;31:1866–1869.

176 Bretagne S, Costa J-M, Fleury-Feith J, et al. Quantitative competitive PCR with bronchoalveolar lavage fluid for diagnosis of toxoplasmosis in AIDS patients. *J Clin Microbiol* 1995;33:1662–1664.

11 Neuropathogenesis of African Sleeping Sickness

CHRISTOPHER A. HUNTER
JOANNE BURKE

THE PARASITE AND THE DISEASE

The Disease

The causative agents of human African trypanosomiasis (HAT) are the protozoan parasites *Trypanosoma brucei rhodesiense* and *T. brucei gambiense*. As their names suggest, these parasites are found in distinct geographic regions, with the former being more common in East Africa and the latter in West Africa. *T. brucei gambiense* is associated with a chronic form of the disease that can last for several years. In contrast, *T. brucei rhodesiense* is a more virulent parasite associated with acute disease that can last from weeks to months. Both of these infections are invariably fatal without chemotherapeutic intervention. In 1986 the World Health Organization (WHO) estimated that there were some 20,000 new cases of HAT annually, with some 50 million people directly at risk from this infection (1). In the last decade, programs to control this infection resulted in the eradication of sleeping sickness in many areas. However, recent outbreaks in Zaire and Uganda highlight the continued risk posed by this infection in rural Africa (2).

Antigenic Variation

One of the most interesting aspects of the biology of *T. brucei* species is their ability to undergo antigenic variation, which allows the establishment of a persistent infection. The basis for this phenomenon is the variable surface glycoprotein (VSG) that covers the entire parasite (Fig 11-1). This coat protects against innate mechanisms of resistance but is highly antigenic and stimulates the production of specific antibody responses. The ability of *T. brucei* to switch surface coat and express another of a different antigenic specificity, and thereby evade the immune response, has resulted in this parasite becoming the paradigm for the study of antigenic variation (3,4). During the course of infection, the majority of the parasites are covered in the same VSG (homotype). Because specific antibodies are produced against the homotype, the parasites are opsonized and rapidly cleared from the circulation, resulting in a dramatic reduction in the number

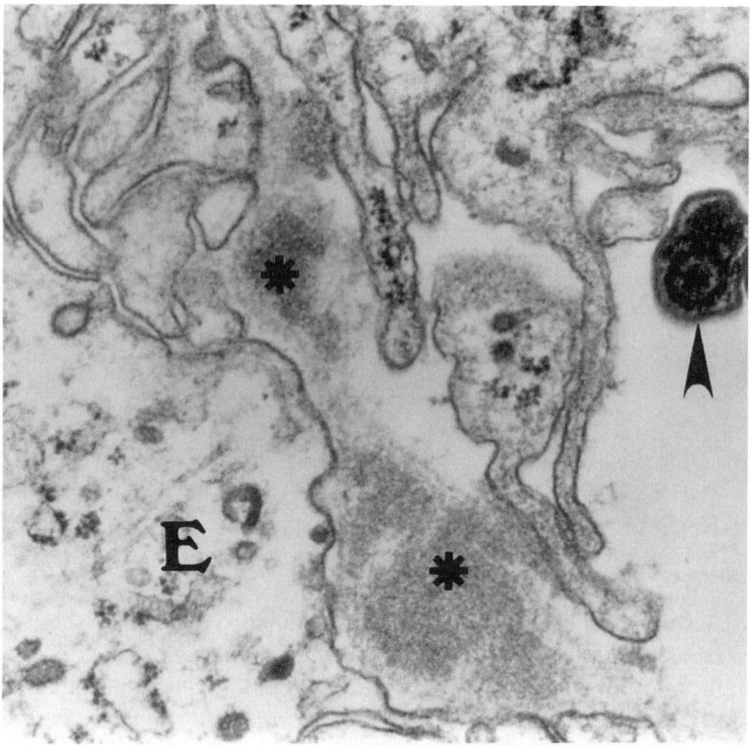

(A)

Figure 11-1. (A) Choroid plexus of the fourth ventricle of a mouse 8 weeks after experimental infection with *Trypanosoma brucei brucei*, demonstrating the subependymal electron-dense immune complexes (asterisk) deposited on the surface of an ependymal cell [E]. A cross section of a flagellum of trypanosome (arrowhead) is also visible. [B] Brain section of a vervet monkey infected with *T. brucei rhodesiense* after treatment with berenil, showing the presence of an interstitial intracerebral trypanosome [T] with the flagella in cross section (large arrowheads). A myelin-sheathed fiber [M] is prominent in this micrograph. Note the presence of the thick coat (the variable surface glycoprotein) on the surface of the trypanosome (small arrowhead). (Courtesy of Dr. A. A. Poltera and Dr. W. Rudin.)

of circulating parasites. However, a small percentage of parasites have changed their surface coat and express VSGs (heterotypes) that are antigenically distinct from the previous homotype. These parasites are not recognized by the humoral immune response and replicate freely, and one of the heterotypes emerges as a new homotype. It needs to be emphasized that expression of the VSG does not protect the parasite from a specific immune response but in fact stimulates an aggressive immune response. The long-term consequences of this continued antigenic insult are, in part, responsible for the extensive immunopathology that is characteristic of this infection and can eventually lead to death of the host.

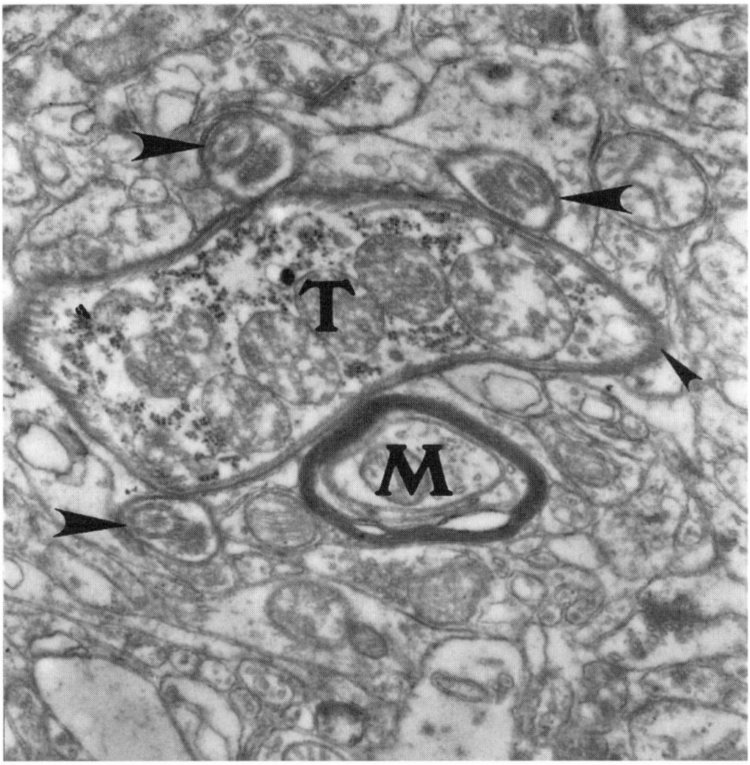

(B)

Figure 11-1. *(continued)*

Course of Infection

Transmission of *T. brucei* is dependent on the tsetse fly, which injects the metacyclic stage of the parasite into the skin. Early events at the site of infection are characterized by the development of a localized inflammatory response (chancre) and the transformation of the parasite to produce the trypomastigote stage. From the skin, parasites enter the draining lymphatics and blood, where they multiply rapidly and invade tissues such as the heart, skeletal muscle, and the brain. During the early course of the infection, disease is characterized by the presence of parasites in the blood, lymphadenopathy, fever, joint pain, and headaches (5). It is during the later stages of the infection in humans that neurologic involvement, associated with the presence of parasites in the central nervous system (CNS), becomes apparent. Interestingly, at this late stage of disease, there may be few parasites in the blood and diagnosis depends on the demonstration of trypanosomes in the cerebrospinal fluid (CSF). Clinically, late-stage disease is characterized by a variety of symptoms including wasting of muscles, lethargy, coma, ataxia, and the disturbed sleep patterns (insomnia at night, drowsiness during the day), which give rise to the name of this disease (5–7). Moreover, there is also evidence of acute and chronic dysfunction of the hypothalamic-pituitary axis that is likely due to parasite infiltration or secondary inflammation, which results in necrosis within the pituitary (8,9). In addition, there are increased numbers of white blood cells, and elevated levels of immunoglobulin and prostaglandin E_2 (PGE_2) in the CSF of patients with late-stage disease (10–12). The finding that PGE_2 is produced is significant since it can suppress many different aspects of the immune response including cytokine production (13) and has been proposed to be involved in the changes in sleep patterns associated with this infection (12).

Chemotherapy of Early- and Late-Stage Disease

During the early stage of infection, patients can be treated with pentamidine or the sulfated napthylamine suramin, which readily clears parasites from the blood and other tissues. However, it is during the chronic stage of the disease that treatment becomes complicated. Suramin and pentamidine do not readily cross the blood-brain barrier (BBB) and fail to eliminate parasites from the brain. Thus, successful drug treatment of late-stage disease is reliant on the arsenical melarsoprol, which is one of the few trypanocidal drugs that can effectively cross the BBB and eradicate parasites established within the brain. However, subcurative chemotherapy with subsequent relapse of the infection can occur in 5% to 30% of patients (10). This situation is further complicated by the occurrence of a fatal posttreatment reactive encephalopathy (PTRE) in approximately 5% to 10% of treated patients with late-stage disease (6,14,15). PTRE is characterized by the development of severe neurologic symptoms, progression to coma, and death approximately 10 to 14 days after treatment (6,14,15). Management of PTRE is a major problem associated with the treatment of late-stage sleeping sickness. Considerable time and effort have been dedicated to the prevention and management of this condition. Supportive treatment with corticosteroids may decrease the incidence of PTRE (11,15). However, in one study, such treatment did not reduce the incidence of PTRE (16). Studies in a murine model suggested that nonsteroidal anti-inflammatory drugs may be of use for the management of this complication of treatment (17). Other workers suggested that a reduction in the total dose of melarsoprol could reduce toxicity without jeopardizing its efficacy (15).

A recent addition to the drugs available for the treatment of early- and late-stage HAT is eflornithine (18,19). This specific irreversible inhibitor of ornithine decarboxylase, an enzyme required for parasite de novo synthesis of polyamines, prevents parasite replication. Thus, it does not directly eliminate the parasite but rather is trypanostatic and is dependent on a functional immune system to clear the parasites (20,21). A notable aspect of eflornithine is the rapid sense of well-being and clinical improvement that it induces in moribund patients with late-stage sleeping sickness, even when it has failed to eliminate the infection. As a consequence, eflornithine has been termed the "resurrection drug" (22). The use of eflornithine is complicated by a requirement for hospitalization and long treatment regimens. Moreover, it is relatively ineffective against *T. brucei rhodesiense* and is expensive for rural Africa (2). Nevertheless, approval of this drug for the treatment of HAT, the first in more than 40 years, provides a suitable alternative to melarsoprol for the treatment of late-stage sleeping sickness caused by *T. brucei gambiense*.

MECHANISMS THAT UNDERLY THE NEUROPATHOGENESIS OF HUMAN AFRICAN TRYPANOSOMIASIS

Immunity and the Brain

Although the African trypanosomes can invade many different tissues, it is their ability to persist within the brain that is an important aspect of this infection. The brain is a unique immunologic site for a number of reasons. The presence of the BBB (which regulates the ability of soluble molecules such as cytokines and immunoglobulins to cross into the brain), the lack of a lymphatic system, low levels of major histocompatibility complex (MHC) expression, and a paucity of resident lymphocytes together ensure that the brain is an immune-privileged site (23). Although it is now recognized that glial cell populations can present antigen and participate actively in immune responses within the brain (23,24) (see also Chapters 6 and 7), the immune response within the brain is limited when compared to other anatomic sites. Thus, infectious organisms within the CNS are likely to be protected from the full consequences of a specific immune response. The combination of antigenic variation and the immune-privileged nature of the brain allow *T. brucei* species to persist within the brain and result in the development of the neuropathology that characterizes this infection.

Neuropathology

Histologically, the neuropathology associated with late-stage sleeping sickness and the development of PTRE in humans is characterized by the presence of prominent perivascular cuffing, a nonspecific lymphoplasmacytic meningoencephalitis of varying intensity, microglial hyperplasia, reactive astrocytes, and infrequent demyelination (6,14,25). Evidence that there are B-cell responses in the brains of patients with late-stage disease is provided by pathology studies showing the presence of Mott cells (immunoglobulin-filled B cells) and by analysis of clinical samples demonstrating intracranial antibody production (26).

The neuropathology observed in clinical cases can also be generated in different simian and rodent models. Studies in rat models showed that invasion of the brain by parasites first occurs in areas in which the BBB is not well developed, that is, the sensory ganglia and circumventricular organs including the area postrema, pineal gland, and median eminence (27). The infiltration of trypanosomes into these areas may relate to the origin of the cardinal symptoms of the disease, for example, sensory disturbances, nausea, disturbed circadian rhythms, and neuroendocrinologic dysfunctions (27). Further studies demonstrated that an early increase in the expression of MHC class I molecules as well as infiltration of macrophages and $CD8^+$ T cells corresponds to areas in which the initial invasion of trypanosomes occurred (28). During chronic infection of rats with *T. brucei gambiense*, there is a mononuclear infiltrate in the leptomeninges and formation of perivascular cuffs. MHC class I– and class II–positive neuroglial cells, B cells, activated T cells, and macrophages are found in these inflammatory lesions and in the white matter. The increased expression of MHC class I and II molecules implies that there is active presentation of parasite antigen within the brain. The presence of T and B cells supports the concept that there is an ongoing antiparasite immune response within the brain and suggests that a T cell–dependent B-cell immune response is initiated within the CNS during this stage of infection (29).

Role of Interferon in Parasite Neurotropism

Studies by Kristenssen et al. (30,31) suggested an important role for interferon (IFN)-γ and an IFN-γ–like molecule in the neuropathogenesis of sleeping sickness. Initial studies with Sprague-Dawley rats infected with *T. brucei* showed a strong and rapid induction of splenocyte IFN-γ production (within 12 hours after infection). This response was shown to be due to $CD8^+$ T cells in experiments in which depletion of the $CD8^+$ T cells in infected animals abrogated IFN-γ production. Surprisingly, depletion of $CD8^+$ T cells also suppressed parasite growth and increased survival of the animals and inhibited the induction of MHC class I molecules in the paraventricular and supraoptic hypothalamic nuclei associated with infection (30). These results suggested that $CD8^+$ T cells are involved directly or indirectly in growth regulation of the parasite and that IFN-γ induced by the parasite during infection may be one of the factors that upregulates expression of MHC molecules in the brain (30). In addition, the authors reported the presence of an IFN-γ–like molecule (as assessed by reaction with IFN-γ–specific monoclonal antibodies and biologic properties similar to those of IFN-γ) localized to small neurons in peripheral sensory ganglia that acts as a growth factor for African trypanosomes (31). These results suggest the development of a tropic mechanism whereby *T. brucei* is attracted to the brain where it will be protected from the full consequences of the immune response and is supplied with an IFN-γ–like growth factor.

Role of CNS-Specific Autoantibodies

As a consequence of the parasite persistence observed during African trypanosomiasis, prolonged antigenic stimulation and continual activation of B cells occur. This results in a hypergammaglobulinemia and polyclonal B-cell activation associated with the production of autoantibodies. Autoantibodies have been implicated in many different aspects of the pathogenesis of African trypanosomiasis including the glomerulonephritis, cardiac involvement, anemia, and neurologic disease. The most suggestive evidence for a role for autoantibodies in the neuropathogenesis of sleeping sickness is the presence of autoantibodies specific for myelin basic protein (MBP) and galactocerebrosides (the major glycolipids of myelin) in the CSF of patients with late-stage sleeping sickness (32,33). Similarly, autoantibodies to the neural specific antigens, MBP, and myelin-specific galactocerebrosides and gangliosides as well as to double-stranded (ds) DNA can be found in the sera of infected mice (34). Moreover, levels of autoantibodies to MBP, gangliosides, and galactocerebrosides in infected mice are positively correlated with the severity of the pathology in the brain. Since titers of dsDNA autoantibodies (a nonneural antigen) do not correlate with the severity of the pathology in the brain, these data suggest that neural-specific autoantibodies may be involved in the development of the neuropathology observed in sleeping sickness.

There are several possible explanations for the high levels of CNS-specific autoantibodies observed during African trypanosomiasis. These autoimmune responses may simply result from the nonspecific polyclonal activation of B cells or could develop owing to a cross-reactivity between parasite antigens and host glial and neuronal antigens, such as have been reported with South American trypanosomes (35). Alternatively, increased titers of brain-specific autoantibodies may be a response to antigens released from the brain as a consequence of the inflammation associated with invasion of the CNS by parasites. Thus, the autoantibodies would not be a direct cause of the immunopathology but instead may be a secondary response to inflammation within the brain.

Posttreatment Reactive Encephalopathy

The basis of PTRE has been controversial. It has been proposed that it is a result of neurotoxicity of the pentavalent antimonials used for drug treatment or an immune complex–mediated disease that results in vascular damage. Previous studies on the neurotoxicity of arsenicals reported hemorrhagic necrosis and the appearance of localized inflammatory lesions in the meninges and choroid plexus and a gliosis in the white matter, a result of an increase in vascular permeability in the CNS and disturbed coagulation. However, in studies with tryparsamide, Hurst (36) found that this arsenical was of low toxicity. Moreover, Haller et al. (6) concluded that, based on clinical and laboratory findings, PTRE was due to a drug-related delayed immune response. Thus, there appears to be an immunologic basis for this phenomena. It should also be noted that histologically PTRE is similar in many ways to the pathology observed in untreated patients who died of late-stage sleeping sickness. Thus, the pathologic processes that occur during the normal progression of the infection are also likely to be involved in the development of PTRE.

Although PTRE is almost exclusively associated with the use of melarsoprol, a reactive encephalitis has developed in some patients after treatment with suramin (37). Furthermore, a murine model of infection was used to demonstrate that PTRE could be induced using the trypanocidal compound berenil (diminazene aceturate), which fails to cross the BBB (38). Thus, the development of PTRE in a murine model was not the result of arsenical toxicity. Pathologically, the lesions observed in the brains of mice treated with berenil were very similar to those in humans and were characterized by the development of perivascular cuffs, encephalitis, meningitis, and activated astrocytes (39) (Fig 11-2). Moreover, the time scale for the development of PTRE was 5 to 14 days, similar to that for PTRE in humans. Importantly, the common feature of the regimens that induced PTRE was that they had to be subcurative, whereas curative regimens failed to induce PTRE (38,40). Although these studies were performed in a murine model, these data suggest that PTRE in humans could be a consequence of subcurative drug treatment. Support for this hypothesis was provided by studies that used the polymerase chain reaction (PCR) to demonstrate the presence of DNA sequences of *T. brucei* in archival brain material from 9 patients who died with PTRE (40). Although parasite DNA may persist after treatment, in the absence of fresh clinical biopsy material from patients with PTRE, these data suggest that patients who died with PTRE were still infected at the time of death.

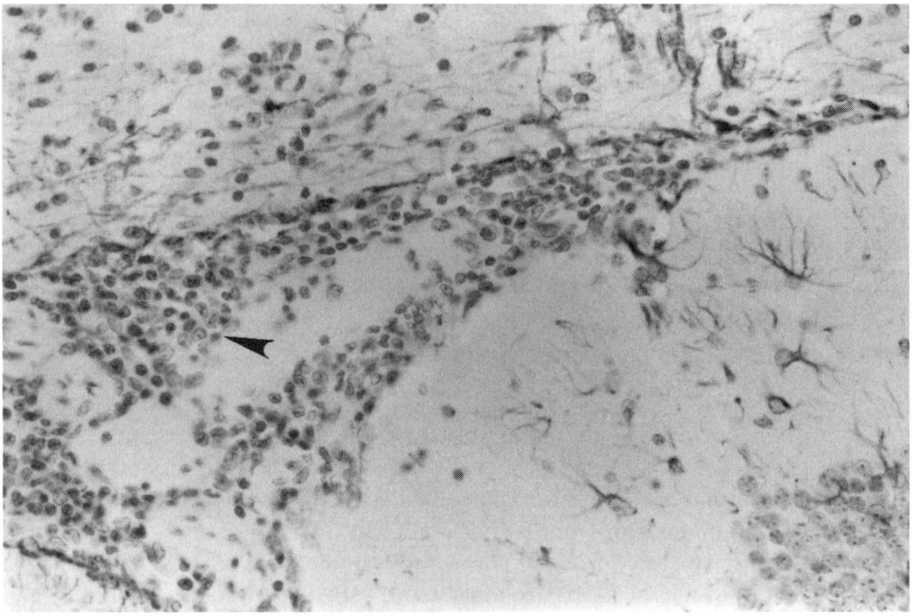

Figure 11-2. Activated astrocytes in the brain of a mouse infected with *T. brucei brucei* and treated with berenil on day 28 after infection. Posttreatment reactive encephalopathy was allowed to develop, and the mouse was killed 2 weeks later. Astrocytes are stained for glial fibrillary acidic protein using immunohistochemistry. Note the large numbers of inflammatory cells in the ventricle (arrowhead).

If PTRE were simply a consequence of subcurative therapy, then there should be a far higher percentage of patients who develop this syndrome. Indeed, PTRE is rarely if ever seen in patients treated with suramin or pentamidine, although a small percentage of these patients would likely have some parasites in the CNS (41). A possible explanation for this finding is that the patients most likely to be treated with melarsoprol are those with late-stage disease and those who probably have a large number of parasites within the brain. Indeed, in the murine model the severity of PTRE in part depends on the parasite load within the brain. This is illustrated by studies in which drug treatment on day 21 after infection (when parasite numbers in the brain are low (42)) results in mild PTRE, whereas drug treatment of mice with relapse infections (with high numbers of parasites in their brains, see Fig11-2) results in more severe PTRE (38). Thus, individuals with a low number of parasites in their CNS when treated with suramin or pentamidine may not develop clinical PTRE.

The findings just described raise the question of why such a violent immune response to parasites within the brain develops after subcurative treatment and not during the normal course of the infection. Studies in patients and murine models previously showed that infection with *T. brucei* results in suppression of the cellular immune response. In murine models this is characterized, in part, by decreased production of interleukin (IL)-2 and reduced expression of the IL-2 receptor by T cells (43) and is associated with macrophage production of nitric oxide, which results in a suppression of T-cell responses (44). Interestingly, infection-induced suppression of the immune system is reversed within hours of treatment with antiparasite drugs (45). It has been proposed that the parasites which persist in the brain after treatment act as a potent stimulus for the restored immune system and stimulate a violent immune response. However, Milord and Pepin (41) highlighted reports that graded doses of melarsoprol decrease the frequency of PTRE in patients with *T. brucei rhodesiense* and questioned the validity of comparing the mouse model with human disease.

Immune Complexes

Elevated levels of immune complexes in the blood and CSF of patients are characteristic of late-stage sleeping sickness and may play a role in the neuropathogenesis of the disease and PTRE (26). Studies with vervet monkeys and infected mice showed elevated levels of circulating immune complexes and the presence of immunoglobulin deposits (see Fig 11-1) and activation of complement in the choroid plexus (46–48). In addition, administration of melarsoprol to infected mice results in an increase in the levels of circulating immune complexes, which decreases within 1 to 2 weeks (46). Based in part on these studies, it was proposed that the development of PTRE may be a consequence of drug-induced lysis of parasites, leading to the rapid release of high levels of parasite antigens within the brain. This would result in the deposition of immune complexes and complement activation, leading to a Jarisch-Herxheimer–type reaction. Pepin and Milord (10) proposed that the killing of parasites in situ releases antigen, which then binds to brain cells and attracts antibodies and T lymphocytes. Thus, aggressive treatment regimens that result in rapid killing of parasites would lead to a sudden release of parasite antigens and subsequent immune reaction. However, treatment of infected mice with a short-term aggressive regimen results in rapid parasitologic cure; PTRE fails to develop and the existing pathology in these mice resolves (38). These results provide no support for the concept that the rapid release of parasite antigens results in the development of PTRE. Instead, these data suggest that viable trypanosomes are required within the brain for the immunopathologic events associated with PTRE to occur. However, these data do not exclude a role for immune complex deposition and subsequent activation of complement in the development of the pathology associated with late-stage disease.

Cytokines and the Inflammatory Response

The important role of cytokines in the regulation of resistance or susceptibility to different parasitic infections suggests that they would also have a major role in the pathogenesis of African trypanosomiasis. However, our knowledge of the role of cytokines in the immune response to African trypanosomiasis is severely limited when compared to our knowledge of the response to other parasitic infections. Studies from patients and animal models indicate an immunologic basis for PTRE and so it is likely that cytokines are involved in these events. The availability of sensitive techniques to detect messenger RNA (mRNA) for different cytokines has allowed the immune events in the brain during PTRE to be characterized. Initial studies that analyzed the immunopathology of PTRE in mice demonstrated the intense activation of astrocytes (as assessed by increased expression of glial fibrillary acidic protein (GFAP)), similar to clinical findings, as well as elevated levels of mRNA for tumor necrosis factor (TNF)-α, IL-1, IL-6, IFN-γ, and IL-4 but not IL-2 (39). These studies were valuable because they gave the first indication that cytokines might be important in the induction of PTRE. In particular, the detection of IL-1, TNF-α, and macrophage inflammatory protein-1 (MIP-1) was of interest because these cytokines cause inflammation in the brain (49,50) and have been implicated in the immunopathology of a number of inflammatory disorders of the CNS (51,52).

Subsequent analyses of the kinetics of cytokine production demonstrated elevated levels of cytokine mRNA, in particular IL-1α and TNF-α, in the brains of infected mice by day 14 of infection (the approximate time when parasites invade the CNS). However, despite the sustained production of these proinflammatory signals, there is little obvious inflammation within the brain, unless the mice are treated with a subcurative drug regimen. This lack of inflammation despite the presence of elevated levels of cytokine mRNA may be related to the suppression of the immune response that accompanies infection (see above). Thus, during infection, the systemic immune system is unable to respond to inflammatory signals from the brain.

Production of Cytokines by Astrocytes

Activation of astrocytes is one of the first pathologic signs of neurologic involvement after infection in mice, and correlates with a time (days 14–21) when parasite invasion of the CNS occurs and levels of mRNA for IL-1α, IL-6, and TNF-α are elevated (53). These results suggest that astrocytes may be important in regulating the immune response within the brain during infection. The concept that astrocytes may regulate an immune response within the brain is not novel (see Chapters 6 and 7). The fact that astrocytes can present antigen (54) and produce cytokines such as IL-1 (55) indicates their ability to participate in an immune response. In addition, astrocytes have other properties that could be important in the control of T-cell responses within the brain. These include the expression of CD44, which is important in T cell–astrocyte adhesion (56); the ability of astrocytes to produce nitric oxide (57) may have a role in the inhibition of T-cell proliferation within the brain (58).

Further studies to characterize the glial cells that produce cytokines during infection were performed using in situ hybridization (ISH) for IL-6 and TNF-α. In the brains of infected mice, prior to the development of significant pathology (day 28 of infection), IL-6 mRNA was localized to individual cells and examination of serial sections revealed that these cells were in areas containing activated astrocytes (Fig 11-3). These data suggest that astrocytes are the source of the elevated levels of IL-6 mRNA observed in the brains of infected mice prior to the development of PTRE. The use of immunohistochemistry revealed that IL-6 protein was only weakly detected in the brains of infected mice but was detected in the brains of mice in which PTRE developed (Burke and

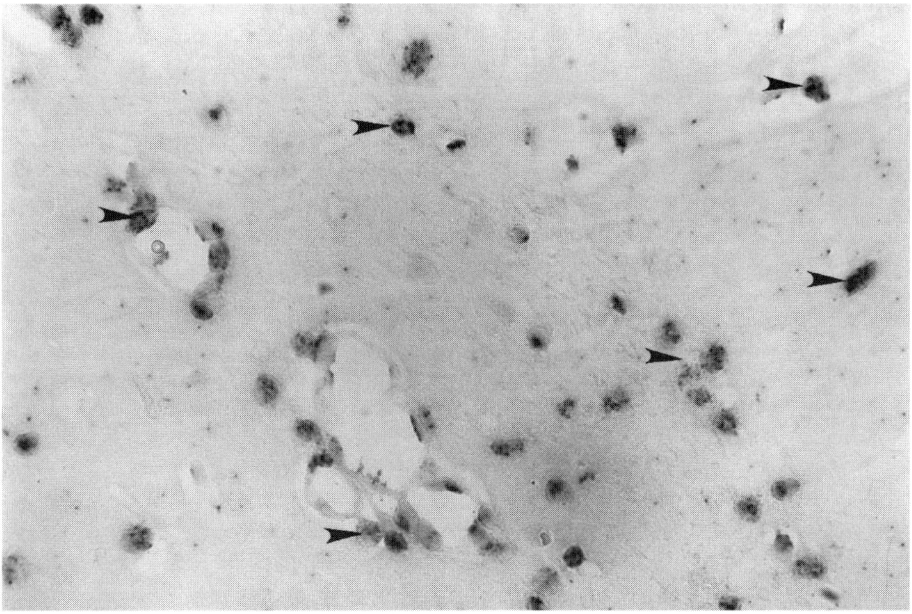

(A)

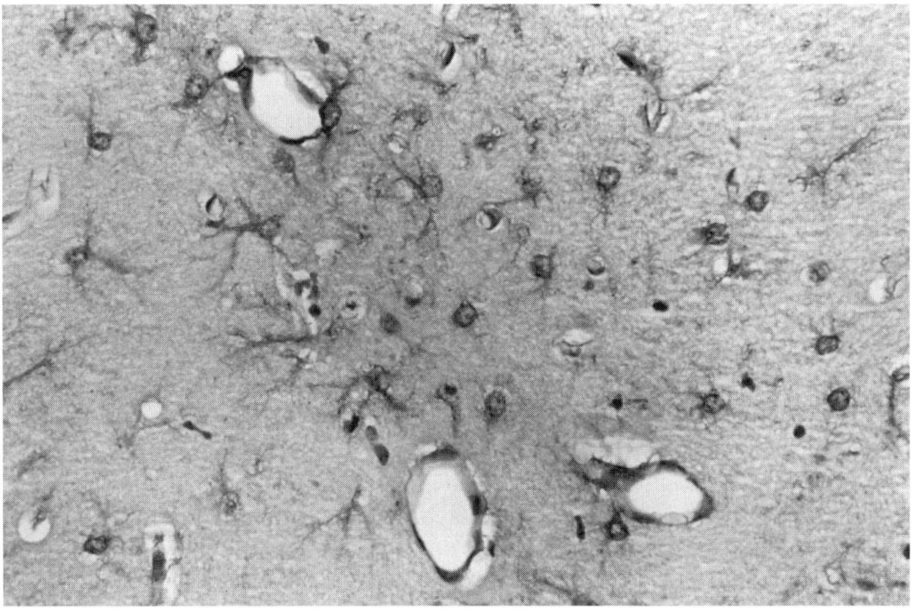

(B)

Figure 11-3. (A) Detection of interleukin (IL)-6 messenger RNA (mRNA) in the brain of a mouse infected with *T. brucei brucei* for 28 days. In the absence of inflammatory cells there are numerous cells positive for IL-6 mRNA (arrowheads). (B) Serial section from the same brain, stained for glial fibrillary acidic protein, demonstrating the presence of activated astrocytes in this site. (C) Brain of a mouse with posttreatment reactive encephalopathy, showing a focus of inflammation that is positive for tumor necrosis factor (TNF)-α mRNA (arrow). Additional cells outside the area of inflammation are also positive. The in situ hybridization was performed using frozen sections and digoxigenin-labeled probes specific for IL-6 and TNF-α mRNA.

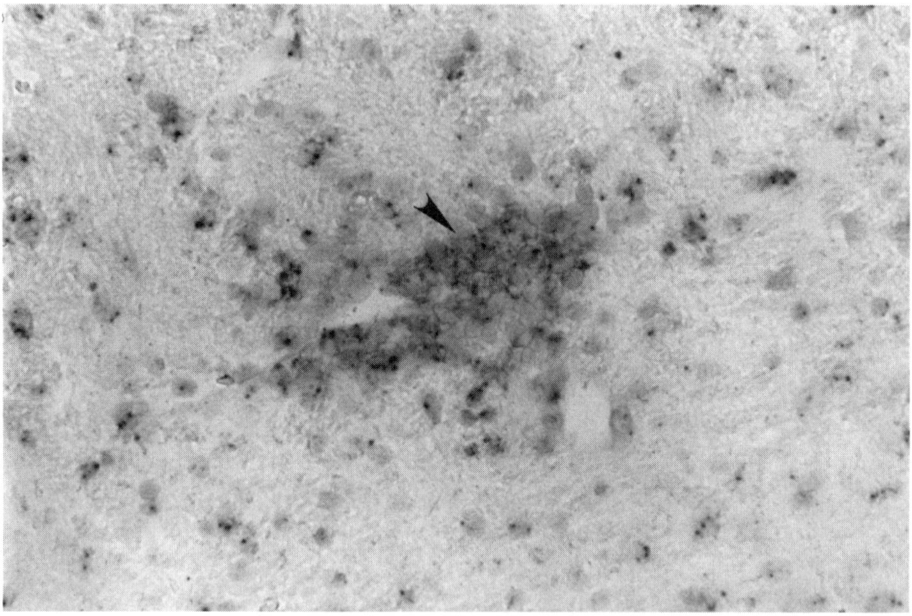

(C)

Figure 11-3. *(continued)*

Rogers, unpublished observations, 1997). These studies demonstrated that IL-6 protein is most prominent at the sites of inflammation and suggested that inflammatory cells are a major source of IL-6 protein during PTRE.

Support for the concept that IL-6 is important in the neuropathogenesis of sleeping sickness is provided by studies of other infections which showed that IL-6 levels are also elevated in the CSF of patients with bacterial or nonbacterial meningitis (59) and that administration of an antibody specific for IL-6 results in a reduction in the severity of toxoplasmic encephalitis (60) (see Chapter 5). Moreover, the generation of transgenic mice with an IL-6 gene under the control of the GFAP promoter resulted in the development of a severe neurologic disease characterized by runting, tremor, ataxia, and seizures (61). In addition, results of studies on IL-6–deficient mice reveal that IL-6 is a necessary component of the fever response to both endogenous IL-1ß and exogenous (lipopolysaccharide) pyrogen in mice (62). Thus, the production of IL-6 in the brain has a number of consequences that may be related to the pathogenesis and clinical symptoms of late-stage sleeping sickness.

ISH revealed that TNF-α mRNA was not readily detected in the brains of infected mice but was detected in those that had PTRE (see Fig 11-3). These studies showed that TNF-α mRNA was most prominent at the sites of inflammation such as the perivascular cuffs that characterize PTRE. Additional immunohistochemical studies confirmed that in mice with PTRE, TNF-α protein can be localized to astrocytes, microglia, and inflammatory cells. Production of TNF-α within the brain could have a number of effects. TNF-α has been reported to directly lyse *T. brucei* (63) and its production within the brain may be important in controlling parasite replication. TNF-α may also be important in the activation of glial cell populations to produce cytokines, the induction of adhesion molecule expression on astrocytes (64), or the stimulation of astrocyte proliferation (65).

The correlation of astrocyte activation in vivo with elevated levels of mRNA for cytokines at the time when parasites first invade the brain suggests that astrocytes may be responding directly to the parasites. In vitro studies demonstrated that cultures of astrocytes, maintained in low endotoxin conditions and exposed to purified trypomastigotes of *T. brucei*, upregulate levels of mRNA for IL-1β and IL-6 (unpublished observations). Previous studies showed that macrophages can produce IL-1 in direct response to the VSG of *T. brucei* (66), which raises the possibility that the VSG may directly stimulate astrocytes to produce cytokines. Interestingly, pretreatment of astrocytes with eflornithine, an inhibitor of polyamine biosynthesis used to treat sleeping sickness, inhibited the ability of lipopolysaccharides or trypanosomes to upregulate levels of IL-1α and IL-6 mRNA in astrocytes. An in vivo correlate of these findings was provided by the use of a stabilate of trypanosomes, which are resistant to eflornithine. Treatment of infected mice with eflornithine prior to or following the development of PTRE ameliorated the inflammatory reaction (67). Because an eflornithine-resistant strain of parasites was used, the effect of eflornithine was independent of its trypanostatic action. These results identify a previously unrecognized anti-inflammatory property of eflornithine and suggest that the remarkable effects of eflornithine reported in patients with late-stage disease may in part be attributable to the anti-inflammatory properties of this drug. This may account for the rare association of PTRE with the use of eflornithine.

FUTURE DIRECTIONS

The results of many of the current studies suggest that there is a significant immunologic component to the neuropathogenesis of sleeping sickness as well as the development of PTRE. Although several reports correlated cytokine production with the development of neuropathology, studies still need to be performed to determine the roles of these different cytokines in the inflammatory processes. In addition, the identification of the parasite components that directly stimulate astrocytes to produce cytokines will be central to our understanding of the events that occur within the brain during sleeping sickness. It will also be important to determine whether the inflammatory reaction within the brain is characterized by an antigen-specific response or simply a nonspecific inflammatory response to parasites within the brain. This information could lead to the development of regimens that will allow successful management or prevention of PTRE. Lastly, the basis of PTRE is a contentious issue. While there is much evidence to suggest an immunologic basis for this reaction, there is still an important question regarding the contribution of melarsoprol to the development of PTRE. As Milord and Pepin (41) highlighted, what is needed "is more aggressive research, with properly designed trials involving large numbers of patients, to answer these very simple questions."

REFERENCES

1 World Health Organization. Epidemiology and control of African trypanosomiasis. Report of a WHO Expert Committee. *World Health Organ Tech Rep Ser* 1986;739:1–125.

2 Kuzoe FAS. Current situation of African trypanosomiasis. *Acta Trop* 1993;54:153–162.

3 Vickerman K. Antigenic variation in trypanosomes. *Nature* 1978;273:613–617.

4 Vickerman K, Myler PJ, Stuart KD. African trypanosomiasis. In: Warren KS, ed. *Immunology and molecular biology of parasitic infections.* 3rd ed. 1993:170–212.

5 Poltera AA. Pathology of human African trypanosomiasis with reference to experimental African trypanosomiasis and infections of the central nervous system. *Br Med Bull* 1985;41:169–174.

6 Haller L, Adams, H, Merowze F, Dago A. Clinical and pathological aspects of human African trypanosomiasis (*T. b. gambiense)* with particular reference to reactive arsenical encephalopathy. *Am J Trop Med Hyg* 1986;5:94–99.

7 Apted FIC. Clinical manifestations and diagnosis of sleeping sickness. In: Mulligan HW, ed. *The African trypanosomes.* New York: Wiley-Interscience, 1970:661–683.

8 Kimata DM, Makawiti DW, Tengekyon KM, et al. Delayed recovery of adrenocortical and testicular function after chemotherapy of human trypanosomiasis. *Acta Trop* 1994;57:69–74.

9 Petzke F, Heppner C, Mbulamberi D, et al. Hypogonadism in Rhodesian sleeping sickness: evidence for acute and chronic dysfunction of the hypothalamic-pituitary-gonadal axis. *Fertil Steril* 1996;65:68–75.

10 Pepin J, Milord F. African trypanosomiasis and drug-induced encephalopathy: risk factors and pathogenesis. *Trans R Soc Trop Med Hyg* 1991;85:222–224.

11 Pepin J, Milord F, Guern C, et al. Trial of prednisolone for prevention of melarsoprol-induced encephalopathy in gambiense sleeping sickness. *Lancet* 1989;1:1246–1250.

12 Pentreath VW, Rees K, Owolabi OA, et al. The somnogenic T lymphocyte suppressor prostaglandin D_2 is selectively elevated in cerebrospinal fluid of advanced sleeping sickness patients. *Trans R Soc Trop Med Hyg* 1990; 84:795–799.

13 Tineke CTM, van der Pouw K, Boeije LCM, et al. Prostaglandin-E2 is a potent inhibitor of human interleukin 12 production. *J Exp Med* 1995;181:775–779.

14 Adams H, Doua A, Dago-Akribi A, et al. Human African trypanosomiasis (*T. b. gambiense*): a study of 16 cases of sleeping sickness with some observations on acute reactive encephalopathy. *Neuropathol Appl Neurobiol* 1996;12:81–94.

15 Pepin J, Milord F, Khonde AN, et al. Risk factors for encephalopathy and mortality during melarsoprol treatment of *Trypanosoma brucei gambiense* sleeping sickness. *Trans R Soc Trop Med Hyg* 1995;89:92–97.

16 Veeken HJGM, Ebeling MCA, Dolmans WMV. Trypanosomiasis in a rural hospital in Tanzania. A retrospective study of its management and the results of treatment. *Trop Geogr Med* 1989;41:113–117.

17 Hunter CA, Jennings FW, Kennedy PGE, Murray M. The use of azathioprine to ameliorate post-treatment encephalopathy associated with African trypanosomiasis. *Neuropathol Appl Neurobiol* 1992;18:619–625.

18 Milord F, Pepin J, Loko L, et al. Efficacy and toxicity of eflornithine for treatment of *Trypanosoma brucei gambiense* sleeping sickness. *Lancet* 1992;340:652–655.

19 Van Nieuwenhove S, Schecter PJ, Declercq J, et al. Treatment of Gambian sleeping sickness in the Sudan with oral DFMO (DL-alpha-difluoromethylornithine), an inhibitor of ornithine decarboxylase: first field trial. *Trans R Soc Trop Med Hyg* 1985;79:692–698.

20 de Gee ALW, McCann PP, Mansfield JM. Role of antibody in the elimination of trypanosomes after DL-alpha-difluoromethylornithine chemotherapy. *J Parasitol* 1983;69:818–822.

21 Bitonti AJ, McCann PP, Sjoerdsma A. Necessity of antibody response with treatment of African trypanosomiasis with alpha-difluoromethylornithine. *Biochem Pharmacol* 1986; 35:331–334.

22 WHO sleeping sickness “resurrection” drug approved. *WHO News* 1990;34:1–3.

23 Fontana A, Frei K, Bodmer S, Hofer E. Immune-mediated encephalitis: on the role of antigen-presenting cells in brain tissue. *Immunol Rev* 1987;100:185–201.

24 Merrill JE. Macroglia: neural cells responsive to lymphokines and growth factors. *Immunol Today* 1987;8:146–150.

25 Poltera AA, Owor R, Cox JN. Pathological aspects of human African trypanosomiasis (HAT) in Uganda. *Virchows Arch A Pathol Anat Histol* 1977;373:249–265.

26 Lambert PH, Berney M, Kazyumba G. Immune complexes in serum and in cerebrospinal fluid in sleeping sickness. Correlation with polyclonal B-cell activation and with intracere-

bral immunoglobulin synthesis. *J Clin Invest* 1981;67:77.

27 Schultzberg M, Ambatsis M, Samuelsson EB, et al. Spread of *Trypanosoma brucei* to the nervous system: early attack on circumventricular organs and sensory ganglia. *J Neurosci Res* 1988;21:56–61.

28 Schultzberg M, Olsson T, Samuelsson EB, et al. Early major histocompatibility complex (MHC) class I antigen induction in hypothalamic supraoptic and paraventricular nuclei in trypanosome-infected rats. *J Neuroimmunol* 1989;24:105–112.

29 Anthoons JAM, Van Marck EAE, Gigase PLJ, Stevens WJ. Immunohistochemical characterization of the mononuclear cells in the brain of the rat with an experimental chronic *Trypanosoma brucei gambiense* infection. *Parasitol Res* 1989;75:251–256.

30 Bakhiet M, Olsson T, Van der meide P, Kristensson K. Depletion of CD8+ T cells suppresses growth of *Trypanosoma brucei brucei* and interferon gamma production in infected rats. *Clin Exp Immunol* 1990;81:195–199.

31 Olsson T, Kelic S, Edlund C, et al. Neuronal interferon-γ immunoreactive molecule: bioactivities and purification. *Eur J Immunol* 1994; 24:308–314.

32 Asonganyi T, Lando G, Ngu JL. Serum antibodies against human brain myelin proteins in Gambian trypanosomiasis. *Ann Soc Belg Med Trop* 1989;69:213–221.

33 Jauberteau PM, Bisser S, Ayed Z, et al. Detection d'autoanticorps anti-galactocerebrosides au cours de la trypanosomose humaine africaine. *Bull Soc Pathol Exot* 1994; 87:333–336.

34 Hunter CA, Jennings FW, Tierney JF, et al. Correlation of autoantibody titres with central nervous system pathology in experimental African trypanosomiasis. *J Neuroimmunol* 1992; 41:143–148.

35 Petry K, Voisin P, Baltz T, Labouesse J. Epitopes common to trypanosomes (*T. cruzi, T. dionisii* and *T. vespertilionis* (Schizotrypanum)): astrocytes and neurons. *J Neuroimmunol* 1987; 16:237–252.

36 Hurst EW. The lesions produced in the central nervous system by certain organic arsenical compounds. *J Pathol Bacteriol* 1959; 77:523–533.

37 de Raadt P. Reactive encephalopathy occurring as a complication during treatment of *Trypanosoma rhodesiense* infections with non-arsenical drugs. In: *East African Trypanosomiasis Research Organization, annual report.* Entebbe, Uganda: Government Printer, 1967:85.

38 Jennings FW, Hunter CA, Kennedy PGE, Murray M. Chemotherapy of *Trypanosoma brucei* infection of the central nervous system: the use of rapid chemotherapeutic regimen and the development of post-treatment encephalopathies. *Trans R Soc Trop Med Hyg* 1993;87:224–226.

39 Hunter CA, Gow JW, Kennedy PGE, et al. Immunopathology of experimental African sleeping sickness: detection of cytokine mRNA in the brains of *Trypanosoma brucei*-infected mice. *Infect Immun* 1991;59:4636–4640.

40 Hunter CA, Jennings FW, Adams JH, et al. Subcurative chemotherapy and fatal post-treatment reactive encephalopathies in African trypanosomiasis. *Lancet* 1992;339:956–958.

41 Milord F, Pepin J. African trypanosomiasis: more aggressive treatment or more aggressive research? *Lancet* 1992;340:250–251.

42 Jennings FW, Gray GD. Relapsed parasitaemia following chemotherapy of chronic *Trypanosoma brucei* infections in mice and its relation to cerebral trypanosomes. *Contrib Microbiol Immunol* 1983;7:147–154.

43 Silghem M, Hamers R, De Baetselier P. Experimental *Trypanosoma brucei* infections selectively suppress both interleukin 2 production and interleukin 2 receptor expression. *Eur J Immunol* 1987;17:1417–1421.

44 Schleifer K, Mansfield JM. Suppressor macrophages in African trypanosomiasis inhibit T cell proliferative responses by nitric oxide and prostaglandins. *J Immunol* 1993;151:5492–5503.

45 Roelants GE, Pearson TW, Morrison WI, et al. Immune depression in trypanosome-infected mice. IV. *Clin Exp Immunol* 1979;37:457–469.

46 Poltera AA, Hochmann A, Lambert PH. *Trypanosoma brucei brucei*: the response to melarsoprol in mice with cerebral trypanosomiasis. An immunopathological study. *Clin Exp Immunol* 1981;46:363–374.

47 Polterea AA. Immunopathological and chemotherapeutic studies in experimental trypanosomiasis with special reference to the heart and brain. *Trans R Soc Trop Med Hyg* 1980;74:706–715.

48 Poltera AA, Sayer PD, Brighouse G, et al. Immunopathological aspects of trypanosomal meningoencephalitis in vervet monkeys after relapse following Berenil® treatment. *Trans R Soc Trop Med Hyg* 1985;79:527–531.

49 Ramilo O, Sáez-Llorens X, Mertsola J, et al. Tumor necrosis factor α-cachectin and interleukin 1β initiate meningeal inflammation. *J Exp Med* 1990;172:497–507.

50 Saukkonen K, Sande S, Cioffe C, et al. The role of cytokines in the generation of inflammation and tissue damage in experimental

gram-positive meningitis. *J Exp Med* 1990; 171:439–448.

51 Jacobs CA, Baker PE, Roux ER, et al. Experimental autoimmune encephalomyelitis is exacerbated by IL-1α and suppressed by soluble IL-1 receptor. *J Immunol* 1991;146:2983–2989.

52 Merrill JE. Effect of lymphokines and monokines on glial cells in vitro and in vivo. In: Goetzl EJ, Spector NH, eds. *Neuroimmune networks: physiology and diseases.* New York: Alan R. Liss, 1989:89–97.

53 Hunter CA, Jennings FW, Kennedy PGE, Murray M. Astrocyte activation correlates with cytokine production in central nervous system of *Trypanosoma brucei brucei*-infected mice. *Lab Invest* 1992;67:635–642.

54 Fontana A, Fierz W, Wekerle W. Astrocytes present myelin basic protein to encephalitogenic T-cell lines. *Nature* 1984;307:273–276.

55 Fontana A, Hensgartner H, de Tribolet N, Weber E. Glioblastoma cells release interleukin 1 and factors inhibiting interleukin 2-mediated effects. *J Immunol* 1984;132:1837–1844.

56 Haegel H, Tolg C, Hofmann M, Ceredig R. Activated mouse astrocytes and T cells express similar CD44 variants. Role of CD44 in astrocyte/Tcell binding. *J Cell Biol* 1993;122:1067–1077.

57 Lee SC, Dickson DW, Brosnan CF, Casadevall A. Human astrocytes inhibit *Cryptococcus neoformans* growth by a nitric oxide-mediated mechanism. *J Exp Med* 1994;180:365–369.

58 Matsumoto Y, Hanawa H, Abo T. In situ inactivation of infiltrating T cells in the central nervous system with autoimmune encephalomyelitis. The role of astrocytes. *Immunology* 1993;79:381–390.

59 Chavanet P, Bonnotte B, Guiguet M, et al. High concentrations of intrathecal interleukin-6 in human bacterial and nonbacterial meningitis. *J Infect Dis* 1992;166:428–431.

60 Suzuki Y, Yang Q, Conley FK, et al. Antibody against interleukin-6 reduces inflammation and numbers of cysts in brains of mice with toxoplasmic encephalitis. *Infect Immun* 1994; 62:2773–2778.

61 Campbell IL, Abraham CR, Masliah E, et al. Neurologic disease induced in transgenic mice by cerebral overexpression of interleukin 6. *Proc Natl Acad Sci USA* 1993;90:10061–10065.

62 Chai Z, Gatti S, Toniatti C, et al. Interleukin (IL)-6 gene expression in the central nervous system is necessary for fever response to lipopolysaccharide or IL-1β: a study on IL-6-deficient mice. *J Exp Med* 1996;183:311–316.

63 Lucas R, Magez S, De Leys R, et al. Mapping the lectin-like activity of tumor necrosis factor. *Science* 1994;263:814–817.

64 Hurwitz AA, Lyman WD, Guida MP, et al. Tumor necrosis factor α induces adhesion molecule expression on human fetal astrocytes. *J Exp Med* 1992;176:1631–1636.

65 Selmaj KW, Farooq M, Norton WT, et al. Proliferation of astrocytes in vitro in response to cytokines. A primary role for tumor necrosis factor. *J Immunol* 1990;144:129–135.

66 Mathias S, Perez R, Diffley P. The kinetics of gene expression and maturation of IL-1α after induction with the surface coat of *Trypanosoma brucei rhodesiense* or lipopolysaccharide. *J Immunol* 1990;145:3450–3455.

67 Jennings FW, Gichuki CW, Hunter CA, et al. The role of the polyamine inhibitor eflornithine in the neuropathogenesis of African trypanosomiasis. *Neuropathol Appl Neurobiol* 1997 (in press).

12

Issues and Controversies in Cysticercosis

THEODORE E. NASH

Cysticercosis is an infection with the larval form of the human tapeworm *Taenia solium* (1). In the usual life cycle, humans become infected with the intestine-dwelling tapeworm following ingestion of a cyst in raw or poorly cooked pork. The adult tapeworm is very long, usually 6 to 20 feet. It consists of a head containing suckers and an armed rostellum by which it anchors itself to the intestinal wall; a neck; and a linear array of increasingly mature proglottids, each containing male and female sexual organs and between 30,000 and 50,000 ova when finally released from the body of the worm. Gravid proglottids are creamy white, motile, and 5 to 7 mm by 20 mm in size and are many times recognizable in the stool or undergarments. In the process of proglottids passing out of the body, eggs are released in the stool, around the perianal area, or the ova remain within the proglottid. When pigs are allowed to feed in areas contaminated with human feces or in some regions are fed human feces, they ingest the ova, which burrow into the intestine, enter the bloodstream, and form cysts in the tissues of the pig (intermediate host) at about 60 days (2). Humans can also act as the intermediate host following ingestion of ova.

Accurate prevalence rates for cysticercosis in endemic regions are generally not available because screening techniques are neither fully sensitive nor specific, or the sample populations are biased. Nevertheless, although the measures of disease and infection are imperfect, it is clear that cysticercosis is a major health concern in endemic countries. In Mexico, for instance, autopsy series have documented cysticercosis in 0.8% to 3.5% (3) and in Mexico City between 4% and 8% of hospitalized neurologic patients are diagnosed with neurocysticercosis (4).

Although fundamental aspects of the clinical manifestations and pathology of cysticercosis were known by the last part of the nineteenth century (5–7), its worldwide presence and relatively high prevalence and associated morbidity in many areas of the world were largely unappreciated. In part, this was due to lack of a sensitive means to diagnose the infection, which included determining the presence of subcutaneous cysticerci, finding the characteristic calcification in tissues, and performing serologic tests that were neither fully sensitive nor specific. The use of newer radiologic methods such as computed tomography (CT) and magnetic resonance imaging (MRI), use of specific serologic assessment, and the development of chemotherapies that kill cysts have revolutionized our knowledge about the disease and the physician's approach to the patient. To some degree, the rapid use of these technical advances has circumvented the implementation of well-controlled studies that may have led to a clearer understanding, for instance, of which patients would best benefit from chemotherapeutic intervention.

Most manifestations of cysticercosis are unique to humans and so the study of disease is primarily limited to humans. However, pigs, the natural intermediate host, under some circumstances can serve as a useful model of infection (2,8). There are difficulties using this model system. The life cycle cannot be maintained in the laboratory because the ova required to infect pigs can only be obtained from tapeworm-harboring humans, who are difficult to find, are only sporadically available, and can usually donate eggs as inocula only once. Standardization of the inocula in repeated or challenge studies is not possible. Production of viable infections is variable and neurologic disease, which is the most common clinical manifestation in humans, is not normally recognized in pigs.

Although much progress has been made, there are a number of important unanswered questions and controversies concerning cysticercosis, and these are discussed here. A more detailed review has been published (9).

TRANSMISSION

Maintenance of the life cycle in nature requires humans who harbor the adult tapeworm; who defecate indiscriminately, allowing unfettered pigs to ingest proglottids or ova; and who ingest raw or inadequately cooked pork. In developed countries the life cycle would be near impossible to maintain because of meat inspection, separation of pigs from human feces, and the practice of cooking pork thoroughly. However, in many regions of the world where sanitation is poor and where pigs are raised, these conditions are readily fulfilled.

The "typhoid Mary" of cysticercosis is the human infected with a tapeworm; all cysticercosis originates either directly or indirectly from tapeworm carriers. Exactly how transmission occurs and who is at risk have only recently been carefully studied. There is reasonable evidence suggesting that the closer persons are associated with a carrier, the more likely they are to be infected. In markedly endemic rural regions, cross-sectional studies show relatively low rates of carriers, from 1% to 3% in most studies (10–15). However, household members have an increased prevalence of seropositivity (10–15) to the parasite and in some studies an increased chance of having symptoms compatible with cysticercosis (10,12–15). Some of these serologically positive family members have been documented to have clinical cysticercosis (16).

Exactly how transmission occurs is not known because there are no documented epidemics of cysticercosis that implicate food or water, for instance, and the time of inoculation is obscured by the usually prolonged incubation periods, often measured in years or even decades (17). There are likely multiple mechanisms. Documented tapeworm carriers (18,19) and Hispanic domestic employees from endemic areas working in households in the United States have been implicated in the transmission of cysticercosis (19). A recent dramatic report documented that four members of an Orthodox Jewish community in New York City were likely infected by Hispanic housekeepers (20). Seven other members from four families were also seropositive, and two had lesions revealed by MRI that were diagnosed as cysticercosis. One housekeeper had *Taenia* eggs in her stool and another was serologically positive. A likely hypothesis is that the carriers contaminate themselves, the environment, and the food they prepare. Contamination occurs when proglottids rupture in the bowel or in the process of passing through the anus, contaminating the perianal region or the undergarments. They can also remain intact in the feces, contaminating the environment.

In the United States, there is an increased awareness and possibly a real increase in the number of persons with known cysticercosis who have never left the United States (21–23). Although close association with persons from endemic areas is found in some cases (22), in others no reasonable explanation exists. Among the possibilities are carriers who contaminate the environment (23) or food in the process of meal preparation, or migrant workers who contaminate vegetables or fruit at the time of harvest. Ingestion of contaminated imported foods is another possible means of transmission (24). The ova of a number of many helminths and protozoan cysts are well suited to survive under conditions in which most bacteria are not able to survive. The occasional contamination of food can lead to infections difficult to detect, and the few ova present can result in sporadic disease with prolonged and varying incubation periods occurring over a wide geographic area. Some parasitic ova are known to remain viable after exposure to disinfectants such as household bleach.

There are a number of biologic and practical implications of cysticercosis transmission within the United States. Since transmission appears to occur from person to person in a household setting, it is probable that low numbers of ova are capable of infecting an individual. This seems at variance with the rather large inocula required to experimentally infect pigs (2,8). Practically, screening or presumptive treatment should be considered for individuals who are potential carriers, particularly those employed in the household setting. Whether migrant workers contaminate fresh foods or whether imported foods are contaminated are questions that should be seriously considered.

THE DISEASE

Variability in incubation and disease manifestations is one of the hallmarks of cysticercosis and has been reviewed (5,9,25–27). Aborted infections almost certainly occur as judged by positive serology without concomitant disease in humans and pigs (see below). Disease can become manifest within months after exposure, averaging about 11 months in persons with a defined period of exposure (22), up to as long as three decades (17). Although they can occur anywhere, lesions are found primarily in the brain, muscle, and subcutaneous tissue and vary in number, size, location, surrounding inflammation and edema, presence of calcification, degree of vascular involvement, and organ location. They can be cystic or nodular in form or the growth of the larvae can be aberrant, occurring as proliferating membranous-vesicular structures (racemose form) or as abnormally large cysts. It is this variability that leads to the diverse clinical symptoms and difficulty in predicting prognosis.

Despite the plethora of manifestations produced by *T. solium* larvae, most patients present with seizures (17,28–31) due to cysts, nodular lesions, or calcifications usually with varying degrees of perilesional edema and enhancement. Hydrocephalus due to obstruction caused by chronic basilar meningitis, or ventricular obstruction due to intravesicular cysts is the second most common presentation (17,28–30,32). Less commonly, patients present with neurologic deficits due to large cysts (33–35) or perilesional edema. Recently, associated infarcts have been found to be relatively common (36,37). In patients with numerous cysts and long-standing disease, multiple stages, pathophysiologic processes, signs, and symptoms are commonplace in the same patient.

It is important to understand that parasites, in order to remain viable, must not incite an inflammatory response. However, for reasons that are unclear, the host does eventually respond to the parasite, and it is reasonable to think that it is the host's immune response that contributes to the death of the cysticercus (5,38,39). This same response, which is at times inordinately intense, is the primary cause of much of the disease (5,38–40). Persisting inflammation leads to continued disease, meningitis due to cysts adjoining the surface or ventricles of the brain, and eventual fibrosis and obstruction.

As will be discussed, cysts killed by chemotherapeutic agents provoke an inflammatory response (early experience reviewed by deAluja and Vargas (39,40,41). One of the major unanswered questions concerning cysticercosis is the following: Is it better to kill cysts all at once by treatment that invokes the predictable inflammatory response and at the same time controls the inflammatory response with corticosteroids, or is it better to let the disease take its own course over months to years?

Despite our increased ability to visualize lesions and diagnose infections, the natural history of cysticercosis is not known. This has led to uncertainty about how to manage patients and to contradictory treatment recommendations. Similar to many chronic diseases, there are recognized clinical and radiologic presentations that represent different stages of the disease. Histologic documentation of radiologic or clinical stages is incomplete. There is near-total agreement, based on histologic and observational studies, that calcified lesions represent dead parasites (5,43–44). However, these may remain as foci (5) for seizures. The presence of perilesional edema around some of these lesions when patients experience seizures (Nash TE, personal observations, 1985) suggests that even dead larvae can provoke vigorous host responses under some circumstances (5). In fact, a continued host response to degenerating cysts may be the cause of many complications of this disease (5). Cystic lesions, particularly those lacking enhancement and accompanying edema, are considered viable cysticerci. During treatment with praziquantel or albendazole, these lesions commonly incite an inflammatory response that eventually involutes to small calcified or noncalcified foci usually accompanied by a small rim of enhancement (42–44). The presence of perilesional enhancement and edema is interpreted as a cyst in the process of involution (45–48). However, at present, except in some defined situations as noted already, it is not possible to predict the clinical course in many patients. For instance, we cannot predict which patients are prone to develop chronic meningitis and hydrocephalus, complications associated with an increased morbidity and mortality (32,48–51). Varying disease manifestations may also be due to geographic differences in strains. It was recently suggested that patients from Central and South America present with few subcutaneous cysts compared to patients with cysticercosis from Asia (52). This may be explained by differences in tropisms among strains of *T. solium* from different geographic regions (52). Because the natural course of cysticercosis is not known, it is unclear when medical intervention is warranted. Long-term observation and controlled studies are necessary to answer the questions.

DIAGNOSIS

The diagnosis is suggested by CT and MRI in conjunction with positive serologic results. Except for biopsy and histologic identification of the cyst, which is usually not possible although definitive, the diagnosis is suggested by a combination of findings (9). The presence of multiple characteristic lesions, either cystic or calcified lesions, is highly suggestive (52–59). Cystic lesions are round, have smooth walls, and may have a typical scolex within the cyst, which when present is practically diagnostic (Fig. 12-1). CT is best for identifying calcifications; the sensitivity in diagnosing intraparenchymal cysticercosis by this technique has been estimated to be approximately 23% to 70% (49,54,55). MRI clearly identifies more noncalcified lesions than does CT, but the sensitivity of this technique, although thought to be high, is not known (48,54–59). Intraventricular cysts are clearly better visualized by MRI and should replace CT-based invasive procedures (56,59). Optimally, both nonenhanced CT and enhanced MRI should be performed.

The recently developed enzyme-linked immunoelectrotransfer blot assay (EITB) for serum antibodies, developed at the Centers for Disease Control, is highly specific and indicates *T. solium* infection (58). Sensitivity is around 94% for patients with two or more brain lesions and 28% for those with single lesions (60) with histologically proved disease. Cerebrospinal fluid (CSF) in this system is not as sensitive as serum (61). Most serologically negative patients have single or only calcified lesions, suggesting a lack of significant antigenic stimulation in these presentations. Other methodologies are less standardized and therefore the sensitivity and specificity vary between testing centers (62). A positive serologic result in a patient with suggestive lesions is considered diagnostic. In endemic regions, positive serology occurs in persons without detectable disease (10,12,63). This most likely represents a failed infection, which is known to occur in experimentally infected pigs (Nash TE, Ballard, unpublished observations, 1989). Patients with tapeworm infections commonly, but not always, have positive serology. Whether this represents occult cysticercosis or is indicative of intestinal tapeworm infections remains unclear (10).

The diagnosis of single lesions can be difficult if the serologic result is negative. There are a number of approaches. Cystic lesions due to cysticercosis will commonly respond to specific therapy, and this can be used as a therapeutic trial. Two studies using this approach demonstrated disappearance of the presumed cysticercosis lesions in most patients (64,65). However, these studies treated enhancing lesions, which were later shown to resolve spontaneously (66); hence, treatment of enhancing or edematous lesions may be unnecessary to effect resolution of these lesions. Symptomatic treatment and waiting for these to resolve might be appropriate. The length of time required before resolution becomes evident is variable, but should be less than 3 months (47). However, there may be clinical benefit from treatment. A retrospective comparison between treated and untreated persons with single enhancing lesions found that although the lesions regressed in both groups, subsequent seizure activity was controlled in all of the treated patients compared to 38% of the untreated patients (46). In another retrospective analysis of patients with epilepsy due to cysticercosis by the same investigators, 83% of all patients with nonenhancing or enhancing cysts who were treated became free of seizures, compared to 26% of untreated patients (67).

Detection of parasite-specific antigen in the CSF has been used to diagnose infection with moderate success (68–70). These procedures are still experimental and trials have not yet compared them to existing diagnostic techniques.

Interpretation of CT and MRI studies can be troublesome for persons not accus-

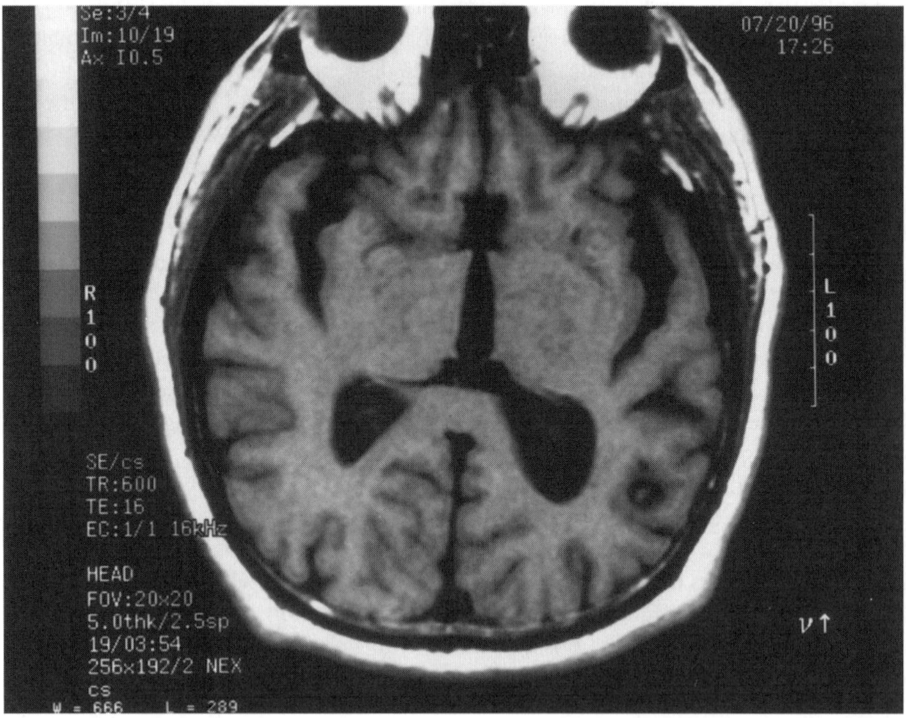

Figure 12-1. A magnetic resonance image of an asymptomatic patient shows a single cystic lesion in the left parietal-occipital region. The intracystic eccentric density is a scolex, which when visualized is highly suggestive, if not pathognomonic, for cysticercosis. Although not well visualized in this image, another cyst is present in the left posterior ventricle.

tomed to seeing these types of patients. Not uncommonly, persons referred with "classic imaging studies" and a "certain" diagnosis of neurocysticercosis have other entities. Usually one of several lesions mimics those of cysticercosis, but the other lesions are so atypical that they should suggest other entities. Most commonly, this happens with the initial presentation of metastatic carcinoma with an occult primary source (personal observations). Tuberculosis, either as single (71) or multiple lesions found in diffuse disease (Hash, personal observations, 1985), and uncommonly, multiple sclerosis can present with suggestive lesions.

Diagnosis of tapeworm infections can be difficult and, until recently, has been exclusively based on detecting single or multiple tapeworm segments, or *Taenia* ova. The finding of *Taenia* ova in stool is only suggestive as *Taenia saginata* ova are identical to *T. solium* (3). A history of passing proglottids is helpful in identifying carriers, but is not sensitive. As mentioned earlier, *Taenia* ova can be found in the stool or perianal area using the cellophane tape method, but this procedure also lacks sensitivity. Treatment and identification of the expelled tapeworm presently comprise the most definitive way of documenting tapeworm carriers. Parasite-specific antigen detection in stools has been used and although the method is sensitive, it cannot distinguish between *T. solium* and *T. saginata* (72,73). However, DNA-based methods have been devised to distinguish *T. solium* from *T. saginata* (74).

TREATMENT

Issues dealing with the treatment of cysticercosis are presently the most contentious. They have arisen because of an imperfect understanding of the natural history of the disease and the lack of suitable controls in treatment trials. With the near-simultaneous development of CT and praziquantel as a cysticidal agent, numerous uncontrolled studies soon documented the resolution of viable cysts (without edema or significant enhancement) following treatment (9,41,75). The temporal association of the resolution of cysts with treatment was so apparent that some believed that randomized, controlled, masked trials were not required (76). Some studies subsequently employed control groups (47,75) whose utility was blunted by biased selection or unblinded assessment. Although there is an occasional report (77) refuting the cysticidal activity of these cysticidal agents, and despite the fact that the studies to date were imperfect, the preponderance of the evidence, both clinical and experimental, indicates that both albendazole and praziquantel are effective cysticidal agents.

Is the clinical course of cysticercosis improved following treatment? Perhaps. In probably the best effort in this regard, Vazquez and Sotelo (47) treated patients with nonenhancing cysts and compared them to an untreated group with nonenhancing cysts and to a group with enhancing cysts. Although the treated groups and the enhancing-cyst group showed resolution of cysts, the treated groups had better control of seizures and less residual lesions than did the enhancing-cyst group. In the control group, the numbers of cysts remained unchanged and the seizure activity remained high. Again, the biased selection of groups and the lack of masked comparisons were flaws in the design. As noted earlier, a retrospective, and therefore less than optimal, study of treated and untreated patients with single enhancing cysts demonstrated a decrease in seizure activity in the treated group (67). Other studies documented the resolution of enhancing cysts (66,78) without specific antiparasitic therapy, and one of these studies in children noted that there were no complications and that subsequent seizures in these patients were easily controlled (78).

Therapy is effective in isolated instances and can result in impressive clinical improvement (34,35,79,80). This has been most clearly documented in patients with large cysts (34,35) or strategically located cysts (80) such as those in the retrobulbar space (79). Anecdotal reports documented remarkable clinical responses in some patients with racemose cysticercosis (54,81,82), a type of cysticercosis usually difficult to treat and associated with a high mortality (9).

There are a number of problems with trying to assess clinical efficacy. First, seizure activity depends on a number of factors unrelated to anticysticidal treatment, including alcohol ingestion and use of antiseizure medication, its optimization, compliance, and degree of follow-up. Second, perhaps more importantly, seizures are only one of several complications that need to be assessed. For instance, the prevention of hydrocephalus, an important complication that leads to an increased mortality, should be assessed. Because hydrocephalus is likely to occur years after the infection developed, follow-up would necessarily be long and therefore difficult.

Two cysticidal drugs are efficacious in the elimination of viable cysts: praziquantel and albendazole. Praziquantel was the first used; has few side effects; is relatively expensive, particularly when given in the recommended 2-week course (50 mg/kg/day in three divided doses for 15 days); and is available in the United States, although it is not licensed for the treatment of cysticercosis by the Federal Drug Administration (FDA) (reviewed by Osler (7)). Albendazole is less expensive, was recently approved for the treatment of neurocysticercosis by the FDA in the United States, and is readily available in many developing countries. However, albendazole is potentially more toxic than praziquantel and is teratogenic. It has been administered as 15 mg/kg in two or three divided doses for 8 to 30 days. Three trials comparing both drugs using optimal dosing have been published (83–85). The trial by Sotelo et al. (83) compared 10 patients in each group against each other and a control group of 5 subjects. Both albendazole and praziquantel were equally efficacious, showing total cyst reductions of 76% and 73%, respectively. There was no change in cyst number in the control group. A second study compared nonconcurrently treated groups with different types of radiologic and clinical presentations, including calcified lesions (84). When only cystic lesions were compared, response rates were practically identical. Seventy-nine percent and 80% of the praziquantel- and albendazole-treated patients, respectively, were cured, and all patients responded after further courses of treatment with the same drug. Responses in the calcified lesion groups differed but the comparisons are likely invalid. In the third study (85), 22 and 21 patients with 178 and 101 cysts initially were treated with praziquantel or albendazole, respectively, yielding total cyst reductions of 50% in the praziquantel group compared to 88% in the albendazole group. However, the groups were not comparable. First, the patients had to purchase their own drug and, because praziquantel is very expensive compared to albendazole, it is not clear whether the patients actually bought and took the drug. Second, 9 of 22 patients in the praziquantel group had more than 5 cysts compared to 2 of 22 in the albendazole group. A fourth study by Sotelo et al. (86) evaluated their total experience from prior studies, including one just reported (83), and found an approximately 60% response rate with praziquantel compared to 85% with albendazole. This study was a compilation of results rather than a randomized study. The results are not in agreement with an earlier above-mentioned report from the same group, possibly owing to the limited number of persons studied in the first study (83), poor study design of the later study, or study-to-study variability (see below). None of the above-mentioned studies were optimally designed for a number of reasons, and furthermore, the results are not in total agreement. These studies, usually referred to as evidence suggesting the greater efficacy of albendazole (87), on closer review fail to fully support this contention. Preferential use of one drug over the other should perhaps be based on other considerations such as availability, cost, potential toxicity, and duration of treatment.

Response rates with either drug vary greatly between reports. One reason for this can be differences in drug metabolism (88,89), although no correlation between drug levels and efficacy has been proved (88,90). Depressed serum levels of praziquantel due to concomitant administration of corticosteroids (91) and the antiseizure medications phenytoin and carbamazepine (92) have been reported, whereas increased levels of albendazole due to corticosteroids have been reported (93). Cimetidine increases the serum level of praziquantel by inhibiting its metabolism and can be used to increase the availability of the drug (94).

The dosage and duration of therapy are still being optimized for both drugs. A 1-day treatment course using praziquantel can be effective (95), whereas an 8-day treatment course of albendazole at 15 mg/day in divided doses can be as effective as a 2-week course (96).

As discussed earlier, reasonable studies support the treatment of patients with viable cysts. The treatment of enhancing cysts is controversial and was discussed earlier. The recommendation not to treat patients with calcified lesions, presumably dead cysts, is poorly studied and based on anecdotal experience (67). The treatment of all persons with epilepsy with all types of cystic lesions led to increased or earlier seizure control (67).

A case can be made for consideration of treatment or critical study of patients who presently are not considered for therapy. The sensitivity of CT ranges from 23% to 70% (49,54,55), and although the sensitivity of MRI is considerably better than that of CT, as noted already, the actual sensitivity is unknown; therefore, a number of patients who might possibly benefit from therapy go untreated. Additionally, the continuous presence of symptoms in untreated patients not uncommonly prompts a re-evaluation to detect new or previously missed lesions. Treatment may be of clinical benefit to a subset of patients and repeated testing in others may be unnecessary. With the availability of relatively safe and easily administered medications as well as the efficacy of a shortened course of therapy, this treatment strategy may be reasonable.

Although corticosteroids are used relatively frequently, there is no consensus as to how they should be used. Host inflammatory responses to lesions, and in the CSF as well, are common following initiation of chemotherapy and occasionally result in death. While some physicians initiate steroid treatment at the beginning (84) or slightly before therapy in most or all patients with viable cysts, others wait for the development of signs or symptoms (76). Most agree that steroids should be used in patients with many cysts, giant cysts, or critically placed cysts. Lesions such as degenerating or calcified cysts that incite an inflammatory response during the course of the disease can also be treated with steroids, with usually rapid reversal of signs and symptoms (personal observations). Corticosteroids are also employed to control the inflammatory responses associated with meningitis and hydrocephalus; one study showed that corticosteroids can prevent clogging of ventriculoperitoneal shunts (97). The duration of treatment is as short as possible, although stopping steroids too soon after the end of chemotherapy is not an uncommon experience (Nash, personal observations, 1985).

NEEDS

Although there are no precise records of the number of persons infected worldwide, from the numerous reports of disease in endemic countries it is obvious that cysticercosis is a disease that produces much morbidity and, not rarely, death. In the United States, cysticercosis is likely the most common invasive helminthic infection recognized, particularly in regions populated with immigrants from endemic regions. Furthermore, infections are more frequently recognized in persons who have been infected in the United States. Despite the importance both here and abroad, few resources are available to study and even document the extent of the disease. Except for some notable exceptions, there is a worldwide malaise in recognizing its importance, and subsequently, in providing financial support for research and control programs. Cysticercosis is a hard disease to study. The life cycle of the tapeworm cannot be maintained in the laboratory and the only model of infection is difficult to use. The course of the disease is measured from years to decades, so that even understanding the natural history of the disease is daunting.

Prevention is the most promising avenue of control. Cysticercosis, like many diseases, spreads by a fecal-oral route and would not exist if only simple hygienic practices were followed. Besides education of the population and possible behavioral changes of tapeworm-infected populations, treatment of tapeworm-harboring populations where rates of transmission are likely highest can decrease and even eliminate transmission (98).

REFERENCES

1 Beaver PC, et al. Cyclophyllidean tapeworms. In: *Clinical parasitology*. Philadelphia: Lea & Febiger 1984:513–543.

2 Herbert V, Berg C. Cysticercosis in pigs due to infection with *Taenia solium* linnaeus, 1758. In: Soulsby EJL, ed. *Parasitic zoonoses*. New York: Academic, 1974:199–211.

3 Woodhouse E, Flisser A, Larralde C. Seroepidemiology of human cysticercosis in Mexico. In: Flisser A et al, eds. *Cysticercosis: present state of knowledge and perspectives*. New York: Academic, 1982:11–23.

4 Schenon H, Villarroel F, Rojas A, Ramírez R. Epidemiology of human cysticercosis in Latin America. In: Flisser A et al, eds. *Cysticercosis: present state of knowledge and perspectives*. New York: Academic, 1982:25–38.

5 Henneberg-Berlin R. Die tierischen parasiten des zentralnerven-system. In: Lewandowsky M, ed. *Handbuch Der Neurologie*. Berlin: Berlag Von Julius Springer 1912:643.

6 Nieto D. Historical notes on cysticercosis. In: Flisser A et al, eds. *Cysticercosis: present state of knowledge and perspectives*. New York: Academic, 1982:1–7.

7 Osler W. *The principles and practice of medicine*. New York: Appleton, 1892.

8 Molinar JL, Meza R, Suárez B, et al. *Taenia soli-*

um: immunity in hogs to the cysticercus. *Exp Parasitol* 1983;55:340–357.

9 Nash TE. Diagnosis and treatment of cysticercosis. *Curr Clin Top Infect Dis* 1986;7:297–310.

10 Sarti E, Schantz PM, Plancarte A, et al. Prevalence and risk factors for *Taenia solium* taeniasis and cysticercosis in humans and pigs in a village in Morelos, Mexico. *Am J Trop Med Hyg* 1992;46:677–685.

11 Allan JC, Velasqueztohom M, Garcianoval J, et al. Epidemiology of intestinal taeniasis in four, rural, Guatemalan communities. *Ann Trop Med Parasitol* 1996;90:157–165.

12 Diaz F, et al. Epidemiology of taeniasis and cysticercosis in a Peruvian village. *Am J Epidemiol* 1992;135:875–882.

13 Sarti Gutierrez EJ, Schantz PM, Lara Aguilera R, et al. *Taenia solium* taeniasis and cysticercosis in a Mexican village. *Trop Med Parasitol* 1988;39:194–198.

14 Diaz Camacho SP, Candil Ruiz A, Suate Peraza V, et al. Epidemiologic study and control of *Taenia solium* infections with praziquantel in a rural village of Mexico. *Am J Trop Med Hyg* 1991;45:522–531.

15 Diaz Camacho S, Candil Ruiz A, Uribe Beltrán M, Willms K. Serology as an indicator of *Taenia solium* tapeworm infections in a rural community in Mexico. *Trans R Soc Trop Med Hyg* 1990;84:563–566.

16 Schantz PM, Sart E, Plancarte A, et al. Community-based epidemiological investigations of cysticercosis due to *Taenia solium*: comparison of serological screening tests and clinical findings in two populations in Mexico. *Clin Infect Dis* 1994;18:879–885.

17 Dixon HBF, Lipscomb FM. Cysticercosis: an analysis and follow up of 450 cases. In: *Medical Research Council special report series, no.* 299. London: Her Majesty's Stationery Office, 1961:1–58.

18 Tasker WG, Plotkin SA. Cerebral cysticercosis. *Pediatrics* 1979;63:761–763.

19 Kruskal BA, Moths L, Teele DW. Neurocysticercosis in a child with no history of travel outside the continental United States. *Clin Infect Dis* 1993;16:290–292.

20 Schantz PM, Moore AC, Muñoz JL, et al. Neurocysticercosis in an Orthodox Jewish community in New York City. *N Engl J Med* 1992;327:692–695.

21 Richards FO, Schantz PM, Ruiz-Tiben E, Sorvillo FJ. Cysticercosis in Los Angeles county. *JAMA* 1985;254:3444–3448.

22 Sorvillo FJ, Waterman SH, Richards FO, Schantz PM. Cysticercosis surveillance: locally acquired and travel-related infections and detection of intestinal tapeworm carriers in Los Angeles county. *Am J Trop Med Hyg* 1992;47:365–371.

23 Locally acquired neurocysticercosis—North Carolina, Massachusetts, and South Carolina, 1989-1991. *MMWR* 1992:41:1–4.

24 Spondola Felix N, Rojas Wastavino G, de Haro Argeaga I, et al. Parasite search in strawberries from Irapuato, Guanajuato and Zamora, Michoacan (Mexico). *Arch Med Res* 1996;27:229–231.

25 Flisser A, et al, eds. *Cysticercosis: present state of knowledge and perspectives*. New York: Academic, 1982.

26 Del Brutto OH, Sotelo J. Neurocysticercosis: an update. *Rev Infect Dis* 1988;10:1075–1085.

27 Webbe G. Human cysticercosis: parasitology, pathology, clinical manifestations and available treatment. *Pharmacol Ther* 1994;64:175–200.

28 McCormick GF, Zee CS, Heiden J, et al. Cysticercosis cerebri, review of 127 cases. *Arch Neurol* 1982;39:534–539.

29 Grisolia JS, Widerholt WC. CNS cysticercosis. *Arch Neurol* 1982;39:540–544.

30 Shandera WX, White AC, Chen JC, et al. Neurocysticercosis in Houston, Texas. *Medicine (Baltimore)* 1994;73:37–52.

31 Sotelo J, Guerrero V, Rubio F. Neurocysticercosis: a new classification based on active and inactive forms. *Arch Intern Med* 1985; 145:442–445.

32 Estañol B, Kleriga E, Loyo M, et al. Mechanisms of hydrocephalus in cerebral cysticercosis: implication of therapy. *Neurosurgery* 1983;13:119–123.

33 Berman JD, et al. Cysticercus of 60-milliliter volume in human brain. *Am J Trop Med Hyg* 1981;30:616–619.

34 Joubert J, Van AS. Rapid and complete resolution of giant cysterical cysts after administration of praziquantel. *S Afr Med J* 1990;77:154–157.

35 Delbrutto OH, Sotelo J, Aguirre R, et al. Albendazole therapy for giant subarachnoid cysticerci. *Arch Neurol* 1992;49:535–538.

36 Cantu C, Barinagarrementeria F. Cerebrovascular complications of neurocysticercosis: clinical and neuroimaging spectrum. *Arch Neurol* 1996;53:233–239.

37 Del Brutto OH. Cysticercosis and cerebrovascular disease: a review. *J Neurol Neurosurg Psychiatry* 1992;55:252–254.

38 Trelles JO, Palomino L. Histopathology of cerebral cysticercosis. In: Bogaert LV, Käfer JP, Poch GF, et al, eds. *Tropical neurology*. Buenos Aires: Libreros Editores 1961:162–181.

39 deAluja AS, Vargas G. The histopathology of porcine cysticercosis. *Vet Parasitol* 1988; 28:65–77.

40 Rabiela-Cervantes MT, Rivas-Hernández A, Rodríguez-Ibarra J, et al. Anatomopathological aspects of human brain cysticercosis. In: Flisser A, Willms K, Laclette JP, Larralde C, eds. *Cysticercosis: present state of knowledge and perspectives.* New York: Academic, 1982:179–200.

41 Groll EW. Chemotherapy of human cysticercosis with praziquantel. In: Flisser A, Willms K, Laclette JP, et al, eds. *Cysticercosis: present state of knowledge and perspectives.* New York: Academic, 1982:207–218.

42 Rodriguez-Carbajal R, Boleaga-Durán. Neuroradiology of human cysticercosis. In: Flissner A et al, eds. *Cysticercosis: present state of knowledge and perspectives.* New York: Academic,1982:139–162.

43 Mazer S, Antoniuv A. The computed tomographic spectrum of cerebral cysticercosis. *Comput Radiol* 1983;7:373–378.

44 Minguetti G, Ferreira MV. Computed tomography in neurocysticercosis. *J Neurol Neurosurg Psychiatry* 1983;46:936–942.

45 Mitchell WF, Snodgrass SR. Intraparenchymal cerebral cysticercosis in children: a benign prognosis. *Pediatr Neurol* 1985;1:151–156.

46 Del Brutto OH. Single parenchymal brain cysticercus in the acute encephalitic phase: definition of a distinct form of neurocysticercosis with a benign prognosis. *J Neurol Neurosurg Psychiatry* 1995;58:247–249.

47 Vazquez V, Sotelo J. The course of seizures after treatment for cerebral cysticercosis. *N Engl J Med* 1992;327:696–701.

48 Martinez HR, Rangelguerra R, Arrredondoestrada JH, et al. Medical and surgical treatment in neurocysticercosis: a magnetic resonance study of 161 cases. *J Neurol Sci* 1995; 130:25–34.

49 Loo L, Braude A. Cerebral cysticercosis in San Diego. *Medicine (Baltimore)* 1982;61:341–359.

50 Sotelo J, Marin C. Hydrocephalus secondary to cysticercotic arachnoiditis. A long-term follow-up review of 92 cases. *J Neurosurg* 1987; 66:686–689.

51 Lobato RD, Lamas E, Portillo JM, et al. Hydrocephalus in cerebral cysticercosis. Pathogenic and therapeutic considerations. *J Neurosurg* 1981;55:786–793.

52 Cruz I, Cruz ME, Teran W, et al. Human subcutaneous *Taenia solium* cysticercosis in an Andean population with neurocysticercosis. *Am J Trop Med Hyg* 1994;51:405–407.

53 Torrealba G, Del Villar S, Tagle P, et al. Cysticercosis of the central nervous system: clinical and therapeutic considerations. *J Neurol Neurosurg Psychiatry* 1984; 47:784–790.

54 Martinez HR, Rangel, Guerra R, et al. MR imaging in neurocysticercosis: a study of 56 cases. *Am J Neuroradiol* 1989;10:1011–1019.

55 Teitelbaum GP, Otto RJ, Lin M, et al. MR imaging of neurocysticercosis. *AJR* 1989;153:857–866.

56 Suss RA, Maravilla KR, Thompson J. MR imaging of intracranial cysticercosis: comparison with CT and anatomopathologic features. *Am J Neuroradiol* 1986;7:235–242.

57 Rhee RS, Kumasaki DY, Sarwar M, et al. MR imaging of intraventricular cysticercosis. *J Comput Assist Tomogr* 1987;11:598–601.

58 Chang KH, Lee JH, Han MH, Han MC. The role of contrast-enhanced MR imaging in the diagnosis of neurocysticercosis. *Am J Neuroradiol* 1991;12:509–512.

59 Zee CS, Segall HD, Destian S, et al. MRI of intraventricular cysticercosis: surgical implications. *J Comput Assist Tomogr* 1993;17:932–939.

60 Wilson M, Bryan RT, Fried JA, et al. Clinical evaluation of the cysticercosis enzyme-linked immunoelectrotransfer blot in patients with neurocysticercosis. *J Infect Dis* 1991;164:1007–1009.

61 Tsang VCW, Brand JA, Boyer AE. An enzyme-linked immunoelectrotransfer blot assay and glycoprotein antigens for diagnosing human cysticercosis (*Taenia solium*). *J Infect Dis* 159:50–59.

62 Diaz JF, Verasteguim M, Gilman RH, et al. Immunodiagnosis of human cysticercosis (*Taenia solium*): a field comparison of an antibody-enzyme-linked immunosorbent assay (ELISA), an antigen-ELISA, and an enzyme-linked immunoelectrotransfer blot (EITB) assay in Peru. *Am J Trop Med Hyg* 1992;46:610–615.

63 Garcia HH, Herrera G, Gilman RH, et al. Discrepancies between cerebral computed tomography and Western blot in the diagnosis of neurocysticercosis. *Am J Trop Med Hyg* 1994;50:152–157.

64 Rawling D, Ferriero DM, Messing RO. Early CT reevaluation after empiric praziquantel therapy in neurocysticercosis. *Neurology* 1989;39:739–741.

65 Del Brutto OH. The use of albendazole in patients with single lesions enhanced on contrast CT. *N Engl J Med* 1993;328:356–357.

66 Padma MV, Behari M, Misra NK, Ahuja GK. Albendazole in single CT ring lesions in epilepsy. *Neurology* 1994;44:1344–1346.

67 Del Brutto OH, Santibañez R, Noboa CA, et al. Epilepsy due to neurocysticercosis: analysis of 203 patients. *Neurology* 1992;42:389–392.

68 Téllez Girón E, Ramos MC, Dufour L, et al. Detection of *Cysticercus cellulosae* antigens in

cerebrospinal fluid by dot enzyme-linked immunosorbent assay (dot-ELISA) and standard ELISA. *Am J Trop Med Hyg* 1987;37:169–173.

69 Estrada JJ, Almon-Estrada J, Kuhn RE. Identification of *Taenia solium* antigens in cerebrospinal fluid and larval antigens from patients with neurocysticercosis. *Am J Trop Med Hyg* 1989;41:50–55.

70 Correa D, Sandoval MA, Harrison LJ, et al. Human neurocysticercosis: comparison of enzyme immunoassay capture techniques based on monoclonal and polyclonal antibodies for the detection of parasite products in cerebrospinal fluid. *Trans R Soc Trop Med Hyg* 1989;83:814–816.

71 Sethi PP, Wadia RS, Kiyawat OP, et al. Ring or disc-enhancing lesions in epilepsy in India. *J Trop Med Hyg* 1994;97:347–353.

72 Allan JC, Velasqueztohom M, Torresalvarez R, et al. Field trial of the coproantigen-based diagnosis of *Taenia solium taeniasis* by enzyme-linked immunosorbent assay. *Am J Trop Med Hyg* 1996;54:352–356.

73 Allan JC, Avila G, Garcia-Noval J, et al. Immunodiagnosis of taeniasis by coproantigen detection. *Parasitology* 1990;101:473–477.

74 Rishi AK, McManus DP. DNA probes which unambiguously distinguish *Taenia solium* from *T. saginata. Lancet* 1987;2:1275.

75 Sotelo J, Escobedo F, Rodriquez, et al. Therapy of parenchymal brain cysticercosis with praziquantel. *N Engl J Med* 1984;310:1001–1007.

76 Sodaro DL. *N Engl J Med* 1984;311:734. Letter.

77 Carpio A, Santillan F, Leon P, et al. Is the course of neurocysticercosis modified by treatment with antihelminthic agents? *Arch Intern Med* 1995;155:1982–1988.

78 Mitchell WG, Crawford TO. Intraparenchymal cerebral cysticercosis in children: diagnosis and treatment. *Pediatrics* 1988;82:76–82.

79 Sihota R, Honavar SG. Oral albendazole in the management of extraocular cysticercosis. *Br J Ophthalmol* 1994;78:621–623.

80 Santoyo H, Corona T, Sotelo J. Total recovery of visual function after treatment for cerebral cysticercosis. *N Engl J Med* 1991;324:1137–1139.

81 Del Brutto OH, Sotelo J. Albendazole therapy for subarachnoid and ventricular cysticercosis. *J Neurosurg* 1990;72:816–817.

82 LaMantia L, Costa A, Eoli M, Savoiardo M. Racemose neurocysticercosis after chronic meningitis: effect of medical treatment. *Clin Neurol Neurosurg* 1995;97:50–54.

83 Sotelo J, Escobedo F, Penagos P. Albendazole vs praziquantel for therapy for neurocysticercosis. *Arch Neurol* 1988;45:532–534.

84 Cruz M, Cruz I, Horton J. Albendazole versus praziquantel in the treatment of cerebral cysticercosis: clinical evaluation. *Trans R Soc Trop Med Hyg* 1991;85:244–247.

85 Takayanagui OM, Jardim E. Therapy for neurocysticercosis: comparison between albendazole and praziquantel. *Arch Neurol* 1992; 49:290–294.

86 Sotelo J, delBrutto OH, Penagos P, et al. Comparison of therapeutic regimen of anticysticercal drugs for parenchymal brain cysticercosis. *J Neurol* 1990;237:69–72.

87 Delbrutto OH. Medical treatment for cysticercosis. *Arch Neurol* 1996;53:295–296. Reply.

88 Jung, H, Hurtado M, Sanchez M, et al. Clinical pharmacokinetics of albendazole in patients with brain cysticercosis. *J Clin Pharmacol* 1992;32:28–31.

89 Na-Bangchang K, Vanijanonta S, Karbwang J. Plasma concentrations of praziquantel during the therapy of neurocysticercosis with praziquantel, in the presence of antiepileptics and dexamethasone. *Southeast Asian J Trop Med Public Health* 1995;26:120–123.

90 Alarcón F, Pérez Y, Banda H, Solelo J. Praziquantel and dexamethasone. *Neurology* 1988;38:997–999.

91 Vazquez ML, Jung H, Sotelo J. Plasma levels of praziquantel decrease when dexamethasone is given simultaneously. *Neurology* 1987; 37:1561–1562.

92 Bittencourt PRM, Gracia CM, Martins R, et al. Phenytoin and carbamazepine decrease oral bioavailability of praziquantel. *Neurology* 1992; 492–496.

93 Jung H, Hurtado M, Medina MT, et al. Dexamethasone increases plasma levels of albendazole. *J Neurol* 1990;237:279–280.

94 Overbosch D. Neurocysticercosis: an introduction with special emphasis on new developments in pharmacotherapy. *Schweiz Med Wochenschr* 1992;122:893–898.

95 Corona T, Lugo R, Medina R, Sotelo J. Single-day praziquantel therapy for neurocysticercosis. *N Engl J Med* 1996;334:125.

96 Garcia HH, Gilman RH, Horton J, et al. Albendazole therapy for neurocysticercosis: a prospective double blind trial comparing 7 vs. 14 days of treatment. *Neurology* (in press).

97 Roman RAS, Sotohernandez JL, Sostelo J. Effects of prednisone on ventriculoperitoneal shunt function in hydrocephalus secondary to cysticercosis: a preliminary study. *J Neurosurg* 1996;84:629–633.

98 Cruz M, Davis A, Dixon H, et al. Operational studies on the control of *Taenia solium* taeniasis/cysticercosis in Ecuador. *Bull World Health Organ* 1989;87:401–407.

13 Cryptococcal Meningitis

JOHN E. BENNETT

Cryptococcosis has only been recognized since 1894 and was considered a rare disease until the incidence of reported cases dramatically increased beginning in the 1940s (1). Increased use of corticosteroid therapy undoubtedly contributed to this rise. Introduction of the first effective therapeutic agent, amphotericin B, in the mid-1950s made recognition important and prompted case reports. During the 1980s, the human immunodeficiency virus type 1 (HIV-1) pandemic brought a surge of new cases and saw introduction of the first effective oral monotherapy, fluconazole. The pace of progress in the study of cryptococcosis is still accelerating.

EPIDEMIOLOGY

Environmental Sources of Exposure

Exposure to cryptococcosis may not be rare, suggesting that most normal persons are not susceptible. *Cryptococcus neoformans* var. *neoformans* (serotypes A and D) is present in weathered pigeon droppings from many parts of the world, with concentrations reaching a million yeast per gram of droppings. *C. neoformans* var. *gattii* (serotypes B and C) has occasionally been isolated from debris under *Eucalyptus calmodulensis* or *Eucalyptus tereticornis* trees in Australia and, rarely, elsewhere. Infected cats may have cryptococcal cervical lymphadenitis, the drainage from which may have numerous cryptococci. Unpasteurized milk from cows with cryptococcal mastitis can be heavily laden with the fungus. And yet, there are no documented point source outbreaks and no convincing epidemiologic connection between a source and a clinical case.

Immunologic Evidence of Exposure

Immune responses suggesting subclinical exposure to *C. neoformans* have been reported. Delayed hypersensitivity reactions to a cryptococcal skin test antigen were detected in 1 (5%) of 21 college students in Maryland, 1 (4%) of 24 normal adults in Kansas, and

13 (81%) of 16 healthy laboratorians working with the fungus (2). The immunoreactive component of the antigen was a 10-kd protein (3). Another cryptococcal skin test antigen elicited a delayed response in 26 (32%) of 82 healthy persons in Oklahoma (4). Normal humans usually have small amounts of serum antibody to the cryptococcal capsular polysaccharide, glucuronoxylomannan (GXM). Among 185 healthy adults, 165 (89%) had antibody to serotype A GXM on radioimmunoassay (5). There was no obvious difference in seropositivity between children and adults. Although a cross-reacting antigen could have elicited either the humoral or the delayed hypersensitivity response, the suggestion remains that exposure to *C. neoformans* can often lead to unrecognized, self-limiting infection.

Portal of Infection

The probable portal of entry for cryptococcosis is the lung. Although a pulmonary focus is detectable on chest x-ray films in only a minority of patients with cryptococcosis, cryptococcal pneumonia can resolve spontaneously and even resolve while the infection disseminates to the central nervous system. Cryptococcosis does not appear to originate in the upper respiratory tract, gastrointestinal tract, or skin. A few laboratory workers accidentally injected cryptococci into their hand while inoculating mice, but no more than a local granuloma resulted.

Predisposing Conditions

Risk factors for clinical disease include adult age, male sex, and underlying conditions that inhibit cell-mediated immunity. At present, well over 90% of patients with cryptococcosis have an underlying disease. The major underlying disease is now advanced HIV-1 infection, the CD4 lymphocyte count usually being less than 200 cells/μL. Infection is rare in children, even those infected with HIV-1, and is less common in normal adult women than men. Among 189 patients not infected with HIV-1 who had cryptococcosis, the male-female ratio was 2:1, the youngest patient was 10 years old, the mean age was 52 years, and 59 (31%) had no underlying disease (data from the Mycoses Study Group). Whether this age and sex predisposition in non-HIV-infected patients is due to differences in immune status or exposure is unknown. Prolonged corticosteroid therapy is present in about half the non-HIV-infected patients, including those with solid organ transplantation and systemic lupus erythematosus. Sarcoidosis, even without corticosteroid therapy, also predisposes to this mycosis. A few patients with cryptococcosis have idiopathic CD4 lymphocytopenia but neutropenia and common variable immunodeficiency are rarely predisposing factors.

A plausible synthesis of the above-mentioned information is that exposure is common, even in children, and results from inhalation of cryptococci living in a saprophytic state in the environment. Infection occurs later as a result of a decline in cell-mediated immunity. If, in fact, long incubation periods are common, as just postulated, then vaccines must be given early if the vaccine is only able to prevent infection and not able to prevent reactivation. For example, HIV-1–infected patients would be immunized when first diagnosed, not when the CD4 count had fallen below 200 cells/μL.

PATHOGENESIS

The neurotropism of C. *neoformans* is a striking but poorly understood phenomenon. In one typical experiment, intravenous injection of 20,000 cryptococci into mice resulted in counts in the lungs, liver, and spleen that reached a stable level of about 10,000 colonies per gram after a few days, but brain colony counts began as low as 10 colonies and rose continuously to 10^7 colony-forming units, largely by expansion of existing foci in the brain (6). Uncontrolled growth and paucity of inflammatory cells in the brain have led to the surmise that host defense is less effective in the brain than in other organs. In support of that concept, intracutaneous and intratracheal inoculation can lead to spontaneously resolving infection, followed by partial immunity. Pulmonary cryptococcosis often heals spontaneously in the previously normal host. Intracerebral infection is not known to resolve spontaneously in humans or experimental animals. Neurotropism then is not the result of tissue tropism, meaning selective localization in the brain, but rather appears to represent the ability of small foci of cryptococci to grow unimpeded within the cerebral cortex.

Death from cryptococcosis begins with progressive loss of cerebral acuity and ends with decerebrate status. Imaging studies usually show small or normal-size ventricles. Opening pressure on lumbar puncture is high. Some patients experience a sudden loss of visual acuity, possibly from compression of blood vessels within the sheath of the optic nerve. The fluid surrounding the optic nerve communicates with the cerebrospinal fluid (CSF) and transmits increased pressure to the delicate rete of vessels surrounding the optic nerve. Autopsy of patients with fatal cryptococcosis reveals massive cerebral edema. Hydrocephalus is uncommon but tends to occur in previously normal patients with extremely indolent infection, few cryptococci in the CSF, and low CSF glucose concentrations. Patients with cryptococcosis who are severely immunosuppressed may die rapidly of disseminated infection, usually with positive blood cultures but few or no organisms in the CSF.

Despite the term *cryptococcal meningitis*, encephalitis is found much more prominently at autopsy. Experimental infection in the mouse mimics the human disease, with death following obvious swelling of the calvarium. Although the swelling of the heads in such mice is commonly ascribed to hydrocephalus, the cerebral ventricles are small and cerebral edema, not hydrocephalus, is obvious on gross inspection of the mouse brain. The cause of cerebral edema in cryptococcosis is unknown but obviously important. Vascular damage is not seen in the brain, at least not with hematoxylin and eosin stain, despite the presence of perivascular cryptococci in the cortical gray matter. Injection of cryptococcal polysaccharide into the brains of living animals can cause cerebral edema. Although the polysaccharide was not checked for endotoxin, GXM may have a role in cerebral edema. Soluble capsular polysaccharide may be seen by immunostaining of human and animal brains, apparently diffusing out of clusters of cryptococci. Sufficient soluble GXM reaches the CSF to make detection of cryptococcal antigen a useful diagnostic test. The possible role of cytokines in causing cryptococcal cerebral edema appears to be an unexplored topic.

In mouse and human brains, cryptococci are most prominent in the perivascular spaces of the cerebral cortex, basal ganglia, and caudate nucleus. It has been postulated that the availability of dopamine may help account for localization in the basal ganglia but the evidence remains tenuous. *C. neoformans* produces a laccase that converts dopamine to melanin and the presence of laccase in this species enhances virulence (7). The mechanism by which melanin on the cryptococcal cell wall might confer virulence is protection against oxidative attack by inflammatory cells (8). Problems with this hypothesis include the facts that few inflammatory cells are present in brain lesions, the stain for melanin is nonspecific, and laccase production is downregulated by growth at 37°C and by glucose. If laccase were shown to be produced within the brain and melanin were shown to be present on the cryptococcal cell wall in vivo, the importance of dopamine in intracerebral growth of cryptococci would be clearer.

Selective Pressure on the Pathogen

Survival of *C. neoformans* in nature is certainly not dependent on virulence, that is, infecting an occasional human or animal. Virulence is likely an accidental result of mechanisms favorable for growing and competing against other microorganisms in certain natural sites. The cryptococcal capsule may not only hinder phagocytosis by mammalian phagocytes but also phagocytosis by soil *Acanthamoebae* organisms. The cryptococcal cell wall may be coated with melanin in nature by the action of laccase on diphenols and aminophenols that are common in plants. Melanin could help shield the fungus from the adverse effects of sunlight, just as the human skin protects itself by tanning. Laccase may also help cryptococci digest plant lignins.

ROLE OF ANTIBODY IN HOST DEFENSE

Naturally Occurring Anticryptococcal Antibody

There is no obvious increased risk of cryptococcosis in patients with low or absent serum IgG, as already pointed out. This does not negate the possibility that antibody may be one of the host defense mechanisms; antibody deficiency alone may not be sufficient to permit clinical disease. IgM antibody against cryptococcal GXM is ubiquitous in serum from normal humans, although in low titer. IgG antibody against GXM is more difficult to detect in normal serum than is IgM antibody, but is often present (9). Normal serum also has IgG antibody to the cryptococcal cell wall glucan. Natural antibody does not appear to be opsonic alone or to accelerate deposition of opsonically active C3b on the capsular surface. Of course, antibody could be protective by other mechanisms. The clinical material is suggestive that anticapsular antibody may have a slight role in normal host defense. IgG antibody against the cryptococcal capsule is present in low but detectable levels in about 40% of non-HIV-infected patients by the time cryptococcosis is diagnosed. Antibody-positive patients have a better prognosis for cure with amphotericin B therapy than do antibody-negative patients. The significance of this correlation is clouded by the fact that antibody-negative patients have higher serum concentrations of cryptococcal capsular antigen. Higher serum antigen concentrations reflect higher tissue burdens of cryptococci and correlate with a poor prognosis (10). One cannot discern whether the patient's serum antibody was the cause or the result of lesser infection. Patients who fail to make IgG serum anticryptococcal antibody during the course of their cryptococcosis fail to respond to vaccination with cryptococcal polysaccharide once they are cured (5). They seem to have long-term tolerance to the antigen. In some studies, patients infected with HIV-1 and not infected with *C. neoformans* have had decreased titers of IgM anticapsular antibody, even early in the course of HIV-1 infection, as well as low levels of κ light chains (9). It is tempting to postulate that the lower IgM anti-GXM titer may be one factor that places these patients at increased risk of developing clinical disease.

Monoclonal and Hyperimmune Polyclonal Anticryptococcal Antibody

In Vitro Effects Antibody concentrations much higher than those present in normal human serum can be raised in experimental animals. Both polyclonal and monoclonal IgG antibody to GXM can opsonize cryptococci for ingestion and killing by phagocytes with an IgG receptor, including human neutrophils, human monocytes, murine macrophages, and murine macrophage-like cell lines. Most of this killing is oxidative and cells that have lost this capacity, such as neutrophils from patients with chronic granulomatous disease, do not kill cryptococci. Both human and murine natural killer (NK) cells and lymphocytes can also kill cryptococci in appropriate systems and this killing can be enhanced by high-titer antibody.

In Vivo Effects The most persuasive argument for the role of humoral immunity comes from the ability of high-titer polyclonal or monoclonal antibody to decrease mortality when given to mice prior to infection. The ability of polyclonal antibody to prolong the life of infected mice was first demonstrated with hyperimmune serum raised in rabbits by injecting whole cryptococci (11) and later with globulin from such rabbits (12). Because both antibody and inocula were injected intraperitoneally in these experiments, the effect of agglutinating the cryptococci was a confounding variable. Active immunization with cryptococcal polysaccharide conjugated to tetanus toxoid was later found to confer incomplete but significant protection against death following administration of a low inoculum (13). Dromer et al. (14) were the first to report that murine monoclonal antibody (IgG1) can delay death in experimental murine cryptococcosis. DBA/2 mice, a strain deficient in the complement component C5, died within 5 days after intravenous injection of a high inoculum, apparently of cryptococcal pneumonia. Mice pretreated with monoclonal antibody died much later from cryptococcal meningitis (15). This effect was not observed in a C5-sufficient mouse strain or with a lower inoculum. Subsequent work by Kozel (16) and Casadevall (17) and their respective coworkers confirmed and extended this observation. Casadevall et al. (17) found that murine monoclonal antibody of IgG1 subclass was superior to IgG3 and that IgM and IgA monoclonal antibody to GXM also prolonged the life of mice experimentally infected with *C. neoformans*. Many, but not all of the experiments by Casadevall et al. were done in A/J mice, a C5-deficient strain. Although the protective effect of IgM antibody might be explained by activation of complement and opsonophagocytosis, the mechanism by which IgA antibody is protective may be entirely different. Receptors for IgA are not known to occur on murine phagocytic cells. IgA antibody should not be opsonically active. As a completely unsupported postulate, one could imagine that limiting the diffusion of GXM away from the cryptococcal cell through deposition of antigen-antibody complexes helps reduce cerebral edema and prolongs life.

COMPLEMENT

Cryptococci readily activate complement in normal human or guinea pig serum. The alternative complement pathway is the major if not the sole pathway. Initially, small foci containing C3 are deposited on the capsular surface. These islands expand until the whole surface is coated with opsonically active C3b. C5a is released, which should stimulate chemotaxis. The increased lethality of a high cryptococcal inoculum injected intravenously into C5-deficient mice may be due to a decreased chemotactic response to cryptococci in this organ. Early after inoculation, the lungs contain twice as many cryptococci, are heavier, have more edema fluid, and have fewer inflammatory cells than do lungs of infected C5-sufficient mice. Insufficient complement components in CSF have been proposed to help explain the markedly less inflammatory response in the brain as compared to the lungs. Cryptococci taken from a patient's spinal fluid have no surface C3. This is not due to insufficient complement components in the patient's serum because incubation of cryptococci from CSF with 10% serum from the same patient results in C3 deposition as detected by direct immunofluorescent antibody. Cryptococci in mouse brains also lack surface complement, as detected by immunofluorescent antibody staining. In one patient whom I studied, cryptococci in skin pus were washed and found to have undetectable C3, but mixing those cells with 10% serum from that patient readily resulted in deposition of C3. The numerous inflammatory cells in the pus may have digested sufficient complement to prevent activation at that site. Depletion of blood complement can occur in cryptococcosis of humans and experimentally infected animals but this is a terminal phenomenon, often accompanied by cryptococcemia (18). Lack of opsonizing complement may help permit cryptococci to circulate within the bloodstream of these patients, just as cobra venom–induced complement depletion appears to do in the guinea pig. Aggregate evidence indicates that at certain sites, notably the lungs and the bloodstream, complement may provide opsonization and chemotaxis that enhances the immune response to cryptococci.

PHAGOCYTES

Neutropenia does not increase the susceptibility of patients or experimental animals to cryptococcosis. Human neutrophils can kill cryptococci in vitro, albeit slowly, provided that the particle is opsonized with IgG antibody or C3b. The presence of relatively few neutrophils in cryptococcal lesions of humans indicates a poor chemotactic response to this stimulus and may help explain the small role of this cell line in host defense. Fresh human monocytes can also kill opsonized cryptococci. When human monocytes are incubated for several days only in culture medium, the monocyte-derived macrophage retains the ability to phagocytose opsonized cryptococci but loses fungicidal capacity, perhaps because the oxidative burst is markedly decreased. Macrophages kill cryptococci at least in part by producing reactive oxygen intermediates. Activated murine macrophages also exert cytostasis on cryptococci by producing oxides of nitrogen using an arginine-dependent pathway (19). Human monocyte-derived macrophages can be activated so that these cells can markedly restrict cryptococcal growth. For example, incubation of normal human peripheral blood mononuclear cells, including lymphocytes and monocytes, with cryptococci will produce cells that can inhibit cryptococcal growth, particularly if antibody to GXM is added (20). Murine resident peritoneal macrophages can be activated to kill cryptococci by incubation with macrophage colony-stimulating factor (21).

LYMPHOCYTES

Predisposition to cryptococcosis has long been associated with conditions that impair responses mediated by thymic-derived lymphocytes, such as HIV-1 infection, Hodgkin's disease, sarcoidosis, and corticosteroid therapy. Athymic nude mice and mice injected with antibody to CD3 are more susceptible to cryptococcal challenge, a finding also consistent with T-cell participation in the immune response. Normal human $CD3^+$ cells bind to cryptococci by broad areas of attachment and this attachment is essential for limiting cryptococcal cell growth in vitro (22). $CD3^+$ cells from immunized mice are more effective than those cells from normal mice in binding cryptococci and limiting fungal growth (23). Among $CD3^+$ cells, both $CD4^+$ and $CD8^+$ cells appear to be essential for immunity. Depletion of either cell line impairs the pulmonary inflammatory response and the ability of mice to clear cryptococci from the lung (6). Depletion of $CD4^+$ cells decreases survival after intravenous administration of inocula and increases dissemination from the lung after intratracheal inoculation (24). Huffnagle et al. (25) provided evidence that $CD4^+$cells play a prominent role in recruiting macrophages and granulocytes to the lung, whereas $CD8^+$ cells increase the numbers of $CD4^+$ cells in the infiltrate and contribute to the local secretion of interferon-γ. Depletion experiments can be criticized for the possible confounding effect of antigen-antibody complexes. However, passive transfer of T cells (26) or $CD4^+$ cells (6) from immune mice into severe combined immunodeficient (SCID) mice improved pulmonary clearance of cryptococci. In vitro, both freshly isolated normal human $CD4^+$ and $CD8^+$ cells can limit cryptococcal growth after activation with interleukin (IL)-2 (27,28). Taken together, there seems little question that $CD4^+$ and $CD8^+$ T cells are important in host defense, particularly in limiting dissemination from the lung to the central nervous system.

NATURAL KILLER CELLS

Both human (27) and murine NK (29) cells inhibit the growth of C. *neoformans* in vitro. A substantial amount of the killing by human NK cells is due to secretion of perforin and can be blocked by antibody to that protein (Horn CA, Washburn RG, personal communication, 1996). Binding of the NK cell to cryptococci occurs by many microvilli; cell contact is essential for growth inhibition (29). Addition of anticryptococcal antibody enhances growth inhibition by murine NK cells (30). The decreased ability of NK cells from HIV-infected patients to kill cryptococci is of interest in that killing was restored to normal by incubation in IL-12 (31). In contrast, NK cells from a small number of previously normal patients with cryptococcosis markedly reduced anticryptococcal activity but incubation with IL-12 had no effect. Although the effect of depleting NK cells in normal mice infected intravenously or intratracheally is extremely modest (32), it may be that these cells assume a more important role in the presence of other defects in host defense.

CONCLUSIONS

The best way of defending the brain against cryptococcosis may be to prevent dissemination beyond the lung. Host defense in the brain is extremely limited, perhaps owing to complement deficiency at that site, contributing to a poor chemotactic stimulus for inflammatory cells. Pulmonary defense relies on complement activation to opsonize cryptococci and recruit macrophages, as well as the anticryptococcal activity of activated macrophages and unstimulated $CD3^+$ cells, and to a lesser extent, NK cells. Humoral immunity likely plays no role during naturally occurring infection, but preexistent high-titer antibody to GXM confers substantial protection, probably through opsonization of the cryptococcal cell and production of chemotactic C5a. By decreasing the number of cryptococci reaching the brain, progressive infection is delayed or averted. Whether sufficient antibody can be produced and maintained in subjects at risk of the disease, such as those infected with HIV-1, can only be determined by clinical trial.

REFERENCES

1 Littman ML, Zimmerman LE. *Cryptococcosis.* New York: Grune & Stratton, 1956.

2 Atkinson AJ, Bennett JE. Experience with a new skin test antigen prepared from *Cryptococcus neoformans. Am Rev Respir Dis* 1968; 97:637–643.

3 Bennett JE. Cryptococcal skin test antigen: preparation variables and characterization. *Infect Immun* 1981;32:373–380.

4 Muchmore HG, Felton FG, Salvin SB, Rhoades ER. Delayed hypersensitivity to cryptococcin in man. *Sabouraudia* 1969;6:285–288.

5 Henderson DK, Bennett JE, Huber MA. Long-lasting, specific immunologic unresponsiveness associated with cryptococcal meningitis. *J Clin Invest* 1982;69:1185–1190.

6 Hill JO, Aguirre KM. CD4+ T cell-dependent acquired state of immunity that protects the brain against *Cryptococcus neoformans. J Immunol* 1994;152:2344–2350.

7 Salas SD, Bennett JE, Kwon-Chung KJ, et al. Effect of the laccase gene, CNLAC1, on virulence of *Cryptococcus neoformans. J Exp Med* 1996;184:377–386.

8 Wang Y, Aisen P, Casadevall A. *Cryptococcus neoformans* melanin and virulence: mechanism of action. *Infect Immun* 1995;63:3131–3136.

9 Houpt DC, Pfrommer GST, Young BJ, et al. Occurrences, immunoglobulin classes, and biological activities of antibodies in normal human serum that are reactive with *Cryptococcus neoformans* glucuronoxylomannan. *Infect Immun* 1994;62:2857–2864.

10 Diamond RD, Bennett JE. Prognostic factors in

cryptococcal meningitis. *Ann Intern Med* 1974; 80:176–181.

11 Gadebush HH. Passive immunization against *Cryptococcus neoformans*. *Proc Soc Exp Biol Med* 1958;98:611–614.

12 Graybill JR, Hague M, Drutz DJ. Passive immunization in murine cryptococcosis. *Sabouraudia* 1981;19:237–244.

13 Devi SJN, Schneerson R, Egan W, et al. *Cryptococcus neoformans* serotype A glucuronoxylomannan-protein conjugate vaccines: synthesis, characterization, and immunogenicity. *Infect Immun* 1991;59:3700–3707.

14 Dromer F, Charreire J, Contrepois A, et al. Protection of mice against experimental cryptococcosis by anti-*Cryptococcus neoformans* monoclonal antibody. *Infect Immun* 1987; 55:749–752.

15 Dromer F, Perronne C, Barge J, et al. Role of IgG and complement component C5 in the initial course of experimental cryptococcosis. *Clin Exp Immunol* 1989;78:412–417.

16 Sanford JE, Lupan DM, Schlageter AM, Kozel TR. Passive immunization against *Cryptococcus neoformans* with an isotype-switch family of monoclonal antibodies reactive with cryptococcal polysaccharide. *Infect Immun* 1990; 58:1919–1923.

17 Mukherjee S, Lee S, Mukherjee J, et al. Monoclonal antibodies to *Cryptococcus neoformans* capsular polysaccharide modify the course of intravenous infection in mice. *Infect Immun* 1994;62:1079–1088.

18 Macher AM, Bennett JE, Gadek JE, Frank MM. Complement depletion in cryptococcal sepsis. *J Immunol* 1978;120:1686–1690.

19 Alspaugh JA, Granger DL. Inhibition of *Cryptococcus neoformans* replication by nitrogen oxides supports the role of these molecules as effects of macrophage-mediated cytostasis. *Infect Immun* 1991;59:2291–2296.

20 Levitz SM, Farrell TP, Mariarz RT. Killing of *Cryptococcus neoformans* by human peripheral blood mononuclear cells stimulated in culture. *J Infect* Dis 1991;163:1108–1113.

21 Brummer E, Stevens DA. Macrophage colony-stimulating factor induction of enhanced macrophage anticryptococcal activity: synergy with fluconazole for killing. *J Infect Dis* 1994; 170:173–179.

22 Murphy JW, Hidore R, Wong SC. Direct interactions of human lymphocytes with the yeast-like organism, *Cryptococcus neoformans*. *J Clin Invest* 1993;91:1553–1566.

23 Muth SM, Murphy JW. Direct anticryptococcal activity of lymphocytes from *Cryptococcus neoformans*-immunized mice. *Infect Immun* 1995;63:1637–1644.

24 Mody CH, Lipscomb MF, Street NE, Toews GB. Depletion of CD4+ (L3T4+) lymphocytes in vivo impairs murine host defense to *Cryptococcus neoformans*. *J Immunol* 1990; 144:1472–1477.

25 Huffnagle GB, Lipscomb MF, Lovchik JA, et al. The role of CD4+ and CD8+ T cells in the protective inflammatory response to a pulmonary cryptococccal infection. *J Leukoc Biol* 1994;55:35–42.

26 Huffnagle GB, Yates JL, Lipscomb MF. T cell-mediated immunity in the lung: a *Cryptococcus neoformans* pulmonary infection model using SCID and athymic nude mice. *Infect Immun* 1991;59:1423–1433.

27 Levitz SM, Dupont MP, Smail EH. Direct activity of human T lymphocytes and natural killer cells against *Cryptococcus neoformans*. *Infect Immun* 1994;62:194–202.

28 Levitz SM, Dupont MP. Phenotypic and functional characterization of human lymphocytes activated by interleukin-2 to directly inhibit growth of *Cryptococcus neoformans* in vitro. *J Clin Invest* 1993;91:1490–1498.

29 Murphy JW, Hidore MR, Nabavi N. Binding interactions of murine natural killer cells with the fungal target *Cryptococcus neoformans*. *Infect Immun* 1991;59:1476–1488.

30 Nabavi N, Murphy J. Antibody-dependent natural killer cell-mediated growth inhibition of *Cryptococcus neoformans*. *Infect Immun* 1986;51:556–562.

31 Horn CA, Washburn RG. Anticryptococcal activity of NK cell-enriched peripheral blood lymphocytes from human immunodeficiency virus-1 infected subjects: responses to interleukin-2, interferon-γ, and interleukin-12. *J Infect Dis* 1995;172:1023–1027.

32 Lipscomb MF, Alvarellos T, Toews GB, et al. Role of natural killer cells in resistance to *Cryptococcus neoformans* infections in mice. *Am J Pathol* 1987;128:354–361.

14
Coccidioides immitis Meningitis

JOHN N. GALGIANI

Coccidioidomycosis is a systemic fungal infection caused by *Coccidioides immitis.* In most persons after respiratory exposure, the infection is controlled without therapy and long-lasting immunity to future infections develops. In a few patients, however, the infection is not confined to the lungs, and lesions develop elsewhere in the body.

Coccidioidal meningitis is the most serious form of extrapulmonary spread, nearly always leading to death if it is not treated. Fortunately, treatments are available, and these include intrathecal amphotericin B or miconazole, and more recently oral therapy with fluconazole or itraconazole. Even though these drugs produce improvement and even remission of symptoms, in a majority of patients cure of infection is usually not possible.

This review begins by briefly describing the epidemiology and therapy for coccidioidal meningitis. The purpose here is to emphasize the scope of the problem that still exists with this complication of coccidioidal infections. From this base, our current understanding of the pathogenesis that leads to central nervous system involvement will be surveyed in an attempt to identify areas where future studies might be particularly productive. Finally, since the immune response in most infected patients is likely responsible for preventing meningitis altogether, recent work toward practical vaccines is considered. A detailed description of the clinical manifestations of coccidioidal meningitis is beyond the scope of this review. However, this information can be found in several other sources (1–5).

EPIDEMIOLOGIC AND CLINICAL OBSERVATIONS

Incidence of Coccidioidal Meningitis

Every year, infection with *C. immitis* occurs in approximately 3% of susceptible persons living within the lower deserts of Arizona (population 3.2 million) or in the southern portions of the Central Valley of California (population 0.8 million) (6). Since one-third to one-half of residents are already immune (7), the number of infections in these areas is likely 60,000 to 80,000 per year. Other parts of California, New Mexico, and Texas also are endemic for coccidioidomycosis but the rates of infection appear to be lower.

Despite the large number of new infections, only a very small proportion of patients have lesions outside of the lungs. In a review of Veterans Administration (VA)–Armed Forces records from 1955 to 1958, 76 (11%) of 699 patients with coccidioidomycosis had disseminated disease and of these, 31 (4.4%) had meningitis (8). In a more recent study of epidemic cases in Kern County, 25 (4.7%) of 536 patients had disseminated lesions and meningitis developed in half of them (2.4%) (9). Both studies overestimate the true frequency of dissemination, as only a fraction of infections result in symptoms warranting medical attention. Moreover, recent evidence suggests that early infection may be undetected by conventional serologic testing (10,11). Population-based studies from the University of Arizona Student Health Center corroborated this impression: The frequency of serologically diagnosed infection was 0.54% of susceptible patients per year, about one-sixth of the rate of skin test conversion (12). Thus, in general terms, of 100,000 patients with new infections, perhaps 200 to 500 patients will have disseminated infection and approximately 100 to 200 of them will develop meningitis.

Natural History of Coccidioidal Meningitis

Meningitis, like most other complications of coccidioidomycosis, usually develops relatively soon after the initial infection occurs. Pappagianis (13) estimated that all of 22 patients who developed meningitis as the result of a specific large dust storm did so at an average of 5.4 weeks from the date of initial infection. In another study, 20 of 25 patients developed meningitis within 6 months (1). Common presenting symptoms are headache, vomiting, and altered mental status. In addition to elevated white blood cell count, elevated protein level, and depressed glucose concentration in the cerebrospinal fluid (CSF), eosinophils are occasionally prominent (14). Hydrocephalus is a common complication, especially in children (15).

If untreated, meningitis is virtually always fatal. Einstein et al. (16) estimated that 95% of patients die within 2 years of diagnosis and the analysis of Vincent et al. (1) corroborated this impression. However, exceptional patients have survived as long as 12 years without treatment (1,17).

Response to Treatment

Amphotericin B Early experience with amphotericin B administered intravenously was unsatisfactory, and this led to trials with intrathecal administration (16,18,19). The exact implementation of this approach and its reported benefit have varied widely among practitioners (for a review, see article by Labadie and Hamilton (20)). Overall, the survival rate of patients treated with intrathecal amphotericin B ranges from 51% to 100%; however, the length of follow-up for the individual studies assessing the survival rate varied widely. Although effective, repeated instillation of deoxycholate-suspended amphotericin B into the ventricular, cisternal, or lumbar spaces causes considerable morbidity and toxicity, and this often limits the use of this therapy. Moreover, in patients with obstructive hydrocephalus, infected portions of the meninges may be isolated entirely from intrathecally administered drug.

Azoles Miconazole, the first imidazole antifungal approved for use in systemic fungal infections in humans, is effective in treating coccidioidal meningitis (15,21). However, although its spectrum of toxicities differs from that of amphotericin B, it also requires parenteral or intrathecal administration and as such has several of the same limitations. Ketoconazole can be administered orally and is effective in some patients using relatively high doses (i.e., 1.0–2.0 g/day orally) (22). More favorable experience has been reported with the newer azoles, itraconazole and especially fluconazole. For example, in one study, 17 (68%) of 25 patients receiving fluconazole (400 mg/day) as initial therapy for coccidioidal meningitis responded for periods of at least 2 years (23). In the same study, fluconazole treatment of 25 patients for whom prior therapy with intrathecal amphotericin B had failed, elicited responses. Another report indicated that maintenance therapy following successful treatment with amphotericin B was even more satisfactory (23a). Similar but more limited experience has been reported with itraconazole (24).

Future Therapies Nikkomycin Z, one of a number of related chitin synthase inhibitors, has both in vitro activity against C. immitis and in vivo efficacy in a meningocerebral model of coccidioidal infection (25,26). Shaman Pharmaceuticals (South San Francisco, CA) has announced its intention to study its efficacy in patients with coccidioidomycosis, and these studies are projected to begin in 1998.

Likelihood of Cure A major drawback to current therapy is the likelihood of relapse if therapy is discontinued. Relapse is common after intrathecal amphotericin B is stopped, although the exact incidence is not documented. Relapse after successful oral azole therapy is also common. Dewsnup et al. (27) recently reported that 14 of 18 patients who discontinued ketoconazole, itraconazole, or fluconazole treatment had recurrent meningeal infections. In that report, relapse was defined as clinical deterioration in combination with worsening CSF indices (protein or glucose concentrations, leukocyte counts, or coccidioidal antibody titers) relative to the last CSF sample available before the end of therapy. Relapses occurred within 1 month or as late as 80 months after azole therapy was stopped. Two patients died and 1 patient developed hydrocephalus as a result of the recurrent infection. Post hoc analysis failed to disclose any specific factors that would predict relapse.

The observation that treatment with current antifungal therapy seldom if ever results in an eradication of the pathogen from the meninges has practical implications. Most obviously, the clinical importance is simply that effective therapy requires treatment to be continued indefinitely. If that is done, then coccidioidal meningitis appears to remain in abeyance. For example, in one study 37 patients were alive after 2 to 4 years of continuous therapy (23). Of these, 27 remained in remission, only 3 subsequently manifest worsening symptoms or CSF abnormalities (27a), and 7 were lost to follow-up 3 years later (unpublished data, NIAID-Mycoses Study Group 17th Annual Meeting, April 10–12, 1996, Bethesda MD).

Another practical consideration is that continued therapy has significant costs. For example, fluconazole therapy at 400 mg/day currently costs approximately $10,000 per year. Thus, if the average life expectancy from the time of initiating treatment were 35 years, the projected cost of treatment would be over one-third of a million dollars per patient. This expense of current therapy lends an additional justification for research into alternative management or prevention strategies, as discussed later.

At the conceptual level, it is of interest that symptoms resolve when fungal proliferation is blocked, and does not require that the organism is not eradicated. The relationship of fungal growth to pathogenesis is discussed in more detail later in this review.

PATHOGENESIS OF COCCIDIOIDOMYCOSIS

Early Events after Infection

Coccidioidomycosis is initiated by inhalation of an arthroconidium, a sporelike structure that evolves from the mature mycelia (28–30). It is difficult to recover cultures of *C. immitis* within the endemic regions by large-volume air sampling (31) and in animal models very small numbers of arthroconidia can be lethal (32). These observations suggest that most naturally acquired human infections are caused by only a single fungal cell. Given its size of approximately 5 microns, an arthroconidium is likely to deposit after inhalation no further into the lung than a bronchiole, and there undergoes a phase transition from its barrel shape to a spherical structure. As the cell enlarges, mitotic division and cell fission are coordinated with internal septation by invagination of the internal layer of the cell wall (33), eventually producing scores of endospores that disperse when the mature spherule ruptures. These events take place within the first 4 days after infection. With growth, an inflammatory response develops. Coccidioidal extracts have been shown to activate complement through both the classic and alternative pathways and could mediate chemotaxis of leukocytes to the site of infection (34,35). Histologically, neutrophils, eosinophils, histiocytes, and other mononuclear cells are represented (36,37). Presumably, when *C. immitis* spreads outside of the chest, such as to the central nervous system, it is hematogenously in the endospore phase.

How an endospore is able to exit the inflammatory lesion within the disrupted lung tissue and enter the bloodstream has not been determined. In tuberculosis and histoplasmosis, two other granulomatous infections, it is reasoned that the mycobacteria or the yeast cells, respectively, are phagocytosed by histocytes that carry the organism via the lymphatic system to the bloodstream and to lesions beyond the lungs (38,30). In *C. immitis* infection, neutrophils and mononuclear leukocytes can phagocytose the endospores (40,41). Moreover, killing of arthospores and young spherules has been demonstrated experimentally with human mononuclear leukocytes (42). However, it is possible that phagocytosis and subsequent intracellular events might not result in the killing of some fungal cells. Those surviving might be carried with phagocytes that move from the infected tissue, through the lymphatic system, and eventually into the vascular space. Another possibility but with less experimental support might be the attachment of a spherule or endospore to the epithelium of a pulmonary venule, with subsequent disruption of the venule and release of endospores directly into the vascular space. Intimate attachment of spherules to human leukocytes has been demonstrated by electron microscopy (43,44), although similar studies have not been performed with epithelial cells of pulmonary veins and no information is available about the role of adhesion molecules or their regulation. Extracellular proteinases have been isolated from *C. immitis* (45–49). These or other proteinases could conceivably be involved in such a process. Further work in this area could yield new directions for antifungal therapy.

Meninges are the most common site within the central nervous system for hematogenously deposited endospores to develop lesions. Basilar more than supracortical meninges are involved, and inflammation is more prominent in the depths of the sulci rather than the peaks of the gyri (50). Exudates contain variable numbers of lymphocytes, plasma cells, macrophages, and encapsulated organisms, often within or near multinucleated giant cells (51). Acute inflammatory reactions are very uncommon. Over time, fibrosis resulting from the inflammatory process within the meninges may interfere with spinal fluid resorption or cause obstruction along its usual course, such as in the aqueduct of Sylvius.

Focal inflammatory lesions can also develop deeper within the brain (52,53). Although vasculitic lesions have been reported in occasional patients for decades, they may be more frequent than previously appreciated. Contemporary noninvasive imaging techniques detect focal lesions consistent with vasculitis in 9% to 40% of patients (54–56). These lesions are characterized by an inflammatory reaction involving the walls of small and medium-size vessels and the adjacent perivascular zones. Within the brain parenchyma, granulomata containing spherules have been observed. Frequently, these lesions produce infarction and serious neurologic impairment or death. Occasionally, larger focal intracranial masses develop. The focal nature of this process is distinguishable from the diffuse leukoencephalopathy described in patients who had received a water-soluble formulation of amphotericin B, amphotericin B methyl ester (57). Furthermore, diffuse leukoencephalopathy was not detected in patients with coccidioidal meningitis who either received no treatment or received conventional formulations of amphotericin B (51).

Whether located on the brain's meningeal surface or in deeper central nervous system lesions, the ineffective inflammatory response to the fungus appears to be the cause of symptoms and later complications of coccidioidal meningitis. As noted already, in many patients with coccidioidal meningitis, the symptoms resolve with therapies that do not eradicate the organism from the brain. In other words, the presence of the fungus per se does not seem to be sufficient to engender inflammation. Rather, it appears that fungal proliferation is required. Exactly what aspect of fungal growth stimulates the destructive inflammatory response is not known. Ampel et al. (58) demonstrated low levels of both tumor necrosis factor and interleukin (IL)-1β in CSF specimens from patients with coccidioidal meningitis. Furthermore, they noted significant correlations of IL-1β with CSF white blood cell counts and clinical symptoms. Dooley et al. (59) found that spherules stimulated human peripheral blood mononuclear cells to secrete tumor necrosis factor, IL-1, and IL-6, and stimulation was equivalent among persons with and those without coccidioidal infection. Mice infected with *C. immitis* exhibited increased levels of these same cytokines (60), and levels were higher in a resistant strain of mouse (DBA/2) than in a strain that was susceptible to lethal infection (BALB/c). These results could be interpreted to suggest that proinflammatory mediators play a role in the control of systemic coccidioidal infections. In other studies, IL-12 treatment of BALB/c mice prior to intraperitoneal challenge resulted in reduced fungal burden in the liver, spleen, and lungs as compared to mice not receiving IL-12 (61). Also, CBA/2 mice treated with anti–IL-12 exhibited increased fungal burden in the liver and spleen, as if IL-12 was an important mediator of control. However, IL-12 treatment of BALB/c mice did not result in a significantly reduced fungal burden in the lungs or the spleen after a respiratory challenge. These results suggest that alveolar macrophages may not be as responsive to IL-12–mediated events such as increased interferon-γ production. Alternatively, other factors might contribute to the respiratory challenge being more difficult for BALB/c mice to control. Since these studies did not address central nervous system involvement, their relevance to coccidioidal meningitis is uncertain. Thus, a detailed understanding of the specific events that trigger and mediate inflammation in coccidioidal infections could afford new opportunities to influence the disease process, and therefore might be a productive avenue for future research.

Control of coccidioidomycosis by cell-mediated immunity is critically dependent on T lymphocytes, both in experimentally produced infections in mice (62–68) and in naturally acquired infections in humans (69–75). Recent work indicated that peripheral blood mononuclear cells from patients with disseminated coccidioidomycosis have virtually no (< 50 μg/mL) interferon-γ response to coccidioidal antigens (76). This is in contrast to the brisk stimulation (average response, 2800 μg/mL) of peripheral blood mononuclear cells from persons in whom coccidioidal infections are competently controlled and who have delayed-type dermal hypersensitivity to coccidioidal skin test antigens (75). This suggests the absence of the Th1-type response described in some experimental animal (77) and human infectious diseases (78) in which cellular immunity plays a role. However, despite the observed depression of interferon-γ, IL-4 and IL-10 levels were not reciprocally elevated (76) as would be indicative of a Th2 response. The reasons for this are not clear, but similar observations were recently made in patients with tuberculosis (79,80). In all of these studies, coccidioidal infections did not specifically involve the central nervous system, and so it is completely unknown whether any of these correlates are associated with meningeal disease.

COCCIDIOIDAL VACCINES

Developing a vaccine to prevent coccidioidomycosis has been an attractive goal for many years (81). The possibility that such a strategy might be useful is rooted in the fact that immunity develops in most persons who are infected naturally. Additional interest was produced by the studies of Charles Smith, Hille Levine, and Demosthenes Pappagianis, which demonstrated durable immunity in mice from intramuscular injections of formalin-killed whole spherules (32,82–86). On the other hand, if immunity depends on a competent T-cell response, then a vaccine that evokes protection by sensitizing T cells may not be of benefit to persons incapable of mounting a competent T-cell response. Such patients might include those with acquired immunodeficiency syndrome (AIDS), those receiving immunsuppressive medications such as corticosteroids, cyclosporine, and methotrexate; and those with hereditary predispositions to progressive infections (87–94). If this were the case, many of the worst consequences of coccidioidal infection may not be prevented. Needless to say, these unresolved issues have stimulated considerable discussion about the ultimate utility of vaccine development for preventing coccidioidomycosis.

Epidemiologic evidence (see above) indicates that approximately half of all patients with coccidioidal meningitis have dissemination at no other sites. Furthermore, most of the patients with the central nervous system as the sole site of dissemination do not have other apparent risk factors or immunosuppressing conditions. Thus, it is possible that perhaps one-third of cases of meningitis occur not because of an inability to develop immunity but rather because of a chance establishment of a meningeal lesion. Under these circumstances, a vaccine that prevents primary infection would significantly reduce the number of new meningeal infections due to *C. immitis*. The high cost of treatment combined with the life-threatening nature of even small numbers of such patients adds justification to efforts in vaccine development.

The original vaccine was a formalin-killed whole spherule preparation. Although highly effective in protecting mice against a lethal coccidioidal challenge, it was unable to diminish the number of new infections detected in a human field trial (95). A possible explanation for this disappointing result is that the amount of antigen used in each dose was inadequate. The dose used in the field trial was 1.75 mg per injection, the maximum possible without unacceptable untoward reactions at the injection site. This dose is 3 logs less than the milligram-per-kilogram dose that had optimally been used in murine studies. Moreover, in dose-ranging murine studies, even a several-fold reduction from the optimal regimens resulted in considerable attenuation of the vaccine's effect (85). Thus, if the explanation for the vaccine's failure was simply an inadequate dose, then identification of the protective antigens and use of them in higher concentration without irrelevant inflammatory cellular components might avoid dose-limiting intolerance.

One antigen that looks attractive as a candidate for subcellular vaccine studies is a proline-rich protein isolated from spherules by toluene treatment and deglycosylation (96,97). Immunoelectron microscopy demonstrated this protein to be located in the spherule cell wall and in the septa among endospores. Peripheral blood mononuclear cells from skin test–reactive patients can be stimulated by this protein under conditions that fail to stimulate subjects nonreactive to skin tests. In addition, patients with both self-limited and progressive coccidioidal infections demonstrate antibodies to this antigen (10,98).

The antigenic analysis of two protective subcellular vaccines—the alkaline-soluble, water-soluble (ASWS) preparation of Cox (99), and the 27 kxg preparation (the supernatant after 27,000g centrifugation of mechanically disrupted formalin-killed spherules) of Pappagianis et al. (100,101)—provides evidence that the proline-rich protein from spherule walls could be a protective antigen. In the ASWS preparation, only two antigenic components have been identified (102). One of these is the tube precipitin antigen (103), predominantly carbohydrate epitopes and reported to be associated with β-1,3-glucanase activity (104,105). The other antigen, designated *antigen* 2 (106), is identical to the proline-rich spherule protein as judged by binding of a monoclonal antibody to both antigen 2 and the proline-rich protein (107).

Regarding the other protective subcellular vaccine, Pappagianis et al. (100,101) reported that the 27 kxg preparation also evokes protection in mice. Analysis of this preparation demonstrated that the proline-rich spherule antigen is the dominant protein in that preparation (Orsborn KI, Galgiani JN, unpublished data, 1994). Taken together, these findings suggest that the proline-rich spherule antigen may likely evoke protection as a vaccine.

The gene that encodes the proline-rich antigen was first cloned and sequenced from a complementary DNA library by Dugger et al. (108). The protein is 194 amino acids in length, and demonstrates a proline-rich repeating motif that is common to some other proteins. However, the remainder of the sequence does not show strong similarity to any other sequences in the Genbank. Subsequently, the identical gene was independently sequenced and reported (109), and its expression product was shown to evoke foot-pad swelling in mice immunized with formalin-killed whole spherules. Thus, it should now be possible to test directly the immunogenicity of the recombinant proline-rich protein in animal studies.

REFERENCES

1 Vincent T, Galgiani JN, Huppert M, Salkin D. The natural history of coccidioidal meningitis: VA-Armed Forces cooperative studies, 1955–1958. *Clin Infect Dis* 1993;16:247–254.

2 Einstein HE, Johnson RH. Coccidioidomycosis: new aspects of epidemiology and therapy. *Clin Infect Dis* 1993;16:349–356.

3 Galgiani JN. Coccidioidomycosis. In: Rakel RE, ed. *Conn's current therapy.* Philadelphia: WB Saunders, 1996;188–190.

4 Galgiani JN. Coccidioidomycosis. *West J Med* 1993;159:153–171.

5 Stevens DA. Current concepts: coccidioidomycosis. *N Engl J Med* 1995;332:1077–1082.

6 Dodge RR, Lebowitz MD, Barbee RA, Burrows B. Estimates of *C. immitis* infection by skin test reactivity in an endemic community. *Am J Public Health* 1985;75:863–865.

7 Lebowitz MD, Johnson WM, Kaltenborn W. Coccidioidin skin test reactivity and cross-reactivity with histoplasmin in a Tucson population. In: Ajello L, ed. *Coccidioidomycosis. Current clinical and diagnostic status.* Miami: Symposia Specialists, 1977:45–61.

8 Reef SE, Galgiani JN, Hutwagner L, et al. Natural history of disseminated coccidioidomycosis. Analysis of Armed Forces-VA collaborative study group records, 1955–1958. In: Einstein HE, Catanzaro A, eds. Coccidioidomycosis. Proceedings of the fifth International Conference. Washington, D.C.: National Foundation for Infectious Diseases, 1996;419.

9 Arsura E, Caldwell J, Johnson R, et al. Coccidioidomycosis epidemic of 1991: epidemiologic features. In: Einstein HE, Catanzaro A, eds. Coccidioidomycosis. Proceedings of the fifth International Conference. Washington, D.C.: National Foundation for Infectious Diseases, 1996;98–107.

10 Wieden MA, Lundergan LL, Blum J, et al. Detection of coccidioidal antibodies by 33-kDa spherule antigen, *Coccidioides* EIA, and standard serologic tests in sera from patients evaluated for coccidioidomycosis. *J Infect Dis* 1996;173:1273–1277.

11 Galgiani JN, Grace GM, Lundergan LL. New serologic tests for early detection of coccidioidomycosis. *J Infect Dis* 1991;163:671–674.

12 Kerrick SS, Lundergan LL, Galgiani JN. Coccidioidomycosis at a university health service. *Am Rev Respir Dis* 1985;131:100–102.

13 Pappagianis D. Coccidioidomycosis. In: Balows A, Hausler WJ Jr, Lennette EH, eds. *Laboratory diagnosis of infectious diseases.* Berlin: Springer, 1988:600–623.

14 Ragland AS, Arsura EL, Ismail Y, Johnson R. Eosinophilic pleocytosis in coccidioidal meningitis: frequency and significance. *Am J Med* 1993;95:154–157.

15 Harrison HR, Galgiani JN, Reynolds AF Jr, et al. Amphotericin B and imidazole therapy for coccidioidal meningitis in children. *Pediatr Infect Dis* 1983;2:216–221.

16 Einstein HE, Holeman CW Jr, Sandidge LL, Holden DH. Coccidioidal meningitis. The use of amphotericin B in treatment. *Calif Med* 1961;94:339–343.

17 Unterharnscheidt F, DeBeukelaer M, Simon

JL. Chronic untreated coccidioidomycosis of the central nervous system: a case of 7½ years duration. *Texas Rep Biol Med* 1969;27:513–531.

18 Winn WA. The treatment of coccidioidal meningitis. The use of amphotericin B in a group of 25 patients. *Calif Med* 1964;101: 78–89.

19 Bouza E, Dreyer JS, Hewitt WL, Meyer RD. Coccidioidal meningitis. An analysis of thirty-one cases and review of the literature. *Medicine (Baltimore)* 1981;60:139–172.

20 Labadie EL, Hamilton RH. Survival improvement in coccidioidal meningitis by high-dose intrathecal amphotericin B. *Arch Intern Med* 1986;146:2013–2018.

21 Deresinski SC, Lilly RB, Levine HB, et al. Treatment of fungal meningitis with miconazole. *Arch Intern Med* 1977;137:1180–1185.

22 Craven PC, Graybill JR, Jorgensen JH, et al. High-dose ketoconazole for treatment of fungal infections of the central nervous system. *Ann Intern Med* 1983;98:160–167.

23 Galgiani JN, Catanzaro A, Cloud GA, et al. Fluconazole therapy for coccidioidal meningitis. *Ann Intern Med* 1993;119:28–35.

23a Perez JA, Johnson RH, Caldwell JW, et al. Fluconazole therapy in coccidioidal meningitis maintained with intrathecal amphotericin B. *Arch Intern Med* 1995;155:1665–1668.

23 Galgiani JN, Catanzaro A, Cloud GA, et al. Fluconazole therapy for coccidioidal meningitis. *Ann Intern Med* 1993;119:28–35.

24 Tucker RM, Denning DW, Dupont B, Stevens DA. Itraconazole therapy for chronic coccidioidal meningitis. *Ann Intern Med* 1990; 112:108–112.

25 Hector RF, Zimmer BL, Pappagianis D. Inhibitors of cell wall synthesis. Nikkomycins. In: Yamaguchi H, Kobayashi GS, Takahashi H, eds. *Recent progress in antifungal chemotherapy.* New York: Marcel Dekker, 1991: 341–353.

26 Hector RF, Zimmer BL, Pappagianis D. Evaluation of nikkomycins X and Z in murine models of coccidioidomycosis, histoplasmosis, and blastomycosis. *Antimicrob Agents Chemother* 1990;34:587–593.

27 Dewsnup DH, Galgiani JN, Graybill JR, et al. Is it ever safe to stop azole therapy for *Coccidioides immitis* meningitis? *Ann Intern Med* 1996;124:305–310.

27a Galgiani JN. Presentation. NIAID—Mycoses Study Group 18th Annual Meeting, April 16–18, 1997.

28 Sun SH, Cole GT, Drutz DJ, Harrison JL. Electron-microscopic observations of the *Coccidioides immitis* parasitic cycle *in vivo. J Med Vet Mycol* 1986;24:183–192.

29 Huppert M, Cole GT, Sun SH, et al. The propagule as an infectious agent in coccidioidomycosis. In: Schlessinger D, ed. *Microbiology.* Washington, DC: American Society for Microbiology, 1983;262–267.

30 Cole GT, Sun SH. Arthroconidium—spherule—endospore transformation in *Coccidioides immitis.* In: Szaniszlo PJ, ed. *Fungal dimorphism.* New York: Plenum, 1985:281–333.

31 Hoggan MD, Ransom JP, Pappagianis D, et al. Isolation of *Coccidioides immitis* from the air. *Stanford Med Bull* 1956;14:190. Abstract.

32 Kong YM, Levine HB, Madin SH, Smith CE. Fungal multiplication and histopathologic changes in vaccinated mice infected with *Coccidioides immitis.* I. *Immunology* 1964; 92:779–790.

33 Hector RF, Pappagianis D. Enzymatic degradation of the walls of spherules of *Coccidioides immitis. Exp Mycol* 1982;6:136–152.

34 Galgiani JN, Isenberg RA, Stevens DA. Chemotaxigenic activity of extracts from the mycelial and spherule phases of *Coccidioides immitis* for human polymorphonuclear leukocytes. *Infect Immun* 1978;21:862–865.

35 Galgiani JN, Yam P, Petz LD, et al. Complement activation by *Coccidioides immitis:* in vitro and clinical studies. *Infect Immun* 1980; 28:944–949.

36 Hungtington RW Jr, Waldmann WJ, Sargent JA, et al. Pathologic and clinical observations on 142 cases of fatal coccidioidomycosis with necropsy. In: Ajello L, ed. *Coccidioidomycosis.* Tucson: University of Arizona Press, 1967:221–225.

37 Echols RM, Palmer DL, Long GW. Tissue eosinophilia in human coccidioidomycosis. *Rev Infect Dis* 1982;4:656–664.

38 Youmans GP. *Tuberculosis.* Philadelphia: WB Saunders, 1979.

39 Sarosi GA, Davies SF. Histoplasmosis. In: Fishman AP, ed. *Pulmonary diseases and disorders.* 2nd ed. New York: McGraw-Hill, 1988:1775–1784.

40 Galgiani JN, Payne CM, Jones JF. Human polymorphonuclear-leukocyte inhibition of incorporation of chitin precursors into mycelia of *Coccidioides immitis. J Infect Dis* 1984;149:404–412.

41 Galgiani JN. Inhibition of different phases of *Coccidioides immitis* by human neutrophils or hydrogen peroxide. *J Infect Dis* 1986; 153:217–222.

42 Ampel NM, Bejarano GC, Galgiani JN. Killing of *Coccidioides immitis* by human pe-

ripheral blood mononuclear cells. *Infect Immun* 1992;60:4200–4204.

43 Drutz DJ, Huppert M. Coccidioidomycosis: factors affecting the host-parasite interaction. *J Infect Dis* 1983;147:372–390.

44 Galgiani JN, Hayden R, Payne CM. Leukocyte effects on the dimorphism of *Coccidioides immitis. J Infect Dis* 1982;146:56–63.

45 Resnick S, Pappagianis D, McKerrow JH. Proteinase production by the parasitic cycle of the pathogenic fungus *Coccidioides immitis. Infect Immun* 1987;55:2807–2815.

46 Yuan L, Cole GT. Characterization of a proteinase inhibitor isolated from the fungal pathogen *Coccidioides immitis. Biochem J* 1989;257:729–736.

47 Yuan L, Cole GT. Isolation and characterization of an extracellular proteinase of *Coccidioides immitis. Infect Immun* 1987;55:1970–1978.

48 Cole GT, Zhu S, Hsu L, et al. Isolation and expression of a gene which encodes a wall-associated proteinase of *Coccidioides immitis. Infect Immun* 1992;60:416–427.

49 Pan S, Zhang M, Cole GT. Isolation and characterization of the arginase-encoding gene (*arg*) from *Coccidioides immitis. Gene* 1995; 154:115–118.

50 Huntington RW. Pathology of coccidioidomycosis. In: Stevens DA, ed. *Coccidioidomycosis. A text.* New York: Plenum Medical, 1980: 113–132.

51 Sobel RA, Ellis WG, Nielsen SL, Davis RL. Central nervous system coccidioidomycosis: a clinicopathologic study of treatment with and without amphotericin B. *Hum Pathol* 1984; 15:980–995.

52 Williams PL, Johnson R, Pappagianis D, et al. Vasculitic and encephalitic complications associated with *Coccidioides immitis* infection of the central nervous system in humans: report of 10 cases and review. *Clin Infect Dis* 1992; 14:673–682.

53 Mischel PS, Vinters HV. Coccidioidomycosis of the central nervous system: neuropathological and vasculopathic manifestations and clinical correlates. *Clin Infect Dis* 1995; 20:400–405.

54 McGahan JP, Graves DS, Palmer PES, et al. *Review.* Classic and contemporary imaging of coccidioidomycosis. *AJR* 1981;136: 393–404.

55 Shetter AG, Fischer DW, Flom RA. Computed tomography in cases of coccidioidal meningitis with clinical correlation. *West J Med* 1985;142:782–786.

56 Dublin AB, Phillips HE. Computed tomography of disseminated cerebral coccidioidomycosis. *Radiology* 1980;135:361–368.

57 Ellis WG, Sobel RA, Nielsen SL. Leukoencephalopathy in patients treated with amphotericin B methyl ester. *J Infect Dis* 1982; 146:125–137.

58 Ampel NM, Ahmann DR, Delgado KL, et al. NIAID Mycoses Study Group. Tumor necrosis factor-α and interleukin-β in cerebrospinal fluid of patients with coccidioidal meningitis during therapy with fluconazole. *J Infect Dis* 1995;171:1675–1678.

59 Dooley DP, Cox RA, Hestilow KL, et al. Cytokine induction in human coccidioidomycosis. *Infect Immun* 1994;62:3980–3983.

60 Cox RA, Magee DM. Production of tumor necrosis factor alpha, interleukin-1α, and interleukin-6 during murine coccidioidomycosis. *Infect Immun* 1995;63:4178–4180.

61 Magee DM, Cox RA. Interleukin-12 regulation of host defenses against *Coccidioides immitis. Infect Immun* 1996;64:3609–3613.

62 Reinhardt TA, Horst RL. Ketoconazole inhibits self-induced metabolism of 1,25-dihydroxyvitamin D_3 and amplifies 1,25-dihydroxyvitamin D_3 receptor up-regulation in rat osteosarcoma cells. *Arch Biochem Biophys* 1989;272:459–465.

63 Beaman L, Pappagianis D, Benjamini E. Mechanisms of resistance to infection with *Coccidioides immitis* in mice. *Infect Immun* 1979;23:681–685.

64 Beaman L, Benjamini E, Pappagianis D. Role of lymphocytes in macrophage-induced killing of *Coccidioides immitis* in vitro. *Infect Immun* 1981;34:347–353.

65 Beaman L, Benjamini E, Pappagianis D. Activation of macrophages by lymphokines: enhancement of phagosome-lysosome fusion and killing of *Coccidioides immitis. Infect Immun* 1983;39:1201–1207.

66 Beaman L. Fungicidal activation of murine macrophages by recombinant gamma interferon. *Infect Immun* 1987;55:2951–2955.

67 Beaman L. Effects of recombinant gamma interferon and tumor necrosis factor on in vitro interactions of human mononuclear phagocytes with *Coccidioides immitis. Infect Immun* 1991;59:4227–4229.

68 Magee DM, Cox RA. Roles of gamma interferon and interleukin-4 in genetically determined resistance to *Coccidioides immitis. Infect Immun* 1995;63:3514–3519.

69 Cox RA, Vivas JR. Spectrum of in vivo and in vitro cell-mediated immune responses in coccidioidomycosis. *Cell Immunol* 1977; 31:130–141.

70 Cox RA, Vivas JR, Gross A, et al. In vivo and in vitro cell-mediated responses in coccidioidomycosis. I. Immunologic responses of persons with primary, asymptomatic infections. *Am Rev Respir Dis* 1976;114:937–943.

71 Cole GT, Kirkland TN, Franco M, et al. Immunoreactivity of a surface wall fraction produced by spherules of *Coccidioides immitis*. *Infect Immun* 1988;56:2695–2701.

72 Deresinski SC, Levine HB, Stevens DA. Soluble antigens of mycelia and spherules in the in vitro detection of immunity to *Coccidioides immitis*. *Infect Immun* 1974;10:700–704.

73 Catanzaro A, Spitler LE, Moser KM. Cellular immune response in coccidioidomycosis. *Cell Immunol* 1975;15:360–371.

74 Barbee RA, Hicks MJ. Clinical usefulness of lymphocyte transformation in patients with coccidioidomycosis. *Chest* 1988;93:1003–1007.

75 Ampel NM, Bejarano GC, Salas SD, Galgiani JN. In vitro assessment of cellular immunity in human coccidioidomycosis: Relationship between dermal hypersensitivity, lymphocyte transformation, and lymphokine production by peripheral blood mononuclear cells from healthy adults. *J Infect Dis* 1992;165:710–715.

76 Corry DB, Ampel NM, Christian L, et al. Cytokine production by peripheral blood mononuclear cells in human coccidioidomycosis. *J Infect Dis* 1996;174:440–443.

77 Mosmann TR, Coffman RL. Heterogeneity of cytokine secretion patterns and functions of helper T cells. *Adv Immunol* 1989; 46:111–147.

78 Yamamura M, Uremura K, Deans RJ, et al. Defining protective responses to pathogens: cytokine profiles in leprosy lesions. *Science* 1991;254:277–279.

79 Zhang M, Lin Y, Iyer DV, et al. T-cell cytokine response in human infection with *Mycobacterium tuberculosis*. *Infect Immun* 1995;63: 3231-3234.

80 Lin YG, Zhang M, Hofman FM, et al. Absence of a prominent Th2 cytokine response in human tuberculosis. *Infect Immun* 1996; 64:1351–1356.

81 Pappagianis D, Levine HB. The present status of vaccination against coccidioidomycosis in man. *Am J Epidemiol* 1975;102:30–41.

82 Pappagianis D. Histopathologic response of mice to killed vaccines of *Coccidioides immitis*. *J Invest Dermatol* 1967;49:71–77.

83 Huppert M, Levine HB, Sun SH, Peterson ET. Resistance of vaccinated mice to typical and atypical strains of *Coccidioides immitis*. *J Bacteriol* 1967;94:924–927.

84 Levine HB, Kong Y, Smith CE. Immunization of mice to *Coccidioides immitis:* dose, regimen and spherulation stage of killed spherule vaccines. *J Immunol* 1965;94:132–142.

85 Levine HB, Miller RL, Smith CE. Influence of vaccination on respiratory coccidioidal disease in cynomolgus monkeys. *J Immunol* 1962;89:242–251.

86 Levine HB, Cobb JM, Smith CE. Immunogenicity of spherule-endospore vaccines of *Coccidioides immitis* for mice. *J Immunol* 1961;87:218–227.

87 Rutala PJ, Smith JW. Coccidioidomycosis in potentially compromised hosts: the effect of immunosuppressive therapy in dissemination. *Am J Med Sci* 1978;275:283–295.

88 Deresinski SC, Stevens DA. Coccidioidomycosis in compromised hosts. Experience at Stanford University Hospital. *Medicine (Baltimore)* 1974;54:377–395.

89 Cohen IM, Galgiani JN, Potter D, Ogden DA. Coccidioidomycosis in renal replacement therapy. *Arch Intern Med* 1982;142;489–494.

90 Jones JL, Fleming PL, Ciesielski CA, et al. Coccidioidomycosis among persons with AIDS in the United States. *J Infect Dis* 1995;171:961–966.

91 Ampel NM, Dols CL, Galgiani JN. Coccidioidomycosis during human immunodeficiency virus infection. Results of a prospective study in a coccidioidal endemic area. *Am J Med* 1993;94:235–240.

92 Pappagianis D. Epidemiology of coccidioidomycosis. *Curr Top Med Mycol* 1988;2:199–238.

93 Pappagianis D, Lindsay S, Beall S, Williams P. Ethnic background and the clinical course of coccidioidomycosis. *Am Rev Respir Dis* 1979;120:959–961. Letter.

94 Deresinski SC, Pappagianis D, Stevens DA. Association of ABO blood group and outcome of coccidioidal infection. *Sabouraudia* 1979; 17:261–264.

95 Pappagianis D, Valley Fever Vaccine Study Group. Evaluation of the protective efficacy of the killed *Coccidioides immitis* spherule vaccine in humans. *Am Rev Respir Dis* 1993; 148:656–660.

96 Dugger KO, Galgiani JN, Ampel NM, et al. An immunoreactive apoglycoprotein purified from *Coccidioides immitis*. *Infect Immun* 1991;59:2245–2251.

97 Galgiani JN, Sun SH, Dugger KO, et al. An arthroconidial-spherule antigen of *Coccidioides immitis:* differential expression during in vitro fungal development and evidence for humoral response in humans after infection or vaccination. *Infect Immun* 1992;60:2627–2635.

98 Galgiani JN, Peng T, Lewis ML, Cloud GA. Cerebrospinal fluid antibodies detected by ELISA against a 33-kDa antigen from spherules of *Coccidioides immitis* in patients with coccidioidal meningitis. *J Infect Dis* 1996;173:499–502.

99 Lecara G, Cox RA, Simpson RB. *Coccidioides immitis* vaccine: potential of an alkali-soluble, water-soluble cell wall antigen. *Infect Immun* 1983;39:473–475.

100 Zimmer BL, Johnson S, Van Hoosear K, Pappagianis D. Immunization of mice with extracts of *Coccidioides immitis*. In: 91st General Meeting of the Program and Abstracts. Washington, D.C. *Am Soc Microbiol* 1991;F26. Abstract.

101 Zimmermann CR, Johnson SM, Zimmer BL, Pappagianis D. Immunization and protection of mice with a soluble, subcellular vaccine of *Coccidioides immitis*. In: *95th General Meeting of the American Society for Microbiology, Program and Abstracts*. 1995:F14. Abstract.

102 Gradon JD, Timpone JG, Schnittman SM. Emergence of unusual opportunistic pathogens in AIDS: a review. *Clin Infect Dis* 1992;15:134–157.

103 Pappagianis D, Zimmer BL. Serology of coccidioidomycosis. *Clin Microbiol Rev* 1990; 3:247–268.

104 Cox RA, Britt LA. Antigenic heterogeneity of an alkali-soluble, water-soluble cell wall extract of *Coccidioides immitis*. *Infect Immun* 1985;50:365–369.

105 Kruse D, Cole GT. A seroreactive 120-kilodalton β-1,3-glucanase of *Coccidioides immitis* which may participate in spherule morphogenesis. *Infect Immun* 1992;60:4350–4363.

106 Huppert M, Spratt NS, Vukovich KR, et al. Antigenic analysis of coccidioidin and spherulin determined by two-dimensional immunoelectrophoresis. *Infect Immun* 1978; 20:541–551.

107 Cox RA, Dolan MJ, Magee DM, Galgiani JN. Production of a murine monoclonal antibody that recognizes an epitope specific to *Coccidioides immitis* antigen 2. *Infect Immun* 1993;61:1895–1899.

108 Dugger KO, Villareal KM, Ngyuen A, et al. Cloning and sequence analysis of the cDNA for a protein from *Coccidioides immitis* with immunogenic potential. *Biochem Biophys Res Commun* 1996;218:485–489.

109 Zhu WF, Yang CM, Magee DM, Cox RA. Molecular cloning and characterization of *Coccidioides immitis* antigen 2 cDNA. *Infect Immun* 1996;64:2695–2699.

15

Rabies: Lessons from the Past and a Glimpse into the Future

HILARY KOPROWSKI
BERNHARD DIETZSCHOLD

Fear, overwhelming fear, has been the instinctive reaction to rabies of humans throughout 43 centuries. Diseases with dramatic onset were always associated with something supernatural, like punishment of mankind for its sins by God or gods. But rabies is something special: the horror of being attacked by a snarling, mouth-foaming, and vicious snapping dog, and the incredible tortures the patient suffered without any possibility of treatment, unable to drink, but conscious to the inevitable end of life.

The great Austrian playwright Ferdinand Raimund, who wrote *Zauberspiele*, "constructs" of the supernatural with the real, was bitten on the hand by a dog during travel from his village to Vienna on August 25, 1836. A day later he shot himself, without even knowing whether the dog had rabies; he was so overwhelmed by his morbid fear of rabies since childhood that he ended his life (1).

Even the Sanskrit word *rabhas* from which *rabies* originates evokes fear since it means "to do violence" (2). In the 1950s in California, a house painter with rabies bit 20 people in one night during an attack of fury. This is a very rare form of the disease in humans, but because it is known to exist, cases of rabies were confused with vampirism, and more often than could be imagined, people with rabies were killed. This happened in Lyon, France, around the year 900 AD when 6 of about 20 people bitten by a rabid bear developed the "mad" form of the disease and were killed by their fellow citizens (3).

Some important dates in the world history of rabies are summarized in Table 15-1. Three dates stand out as important historical facts. The twenty-third century BC discovery of the Pre-Mosaic Eshmuna Code of Babylon provided the first concrete evidence of the existence of rabies as a disease. In 1584 AD, Girolamo Fracastoro published his "incurable wound" treatise (4). Fracastoro, confirming that humans acquire rabies by bite, established the limits of the incubation period (correct until recent times) and described in detail the clinical symptoms of the disease in humans. He also stated categorically that no one survives the disease. The year 1885 is another milestone in the history of rabies: Pasteur developed the first antirabies vaccine.

Table 15-1. Myths and Facts about the History of Rabies

Date	*Source*	
30th century BC	Dog as emissary of death of accompanying God of Death in India	*Rabbhas* in Sanskrit means "to do violence"
23rd century BC	Pre-Mosaic Eshmuna Code of Babylon	Lethal outcome of rabies in dogs
7th century BC	Iliad	Teucer calls Hector a "rabid dog"
4th century BC	Aristotle—"Natural History of Animals"	Transmission of canine rabies by bite
1st century AD	Celsus	Term *hydrophobia* first used; transmission by saliva
11th century AD	Avicenna	Description of human cases
Early 16th century	Petrus Martyr-Anglerius	Transmission by vampire bats
1584	Fracastoro—"The Incurable Wound"	Lethal outcome of the disease
1804	Zinke	Transmission to rabbits and roosters
1879	Galtier	Serial transmission in rabbits
1885	Pasteur	Development of first rabies vaccine

THE NATURE OF THE BEAST: STRUCTURE, PROTEINS, AND THEIR FUNCTION

Rabies virus is a bullet-shaped particle, 270 nm long and 70 nm in diameter on average, with one rounded and one flat end (4). It is an enveloped virus with the outer surface covered by spikes composed of trimers of the virus glycoprotein (G protein). The ribonucleoprotein (RNP) core exhibits helical symmetry with a diameter of 50 nm.

The rabies (G) protein is the serotype-specific antigen and the only antigen that can induce and react with virus-neutralizing antibodies. Reactivity with anti-G monoclonal antibodies (MAbs) has permitted delineation of five antigen sites on the G protein. A linear determinant is located between residues 258 and 275 of the G protein and a synthetic fragment comprising these amino acids induces formation of rabies-neutralizing antibodies and protection against challenge with virulent rabies virus.

The nucleocapsid (N) protein is the major rabies virus antigen responsible for the induction of virus-specific helper T cells. Comparisons of amino acid sequences revealed great similarity between different N proteins of various fixed strains of rabies. The use of overlapping peptides encompassing the N protein sequence (5) has served to identi-

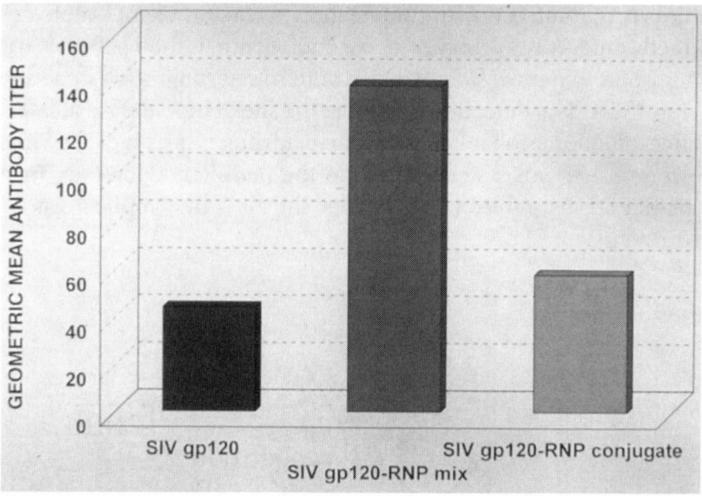

Figure 15-1. Ribonucleoprotein (RNP)-mediated potentiation of antibody response to simian immunodeficiency virus (SIV) gp120.

fy several T-cell epitopes on the N protein. The rabies RNP, which has an adjuvant function, can enhance immunity not only to homotypic antigen but also to other unrelated antigens (6). Figure 15-1 shows the capacity of RNP to potentiate the antibody response against the gp120 antigen of simian immunodeficiency virus (SIV).

The three other proteins of rabies virus, the nominal phosphoprotein (NS), the matrix protein (M), and the L protein, are of lesser immunogenic importance. Although the NS protein induces a strong cytotoxic T-lymphocyte (CTL) response in H-2K mice, the importance of CTLs in the immune defense against rabies is not clear. In contrast to the G and N proteins, there is a high degree of amino acid sequence homology between NS proteins from various strains of rabies. The antigenic structure of the M protein has not been studied, but it may play a role in the interaction with the G and N proteins during virus assembly. The L protein is the largest rabies protein and it functions in synthesis, capping, methylation, and polyadenylation of viral RNA.

RABIES VIRUS ENTRY AND SPREAD IN THE HOST (LIFE CYCLE OF RABIES)

Following inoculation of mouse-adapted neurotropic rabies virus into peripheral tissue (skin or muscle), the virus disappears from the inoculation site within 6 hours and can be detected in neurons of the brain or spinal cord 18 to 24 hours after the time of infection. In animals infected intranasally, virus RNA can be detected in the brain 6 to 12 hours after the time of infection. These findings suggest that (at least) in the mouse-adapted rabies virus, there is no virus replication in the muscle or skin tissue. The virus probably directly enters unmyelinated nerve endings and is then passively carried by fast retrograde transport to neurons of the brain or to spinal ganglia where virus replication can occur (Fig 15-2). The detection of virus at the site of inoculation at later times (e.g., 30 hours) after infection probably reflects the centrifugal spread of the virus from neurons of the central nervous system (CNS) to the periphery. However, in street rabies viruses, in particular, bat rabies virus variants, the virus may replicate at the site of inoculation (e.g., skin).

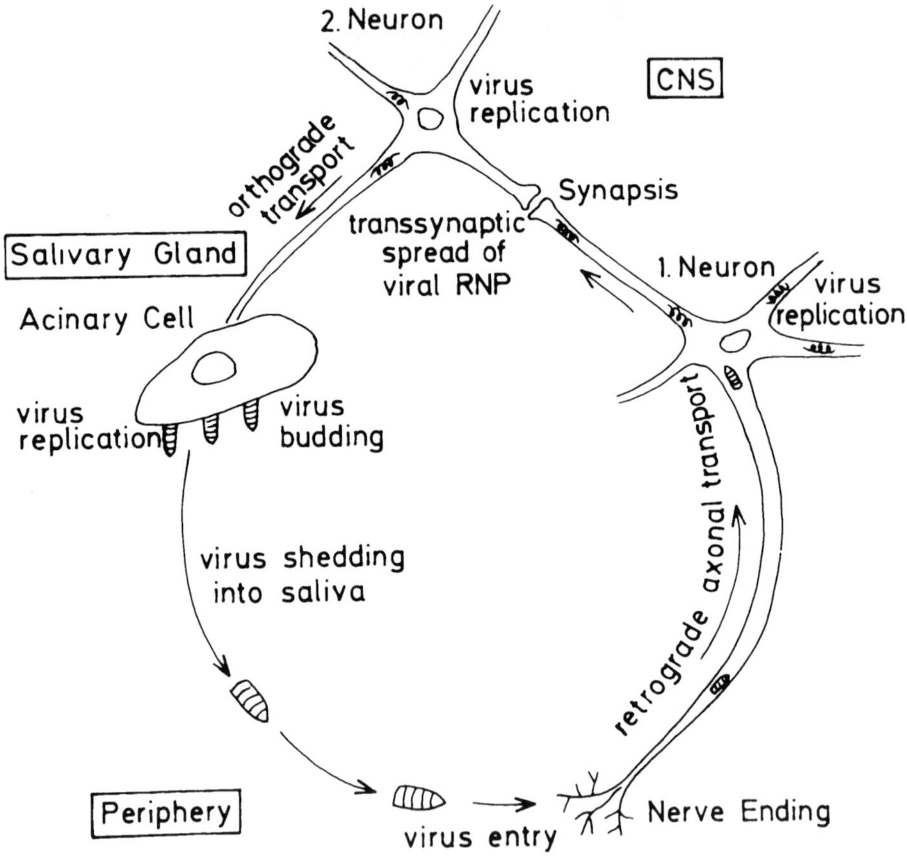

Figure 15-2. Rabies virus infection cycle. The virus, after infection of the nerve endings, enters spinal ganglion neurons through retrograde axonal transport and then moves on to the central nervous system (CNS) as viral ribonucleoprotein (RNP) through transsynaptic spread. After further replication in neurons of the central nervous system, the virus moves to salivary glands and is finally shed in the saliva.

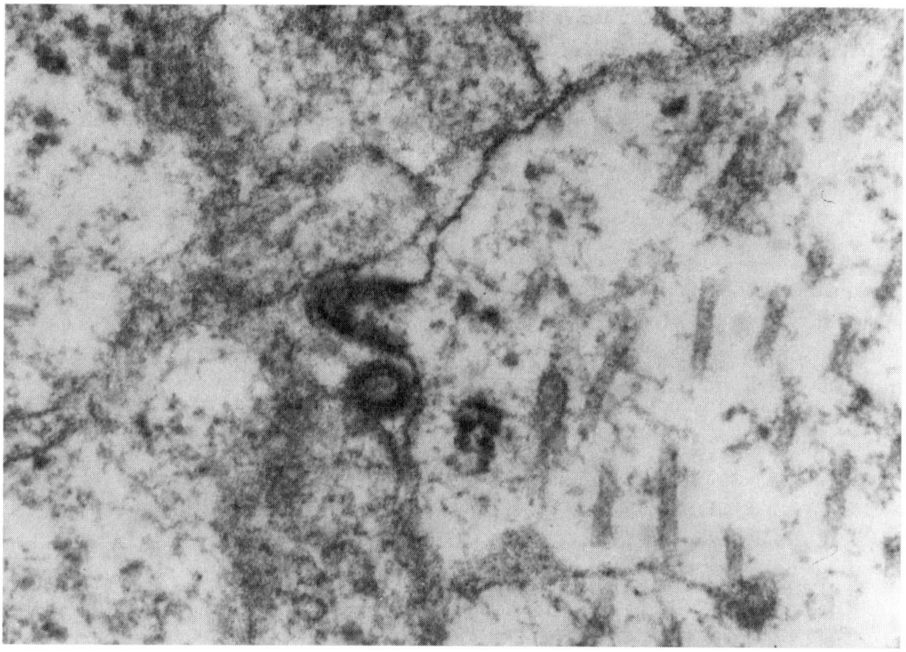

Figure 15-3. Rabies virus particles budding from infected cells in mouse brain.

It is not absolutely clear how rabies virus spreads transsynaptically within the CNS. Electron microscopic studies revealed that rabies RNPs rather than intact virus particles are transported across synapses (7), although studies with G protein variant viruses indicated that the G protein must also be involved in transsynaptic spread (8). In the late stages of infection, virus assembly occurs and budding virus particles can be observed in neurons (Fig 15-3) and acinar cells of the salivary glands.

The life cycle of rabies virus in vivo shows great economy in terms of virus spread in the CNS, as it scrupulously avoids formation of complete virus particles and their budding until the last stages of the disease.

HOW DOES THE VIRUS CAUSE NEUROLOGIC DISEASE AND DEATH?

There are two approaches to answering this question. One is based on the assumption that the symptoms of rabies infection are a direct consequence of virus replication in the CNS. The other approach assumes that the inflammatory response of the host to rabies infection accounts for most of the symptomatology of the disease.

Neuronal Dysfunction as a Direct Consequence of Virus Replication in the CNS

The initial virus infection of the CNS in experimental rodents is followed by a relatively long incubation time (eclipse period) during which no viral RNA can be detected in the CNS by Northern blot analysis (9). The eclipse phase lasts approximately 72 hours and is followed by a rapid exponential increase in viral RNA synthesis between 96 and 120 hours. Although virus RNA levels reach a maximum at 120 hours after the time of infection, rats show the first signs of disease at 144 hours after infection and most of the animals die at 168 hours after infection. At the peak of infection, rabies virus RNA can be detected in all areas of the brain except the dentate gyrus. The appearance of rabies virus messenger RNA (mRNA) is accompanied by increased mRNA expression of host immediate early-response genes such as *egr-1*, and rabies virus mRNA is codistributed

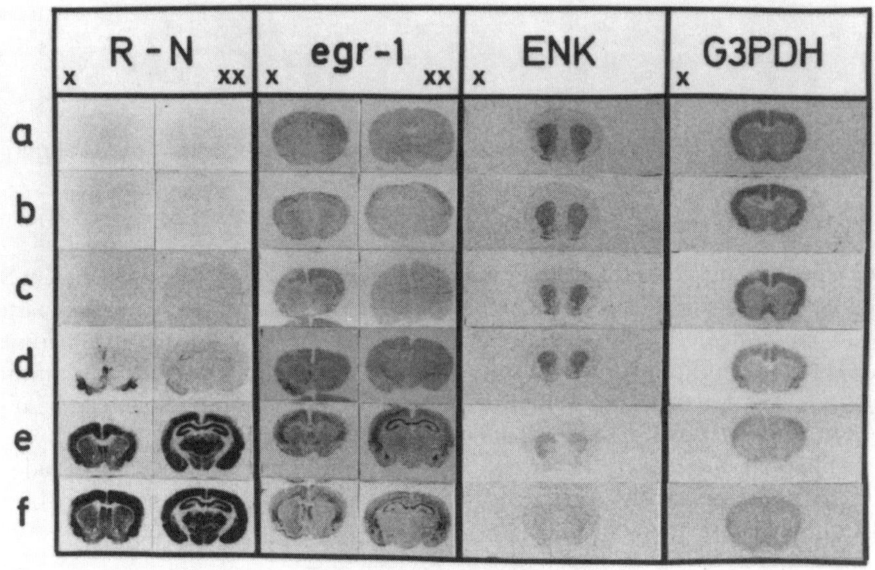

Figure 15-4. Distribution of rabies virus N RNA (R-N), *egr-1* messenger RNA (mRNA), proenkephalin (ENK) mRNA, and glyceraldehyde-3-phosphate dehydrogenase (G3PDH) mRNA in adjacent coronal sections through the caudate putamen (X) and hippocampus (XX) of normal rats (a) and rabies virus–infected rats at 48 (b), 72 (c), 96 (d), 120 (e), and 144 (f) hours after the time of infection. Hybridization was performed on slide-mounted tissue sections. p.i. = postinfection. Source: Fu ZF, Weihe E, Zheng YM, et al. Differential effects of rabies and Borna disease on immediate-early- and late-reponse gene expression in brain tissues. J Virol 1993;67:6674–6681.

with *egr-1* mRNA in the hippocampus and the cortex (Fig 15-4). The correlation between activated *egr-1* mRNA expression and the strong increase in viral RNA raises the possibility that the activation of certain immediate early-response genes that encode transcription factors may actually be a prerequisite for exponential virus replication.

In contrast to the induced expression of immediate early-response genes, the expression of mRNAs transcribed from host late-response genes, such as proenkephalin (ENK) (see Fig 15-4) and neuronal constitutive nitric oxide (NO) synthase (not shown), is significantly decreased by rabies virus infection (9). The expression of the housekeeping gene glyceraldehyde-3-phosphate dehydrogenase (G3PDH) mRNA is also dramatically decreased in rabies virus–infected rat brain (see Fig 15-4). These data suggest that rabies virus replication in neurons may lead to a general inhibition of host gene expression. The decreased expression of important neurotransmitters and neuropeptides, such as ENK and tyrosine hydroxylase, must result in a breakdown of vital neuronal functions in the infected host.

Role of Inflammation in the Pathogenesis of Rabies

Results of studies with rabies virus–infected human brains and brains from experimentally infected animals suggest involvement of inflammatory reactions in the neuropathogenesis of rabies. However, the inflammatory response in the CNS to rabies virus infection depends largely on the route of infection, the host species, and the virus strain. In mice and rats, less neuroinvasive rabies strains often cause more extensive inflammation than do highly neurovirulent strains. In experiments with intranasal infection of fixed virus, inflammatory infiltration in the olfactory bulb and degeneration of mitral neurons are observed. There is evidence that inflammatory cells, mostly monocytes, produce NO in viral and allergic diseases of CNS (10). NO or its product peroxynitrite can cause damage to neurons and astrocytes. Electron paramagnetic resonance methodology to detect NO in the brain of rabies-infected mice (11) revealed peak NO levels on day 6 after infection, when virus production was at a maximum (Fig 15-5). Double staining of neurons (panneuronal marker 9.5) and inducible NO synthase (iNOS) in sections of rabies virus–infected rat brains demonstrated neuronal destruction in the presence of NO (data not shown). However, it is not certain whether inflammation and the production of free radicals associated with inflammatory processes play a decisive role, as in the case of some other CNS infections, in the outcome of a rabies virus infection because it is not clear that immunosuppression has major effects on the clinical course of rabies.

VIRUS CLEARANCE AND PERSISTENCE

Role of Inflammatory Cytokines in Virus Clearance from the CNS

An attenuated rabies virus (12) with arginine in position 333 replaced by glutamine and injected intranasally into rats can be first detected on day 3 after injection and persists in the brain for 10 days, when it spontaneously disappears (Fig 15-6A). By contrast, ra-

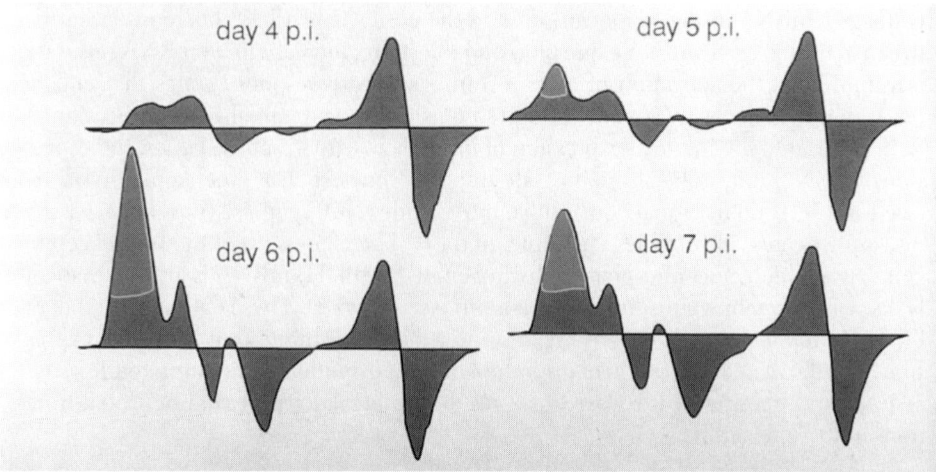

Figure 15-5. Detection of nitric oxide production in the brain during infection with rabies challenge virus standard (CVS) virus using electron paramagnetic resonance spin trapping.

bies virus RNA can be detected in the brain tissue of rats infected with the pathogenic strain from day 4 after injection until the animals die from infection at day 7 (Fig 15-6B). Analysis of cytokine expression in the brain tissue of rats injected with the attenuated virus (see Fig 15-6A) revealed the presence of interferon (IFN)-γ at day 4 after injection, at about the same time rabies mRNA is detected, whereas interleukin (IL)-6 and TNF-α appear at a later stage after infection. In the case of infection with virulent virus (see Fig 15-6B), IFN-γ appears in the brain of rats very late (day 6 after injection) at a time when the animals are sick or dying. Thus, clearance of the virus seems to be associated with the early appearance of IFN-γ, a cytokine that may play a role in suppressing virus replication in brain tissue.

Role of Rabies Virus–Neutralizing Antibody in Virus Clearance from the CNS

Animals infected with either lethal or nonpathogenic rabies virus strains also show remarkable differences in the production of rabies virus–neutralizing antibody. In animals infected with nonpathogenic rabies virus strains, the production of virus–neutralizing antibody is faster and reaches much higher levels than that in animals infected with pathogenic viruses (Table 15-2). The role of antibodies in virus clearance was confirmed by experiments in which rats were treated with a virus neutralizing MAb after infection; reverse transcriptase–polymerase chain reaction analysis revealed that rabies virus had invaded the CNS by 12 hours after infection, but that rabies virus RNA was completely cleared after the animals were treated intramuscularly with a virus-neutralizing MAb

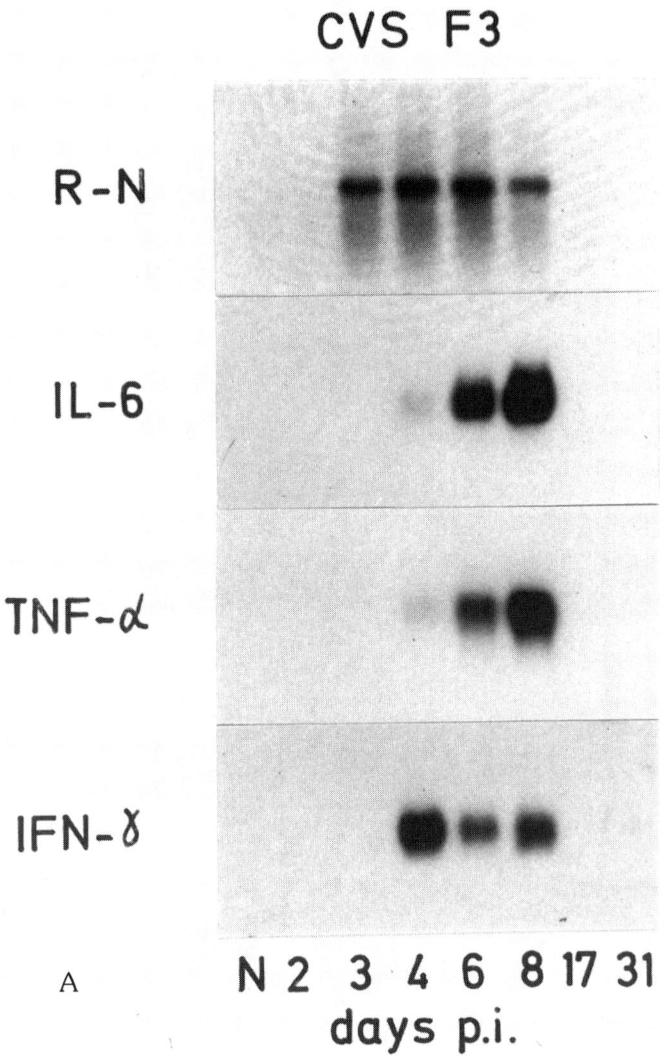

Figure 15-6. Effects of nonpathogenic F3 (A) and pathogenic CVS-11 virus (B) on expression of cytokines. Rats were infected with rabies virus variant CVS-F3 or CVS-11. At indicated times after infection (p.i.), rats were killed and perfused with phosphate-buffered saline solution. Brains were removed and RNA was isolated from the cerebrum. Reverse transcriptase–polymerase chain reaction was performed on these samples using primers specific for rabies virus nucleocapsid (R-N) and for the cytokines interleukin (IL)-6, tumor necrosis factor (TNF)-α, interferon (IFN)-γ, and IFN-α. Amplified complementary DNA was resolved in agarose gels and analyzed by Southern blotting. Source: Fu ZF, Dietzschold B. Recent advances in the study of rabies. In Koprowski HK, Oldstone MBA, eds. Microbe Hunters: Then and Now. Bloomington, IL: Medi-Ed Press 1996:47–55.

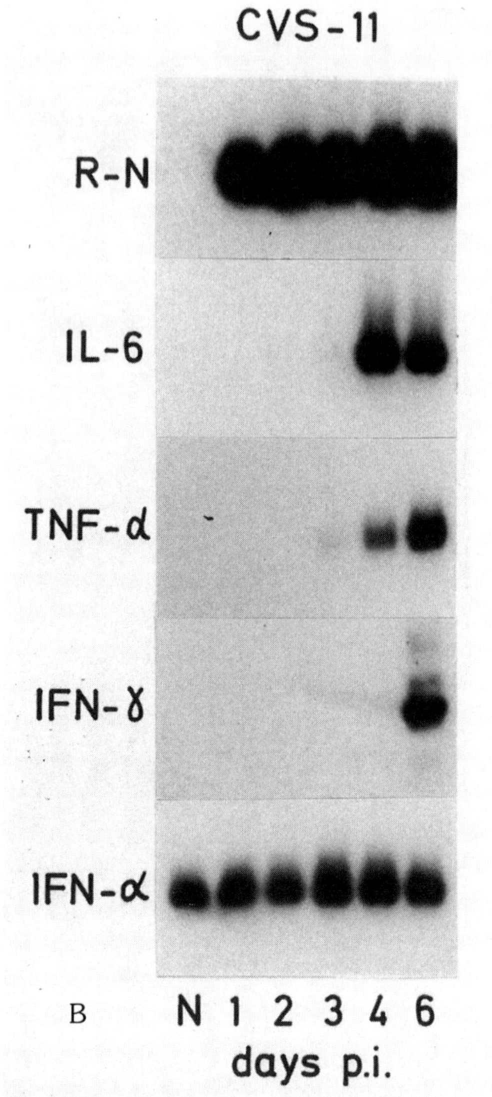

Figure 15-6. *(continued)*

24 hours after infection (13). This experiment clearly demonstrated that virus-neutralizing antibodies are involved in the clearance of rabies virus infection from the CNS.

The protective activity of virus-neutralizing antibody was further demonstrated in postexposure treatment experiments in hamsters. Eighty percent of the hamsters were protected when a cocktail of rabies virus–neutralizing MAbs was administered intra-

Table 15-2. Virus-Neutralizing Antibody (VNA) Titers after Infection of Mice with Pathogenic or Apathogenic Rabies Virus

	VNA Titers	
Days after Infection	*Rabies CVS strain (Pathogenic)*	*Rabies F3 strain (Apathogenic)*
3	90	80
4	80	200
6	200	740
10	—	4860
17	—	10,940
30	—	10,940

muscularly 36 hours after the time of infection with a highly pathogenic rabies virus strain, whereas 100% of the untreated animals died from rabies (14).

Figure 15-7 outlines the putative mechanism involved in the clearance of rabies-infected brain tissue by an antibody. During rabies infection, vasoactive substances such as bradykinin and prostaglandin (15) may be produced in rabies-infected brain

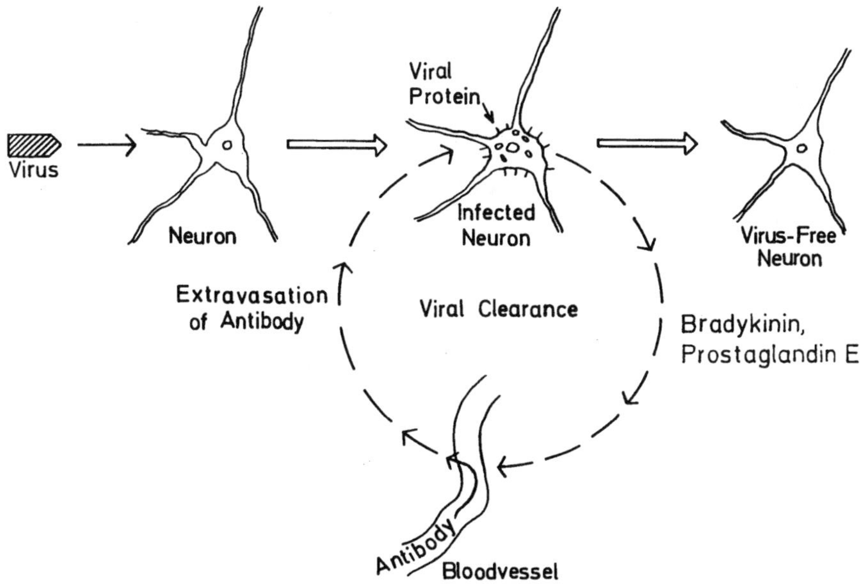

Figure 15-7. Model for clearance of rabies virus from infected neurons with rabies virus–neutralizing antibody. Source: Dietzschold B. Antibody-mediated clearance of viruses from the mammalian central nervous system. Trends in Microbiology 1993;63–66.

tissue, as they are in Borna disease virus infection (16). The permeability of the blood-brain barrier to the rabies antibody permits it to clear the virus infection from the neurons.

Internalization of the antibody into the infected cells has been shown in a tissue culture model (Fig 15-8) wherein rabies-infected neuroblastoma cells were exposed to antibody at 0°C for 1 hour and then for 2 hours at 37°C. The results indicate penetration of antibody into the cells (13).

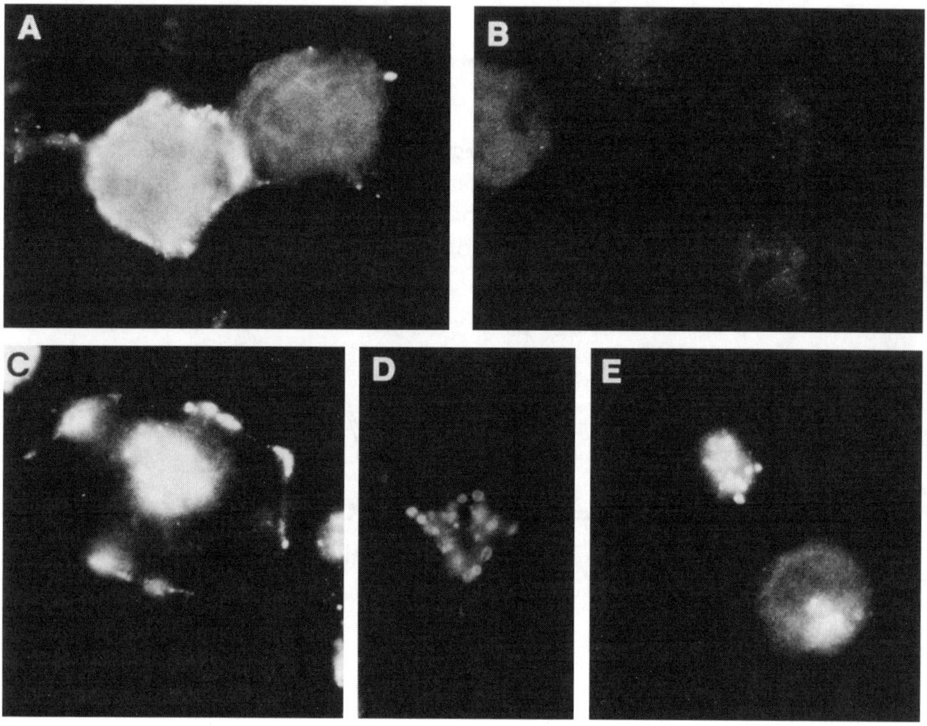

Figure 15-8. Adsorption and internalization of monoclonal antibody (MAb) 1112-1 by rabies virus–infected neuroblastoma (NA) cells. NA cells were infected with CVS-11 virus at a moi of 1. (A, B) Twenty-four hours after infection, cells were treated for 1 hour at 4°C with MAb 1112-1 and then the antibody was washed off with 0.25 M sodium acetate (pH 4) for 2 minutes. (C–E) Cells were incubated with the MAb for 1 hour at 4°C and then for 2 hours at 37°C before the antibody was washed off. Adsorbed or internalized MAb was detected by fluorescent staining techniques. After adsorption at 4°C, antibody can be removed completely (B); after additional incubation at 37°C, antibody is present in the cytoplasm (D, E). Source: Dietzschold b, Kao M, Zheng YM. Delineation of putative mechanisms involved in antibody-mediated clearance of rabies virus from the central nervous system. *Proc Natl Acad Sci USA* 1992;89:7252–7256.

NEW PATTERNS OF RABIES INFECTION (EMERGING INFECTION)

Girolamo Fracastoro in his treatise on incurable wounds (14) established certain tenets of rabies infection that remained valid for centuries. One tenet referred to the transmission of rabies by a bite and the second, that the incubation period of rabies in humans extended up to 4 months. However, the data collected in the last 10 years have called for revision of these tenets.

Between 1986 and 1995, there were 18 human cases of rabies in the United States, but in only 4 was the exposure source known (17). In 1995 and 1996, the two cases of rabies were in children who denied having direct contact with a rabid bat that was found in their bedrooms (i.e., rabies without visible bite wounds).

The second revision of Fracastoro's tenets refers to the incubation period. Recent data (Table 15-3) now indicate that the incubation period may be as long as 6 years (18). Although the three immigrants described by Smith et al. (18) died of rabies in the United States, there was no known source of exposure to the disease in America. Contrariwise, rabies variants with antigenic characteristics identical with the isolates from the immigrants were found in the country or near the country where the immigrant lived prior to coming to the United States. Attempts were made to establish a model in which rabies disease would be fatal in a certain proportion of the animals, whereas the rest would recover. Mice infected intranasally with the attenuated F3 strain of rabies developed clinical disease between days 12 and 16 after the time of infection; 40% died and the rest recovered. Virus mRNA in the brains of these mice increased between days 8 and 11 after infection and then declined but never became completely absent. Virus remained in the brain tissue of these seemingly recovered animals for more than 40 days in the presence of circulating antibody that could neutralize the virus in vitro at a dilution of 1:100,000 (Fig 15-9). Thus, in mild infection of the CNS, the blood-brain barrier might remain intact and impenetrable to the circulating antibody. There is still the problem of explaining the persistence of the rabies virus for 6 years in the human body before it becomes virulent enough to cause the disease. Perhaps only a small number of neurons are infected with the virus and its spread is limited to a rate that will result in the dysfunction of a mass of neurons only many years after infection.

Table 15-3. Prolonged Incubation Period in Humans Exposed to Rabies

Country of Exposure to Rabies	*Incubation Period*
Laos	$>$ 6 years
Philippines	6 years
Mexico	9 months

SOURCE: Data from Smith JS, Fishbein DB, Rupprecht CE, Clark K. Unexplained rabies in three immigrants in the United States. *N Engl J Med* 1991;324:205–211.

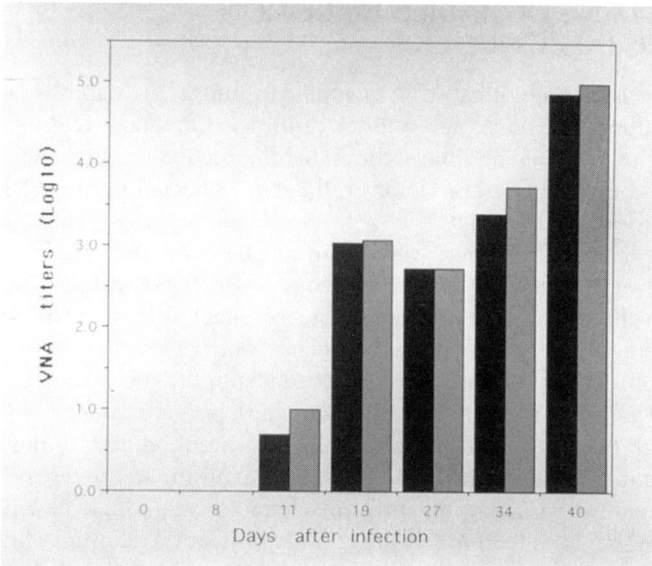

Figure 15-9. Virus-neutralizing antibody titers in C3H mice infected with CVS-F3. Six- to 8-week-old female C3H mice were intranasally infected with either pathogenic CVS-F3. At each time point, two animals were killed, blood was collected, and virus-neutralizing antibody titers were determined. Black bar = mouse 1; gray bar = mouse 2.

Turning to the unusual cases of rabies without known exposure, viruses isolated from the patients were classified as originating from the silver-haired bat (*Lasionycteris noctivagans*). The association of the silver-haired bat with human rabies is rather puzzling because although rabid bats were found in every state in the United States (Fig 15-10), in the survey of the population of bats in New York State, only 0.4% were silver-haired bats (19). Since all bat isolates in the United States belong to genotype 1 rabies virus common to many terrestrial animals and dogs, more subtle characteristics of the silver-haired bat isolates might explain its unusual role in causing rabies in humans.

For comparative purposes, the viruses isolated from humans who died in the presence of either the silver-haired bats (SHBRV) without being bitten were studied together with a virus of coyote origin (COSRV), representing the canine strains of the United States (20). As shown in Figure 15-11, the COSRV was much more pathogenic than the SHBRV in intramuscularly injected mice. When mice were injected intradermally, the SHBRV was slightly more pathogenic than the COSRV.

More striking differences between the two viruses relate to their temperature sensitivity. Whereas the two viruses grow to approximately the same titers in neuroblastoma cultures (Fig 15-12), the yield of SHBRV in nonneuronal cultures of BHK-21 fibro-

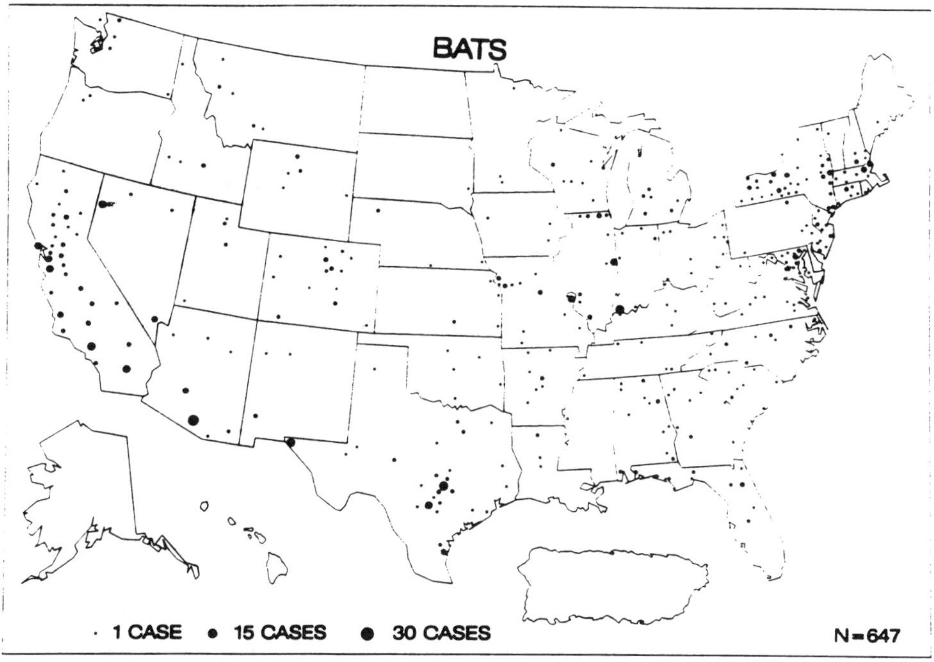

Figure 15-10. Reported cases of rabies in bats by county, 1992. Dot size is proportional to the number of cases in the county. Source: Krebe JW, Strine TW, Smith JS, et al. Rabies surveillance in the United States during 1994. JAVMA 1995; 207:1562–1575.

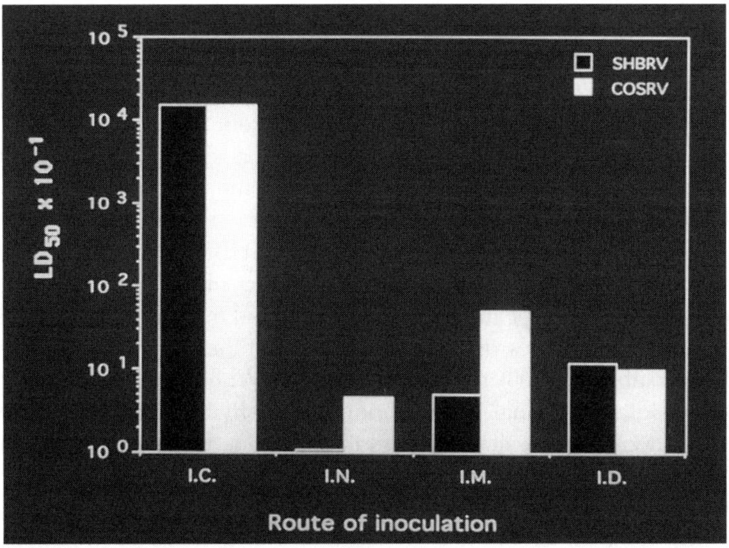

Figure 15-11. Pathogenicity of silver-haired bat rabies virus (SHBRV) and coyote strain of rabies virus (COSRV) in mice. I.C. = intracranially; I.N. = intranasally; I.M. = intramuscularly; I.D. = intradermally.

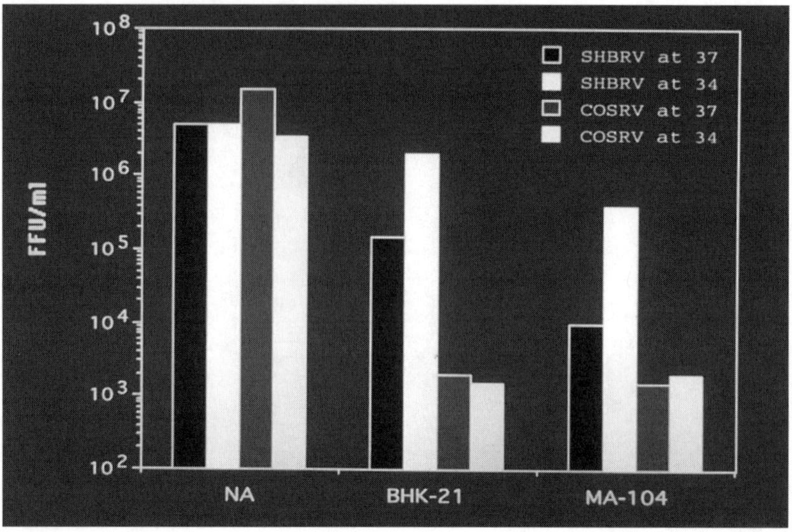

Figure 15-12. Virus titers of silver-haired bat rabies virus (SHBRV) and coyote strain of rabies virus (COSRV) stocks in neuroblastoma (NA) cells, BHK-21 fibroblasts, and MA-104 epithelial cells. FFU = fluorescent focus forming units.

blasts and MA 104 epithelial cells is much higher than that of COSRV, particularly when the cultures are kept at 34°C. Fusiogenic activity of SHBRV in nonneuronal cultures at 34°C is much higher than that of COSRV. Amino acid sequences of the glycoprotein (Fig 15-13) of SHBRV are considerably different from the COSRV sequences, particularly in the toxic loop region, which is the area responsible for the attachment of the virus to the putative receptor on the cell membrane. Similar results were obtained with the human isolates of Mexican Freetail bat virus.

Table 15-4 summarizes the results of the study of SHBRV and COSRV. SHBRV belongs to the same serotype as all other isolates of rabies in the United States. However, it shows a different phenotype than the coyote virus and may have a selective advantage over the classic canine rabies virus strains by virtue of the capacity to replicate in nonneuronal cells subject to lower body temperature. Whether these phenotypic differences account for the unusual phenomenon linking the presence of the silver-haired bat with the fate of a rabies victim is hard to determine without engaging in the wild speculation of human infection by "microscopic" bat bites, with the virus replicating at some lower temperature ments of the skin cellular elements such as Langerhans cells. It is absolutely essential to continue investigations of viruses isolated from a variety of bats and of their human victims. Such studies and in-depth investigations of the long incubation period are necessary in light of the potential menace of the virus because of its changing character.

```
          |-signal  peptide-|
SHBRV  -19:MIPQALQFVPLLIPSLCFGKFPIYTIPDKLGPWSPIDIHHLSCP
COSRV  -19:.V...L...I.VF........H.......................

SHBRV   26:NNLVAEDEGCTSLSGFSYMELKVGYISAIKVNGFTCTGVVTEAET
COSRV   26:....V......N.................E.A.............

SHBRV   71:YTNFVGYVTTTFKRKHFRPMPDACRAAHDWKMAGDPRYEDSLQNP
COSRV   71:...S.....A..R......T.....S.YN..........E..H..

SHBRV  116:YPDYHWLRTVKTTKESLVIISPSVADLDPYDKSLHSRVFPSGKCL
COSRV  116:.A.......R...A..........................I...S

                                ___________________________
SHBRV  161:GITVSSTYCSTNHDYTIWMPVEARLGTSCDIFTNSKGKKASKGGR
COSRV  161:....................ENP....W....V..R..R....SK

           __
SHBRV  206:TWGFVDERGLYKSLKGACKLKLCGVPGLRLMDGTWVSIQTSDDIK
COSRV  206:IC.......................L..........AM...EET.

SHBRV  251:WCPPDQLVNLHDFHSDEIEHLVVEELIKKREGCLDALESIMTTKS
COSRV  251:.............R............V...E..............

                                                  *
SHBRV  296:VSFRRLSHLRKLVPGFGKAYTIFNNTLMEADAHYKSVRTWNEVIP
COSRV  296:........................K.S...............I..

SHBRV  341:SKGCLKVGGRCHPPVNGVFFNGIILGPDGNVLIPEMQSSLLQQHM
COSRV  341:.....R.......H..............DH...............

SHBRV  386:ELLESSVIPLTHPLADPSTVFKDGDEAEDFVEVHLPDVHKQVSEI
COSRV  386:..........M...G.......E......................GV

                       |transmembrane domain|-------------
SHBRV  431:DLGLPSWGKYLLMSAGVLATLILAIFLITCCRRANRTESTQRGRR
COSRV  431:.....N....V.......IS.M.L...M.....V..P.....SPG

          cytoplasmic  domain----------|
SHBRV  476:ESGGKVSVAPQNGKIISSWELYKSGSETGL
COSRV  476:GA.R....TS.S..V.....S....G..R.
```

Figure 15-13. Amino acid sequences of rabies virus G proteins of silver-haired bat rabies virus (SHBRV) and coyote strain of rabies virus (COSRV). Total RNA was isolated from virus-infected suckling mouse brains and subjected to polymerase chain reaction cloning and sequencing. Dots indicate conserved sequences between the two viruses. Underlined are the putative glycosylation signals at positions 37 and 319. The line above positions 181 to 207 represent a highly variable region. The asterisk denotes the arginine residue at position 333. Source: Morimoto K, Patel M, Corisdeo S, et al. Characterization of a unique variant of bat rabies responsible for newly emerging human cases in North America. *Proc. Natl Acad Sci USA* 1996; 93:5653–5658.

Table 15-4. Summary

Silver-haired bat rabies virus (SHBRV) has unique properties compared to the coyote strain of rabies virus (COSRV), a representative of the classic canine rabies strains:

1 SHBRV infects and replicates more efficiently than COSRV in nonneuronal cells.

2 Infectivity and fusiogenic activity of SHBRV in nonneuronal cells are superior at a lower temperature (34°C versus 37°C).

3 The amino acid sequence of the G protein of SHBRV differs considerably from that of COSRV, particularly in the toxic loop region, which is considered to be important for virus attachment.

ENVOI

Rabies disease has been known for 43 centuries and the virus has been studied extensively for more than a hundred years. Although once considered unique in its homogeneity as representing one genotype and one phenotype, research in the past few decades has changed our views about rabies. Rabies is still represented by one serotype that consists of many variants. Characterization of the phenotypes of these variants has permitted determination of their prevalence in a given species in a given locality. Other surprises included the discovery of nine species belonging to the *Lyssavirus* genus (Table 15-5), which except for Duvenhage and European bat type 2 do not appear to be human pathogens. However, as our knowledge of rabies increases, so too does our ignorance. Until now, it was not clear whether the inflammatory response (if present) plays any role in rabies pathogenicity for the CNS. We know that such a response causes dysfunction of the neurons, but it remains unknown whether this can account for the unfortunately lethal outcome of the disease. Finally, although analyses of the variants involved in rabies deaths without apparent exposure have begun, much remains to be determined before all facts are assembled and properly interpreted. The task ahead will be difficult but undoubtedly rewarding.

Table 15-5. Lyssaviruses

Rabies Serogroup	
Rabies (RAB)	Lagos bat (LB)
Mokola (MOK)	Kotonkan (KOT)
Duvenhage (DUV)	Obodhiang (OBD)
European bat type 1 (EB-1)	Rochambeau (RBU)
European bat type 2 (EB-2)	

REFERENCES

1 Kaplan MM, Koprowski H. Rabies. *Sci Am* 1980;242:120–134.

2 Koprowski H. Visit to an ancient curse. *Sci Am Sci Med* 1995;2:48–57.

3 Steel JH, Fernandez PJ. History of rabies and global aspects. In: Baer GM, ed. *The natural history of rabies*. Boca Raton, FL: CRC Press, 1991:3–24.

4 Fracastoro H. *Veronensis Opera Omnia*, Venetiis, MDLXXXIIII (1584).

5 Dietzschold B, Rupprecht CE, Fu ZF, Koprowski H. Rhabdoviruses. In: Fields BN, Knipe DM, Howley PM, et al, eds. *Fields virology*. 3rd ed. Philadelphia: Lippincott-Raven, 1996:1137–1159.

6 Hooper DC, Pierard I, Modelska A, et al. Rabies ribonucleocapsid as an oral immunogen and immunological enhancer. *Proc Natl Acad Sci USA* 1994;91:10908–10912.

7 Gosztonyi G, Dietzschold B, Kao M, et al. Rabies and Borna disease. A comparative pathogenetic study of two neurovirulent agents. *Lab Invest* 1993;68:285–295.

8 Dietzschold B, Wiktor TJ, Trojanowski JQ, et al. Differences in cell-to-cell spread of pathogenic and apathogenic rabies virus in vivo and in vitro. *J Virol* 1985;56:12–18.

9 Fu ZF, Weihe E, Zheng YM, et al. Differential effects of rabies and Borna disease viruses on immediate-, early- and late-response gene expression in brain tissues. *Virology* 1993; 67: 6674–6681.

10 Koprowski H, Zheng YM, Heber-Katz E, et al. *In vivo* expression of inducible nitric oxide synthase in experimentally induced neurological diseases. *Proc Natl Acad Sci USA* 1993; 90:3024–3027.

11 Hooper DC, Ohnishi ST, Kean R, et al. Local nitric oxide production in viral and autoimmune diseases of the central nervous system. *Proc Natl Acad Sci USA* 1995;92:5312–5316.

12 Dietzschold B, Wunner WH, Wiktor TJ, et al. Characterization of an antigenic determinant of the glycoprotein that correlates with pathogenicity of rabies virus. *Proc Natl Acad Sci USA* 1983;80:70–74.

13 Dietzschold B, Kao M, Zheng YM, et al. Delineation of putative mechanisms involved in antibody-mediated clearance of rabies virus from the central nervous system. *Proc Natl Acad Sci USA* 1992;89:7252–7256.

14 Schumacher CL, Dietzschold B, Ertl HCJ, et al. Use of mouse anti-rabies monoclonal antibodies in postexposure treatment of rabies. *J Clin Invest* 1989;84:971–975.

15 Williams TJ, Peck MJ. Role of prostaglandin mediated vasodilation in inflammation. *Nature* 1977;270:215–217.

16 Morimoto K, Hooper DC, Bornhorst A, et al. Intrinsic responses in Borna disease virus (BDV) infection of CNS. *Proc Natl Acad Sci USA* 1996 (in press).

17 Rupprecht CE, Smith JS, Fekadu M, Child JE. The ascension of wildlife rabies: a cause for public health concern or intervention. *Emerging Infect Dis* 1995;1.

18 Smith JS, Fishbein DB, Rupprecht CE, Clark, K. Unexplained rabies in three immigrants in the United States. *N Engl J Med* 1991; 324:205–211.

19 Warrell M. Human deaths from cryptic bat rabies in the USA. *Lancet* 1995;346:65–66.

20 Morimoto K, Patel M, Corisdeo S, et al. Characterization of a unique variant of bat rabies virus responsible for newly emerging human cases in North America. *Proc Natl Acad Sci USA* 1996;93:5653–5658.

16 Herpes Simplex Infections of the Central Nervous System

RICHARD J. WHITLEY
ANN ARVIN

Herpes simplex virus (HSV) infections of the central nervous system (CNS) are associated with significant morbidity and mortality, even when appropriate antiviral therapy is provided. Infection of the brain by HSV can occur from birth throughout life. Life-threatening HSV infections of the brain are subdivided into those attributable to neonatal HSV infection and those occurring beyond the age of 3 months, which are generally identified as herpes simplex encephalitis (HSE). Both forms of HSV infections of the CNS are associated with significant neurologic sequelae, irrespective of virus type (HSV-1 versus HSV-2) and, surprisingly, the time of introduction of antiviral therapy. The pathogenesis, etiologic viral type, diagnostic dilemmas, and outcome with therapy vary for each of these two entities. Of note, benign HSV infections of the CNS have been reported and present as either aseptic meningitis or Mollaret's syndrome.

Neonatal HSV infection occurs in 1 of 3500 to 5000 deliveries in the United States. Infection can be subdivided into three disease classifications: 1) skin, eye, and mouth; 2) encephalitis; and 3) disseminated disease. For babies with skin, eye, and mouth disease, accounting for approximately 45% of all babies with neonatal herpes, the CNS is not apparently involved as predicated on clinical, neurodiagnostic, and laboratory evaluation. However, as many as 10% have neurologic impairment at long-term follow-up, implying subclinical infection of the CNS and then insidious reactivation later in life. Babies with encephalitis account for 35% of cases of neonatal herpes, whereas the remaining 20% of babies have disseminated disease and three of four of them will have CNS involvement. Thus, of all babies with neonatal HSV infection, approximately 50% will have CNS disease. Likely, the pathogenesis of CNS disease differs for those babies with encephalitis versus those with disseminated disease. The diagnosis of HSV disease in the newborn is straightforward if skin vesicles are present; however, in many infants these pathognomonic lesions are absent. Neonatal herpes and the associated problems of diagnosis and perinatal transmission have been discussed at length elsewhere (1–4). The estimated costs for the direct and indirect management of babies with neonatal HSV infection is $500 million per year (5).

In children over the age of 3 months and adults, HSE remains the most common cause of sporadic fatal encephalitis in the Western world (6–9). This disease was definitively recognized in 1941 as the cause of rapidly progressive encephalitis (10). While the literature is replete with case reports that describe HSE, the method of unequivocal diagnosis has remained controversial until recent years (6,11–14). Currently, HSE is estimated to occur in 1 in 250,000 to 500,000 individuals per year. The projected costs (direct and indirect) for the management of all patients with presumed HSE in the United States are estimated to be $500 million (15).

The National Institute of Allergy and Infectious Diseases (NIAID) Collaborative Antiviral Study Group (CASG) has defined the clinical presentation, diagnosis, and outcome of patients with HSV infections of the CNS. Over the past 20 years, clarification of these issues was possible because of uniform diagnostic approaches, namely, isolation of HSV from clinical specimens obtained from newborns or brain tissue at biopsy, a procedure not routinely employed in other studies. Through these trials, clinical presentation, sites of viral excretion, role of diagnostic brain biopsy, effectiveness of treatment, and prognostic factors were identified. Furthermore, diseases that mimic HSE were recognized and reported (16). These data provide the basis for much of the discussion below.

PATHOGENESIS OF HUMAN DISEASE AND OUTCOME

Neonatal HSV infection is usually acquired either in utero (intrauterine infection—5% of cases) or as a consequence of intrapartum contact of the fetus with infected maternal secretions (85% of cases). The remaining cases occur following postpartum exposure to HSV during the first 4 weeks of life. As noted above, three forms of infection have been defined. In the United States, most cases of genital herpes are caused by HSV-2; however, in Japan, most cases of genital herpes are caused by HSV-1. The differences in virus type influence the outcome, particularly of the CNS, as will be discussed.

Because the mother is the usual source of infection of the newborn, a few comments are in order. The risk of neonatal HSV infection is significantly higher following the mother's first episode of genital infection (30%–50%) as compared to recurrent genital infection (< 5%) (17,18). Thus, virus load associated with first-episode infection, transplacental immune globulin, or localized immune responses may well confer a degree of protection for the newborn. It should be recognized that discordance in infection status between sex partners is a risk factor for transmission of infection between individuals. If the male sex partner has HSV-2 infection, there is 5% risk of transmission to the baby's mother during gestation (19). Thus, careful counseling of sexually active adults wishing to conceive is essential. Routine condom use and consideration of paternal suppressive acyclovir may be warranted to decrease the risk of transmission.

In relation to the time of presentation of encephalitis during the neonatal period of life, babies with CNS infection present with disease on average at the age of 2 weeks. In contrast, newborns with disseminated disease with brain involvement present with encephalitis at the age of 7 to 9 days or earlier. The difference in age at presentation suggests a variation in the pathogenesis of these two forms of neonatal HSV disease. For babies with encephalitis alone, HSV accession to the CNS is thought to be by intraneuronal routes. The majority—60%—of these babies do not develop skin lesions. At the outset, brain disease is often localized to one or both temporal lobes, but can progress to involve all regions of the brain. In contrast, disseminated disease is usually associated with viremia and, as a consequence, multiorgan involvement. Thus, CNS infection in this subgroup of babies is usually diffuse, implying blood-borne spread of virus to the brain.

As noted already, babies with disease localized to the skin, eye, or mouth are at risk for CNS impairment. While such findings appear to contradict initial disease classification, only recently has insight into this perplexing observation been provided. Specifically, the application of polymerase chain reaction (PCR) to the cerebrospinal fluid (CSF) from these babies revealed the presence of HSV DNA, implying subtle involvement of the CNS (20).

In the absence of therapy, the mortality following encephalitis or disseminated disease in the newborn is 50% and 90%, respectively. The majority of survivors, namely more than 50% of each subgroup, have significant neurologic impairment in spite of antiviral therapy.

The pathogenesis of HSE in older children and adults remains poorly understood. Virtually in all patients, HSE is caused by HSV-1, although there are a few patients with proven HSV-2 infection of the brain parenchyma (21). In contrast, HSV-2 infection is a common cause of aseptic meningitis following first-episode genital disease, particularly in women (22). While HSV-2 is a known cause of severe encephalitis in the newborn, similar disease in older children and adults has not been documented.

Both primary and recurrent HSV infections can result in HSE. Approximately one-third of cases are the consequence of primary infection whereas the remaining ones are the result of reactivation of HSV (23). Whether reactivation of HSV occurs directly in the brain or is the consequence of intraneuronal spread of virus from peripheral sites to the CNS remains debated (24); however, HSV DNA has been detected in the brain tissue, and at multiple sites (not just the temporal lobe) of individuals dying from other causes, suggesting that direct reactivation is a possibility (25).

The route of access of virus to the CNS in humans with *primary* infection is the subject of discussion. Studies have defined pathways of HSV access to the brain in animals, including both olfactory and trigeminal tracts, among others (26). Animal model data indicate that the olfactory tract can provide one neurologic avenue for virus to reach the CNS, with subsequent localization of infection to the orbitofrontal region of the brain (27,28). Olfactory bulb and nerve involvement in human disease associated with primary infection has been documented in a few patients (29–32).

Recurrent infection leading to HSE is similarly confusing pathogenetically. Latent virus can be demonstrated within the brain tissue of animals (33); however, the occurrence of reactivation in human brains is hypothetical, in spite of the PCR data noted previously (25). It has been suggested that reactivation of virus occurs peripherally, namely, in the olfactory bulb or the trigeminal ganglia, resulting in subsequent neuronal transmission (24,25,28,34). These questions remain the subject for future investigation, particularly in relevant animal models.

Ten percent to 20% of patients with HSE shed HSV from a peripheral site, such as the oropharynx or nasopharynx (23). In one study using brain biopsy as a method of diagnosis, CNS and peripheral isolates were compared by restriction enzyme analyses.

Following primary infection, both the brain and peripheral isolates appeared identical when evaluated by restriction enzyme cleavage with multiple enzymes. However, with recurrent infection, in one-third of subjects, the virus isolated from the peripheral site was different from that found in the CNS (13). Thus, the issues of reactivation of virus within the CNS, the potential for enhanced neurotropism of certain viruses, and the selective reactivation and access of HSV by the trigeminal route or other routes to the CNS require further investigation.

The severity of HSE in older children and adults is illustrated by early studies with ineffective antiviral drugs or placebo-controlled trials. In the absence of therapy or following the administration of an ineffective therapeutic agent (idoxuridine or cytosine arabinoside), mortality was in excess of 70% and only approximately 2.5% of patients overall (11% of survivors) returned to normal function (35–39). Brain biopsy and the isolation of HSV from brain tissue comprised the diagnostic method employed in our historical studies; however, now a far broader spectrum of disease is becoming clear as PCR is used to evaluate CSF specimens obtained from patients with altered mentation. It is clear that HSV meningitis, oftentimes caused by HSV-2, is usually a benign infection of the meninges, in contrast to HSE, which involves active viral replication in the brain cortex.

MOLECULAR PATHOGENESIS

For some time, several investigators (40–43) suggested a molecular basis for the neurovirulence of HSV. Laboratory investigations utilized many different strains of HSV to assess both phenotypic and genotypic characteristics of neurovirulence. The biologic relevance of strains that have been passed several times in vitro to human disease is questionable.The results of recent studies of gene function have been illuminating. As summarized in Table 16-1, several genes, when deleted, reduce neurovirulence. One gene appears to significantly influence neurovirulence in animal model systems. This diploid gene maps to the inverted repeats of the unique long segment of HSV DNA and has been identified as the $\gamma_1 34.5$ gene. When both copies of this gene are deleted in toto

Table 16-1. Deletions with Decreased Neurovirulence

$U_S 1$	Regulatory protein
(ICP22)	—
$U_S 2$	Protein kinase
$U_S 3$	? Protein kinase
$U_L 13$	—
$U_L 16$	—
$U_L 24$	—
Glycoproteins: gE, gG, gl, gJ	—
Ribonucleotide reductase	—
Thymidine kinase	—
$\gamma_1 34.5$ (ICP34.5)	Blocks apoptosis
$U_L 55\text{-}56$	—

Table 16-2. Deletions with No Effect on Neurovirulence

Glycoproteins: gC cells	Attachment to polarized cells
U_S9	—
U_S10	—
U_S11	—
U_S12 (α 47)	Blocks class I MHC presentation

or a stop codon is inserted into the carboxyl terminus of the gene, neurovirulence is completely abated (44). Specifically, when these genetically engineered viruses are inoculated intracerebrally into BALB/c mice, the PFU/LD_{50} ratio is higher than 10^6 whereas wild-type virus and the restored constructs have similar ratios of 10^3. The $\gamma_1 34.5$ gene product precludes a host cell host stress response, which would normally result in cell death. This effect is mediated by eIF-2 and protein kinase (45). The implications of these observations are significant. Because the genetically engineered HSVs are incapable of producing progeny virus on inoculation into the CNS, their potential application to the treatment of brain tumors as well as for vaccine development becomes apparent (46–49). Differential expression of the $\gamma_1 34.5$ gene in wild-type isolates from a variety of clinical illnesses has not yet been assessed. Notably, deletion of other genes, as noted in Table 16-2, do not appear to influence neurovirulence.

PATHOLOGY

The histopathologic changes represent a combination of virally mediated cellular death and associated inflammatory response. Changes induced by viral infection include ballooning of infected cells and the appearance of condensed chromatin within the nuclei of cells, followed by subsequent degeneration of the cellular nuclei, generally within parabasal and intermediate cells of the epithelium. Cells lose intact plasma membranes and form multinucleated giant cells.

Vascular changes in the area of infection include perivascular cuffing and areas of hemorrhagic necrosis. Widespread areas of hemorrhagic necrosis, mirroring the area of infection, become most prominent. When the brain is involved, oligodendrocytic involvement and gliosis are common, as is astrocytosis, but these changes develop very late in the disease course. Local lymphatics can show evidence of infection with intrusion of inflammatory cells, which allows for the draining of infected secretions from the area of viral replication. The intensity of the inflammatory response is significantly less with recurrent disease. As host defenses develop, an influx of mononuclear cells can be detected in infected tissue.

HOST IMMUNE RESPONSE

The cell-mediated immune response is considered critical in the control of infections caused by HSV types 1 and 2. Clinical evidence for this important role in host defense is suggested by the severe disease caused by HSV infection in persons whose cellular immune function is compromised (50–52). T-lymphocyte proliferation to HSV antigens in vitro has been studied extensively as a measure of cell-mediated immunity to the virus in persons with oral and genital HSV infections. Changes in T-cell recognition of HSV antigens, quantitated by the magnitude of the stimulation index (SI), correlate with the temporal course of recurrences, duration of virus excretion, and severity and duration of symptoms (53–62).

A recent study measured T-cell recognition of common and type-specific HSV glycoproteins in 72 subjects. T cells were stimulated with whole HSV-2 antigen and glycoproteins gB2, gD2, and gG2. T-cell proliferation in response to HSV-2 antigen and gG2 was significantly higher in subjects with HSV-2 infection than in those with HSV-1 infection only: Responses to gB2 and gD2 were the same. Helper T-cell (Th) type 1 and Th2 cytokine production in response to whole HSV-2 antigen, gB2, and gD2 was evaluated in 33 subjects. Interleukin (IL)-2 and interferon-γ responses to most antigens were significantly higher among HSV-2–seropositive subjects than seronegative subjects. IL-4 synthesis was negligible: IL-10 was produced in seronegative and seropositive persons, but HSV-2 antigen responses were significantly higher in HSV-2–seropositive persons. Naturally acquired immunity to HSV involves T-cell recognition of common and type-specific glycoproteins, prominent Th1 responses, and discordant Th2 responses with little IL-4 and substantial IL-10 production.

Antibody responses in HSE correlate with disease severity. Cytotoxic T-lymphocyte responses are depressed in HSE, at least in adults, but the contribution of cell-mediated immune responses to the disease pathogenesis is unknown.

Humoral immune responses in the newborn are not totally protective against neonatal HSV encephalitis (63,64). The presence of antibody at the onset of the disease appears to restrict disease to the skin or CNS (18). Neonates with encephalitis demonstrate delayed T-cell proliferation as compared to older children with disease (52). Disease progression may be more extensive in neonates with severely impaired T-cell responses. Levels of interferon-α and -γ are depressed in neonates with encephalitis, whereas tumor necrosis factor (TNF)-α levels are unchanged (52,65).

The detection of antibodies in the CSF of older children and adults has been used for diagnostic purposes (seroconversion in the CSF). However, humoral immune responses do not occur promptly enough to assist in making decisions on the institution of antiviral therapy (23).

Diagnosis

To properly evaluate any therapeutic agent, the correct diagnosis is essential. Most published studies of HSE in older children and adults indicated that the clinical presentation is one of a focal encephalopathic process associated with altered levels of consciousness, fever, focal seizures, and hemiparesis (approximately one-third of patients) (21). While the clinical presentation of patients allows some physicians to treat empirically, these symptoms can hardly be considered pathognomonic for HSE (8,14,21,66). Furthermore, the recognition of unusual neurologic findings (namely, a subacute or chronic encephalitis) in patients with HSE who also have acquired immunodeficiency syndrome (AIDS) emphasizes diagnostic dilemmas in unique patient populations (67). In the newborn, diagnosis can be difficult. Many newborns, as many as 60%, with encephalitis may not have evidence of skin vesicles, the hallmark of neonatal HSV infection. Furthermore, disease presents at a time when other infections of the CNS, including group B streptococcal meningitis, are common. Because of the lack of a pathognomonic clinical presentation and a growing reluctance to perform brain biopsies, efforts to develop alternative diagnostic procedures have progressed. These diagnostic procedures can be divided into 1) neurodiagnostic studies and 2) evaluation of biologic specimens.

Neurodiagnostic studies performed on patients with presumed HSE include electroencephalography (EEG) (spike and slow wave activity localized to the temporal region of the brain) (68–72), computed tomography (CT) (radiolucent lesion, edema, or hemorrhage) (73–76), technetium brain scanning (localized uptake) (77), or more recently, magnetic resonance imaging (MRI). Each of these procedures has varying sensitivity and specificity for diagnosis but none, including MRI, have sufficiently high values to be uniformly useful (78). Parenthetically, CT evidence of a focal lesion at the time of onset of therapy for proven HSE is indicative of severe morbidity in the long term (79). Thus, if neurodiagnostic tests are to be of utility, localization by EEG prior to the development of CT or MRI evidence of a lesion would have to establish the etiology of disease; however, the specificity would likely remain unacceptable. The utility of MRI for the diagnosis of HSE appears the most sensitive of the neurodiagnostic studies; however, it has not been compared to PCR confirmation of disease (80,81).

Because of the lack of uniform predictability of these diagnostic tests, research efforts have focused on the assessment of serum and CSF specimens (23,82–86). For some of the studies performed by our group, the gold standard has been the isolation of HSV from the brain tissue. Without properly classified specimens, the definition of sensitivity and specificity of noninvasive diagnostic assays can be misleading. This is especially the case for HSE, because in patients with altered mentation and fever, reactivation of labial HSV can lead to a significant increase in the quantity of both CSF and serum antibodies (23). With increasing CSF HSV antibody titers or serum-CSF antibody ratios (≤ 20), a diagnosis can be established retrospectively, but in only 80% of patients (23,83–85,87–92). Antibodies may appear in the CSF as the consequence of a breakdown in the blood-brain barrier; therefore, appropriate controls for leakage of serum antibodies must be employed, a requirement that has been absent in many of the reported trials. The aforementioned approaches have a sensitivity and specificity that vary between 75% and 85%, and 60% and 90%, respectively (23).

Recently, immunoblot analysis and enzyme-linked immunosorbent assay (ELISA) have been used to test CSF for evidence of HSV (86,93–95). Specimens obtained early in the disease course, namely within 7 days of disease onset, are associated with a high sensitivity ($> 90\%$) and specificity ($> 90\%$) for each of these assays, particularly if specimens have not been frozen and thawed on multiple occasions, as will be discussed. These assays are generally not useful for decisions regarding the initiation of antiviral therapy.

POLYMERASE CHAIN REACTION

Significant experience with PCR indicates that it currently is a useful tool for the diagnosis of HSE (95). Utilizing primers from an HSV DNA sequence that was common to both HSV types 1 and 2 (either the glycoprotein B domain or HSV DNA polymerase), several investigators successfully identified HSV DNA in the CSF. Reports from two large studies support the utility of this assay. First, a Scandinavian study evaluated CSF specimens from 43 consecutive patients with HSV verified either by virus isolation (13 patients) or by intrathecal antibody production (30 patients). The control subjects for these studies included patients with other identifiable diseases (96). HSV DNA was detected in 42 of 43 patients with proven HSE. All control subjects were negative for HSV DNA as evaluated by this assay system. The second series was that of the NIAID CASG, which evaluated CSF specimens from patients with brain biopsy–proved HSE (97). The sensitivity and specificity of the assay used were 98% and 94%, respectively. Notably, all CSF specimens tested were positive for HSV DNA at the time of clinical presentation. The validity of this assay has also been established in newborns with CNS infections (20,98). As an increasing number of specimens are analyzed, it is becoming apparent that the CSF in a small but not insignificant proportion (5%–10%) of patients remains HSV DNA positive at the end of therapy. The implications for clinical relapse are obvious but have not been adequately analyzed.

As laboratories worldwide become more familiar with the application of PCR, the spectrum of HSV infections of the CNS is being redefined (99,100). A word of caution is indicated, however. The application of PCR to the study of human specimens must be done with extreme care. Knowledge of potential sources of contamination and interference is essential. Thus, careful attention to the selection of controls with each assay run is mandatory.

TREATMENT

Acyclovir is the treatment of choice for both neonatal HSV infections of the CNS and HSE. It is a selective inhibitor of HSV replication, representing one of the most important advances in antiviral therapy. Acyclovir is a synthetic acyclic purine nucleoside analog that selectively inhibits HSV-1 and HSV-2 (101,102). Acyclovir is converted to its monophosphate derivative by virus-encoded thymidine kinase, an event that does not occur to any significant extent in uninfected cells. Subsequent diphosphorylation and triphosphorylation is catalyzed by cellular enzymes and results in acyclovir triphosphate concentrations 40- to 100-fold higher in HSV-infected cells than in uninfected cells. Acyclovir triphosphate inhibits viral DNA synthesis by competing with deoxyguanosine triphosphate as a substrate for viral DNA polymerase (103,104). DNA synthesis is then terminated because acyclovir triphosphate lacks the three hydroxyl required for DNA chain elongation. The viral polymerase has greater affinity for acyclovir triphosphate than does cellular DNA polymerase, resulting in little incorporation of acyclovir into cellular DNA. In vitro, acyclovir is active against HSV-1 (average ED_{50} = 0.04 mg/mL), HSV-2 (0.10 mg/mL), and varicella-zoster virus (0.50 mg/mL).

In the treatment of neonatal HSV infections of the brain, acyclovir is as effective as vidarabine, but it is not superior (105). No infant with disease localized to the skin, eye, or mouth died, but the mortality rates of infants with encephalitis and those with disseminated infection overall were 18% and 55%, respectively. Importantly, even though HSV infection appeared to be localized to the skin, eye, and mouth, neurologic impairment developed beyond 2 years in children who received vidarabine and acyclovir, accounting for morbidity in 10% and 2% of patients, respectively. Following the development of encephalitis, 50% of survivors treated with vidarabine and 43% of survivors treated with acyclovir developed normally. Infants who survived disseminated infection developed normally at rates of 62% and 57% following vidarabine and acyclovir treatment, respectively. The dosage of acyclovir employed in these studies was 10 mg/kg every 8 hours for 10 to 14 days. Unlike other studies comparing vidarabine and acyclovir, in the study being discussed, these two drugs had identical effects on the outcome of this disease. Nevertheless, viral clearance in infants who received acyclovir was accelerated compared to that in vidarabine recipients. Parenthetically, approximately 10% of babies with either encephalitis or disseminated disease with brain involvement relapsed 5 to 15 days after completing a course of antiviral therapy. Unfortunately, CSF was not available for PCR detection of HSV DNA at the completion of therapy, as opposed to the time of relapse (105).

To improve outcome, more active drugs that have greater activity in the CNS must be developed. Importantly, therapy must prevent progression of infection to the CNS or disseminated disease. Ideally, prevention of neonatal HSV infection, including CNS involvement, by either immunization of the mother at risk or immunoprophylaxis and therapy of the newborn delivered to the mother with asymptomatic primary or initial infection would be far more desirable. While the currently recommended dose is 10 mg/kg three times daily, higher doses and longer periods of treatment are being investigated.

Acyclovir therapy of HSE in older individuals is administered at similar dosages as those employed for neonatal HSV infection. When acyclovir and vidarabine were compared for the treatment of biopsy-proved HSE, the mortality at 3 months was 19% for acyclovir recipients compared with approximately 50% for vidarabine recipients. Over time, the mortality attributable to HSV increased to approximately 30% overall in acyclovir recipients. Normal function was re-established in 38% of patients who received acyclovir. However, detailed neurologic examinations years after the onset of HSE have yet to be performed. Parenthetically, the use of brain biopsy should be reserved for patients for whom the diagnosis is still unclear and in the presence of progressive neurologic deterioration despite acyclovir therapy.

Drugs with enhanced capability of penetrating the blood-brain barrier, with greater potency against HSV, and with good oral bioavailability that can be administered following intravenous therapy will be evaluated in the future. Clinical relapse remains problematic for patients with HSE, as well as patients who have neonatal herpes infection. Approximately 5% to 10% of patients with HSE have clinical relapse.

PROGNOSTIC FACTORS FOR NEUROLOGIC IMPAIRMENT

As shown in Table 16-3, the risk factors for neurologic impairment in babies with encephalitis or disseminated disease are identified (106). Knowledge of these risk factors provides insight into disease pathogenesis as well as a basis for counseling families of children with such a high probability for neurologic impairment. Surprisingly, disease

Table 16-3. Prognostic Factors Identified by Multivariate Analyses for Neonates with HSV Infection

	Relative Risk	
	Mortality	***Morbidity***
Total group (n = 202)		
Extent of disease		
Skin, eyes, or mouth	1	1
CNS	5.8[a]	4.4[a]
Disseminated	33[a]	2.1[a]
Level of consciousness		
Alert or lethargic	1	NS
Semicomatose or comatose	5.2[a]	NS
Disseminated intravascular coagulopathy	3.8[a]	NS
Prematurity	3.7[a]	NS
Virus type		
HSV-1	2.3[b]	1
HSV-2	1	4.9[a]
Seizures	NS	3.0[a]
Infants with disseminated disease (n = 46)		
Disseminated intravascular coagulopathy	3.5[a]	NS
Level of consciousness		
Alert or lethargic	1	1
Semicomatose or comatose	3.9[a]	4.0[a]
Pneumonia	3.6[a]	NS
Infants with CNS involvement (n = 71)		
Level of consciousness		
Alert or lethargic	1	NS
Semicomatose or comatose	6.1[a]	NS
Prematurity	5.2[a]	NS
Seizures	NS	3.4[a]
Infants with infection of the skin, eyes, or mouth (n = 85)		
No. of skin vesicle recurrences		
< 3	NA	1
≥ 3	NA	21[a]
Virus type		
HSV-1	NA	1
HSV-2	NA	14[bc]

[a] $p < 0.01$.
[b] $p < 0.05$.
[c] Because of the correlation between virus type and skin vesicle recurrence, virus type was not significant in the multivariate model; however, it was significant as a single factor.
CNS = central nervous system; NS = not statistically significant ($p > 0.05$); NA = not applicable (no baby with disease confined to the skin, eyes, or mouth died).
SOURCE: Adapted by permission of the New England Journal of Medicine, from Whitley RJ, Arvin A, Prober C, et al. Predictors of morbidity and mortality in neonates with herpes simplex virus infections. *N Engl J Med* 1991;324:450–454.

duration did not prove a statistically significant risk factor for morbidity but it did predict mortality.

For HSE in older children and adults, only three factors proved to correlate with long-term neurologic outcome. These characteristics are a Glasgow Coma Score lower than 6, age older than 30 years, and encephalitis for longer than 4 days. The presence of any combination of these factors predicted a significantly poorer neurologic outcome. Thus, to ensure the most favorable outcome, therapy must be instituted before semicoma or coma develops. These data stress the need for improved therapeutic regimens for HSE so that accurate prognostic information can be obtained.

CONCLUSIONS

HSV infections of the CNS remain both common and morbidity-inducing diseases. Adequate therapy remains to be established for this infection because many individuals treated appropriately with acyclovir still develop significant neurologic impairment (36,107,108). Essential to improved outcome will be the development of drugs with the enhanced capability of penetrating the CNS as well as increased activity against HSV. Furthermore, the obvious need for early diagnosis is essential. Current diagnostic approaches have successfully utilized PCR in the identification of individuals with probable HSE. The quantitation of PCR and its comparison to neurologic outcome in patients with HSE will attract increased attention. The spectrum of HSV infections of the CNS will be further clarified if PCR is used appropriately, including the employment of proper controls.

REFERENCES

1. Prober CG, Corey L, Brown ZA, et al. The management of pregnancies complicated by genital infections with herpes simplex virus. *Clin Infect Dis* 1992;15:1031–1038.
2. Whitley RJ, Arvin A. The natural history, pathogenesis, and treatment of neonatal herpes simplex virus infections. *Semin Pediatr Infect Dis* 1994;5:56–64.
3. Whitley RJ, Arvin A. Herpes simplex virus infection. In: Remington J, Klein J, eds. *Infectious diseases of the fetus and newborn infant*. Philadelphia: WB Saunders, 1995:354–376.
4. Whitley RJ. Herpes simplex virus. In: Fields BN, Knipe DM, Howley PM, et al, eds. *Fields virology*. Philadelphia: Lippincott-Raven, 1996: 2297–2342.
5. Mennemeyer ST, Cyr LP, Whitley RJ. Acyclovir therapy for neonatal herpes simplex virus: A cost effectiveness analysis. *J Health Econ* (submitted).
6. Meyers HM Jr, Johnson RT, Crawford IP, et al. Central nervous system syndromes of "viral" etiology: a study of 713 cases. *Am J Med* 1960;29:334–347.
7. Olson LC, Buescher EL, Artenstein MS. Herpesvirus infections of the human central nervous system. *N Engl J Med* 1967; 277:1271–1277.
8. Johnson RT, Mims CA. Pathogenesis of viral infections of the nervous system. *N Engl J Med* 1968;278:23–30, 84–92.
9. Goldsmith SM, Whitley RJ. Herpes simplex encephalitis. In: Lambert HP, eds. *Infections of the central nervous system*. Philadelphia: BC Decker, 1991:283–299.
10. Smith MG, Lennette EH, Reames HR. Isolation of the virus of herpes simplex and the demonstration of intranuclear inclusions in a case of acute encephalitis. *Am J Pathol* 1941;17:55–68.
11. Rappel M, Dubois-Dalcq M, Sprecher S, et al. Diagnosis and treatment of herpes encephali-

tis: a multidisciplinary approach. *J Neurol Sci* 1971;12:443–458.

12 Johnson RT, Olson LC, Buescher EL. Herpes simplex virus infections of the nervous system: problems in laboratory diagnosis. *Arch Neurol* 1968;18:260–264.

13 Whitley RJ, Lakeman AD, Nahmias AJ, Roizman B. DNA restriction-enzyme analysis of herpes simplex virus isolates obtained from patients with encephalitis. *N Engl J Med* 1982;307:1060–1062.

14 Hanley DF, Johnson RT, Whitley RJ. Controversies in neurology: yes, brain biopsy should be a prerequisite for herpes simplex encephalitis treatment. *Arch Neurol* 1987; 44:1289–1290.

15 Institute of Medicine, Committee on Issues and Priorities for New Vaccine Development. Appendix I. Prospects for immunizing against herpes simplex virus 1 and 2. In: eds. *New vaccine development establishing priorities: disease of importance in the United States.* Washington, DC: National Academy Press, 1985:280–312.

16 Whitley RJ, Cobbs CG, Alford CA Jr, et al. Diseases that mimic herpes simplex encephalitis: diagnosis, presentation and outcome. *JAMA* 1989;262:234–239.

17 Brown ZA, Benedetti J, Ashley R, et al. Neonatal herpes simplex virus infection in relation to asymptomatic maternal infection at the time of labor. *N Engl J Med* 1991;324:1247–1252.

18 Prober CG, Sullender WM, Yasukawa LL, et al. Low risk of herpes simplex virus infections in neonates exposed to the virus at the time of vaginal delivery to mothers with recurrent genital herpes simplex virus infections. *N Engl J Med* 1987;316:240–244.

19 Kulhanjian JA, Soroush V, Au DS, et al. Identification of women at unsuspected risk of primary infection with herpes simplex virus type 2 during pregnancy. *N Engl J Med* 1992;326:916–920.

20 Kimberlin DK, Lakeman FD, Arvin AM, et al. Application of the polymerase chain reaction to the diagnosis and management of neonatal herpes simplex virus disease. *J Infect Dis* 1996; 174:1162–1167.

21 Whitley RJ, Tilles J, Linneman C Jr, et al. Herpes simplex encephalitis: clinical assessment. *JAMA* 1982;247:317–320.

22 Corey L. The diagnosis and treatment of genital herpes. *JAMA* 1982;248:1041–1049.

23 Nahmias AJ, Whitley RJ, Visintine AN, et al, the NIAID Collaborative Antiviral Study Group. Herpes simplex encephalitis: laboratory evaluations and their diagnostic significance. *J Infect Dis* 1982;145:829–836.

24 Davis LE, Johnson RT. An explanation for the localization of herpes simplex encephalitis. *Ann Neurol* 1979;5:2–5.

25 Baringer JR, Pisani P. Herpes simplex virus genomes in human nervous system tissue analyzed by polymerase chain reaction. *Ann Neurol* 1994;36:823–829.

26 Johnson RT. The pathogenesis of herpes virus encephalitis. I. Virus pathways to the nervous system of suckling mice demonstrated by fluorescent antibody staining. *J Exp Med* 1984;119:343–356.

27 Schlitt M, Lakeman FD, Wilson ER, et al. A rabbit model of focal herpes simplex encephalitis. *J Infect Dis* 1986;153:732–735.

28 Stroop WG, Schaefer DC. Production of encephalitis restricted to the temporal lobes by experimental reactivation of herpes simplex virus. *J Infect Dis* 1986;153:721–731.

29 Dinn J. Transolfactory spread of virus in herpes simplex encephalitis. *Br Med J* 1980;281:1392.

30 Whitley RJ. Therapeutic advances for severe and life-threatening herpes simplex virus infections. In: Lopez C, Roizman B, eds. *Human herpesvirus infections.* New York: Raven, 1986:153–164.

31 Ojeda VJ, Archer M, Robertson TA, Bucens MR. Necropsy study of olfactory portal of entry in herpes simplex encephalitis. *Med J Aust* 1983;1:79–81.

32 Twomey JA, Barker CM, Robinson G, Howell DA. Olfactory mucosa in herpes simplex encephalitis. *J Neurol Neurosurg Psychiatry* 1979;42:983–987.

33 Rock DL, Frasher NW. Detection of HSV-1 genome in central nervous system of latently infected mice. *Nature* 1983;302:523–531.

34 Griffith JR, Kibrick S, Dodge PR, Richardson EP. Experimental herpes simplex encephalitis: electroencephalographic, clinical, virologic, and pathologic observations in the rabbit. *Electroencephalogr Clin Neurophysiol* 1967; 23:263–267.

35 Boston Interhospital Virus Study Group and the NIAID Sponsored Cooperative Antiviral Clinical Study. Failure of high dose 5-deoxyuridine in the therapy of herpes simplex virus encephalitis: evidence of unacceptable toxicity. *N Engl J Med* 1975;292:600–603.

36 Whitley RJ, Soong S-J, Dolin R, et al. Adenine arabinoside therapy of biopsy-proved herpes simplex encephalitis: National Institute of Allergy and Infectious Diseases Collaborative

Antiviral Study. *N Engl J Med* 1977; 297:289–294.

37 Whitley RJ, Soong S-J, Hirsch MS, et al. Herpes simplex encephalitis: vidarabine therapy and diagnostic problems. *N Engl J Med* 1981;304:313–318.

38 Longson M. Le defi des encephalitis herpetiques. *Ann Microbiol (Paris)* 1979;130:5.

39 Longson MM, Bailey AS, Klapper P. Herpes encephalitis. In: Waterson AP, ed. *Recent advances in clinical virology*. New York: Churchill Livingstone, 1980:147–157.

40 Centifanto-Fitzgerald YM, Yamaguchi T, Kaufman HE, et al. Ocular disease pattern induced by herpes simplex virus is genetically determined by a specific region of viral DNA. *J Exp Med* 1982;155:475–489.

41 Javier RT, Izumi KM, Stevens JG. Localization of herpes simplex virus neurovirulence gene dissociated from high-titer virus replication in the brain. *J Virol* 1988;62:1381–1387.

42 Javier RT, Thompson RL, Stevens JG. Genetic and biological analyses of a herpes simplex virus intertypic recombinant reduced specifically for neurovirulence. *J Virol* 1987;61:1978–1984.

43 Thompson RL, Rogers SK, Zerhusen MA. Herpes simplex virus neurovirulence and productive infection of neuro cells is associated with a function which maps between 0.82 and 0.832 map units on the HSV genome. *Virology* 1989;172:435–450.

44 Chou J, Kern ER, Whitley RJ, Roizman B. Mapping of herpes simplex virus-1 neurovirulence to 34.5, a gene nonessential for growth in culture. *Science* 1990;250:1262–1266.

45 Chou J, Chen J-J, Gross M, Roizman B. Association of a novel $M_1$90,000 phosphoprotein with PKR kinase in cells exhibiting enhanced phosphorylation of eIF-2alpha and premature shutoff of protein synthesis after infection with gamma 134.5^- mutants of herpes simplex virus 1. *Proc Natl Acad Sci USA* 1995.

46 Chambers R, Gillespie GY, Soroceanu L, et al. Comparison of genetically engineered herpes simplex viruses for the treatment of brain tumors in a scid mouse model of human malignant glioma. *Proc Natl Acad Sci USA* 1995;92:1411–1425.

47 Markert JM, Malick A, Coen D, Martuz RL. Reduction and elimination of encephalitis in an experimental glioma therapy model with attenuated herpes simplex mutants that retain susceptibility to acyclovir. Neurosurgery 1993;32:597–603.

48 Andreansky SS, He B, Gillespie GY, et al. Application of genital engineered herpes simplex viruses to the treatment of experimental brain tumors. *Proc Natl Acad Sci USA* 1996; 93:11313–11318.

49 Andreansky S, Soroceanu L, Flotte ER, et al. Evaluation of genetically engineered herpes simplex viruses as oncolytic agents for human malignant brain tumors. *Cancer Res* (in press).

50 Pollard RB, Arvin AM, Gamberg P, et al. Specific cell-mediated immunity and infections with herpes viruses in cardiac transplant recipients. *Am J Med* 1982;73:679–687.

51 Ramsey PG, Fife KH, Hackman RC, et al. Herpes simplex virus pneumonia: clinical, virologic, and pathologic features in 20 patients. *Ann Intern Med* 1982;97:813–820.

52 Sullender WM, Miller JL, Yasukawa LL, et al. Humoral and cell-mediated immunity in neonates with herpes simplex virus infection. *J Infect Dis* 1987;155:28–37.

53 Burchett SK, Corey L, Mohan KM, et al. Diminished interferon-gamma and lymphocyte proliferation in neonatal and postpartum primary herpes simplex virus infection. *J Infect Dis* 1992;165:813–818.

54 Cauda R, Laghi V, Tumbarella M, et al. Immunological alterations associated with recurrent herpes simplex genitalis. Clin Immunol Immunopathol 1989;51:294–302.

55 Corey L, Reeves WC, Holmes KK. Cellular immune response in genital herpes simplex virus infection. *N Engl J Med* 1978; 299:986–991.

56 LI A II, Chernesky MA, Rawls WE, RB DP. Depressed herpes simplex virus-induced lymphocyte blastogenesis in individuals with severe recurrent herpes infections. *Clin Immunol Immunopathol* 1978;9:253–263.

57 Kalimo KOK, Joronen IA, Havu VK. Cell-mediated immunity against herpes simplex virus envelope, capsid, excreted, and crude antigens. *Infect Immun* 1983;39:24–28.

58 Lopez C, O'Reilley RJ. Cell-mediated immune responses in recurrent herpesvirus infections. I. Lymphocyte proliferation assay. *J Immunol* 1977;118:895–902.

59 Rattray MC, Peterman GM, Altman IC, et al. Lymphocyte-derived chemotactic factor synthesis in initial genital herpesvirus infection: correlation with lymphocyte transformation. *Infect Immun* 1980;30:110–116.

60 Rasmussen L, Merigan TC. Role of T-lymphocytes in cellular immune responses during herpes simplex virus infection in humans. *Proc Natl Acad Sci USA* 1978;75:3957–3961.

61 Shillitoe EJ, Wilton JMA, Lehner T. Sequen-

tial changes in cell-mediated immune responses to herpes simplex virus after recurrent herpetic infection in humans. *Infect Immun* 1977;18:130–137.

62 Vestey JP, Norval M, Howie SEM. Lymphoproliferative responses in recrudescent orofacial herpetic infections. *J R Soc Med* 1990;83:308–311.

63 Kahlon J, Whitley RJ. Antibody response of the newborn after herpes simplex virus infection. *J Infect Dis* 1988;158:925–933.

64 Kohl S, West MS, Prober CG, et al. Neonatal antibody-dependent cellular cytoxic antibody levels are associated with the clinical presentation of neonatal herpes simplex virus infection. *J Infect Dis* 1989;160:770–776.

65 Burchett SK, Corey L, Mohan KM, et al. Diminished interferon-gamma and lymphocyte proliferation in neonatal and postpartum primary herpes simplex virus infection. *J Infect Dis* 1992;165:813–818.

66 Adam JH, Jennett WB. Acute necrotizing encephalitis: a problem in diagnosis. *J Neurol Neurosurg Psychiatry* 1967;30:248–260.

67 Levy RM, Bredesen DE, Rosenblum MC. Neurological manifestations of the acquired immunodeficiency syndrome (AIDS): experience at UCSF and review of the literature. *J Neurosurg* 1985;62:475–595.

68 Radermecker J. Systematique its electrocencephalographic des encephalitis it encephalopathies. *Electroencephalography* 1956; suppl 5:1–243.

69 Upton A, Grumpert J. Electroencephalography in diagnosis of herpes simplex encephalitis. *Lancet* 1970;1:650–652.

70 Smith JB, Westmoreland BF, Reagan TJ, Sandok BA. A distinctive clinical EEG profile in herpes simplex encephalitis. *Mayo Clin Proc* 1975;50:469–474.

71 Miller JHD, Coey A. The EEG in necrotizing encephalitis. *Electroencephalogr Clin Neurophysiol* 1959;2:582–585.

72 Chien LT, Boehm RM, Robinson H, et al. Characteristic early electroencephalographic changes in herpes simplex encephalitis. *Arch Neurol* 1977;34:361–364.

73 Enzmann DR, Ransom B, Norman D. Computed tomography of herpes simplex encephalitis. *Radiology* 1978;129:419–425.

74 Zimmerman RD, Russell EJ, Leeds NE, Kaufman D. CT in the early diagnosis of herpes simplex encephalitis. *AJR* 1980;134:61–66.

75 Sage MR, Dubois PJ, Oakes J, et al. Rapid development of cerebral atrophy due to perinatal herpes simplex encephalopathy. *J Comput Assist Tomogr* 1961;5:763–766.

76 Kaiser MC, Veiga-Pires JA. Sequential CT appearance in herpes simplex encephalopathy (HSE) sequelae complicated by trauma. *Fortschr Rontgenstr* 1983;139:692–694.

77 Karlin CA, Robinson RG, Hinthorn DR. Radionuclide imaging in herpes simplex encephalitis. *Radiology* 1978;126:181–814.

78 Zimmerman RA. Imaging of intracranial infections. In: Scheld WM, Whitley RJ, Durack DT, eds. *Infections of the central nervous system*. New York: Raven, 1991:887–907.

79 Morawetz RB, Whitley RJ, Murphy DM. Experience with brain biopsy for suspected herpes encephalitis—a review of forty consecutive cases. *Neurosurgery* 1983;12:654–657.

80 Bakken JS, Camenga DL, Glazier MC, Coughlan JD. Herpes simplex 1 virus encephalitis: early diagnosis with magnetic tomography (MT). *Tidsskr Nor Laegeforen* 1989;109:2430–2432.

81 Zimmerman RD, Haimes AB. The role of MR imaging in the diagnosis of infection of the central nervous system. *Curr Clin Top Infect Dis* 1989;10:82–108.

82 Dayan AD, Stokes ML. Rapid diagnosis of encephalitis by immunofluorescent examination of cerebrospinal fluid cells. *Lancet* 1973;I:177–179.

83 Lerner AM, Bailey EJ, Nolan DC. Complement-requiring neutralizing antibodies in herpes virus hominis encephalitis. *J Immunol* 1970;104:607–615.

84 Lerner AM, Lawter CB, Nolan DC, Shippey MJ. Passive hemagglutinating antibodies in cerebrospinal fluids in herpesvirus hominis encephalitis. *Proc Soc Exp Biol Med* 1972; 140:1460–1466.

85 Levine DP, Lauter CB, Lerner AM. Simultaneous serum and CSF antibodies in herpes simplex virus encephalitis. *JAMA* 1978; 240:356–360.

86 Lakeman FD, Koga J, Whitley RJ, the NIAID Collaborative Antiviral Study Group. Detection of antigen to herpes simplex virus in cerebrospinal fluid from patients with herpes simplex encephalitis. *J Infect Dis* 1987; 155:1172–1178.

87 Vandvik B, Skoldenberg B, Forsgren M, et al. Long-term persistence of intrathecal virus-specific antibody responses after herpes simplex virus encephalitis. *J Neurol* 1985; 231:307–312.

88 Skoldenberg B, Kalimo K, Carlstrom A, et al. Herpes simplex encephalitis: a serological follow-up study. *Acta Neurol Scand* 1981; 63:273–275.

89 Klapper PE, Laing I, Longson M. Rapid non-

invasive diagnosis of herpes encephalitis. *Lancet* 1981;2:607–608.

90 Koskiniemi ML, Vaheri A. Diagnostic value of cerebrospinal fluid antibodies in herpes simplex virus encephalitis. *J Neurol Neurosurg Psychiatry* 1982;45:239–242.

91 MacCallum OF, Chinn IJ, Gostling JVT. Antibodies to herpes simplex virus in the cerebrospinal fluid of patients with herpetic encephalitis. *J Med Microbiol* 1974;7:325–331.

92 Koskiniemi M, Vaheri A, Taskinen E. Cerebrospinal fluid alterations in herpes simplex virus encephalitis. *Rev Infect Dis* 1984; 6:608–618.

93 Kahlon J, Lakeman FD, Ackerman M, Whitley RJ. Human antibody response to herpes simplex virus specified polypeptides following primary and recurrent infection. *J Clin Microbiol* 1985;23:725–730.

94 Kahlon J, Chatterjee S, Lakeman F, et al. Detection of antibodies to herpes simplex virus in the cerebrospinal fluid of patients with herpes simplex encephalitis. *J Infect Dis* 1987;155:38–44.

95 Rowley A, Lakeman F, Whitley R, Wolinsky S. Rapid detection of herpes simplex virus DNA in cerebrospinal fluid of patients with herpes simplex encephalitis. *Lancet* 1990; 335:440–441.

96 Aurelius E, Johansson B, Skoldenberg B, et al. Rapid diagnosis of herpes simplex encephalitis by nested polymerase chain reaction assay of cerebrospinal fluid. *Lancet* 1991; 337:189–192.

97 Lakeman FD, Whitley RJ, National Institute of Allergy and Infectious Disease Collaborative Antiviral Study Group. Diagnosis of herpes simplex encephalitis: application of polymerase chain reaction to cerebrospinal fluid from brain biopsied patients and correlation with disease. *J Infect Dis* 1995;171:857–863.

98 Kimura H, Futamura M, Kito H, et al. Detection of viral DNA in neonatal herpes simplex virus infections: frequent and prolonged presence in serum and cerebrospinal fluid. *J Infect Dis* 1991;164:289–293.

99 Schlesinger Y, Storch GA. Herpes simplex meningitis in infancy. *Pediatr Infect Dis J* 1994;13:141–144.

100 Schlesinger Y, Tebas P, Gaudreault-Keener M, et al. Herpes simplex type 2 meningitis in the absence of genital lesions: improved recognition using the polymerase chain reaction. *Clin Infect Dis* 1995;20:842–848.

101 Schaeffer HJ, Beauchamp L, deMiranda P, et al. 9-(2-Hydroxyethoxymethyl) guanine activity against viruses of the herpes group. *Nature* 1978;272:583–585.

102 Elion GB, Furman PA, Fyfe JA, et al. Selectivity of action of an antiherpetic agent, 9-(2-hydroxyethoxymethyl) guanine. *Proc Natl Acad Sci USA* 1977;74:5716–5720.

103 Fyfe JA, Keller PM, Furman PA, et al. Thymidine kinase from herpes simplex virus phosphorylates the new antiviral compound, 9-(2-hydroxyethoxymethyl)guanine. *J Biol Chem* 1978;253:8721–8727.

104 Derse D, Chang Y-C, Furman PA, Elion GB. Inhibition of purified human and herpes simplex virus-induced DNA polymerase by 9-(2-hydroxyethoxymethyl)guanine [acyclovir] triphosphate: effect on primer-template function. *J Biol Chem* 1981;256:11447–11451.

105 Whitley RJ, Arvin A, Prober C, et al. A controlled trial comparing vidarabine with acyclovir in neonatal herpes simplex virus infection. *N Engl J Med* 1991;324:444–449.

106 Whitley RJ, Arvin A, Prober C, et al. Predictors of morbidity and mortality in neonates with herpes simplex virus infections. *N Engl J Med* 1991;324:450–454.

107 Whitley RJ, Alford CA Jr, Hirsch MS, et al. Vidarabine versus acyclovir therapy in herpes simplex encephalitis. *N Engl J Med* 1986; 314:144–149.

108 Whitley RJ. Herpes simplex virus infections of the central nervous system: a review. *Am J Med* 1988;85:61–67.

17

Viral Persistence in the Central Nervous System

GLENN F. RALL
MICHAEL B. A. OLDSTONE

The features that distinguish resident brain cells from other differentiated cells probably also contribute to the ability of many neurotropic viral infections to establish persistent infections in the central nervous system (CNS). For example, though CNS neurons are essential for host survival, they are terminally differentiated and cannot be replaced once destroyed (1). Consequently, a viral infection that results in neuronal death would deplete a vital pool of cells, unlike an infection of, for example, hepatocytes, in which cell division compensates for virus-induced cell death. Since massive neuronal dropout caused by lytic viral infection would kill both host and virus, it is likely that neurons and viruses have adapted to coexist, allowing an infection to persist in a viable host.

Viruses enter the CNS by two major routes. Many blood-borne viruses bypass the blood-brain barrier by the so-called Trojan horse approach (2). In this case, viruses such as human immunodeficiency virus type 1 (HIV-1), measles virus, and lymphocytic choriomeningitis virus (LCMV) infect cells, including activated lymphocytes and macrophages, which routinely cross the barrier and percolate through the CNS. Once in the CNS, these infected hematogenous cells can produce progeny virus that can then infect resident brain cells. Other viruses such as the herpesviruses and rabies virus are transported along axon processes from the peripheral nervous system into the CNS, presumably by crossing synaptic junctions (3).

Regardless of their mechanism of entry, many viruses that can access the CNS undergo a switch to a persistent phenotype upon infection of resident brain cells. In these infections, viral nucleic acids and proteins are readily detected in the absence of direct cell death or induction of the immune response, and often in the absence of production of extracellular infectious progeny. While the detailed mechanisms by which viruses establish and maintain long-term persistent infections are largely unknown, both viral genes (4–6) and host cellular genes (7) cooperatively promote viral persistence. Some of these mechanisms are addressed later in this chapter.

Thus, the establishment of viral persistence (and in some instances, the initiation of disease) depends on a complex interaction between the viral genome, the susceptible host cells, and the immune response. By definition, a persistent infection is one in which some level of viral replication and gene expression occurs. Thus, for a replicating virus to maintain a long-term infection within its host, it must meet two prerequisites: it must be noncytopathic, and it must evade recognition and elimination by the host immune response. As one might predict, the strategies that viruses employ to establish persistence are varied, but some fundamental principles that have recently surfaced shed light both on the dynamics of viral replication in resident brain cells and on the factors that govern the profile and extent of the immune response in the infected CNS.

How neurons block the production of infectious virus despite viral gene expression remains largely unknown, and is relevant to the human infections caused by the measles virus (8), rabies virus (9), influenza virus (10), poliovirus (11), and mumps virus (12), and to the animal infections caused by the Borna virus (13), the coronaviruses (14), and the arenaviruses (15), among others. Since each of these viruses can establish productive infections in other differentiated cells, the dramatic reduction in infectious virus production within the brain suggests that the neuronal environment, in some way, is inhospitable for viral propagation. A major unresolved issue is whether the inhibition or expression of a specific neuronal gene (or genes) may be responsible for reduced infectious viral yields. Interestingly, despite a paucity of cell-free virus in the brain, most neurotropic viruses spread through the CNS with remarkable efficiency, suggesting that alternatives to the large-scale production of cell-free infectious virus are used to disseminate throughout the CNS.

While some persistent neurotropic viruses do not induce substantial CNS damage, many infections do lead to CNS diseases and are accompanied by neuronal dropout, gliosis, blood-brain barrier dysfunction, and immune cell recruitment into the parenchyma. These syndromes include subacute sclerosing panencephalitis (SSPE) following acute measles infection, the spongiform encephalopathies caused by lentiviral infections such as with the Visna virus, the demyelination caused by mouse hepatitis virus (MHV) and Theiler's murine encephalomyelitis virus (TMEV), the chronic neurodegenerative disease following Borna virus infection, postinfluenza encephalitis, mumps meningoencephalitis, and CNS neoplasms possibly resulting from the human polyomaviruses JC and BK. Moreover, the recent finding that Borna disease virus is associated with CNS disorders such as schizophrenia and clinical depression (13) indicates that viral infection may also play a role in a number of CNS disorders with ambiguous etiology.

What triggers a neurotropic virus to initiate CNS disease remains unresolved but at least two possibilities exist. In one scenario, infection may not induce overt cell death, but may impair cellular functions, leading to the generation of neurotoxins, such as excitatory amino acids and free radicals. For example, mice persistently infected with LCMV show neurologic deficits (16), despite the absence of inflammation and necrosis within the CNS. These deficits correlate with neurochemical abnormalities, including a virus-specific suppression of the neurotransmitter somatostatin (17) or growth-associated protein (GAP-43), a protein involved in cognitive function (18). Moreover, neuronal dropout as a consequence of HIV-1 infection of microglia in the CNS may be due to the production of glutamate or nitric oxide within the CNS (19). These data suggest that infection and the onset of pathology occur simultaneously, and the apparent delay between infection and clinical signs of disease may reflect the requirement for a threshold level of CNS damage.

In another scenario, persistent infections may remain noncytopathic for extended periods. Restrictions imposed by the host cell on viral production could result in the spontaneous generation of neurovirulent variants that then initiate a rapid disease course. As a possible example of a shifting virus-host relationship, a recent study showed that as many as 20% of all individuals acutely infected with measles virus have a persistent measles virus infection within the CNS (20). However, only 1 of 100,000 patients with acute infection go on to develop the lethal neurodegenerative disease SSPE, which often appears months or years after the primary infection. Viral RNA isolated from SSPE brain tissues consistently contain biased hypermutations in the envelope-associated genes (21). No such changes have been found in persistently infected, non-SSPE isolates. While this suggests that cytopathic variants arise following neuronal infection, the role of these "defective virions" in measles-associated neuropathology is not known.

One of the contributing factors that allows for the long incubation period between the time of infection and presentation of disease is the relative paucity of the immune response within the CNS. Both anatomic (blood-brain barrier) and molecular (restricted major histocompatibility complex (MHC) gene expression) factors contribute to the "immune privilege" of the CNS. Nevertheless, antiviral lymphocytes can gain entry to the brain parenchyma (22–24) and may also be a component of virus-induced CNS disease.

In this chapter, we review how these "prerequisites of persistence"—noncytopathicity and immune avoidance—feature in persistent CNS viral infections. We also address recent work with animal models, to understand concepts that underlie demyelinating and neurodegenerative diseases, and how these animal model systems may shed light on human disease. We conclude the chapter with a brief discussion of some of the remaining challenges in this field, and how some recently reported evidence may help to direct the course of such work.

REQUIREMENTS FOR VIRAL PERSISTENCE

Emergence of Viral Variants Associated with the Persistent Phenotype

Measles Measles virus can establish persistent infection of neurons and glia in the human CNS, resulting in diseases such as SSPE and measles inclusion body encephalitis (MIBE) months to years after the onset of acute infection (reviewed elsewhere (8)). SSPE occurs in children and young adults; the mean age at onset is between 7 and 8 years. The initial presenting symptom is cognitive dysfunction, followed by seizures and clumsiness. The final stages consist of progression from a vegetative state to coma and death. Histologically, large numbers of viral core particles are seen in infected cells, but no infectious virus is produced. The restrictions to productive measles virus infection have been determined from viral RNA isolated from brain material of autopsied SSPE patients. Expression of the viral envelope proteins matrix, fusion, and hemagglutinin

(M, F, and H, respectively) is reduced owing to the presence of a low abundance of the corresponding messenger RNAs (mRNAs) or the incorporation of point mutations in these genes that lead to absent or defective protein expression. Transcriptional attenuation of measles virus appears to be particularly pronounced in differentiated brain cells, since treatment of neuroblastoma cells with differentiation agents increases the attenuation of transcription (25). In addition, viral RNA purified from infected brain homogenates reveals an abundance of scattered point mutations and clustered transitions of uridine residues to cytidine, or more rarely, of adenine to guanidine (21). These "biased hypermutations" can be attributed to a cellular enzyme called *double-stranded RNA–specific adenosine-deaminase activity* (DRADA), which targets the double-stranded RNAs that form accidentally when the nascent transcripts fold back onto the genomic template. DRADA activity results in the replacement of an A-U pair with a G-C pair (8,26). Defective measles virus genomic RNAs of the 5′ copy-back type have also been identified in brain cells of patients with SSPE (27). Thus, persistent measles infection of the CNS is characterized not only by the presence of mutant, full-length genomes, but also by small deleted genomes that may limit replication and transcription by nonproductively binding polymerase and transcription complexes.

As a consequence, these mutated viruses lack components that are essential for the assembly and budding of the mature infectious particles. An important yet unresolved issue is whether these changes occur once the virus is present within resident brain cells, or whether such changes facilitate entry into CNS cells. The presence of wild-type measles virus sequences in SSPE brain material argues in favor of nonmutated virions initially infecting the CNS. If this is the case, then factors in the neuronal cytoplasm must hasten the attenuation of viral gene functions and favor the establishment of a persistent infection over a lytic, productive infection.

Theiler's Murine Encephalomyelitis Virus TMEV infection occurs naturally in mice and has been used as a model system to study demyelinating diseases such as multiple sclerosis. Viral isolates are classified into two groups based on their neurovirulence. The highly neurovirulent group, which includes isolates GDVII and FA, cause a rapidly fatal encephalitis that kills the mouse in a matter of days (28,29). The less neurovirulent, "persistent" strains, such as DA and BeAn, induce a biphasic disease in which an infection of neurons causes an early mild encephalitis, followed by a migration of virus to the spinal cord where it establishes a lifelong infection of oligodendrocytes (30) and macrophages (31). This second phase of infection precipitates an inflammatory response and induces demyelination. The differences in lethality between the virulent and persistent strains is remarkably high: greater than 10^5 plaque-forming units/lethal dose $(PFU/LD)_{50}$ (32). What are the molecular differences between these strains that result in such dramatically different pathogenic outcomes?

Both the highly neurovirulent GDVII and the persistent DA and BeAn strains have been completely sequenced, and recombinant chimeras between parental complementary DNAs (cDNAs) have been inoculated into mice. Neurovirulence has been mapped to the leader and coat proteins (33–35) while persistence can be mapped even more specifically to the sequences encoding the VP1 region (36). Thus, replacing the capsid of a neurovirulent strain with the persisting strain results in the complete attenuation of virulence, and vice versa. These findings suggest that the mechanism for pathogenesis by these strains involves the exterior surface of the virus, and implies that immune or receptor-mediated events may be involved (32). A discrepancy in the literature regarding the ability of one such chimera, R4, to cause persistence and demyelination led to the finding that a single amino acid, located at the tip of the loop that spans the twofold axis of the capsid, could confer the ability of a chimeric virus to persist and demyelinate or to result in the rapidly fatal neurovirulent phenotype (37).

In addition to the capsid, it has also been suggested that the "L" region of the genome may contribute to persistence, since persisting strains contain an alternate open reading frame that codes for an 18-kd protein called *I* (38), or *L** (39). Sequence analysis of neurovirulent and persistent isolates led to the surprising finding that the neurovirulent strains may have evolved from the persistent strains, since the major difference between the two groups at this site is the ablation of the methionine in the virulent strain, and therefore an inability to synthesize the protein. This suggests that the I protein might be a determinant of persistence, and that its absence may allow for the outgrowth of neurovirulent strains.

Mouse Hepatitis Virus As the name implies, MHV, a member of the coronaviruses, can infect the liver and result in hepatitis in the natural mouse host. However, MHV has also been used as a model of CNS infection, since a number of strains, JHM and A59 among them, can infect the CNS and produce a demyelinating encephalomyelitis similar to multiple sclerosis. Like TMEV, MHV causes both acute and chronic disease, and the distribution and type of infected cells within the CNS shift between these phases (40). During the acute infection, MHV strain JHM (hereafter, JHMV) has tropism for neuroectodermal cells including neurons, glial cells, and ependymal cells, although neurons have been identified as the primary targets in acute encephalomyelitis (41–43). Some investigators argued that infection of neurons may actually be a prerequisite for infection of glia, a hypothesis that is supported by in vitro studies (44). Spread of JHMV in infected mice occurs via well-defined neuroanatomic tracts, particularly the olfactory, trigeminal, and limbic pathways (reviewed elsewhere (40)). Conversely, the delayed chronic form of the infection, during which time the demyelination occurs, is characterized by infection of white matter, predominately oligodendrocytes (45) and astrocytes (46,47).

A variety of hemagglutinin-esterase (HE) protein–defective mutants arise during infection, demonstrating the extreme variability and rapid evolution of HE gene expression in contrast to other virus structural proteins (48). Interestingly, the timing of their appearance coincides with the localization of viral antigens to glial cells and the onset of demyelination, in contrast to infection of neurons during the acute phase (49). Thus, the possibility exists that HE mutations allow MHV to infect other resident brain cells, and that selection of HE-defective mutants might be associated with persistent viral infection and/or demyelination.

Lymphocytic Choriomeningitis Virus

Influence of Infected Host Cells on Viral Mutations The emergence of variants during persistent infection is not surprising, especially for RNA viruses that undergo rapid mutation. As the examples described previously illustrate, some mutations in the genome can dramatically influence viral pathogenicity. Do changes in the viral genome impact an infection equally, regardless of the cell type infected, or do some changes mediate cell-specific effects?

For LCMV, which causes a natural infection of mice, it has been firmly established that a profound influence of host cells exists for the selection of viral variants (50–53). For example, most CNS isolates cause acute infections in mice following intraperitoneal inoculation that resolve in 2 weeks as a result of the LCMV cytotoxic T-lymphocyte (CTL) response. In contrast, many of the splenic isolates cause chronic infections, associated with a decreased T-cell response. Very few nucleotide changes leading to amino acid changes mediate these disparate effects. One common change in the spleen isolates is a phenylalanine to leucine (F to L) change at residue 260 in the viral glycoprotein (54,55). Two groups independently (56,57) demonstrated that the leucine mutants arise rapidly from the parental strain in tissues such as spleen and liver, but that the parental sequence is retained in the majority of brain isolates. Furthermore, the parental strain replicates more efficiently and outcompetes the persisting leucine mutants in the cultured neuronal cell lines PC12 and GT1-7 (57), confirming that there is a strong molecular association between the ability to grow in neuronal cells and the retention of phenylalanine residue at position GP_{260}. The viral glycoprotein (GP-C) is posttranslationally cleaved to generate GP-1 and GP-2, which associate on the virion and cell surface. Amino acid GP-260 is located only six residues from the glycoprotein cleavage site. This position may be important for association of GP-1 and GP-2 on the surface of the virion, it may affect processing of the glycoprotein precursor to GP-1 and GP-2, or it may govern receptor recognition. Earlier studies had shown that the presence of a leucine at position 260 was necessary for enhanced infection of macrophages (51,58), while LCMV isolates with a phenylalanine at position 260 replicate more efficiently in neurons (56,57,59). Thus, a rather conservative amino acid change contributes significantly to the ability of a virus to infect various cell types: tropism for macrophages is a critical determinant in selection of the "L" genotype in the spleen and liver, and tropism for neurons is important in retention of the "F" genotype in the CNS.

The organ-specific selection of viral variants is likely to be a general finding for other chronic viral infections. For example, persistent infection with HIV results in the emergence of variants in the CNS that consistently differ from those found in peripheral blood (60,61).

Influence of Infected Host Cells on Viral Growth It is becoming clear that the neuron provides a unique environment for many viruses, particularly since infection of neurons by many viruses is accompanied by a dramatic decline in gene expression. The mechanisms that enable viruses to infect and persist in differentiated cells, and the specific interactions established between the persisting virus and the neuron, are issues of paramount importance for the understanding of neuroviral pathogenesis.

One might assume that the decrease in viral gene expression is due to the absence of proliferation of mature neurons, since some reports showed that decreased cell growth also decreases the replication rate of infecting viruses. However, it is probably incorrect to assume that reduced viral gene expression is due solely to the absence of cell division: a recent report using the neuronal cell line PC12 and LCMV infection revealed that both the lack of cell division and the "differentiated status" of the neuron-like PC12 cells impact on the rate of viral gene expression (62). PC12 cells are a pheochromocytoma clone that has been used extensively as a model of neuronal differentiation. These cells can be induced to undergo morphologic and physiologic differentiation characterized by a lack of cell division, extension of functional processes, and expression of a variety of neuron-specific markers following low-dose exposure to nerve growth factor (NGF). Infection of undifferentiated cultures with LCMV resulted in high-titer infections, while infection of NGF-differentiated cells produced 3- to 4-log less infectious virus (62). The reduction in viral yield could be attributed to decreased viral transcription, and not to a reduced ability of LCMV to infect the cells. This result, however, did not indicate whether the "differentiated" aspect of these cells, or the fact that they are nondividing, was responsible for the reduced viral yields. Starvation of these cells by serum depletion stops the cells from dividing, but does not induce differentiation. Infection of these cells with LCMV resulted in a decreased viral yield of approximately 1 log, suggesting that whatever intracellular changes are induced by the differentiation of these cells to a neuron-like phenotype were predominately responsible for the 3- to 4-log decrease in viral yields as well.

What neuron-specific features could be responsible for a reduced ability to replicate in differentiated PC12 cells? Levels of intracellular cyclic adenosine monophosphate (cAMP) vary with the state of cell growth and differentiation, being relatively high in quiescent and terminally differentiated neural cells, and cAMP can exert a variety of effects on viral replication (63–65). In particular, it has been proposed that the shift from acute to persistent measles virus infection may depend on the intracellular level of cyclic nucleotides (64). Additionally, levels of 2′-5′ adenylate (2-5A)–dependent ribonuclease (RNase) and 2-5A synthetase, both members of the 2-5A system, are elevated in growth-arrested cells (66,67). Because several reports implicated the 2-5A system as the mechanism by which interferon inhibits the replication of picornaviruses (68,69), it is conceivable that the 2-5A system may also contribute to the reduced yields of LCMV in NGF-treated PC12 cells.

Viral Evasion of the Immune Response

The Blood-Brain Barrier and the Lack of Class I MHC Expression on Resident Brain Cells To establish persistent infections, noncytolytic viruses must also evade host immune response recognition. This can be accomplished in two ways. Viruses with large genomes, such as the DNA viruses herpes simplex virus types 1 and 2 (HSV-1 and -2), the poxviruses, and the adenoviruses, can reduce immune recognition of infected target cells by synthesizing viral proteins that actively interfere with the host cell antigen-processing pathway. RNA viruses, which typically have smaller genomes and cannot encode the array of immune response–altering proteins, may bypass immune detection by infecting naturally "immune-privileged" cells. Resident brain cells within the parenchyma, including neurons, oligodendrocytes, microglia, and astrocytes, are considered among these immunologically privileged cells for two reasons. The blood-brain barrier, the densely packed endothelial cells that comprise the capillary walls of most regions of the brain (70), restricts the passage of blood-borne proteins and cells (including naive lymphocytes) into the brain, while nutrients and oxygen either readily diffuse or are transported across the endothelial barrier. The restriction is due to both the tight junctions between the capillary endothelia and a lack of active transport by the endothelial cells themselves (70). Thus, essential components of the immune system often cannot respond to CNS infections unless they are synthesized intrathecally. As a result, the degree of immunologic surveillance and the vigor of the immune response are significantly restricted in the brain compared to non-CNS tissues.

Furthermore, neurons have a defense to prevent cytolysis caused by the cytotoxic arm of the immune response: an inability to be "seen" by antiviral CTLs. Even though the blood-brain barrier restricts access of many immune response modulators into the parenchyma, including cytokines and antibodies, activated T lymphocytes can traverse the barrier and percolate through the brain parenchyma (71,72). These infiltrating, activated T cells are restricted from recognizing virally infected neurons, however, because neurons lack the ability to synthesize class I MHC glycoproteins that are required for CTL–target cell interaction (73). These cell surface molecules, present on virtually all cells but neurons and trophoblasts, present processed viral proteins to the T-cell receptor of $CD8^+$ CTLs. Neurons, both in vivo (73–75) and in vitro (73,76–78), do not transcribe the class I MHC heavy chain and, hence, despite being infected and expressing viral proteins on their surfaces, do not serve as targets for CTL-mediated lysis.

To confirm that neuronal MHC expression could result in a deleterious, antineuron immune response, investigators established transgenic mice in which a functional class I MHC molecule was expressed on CNS neurons (79). These mice are referred to as NSE-D^b; the promoter used was the neuron-specific enolase (NSE) promoter, and the specific class I MHC molecule expressed was the D^b molecule. Infection of both normal and NSE-D^b transgenic neonatal mice with LCMV established a lifelong persistent infection. Inoculation of neonates results in infection of virtually all organs; however, the only cells in the CNS parenchyma that are infected are neurons (80,81). Virus and viral nucleic acid can be cleared from normal (nontransgenic) persistently infected mice by an adoptive transfer of haplotype-matched CTLs derived from an immunized mouse, and viral clearance from the CNS occurs within 60 to 120 days (80). Animal sickness or death does not occur. However, adoptive transfer of the same antiviral H-2^b restricted CTLs into NSE-D^b transgenic mice persistently infected with LCMV resulted in significant morbidity and mortality (79), coupled with an increase in the number of $CD8^+$ T lymphocytes within the brain parenchyma, an increased rate of clearance of infectious virus from infected neurons, and an increased permeability of the blood-brain barrier. Interestingly, the permeability of the barrier remained altered, even once virus was completely cleared from surviving mice (79).

In the NSE-D^b transgenic mice, neuronal clearance was not accompanied by neuronal lysis, suggesting that intraparenchymal cytokine production may participate in the clearance of infectious virus from transgenic brains. Inhibition of viral synthesis in the absence of cell death has been documented in the CTL response to hepatitis B virus infection of hepatocytes (82) and in HIV (83). In these systems, CTL production of inflammatory cytokines such as interferon (IFN)-γ and tumor necrosis factor (TNF)-α can downregulate viral expression without concomitant cell death. An alternative explanation for the lack of neuronal dropout in the NSE-D^b transgenic mice is the mature neurons can express "antideath" genes, such as *bcl-2*, that protect neurons from apoptosis (reviewed elsewhere (84)), which may prevent their destruction by CTLs.

The protracted effect of neuronal MHC expression on blood-brain barrier permeability could also be explained by soluble CTL products such as cytokines. Several CNS diseases have been associated with transient or permanent changes in blood-brain barrier permeability, including those associated with CNS infection, demyelinating diseases, and tumors. The finding that abnormal permeability of the blood-brain barrier and clinical illness were present long after virus had been cleared from infected mice indicates that viral infections and CTL-CNS interactions may induce blood-brain barrier disruptions and neurologic disease by a "hit-and-run" mechanism, triggering a cascade of pathogenic events that proceed in the absence of continual viral stimulation.

Incompleteness of Immune-Mediated Viral Clearance Despite the physical and molecular pressures that restrict the immune response within the CNS, activated CTLs cross the intact blood-brain barrier (22–24). However, in a number of cases, the immune response cannot completely eliminate the virus, allowing the virus to persist in the CNS. Below are two examples which suggest that viruses may have developed ways to persist even in the face of immune recognition, and that an antiviral immune response may actually contribute to the transition to a persistent CNS infection.

Sindbis Several arthropod-borne viruses, including the alphaviruses, flaviviruses, and bunyaviruses, can cause an acute encephalitis that is characterized by the development of an effective immune response and viral clearance without induction of a fatal disease in the host. Sindbis virus, a member of the alphavirus family, replicates rapidly in neurons of the brains of both newborn and adult mice, but the outcome of infection is dramatically different: Newborns die within 3 to 4 days after infection, whereas adults begin clearing virus within 4 to 5 days after infection (84). Although a perivascular cellular response consisting of T cells, B cells, and macrophages can be found in mice actively clearing a Sindbis infection, clearance of infectious virus can be mediated by passive transfer of antibodies to the surface glycoprotein, E2 (85), presumably by restricting viral gene expression rather than by lysing infected neurons.

However, this "clearance" is not complete. With reverse transcriptase–polymerase chain reaction (PCR) methods, Sindbis RNA was detected in brain samples more than 17 months after infection (86). As long as antibody was present (e.g., in normal mice, or in severe combined immunodeficiency (SCID) mice treated with high doses of the anti-E2 antibody), virus remained quiescent. However, removal of antibody "surveillance" allowed for the rapid reactivation of infectious Sindbis virus. Thus, it appears that the expression of genes, including *bcl-2*, within mature neurons prevents virus- or immune-induced apoptosis, protecting infected neurons from lysis (84). Antibody produced in response to the infection can clear infectious virus from persistently infected brains (85), but cannot completely eliminate viral nucleic acid from infected neurons (86). Without the continuous presence of antibody in the CNS, these "latent" viruses can become reactivated. Thus, while antibody eliminates infectious virus by a noncytolytic mechanism—obviously important for a nondividing and essential pool of cells—the price that is paid is that neurons remain persistently infected, and that antibody must be continuously present to keep the latent virus from reactivating (84).

While there does not appear to be an overt consequence of Sindbis RNA persistence in neurons, specific alterations in certain neuronal genes occurs with other persistent viral infections of neurons. For example, persistent infection of neurons with LCMV depresses neurotransmitter and GAP-43 synthesis, without inducing neuronal injury (18,87).

Mouse Hepatitis Virus Infection with neurotropic MHV results in an acute encephalitis with primary demyelination (88,89). Survivors of the acute infection do not clear the infection from the brain and exhibit ongoing demyelination (89).

The host's antiviral response, both humoral and cell mediated, is the critical component in determining the clinical outcome of acute MHV infection and the establishment of persistent infection. Both $CD8^+$ and $CD4^+$ Th1 cells provide protection from acute illness, but they also contribute to virus-induced immunopathology. Thus, an immune response that allows animals to survive the initial, virus-induced encephalitis also results in the development of demyelinating disease, suggesting that while a broad host immune response may protect a mouse from MHV-induced acute disease, it cannot clear virus completely from the CNS. Subsequently, elements of the residual infection, the intrathecal immune response, or a combination of the two then go on to result in the demyelination associated with the chronic infection.

MODELS OF HUMAN DISEASE

While some viruses that establish persistent CNS infections do not induce disease, many others can. Owing in part to the complexity of the CNS, the etiology of these diseases is complex: Viral infection of one cell type may lead to dysfunction of another, uninfected resident brain cell. For example, HIV-1 is thought to infect only resident brain macrophages (microglia), yet a major neuropathologic lesion in patients who have AIDS dementia complex is neuronal dropout.

Furthermore, persistent viral infections have been considered to be potentiating agents of human CNS diseases, including multiple sclerosis and schizophrenia. While there is no direct evidence for a viral role in these diseases, one must bear in mind two considerations: 1) Viruses do not need to cause tissue damage to cause disease (17,18), and 2) viruses may initiate a cascade of events leading to disease that can continue in the absence of the infection (79).

To understand the complex events by which viruses or the antiviral immune responses cause CNS disease, animal models are particularly useful. Below, two models currently in use are discussed to better understand demyelinating diseases such as multiple sclerosis, and neurodegenerative diseases such as those associated with chronic measles virus infection of the CNS.

Demyelinating Diseases: The Theiler's Murine Encephalomyelitis Virus System

As described earlier, certain strains of TMEV can induce a biphasic CNS disease. The acute CNS infection occurs 2 to 20 days after intracranial inoculation and the resultant disease is clearly a consequence of viral damage. Surviving animals go on to develop a chronic CNS disease with inflammatory demyelinating lesions that are confined to the white matter. It is this latter form of disease that is discussed here. The parallels between TMEV-induced demyelination and human demyelinating diseases such as multiple sclerosis make TMEV an attractive murine model to study the pathogenesis of virus-induced demyelination. These similarities include the following: 1) Chronic pathologic involvement is limited to white matter; 2) myelin breakdown is accompanied by immune cell infiltration, and disease is immune mediated; 3) demyelination results in a neurologic disease; and 4) the disease is under multigenic control with a strong linkage to certain MHC loci.

Similar to the acute disease, the chronic CNS disease could be induced by the virus itself: Virus persists in the CNS, and both oligodendrocytes (90) and microglia (31) are the principal cell types infected. However, direct oligodendrocyte lysis or virus-induced alterations of oligodendrocyte myelin production is unlikely since no abnormalities in oligodendrocyte number or integrity appear during myelin breakdown. Rather, it appears that myelin breakdown is associated with the presence of mononuclear cells, since immunosuppressive therapies reduce both the incidence and the severity of the chronic disease (91).

Inflammatory lesions associated with the demyelination and neurologic disease consist of macrophages, and $CD4^+$ and $CD8^+$ T lymphocytes (32). Recent studies dissected the individual contributions made by both the CD4 and the CD8 arms of the cellular immune response, using both in vivo $CD4^+$ and $CD8^+$ cell depletion approaches with monoclonal antibodies and genetically deficient mice (knockout mice) that lack CD4 or CD8 cells.

When $CD4^+$ cells are depleted prior to infection, mice die 3 to 5 weeks after the onset of infection, implying that $CD4^+$ cells play a major protective role in the early stages of the CNS infection, perhaps by providing help for antibody production by B cells (92). Conversely, administration of anti-CD4 antibody to chronically infected mice effectively reduces the incidence of demyelinating lesions, implying a role of helper T cells in the progression of the demyelinating disease (32). Thus, $CD4^+$ cells protect during the early phases of infection, but ultimately play a major part in the demyelinating phenotype associated with later stages of TMEV infection, likely by mediating a delayed-type hypersensitivity (DTH) response (93).

By what mechanism do $CD4^+$ Th1-type T cells demyelinate? It has been proposed (31,93) that persistent infection with TMEV triggers clonal expansion of TMEV-specific, DTH (Th1) class II–restricted T cells. The production of proinflammatory cytokines, such as IFN-γ and TNF, leads to the recruitment of additional monocytes and lymphocytes to sites of demyelination. The collective impact of this accumulation of activated immune cells may result in the nonspecific "bystander" response that causes the demyelinating phenotype. Production of cytokines may exacerbate this effect, and myelin damage may result from the release of macrophage proteases, cytokines, or free radicals (32).

However, it is also important to bear in mind that at least one locus involved in the susceptibility of some strains maps to the H-2D gene, implying that a class I MHC/CD8 component may also contribute to this disease (94,95). β_2-Microglobulin knockout mice on an otherwise resistant background develop inflammatory demyelinating lesions, whereas control mice are resistant (96,97). In vivo depletion of $CD8^+$ T cells prior to infection with TMEV results in mice that are less efficient at clearing virus from the CNS, and interestingly, that develop the demyelinating disease at an earlier onset. These data suggest that $CD8^+$ cells actually protect the CNS by eliminating virus and downregulating the severity of the demyelination (98). Interestingly, the class I–deficient mice with demyelinating lesions do not develop the neurologic impairment seen in susceptible strains of mice, despite the presence of "demyelination, virus replication, $CD4^+$ cells, macrophages, immunoglobulins, virus-specific antibodies, virus-specific DTH responses, and cytokines" (99). Thus, the development of chronic disease with neurologic impairment may require the presence of class I MHC and $CD8^+$ T cells.

It is important to note that viral persistence does not always correlate with demyelination. Viral persistence does seem to be a prerequisite, but the development of disease is clearly multifactorial, depending on factors such as the genetic background of the host and the site of infection within the brain. Thus, while the TMEV system affords the opportunity to address, for example, the role of T-cell subsets, it also serves as a reminder of the difficulty in completely understanding the chain of events that leads to a human CNS disease.

Neurodegenerative Diseases: A Transgenic Model for Measles Virus Infection of the CNS

Humans are the only natural host for measles virus infection, and the unavailability of susceptible small animals has limited our understanding of the pathogenesis of the acute infection and its potential complications, which include transient immunosuppression and persistent infection of the CNS. In approximately 1 in 100,000 patients with acute measles, persistent CNS infection leads to the fatal neurodegenerative disease SSPE (100). A recent study, however, indicated that long-term infection of the CNS occurs in approximately 20% of apparently healthy individuals, suggesting that measles virus persistence is more common than previously thought, and that chronic CNS infection does not irrevocably lead to SSPE (21).

While mice are not susceptible to infection with human measles virus strains, murine fibroblast and lymphoid cell lines can be rendered permissive for measles virus by expression of the human measles virus receptor, CD46 (101,102). CD46 is a complement regulatory protein that protects host tissue from complement deposition by binding to complement components C3b and C4b. The expression of CD46 on primate cells parallels the clinical tropism of measles virus infection in humans and nonhuman primates (103).

To test whether expression of CD46 in mouse neurons could confer susceptibility to human measles virus infection, transgenic mice were generated that expressed human CD46 under the transcriptional control of the NSE promoter, which restricts expression to CNS neurons in the brains of transgenic mice. NSE-CD46 mice were inoculated intracerebrally with 1×10^5 PFUs of measles virus–Edmonston as adults and as neonates (104). Immunohistochemical staining of brain sections using human SSPE serum revealed no staining for measles virus antigens in either nontransgenic neonates or nontransgenic adults. In infected adults, measles virus antigen was found in the cytoplasm and neuronal processes of neurons, primarily in the neuron-dense hippocampus. The low-level infection of transgenic adults did not result in any clinical illness. However, infection of neonates (< 48 hours postnatally) with a similar dose and route resulted in widespread infection of neurons, predominately but not exclusively within the hippocampus, thalamus, hypothalamus, and cerebellum. Viral antigen was detected as early as 2 days after infection, and the extent of viral infection in the CNS increased as the animal aged, indicating viral replication and spread. By 3 weeks after the onset of infection, the mice developed obvious tremors and seizures, accompanied by a ruffled appearance, lack of motility, and hunched posture. Infected mice died within 3 days of the onset of symptoms. In this model system, the role of CD46 is clearly to allow viral infection to occur, since none of the nontransgenic mice, infected similarly and housed with infected transgenic mice, showed neuronal infection or clinical disease. Furthermore, the dependence of infection and disease on the age of the mouse suggests that the developing CNS is perhaps more susceptible to measles infection than the mature CNS.

CONCLUDING REMARKS

Multiple host and viral factors influence the final outcome between a virus–CNS cell interaction. This chapter described some of these host factors, and identified specific viruses, their genes, and gene products that play a role in the interaction. Interestingly, immunocytotherapy can remove viral sequences and proteins from infected neurons. Whether this will also cure the associated disease and restore normal homeostasis remains to be determined. The advent of techniques to place and express specific host or viral genes in specific CNS cells and the availability of gene knockout technology promise to uncover many of the remaining puzzles of virus-induced CNS diseases.

REFERENCES

1 Esiri MM, Kennedy PGE. Virus diseases. In: Fields BN, Knipe DM, eds. *Field's virology*. New York: Raven, 1992:241–266.

2 Meltzer MS, Gendelman HE. Mononuclear phagocytes as targets, tissue reservoirs, and immunoregulatory cells in human immunodeficiency virus disease. *Curr Top Microbiol Immunol* 1992;181:239–263.

3 Enquist LW. Circuit-specific infection of the mammalian nervous system. *ASM News* 1995;61:633–638.

4 Chou J, Roizman B. The gamma 1 (34.5) gene of herpes simplex virus 1 precludes neuroblastoma cells from triggering total shutoff of protein synthesis characteristic of programmed cell death in neuronal cells. *Proc Natl Acad Sci USA* 1992;89:3266–3270.

5 Clem RJ, Fechmeimer M, Miller LK. Prevention of apoptosis by a baculovirus gene during infection of insect cells. *Science* 1991; 254:1388–1390.

6 Gregory CD, Dive C, Henderson S, et al. Activation of Epstein-Barr virus latent genes protect human B cells from death by apoptosis. *Nature (London)* 1991;349:612–614.

7 Levine B, Huang Q, Isaacs JT, et al. Conversion of lytic to persistent alphavirus infection by the bcl-2 cellular oncogene. *Nature (London)* 1993;361:739–742.

8 Johnston ICD, Dunster LM, Schneider-Schaulies J, et al. Measles virus replication in neural cells. *Trends Microbiol* 1995; 3:361–365.

9 Gosztonyi G, Dietzschold B, Kao M, et al. Ra-

bies and Borna disease. A comparative pathogenetic study of two neurovirulent agents. *Lab Invest* 1993;68:285–295.

10 Louria DB, Blumenfeld HL, Ellis JT, et al. Studies on influenza in the pandemic of 1957-1958. II. Pulmonary complication of influenza. *J Clin Invest* 1993;38:213–265.

11 Singh IP, Chopra AK, Coppenhaver DH, et al. Vertebrate brains contain a broadly active antiviral substance. *Antiviral Res* 1995; 27:375–388.

12 Sindic CJ, Monteyne P, Laterre EC. The intrathecal synthesis of virus-specific oligoclonal IgG in multiple sclerosis. *J Neuroimmunol* 1994;54:75–80.

13 Gosztonyi G, Ludwig H. Borna disease—neuropathology and pathogenesis. *Curr Top Microbiol Immunol* 1995;190:39–73.

14 Pasick JMM, Kalicharran K, Dales S. Distribution and trafficking of JHM coronavirus structural proteins and virions in primary neurons and the OBL-21 neuronal cell line. *J Virol* 1994;68:2915–2928.

15 Buchmeier MJ, Welsh RM, Dutko FJ, Oldstone MBA. The virology and immunobiology of lymphocytic choriomeningitis virus infection. *Adv Immunol* 1980;30:275–331.

16 Hotchin J, Seegal R. Virus-induced behavioral alteration of mice. *Science* 1976;196:671–674.

17 Lipkin WI, Battenberg ELF, Bloom FE, Oldstone MBA. Viral infection of neurons can depress neurotransmitter mRNA levels without histologic injury. *Brain Res* 1988; 451:333–339.

18 de la Torre J, Mallory M, Brot M, et al. Viral persistence in neurons alters synpatic density and cognitive functions without destruction of neural cells. *Virology* 1996;220:508–515.

19 Lipton SA. Neuronal injury associated with HIV-1 and potential treatment with calcium-channel and NMDA antagonists. *Dev Neurosci* 1994;16:145–151.

20 Katayama Y, Hotta H, Nishimura A, et al. Detection of measles virus nucleoprotein mRNA in autopsied brain tissues. *J Gen Virol* 1995;76:3201–3204.

21 Billeter MA, Cattaneo R, Spielhofer R, et al. Generation and properties of measles virus mutations typically associated with subacute sclerosing panencephalitis. *Ann NY Acad Sci* 1994;724:367–377.

22 Wekerle H, Linington C, Lassmann H, Meyermann R. Cellular immune reactivity within the CNS. *Trends Neurosci* 1986;9:271–277.

23 Hickey WF, Kimura H. Graft versus host disease elicits expression of class I and II MHC antigens and presence of scattered T lymphocytes in the rat CNS. *Proc Natl Acad Sci USA* 1987;84:2082–2086.

24 Hickey WF, Hsu BL, Kimura H. T lymphocyte entry into the central nervous system. *J Neurosci Res* 1991;28:254–260.

25 Yoshikawa Y, Yamanouchi K. Effect of papaverine treatment on relication of measles virus in human neural and non-neural cells. *J Virol* 1984;50:489–495.

26 Kim U, Nishikura K. Double-stranded RNA adenosome deaminase as a potential mammalian RNA editing factor. *Semin Cell Biol* 1993;4:285–293.

27 Sidhu M, Crowley J, Lowenthal A, et al. Defective measles virus in human subacute sclerosing panencephalitis. *Virology* 1994; 202:631–641.

28 Theiler M. Spontaneous encephalomyelitis of mice, a new virus disease. *J Exp Med* 1937; 65:705–719.

29 Brahic M, Bureau J, McAllister A. Genetic determinants of the demyelinating disease caused by Theiler's virus. *Microb Pathog* 1991; 11:77–84.

30 Aubert C, Chamorro M, Brahic M. Identification of Theiler's virus infected cells in the central nervous system of the mouse during demyelinating diseases. *Microb Pathog* 1987; 3:319–326.

31 Clatch R, Miller S, Metzner R, et al. Monocytes/macrophages isolated from the mouse central nervous system contain infectious Theiler's murine encephalomyelitis virus (TMEV). *Virology* 1990;176:244–254.

32 Litpon H. Theiler's murine encephalomyelitis virus: animal models. In: McKendall R, Stroop W, eds. *Handbook of neurovirology*. New York: Marcel Dekker, 1994:521–528.

33 Calenoff MA, Faaberg KS, Lipton HL. Genomic regions of neurovirulence and attenuation in Theiler's murine encephalomyelitis. *Proc Natl Acad Sci USA* 1990;87:978–982.

34 Fu J, Stein S, Rosenstein L, et al. Neurovirulence determinants of genetically engineered Theiler's viruses. *Proc Natl Acad Sci USA* 1990;87:4125–4129.

35 McAllister A, Tangy F, Aubert C, et al. Genetic mapping of the ability of Theiler's virus to persist and demyelinate. *J Virol* 1990; 64:4252–4257.

36 Tangy F, McAllister A, Aubert C, et al. Determinants of persistence and demyelination of the DA strain of Theiler's virus are found only in the VP1 gene. *JNL* 1991;65:1616–1618.

37 Jarousse N, Grant RA, Hogle JM, et al. A sin-

gle amino acid change determines persistence of a chimeric Theiler's virus. *J Virol* 1994; 68:3364–3368.

38 Kong W-P, Roos RP. Alternative translation initiation site in the DA strain of Theiler's murine encephalomyelitis virus. *J Virol* 1991; 65:3395–3399.

39 Chen H-H, Kong W-P, Zhang L, et al. A picornaviral protein synthesized out of frame with the polyprotein plays a key role in virus-induced immune-mediated demyelinating disease. *Nat Med* 1995;1:927–931.

40 Pasick J, Dales S. Coronavirus diseases. In: McKendall R, Stroop W, eds. *Handbook of neurovirology.* New York: Marcel Dekker, 1994:649–661.

41 Zimprich F, Winter J, Wege H, Lassmann H. Coronavirus induced primary demyelination: indications for the involvement of a humoral immune response. *Neuropathol Appl Neurobiol* 1991;17:469–484.

42 Knobler RL, Haspel MV, Oldstone MBA. Mouse hepatitis virus type 4 (JHM strain)-induced fatal central nervous system disease I. Genetic control and the murine neuron as the susceptible site of disease. *J Exp Med* 1981;153:832–843.

43 Buchmeier MJ, Lewicki HA, Talbot PJ, Knobler RL. Murine hepatitis virus-4 (strain JHM)-induced neurologic disease is modulated *in vivo* by monoclonal antibody. *Virology* 1984;132:261–270.

44 Pasick JMM, Dales S. Infection by coronavirus JHM of rat neurons and oligodendrocyte-type-2 astrocyte lineage cells during distinct development stages. *J Virol* 1991; 65:5013–5028.

45 Lambert PW, Sims JK, Kniazeff AJ. Mechanism of demyelination in JHM virus encephalomyelitis. *Acta Neuropathol (Berl)* 1973;24:76–85.

46 Massa PT, Wege H, ter Meulen B. Analysis of murine hepatitis virus (JHM strain) tropism toward Lewis rat glial cells *in vitro*. *Lab Invest* 1986;55:318–327.

47 Pearlman S, Ries D. The astrocyte is a target cell in mice persistently infected with mouse hepatitis virus, strain JHM. *Microb Pathog* 1987;3:309–314.

48 Yokomori K, Stohlman SA, Lai MMC. The detection and characterization of multiple hemagglutinin-esterase (HE)-defective viruses in the mouse brain during subacute demyelination induced by mouse hepatitis virus. *Virology* 1993;192:170–178.

49 Yokomori K, Baker SC, Stohlman SA, Lai MMC. Hemagglutinin-esterase-specific monoclonal antibodies alter the neuropathogenicity of mouse hepatitis virus. *J Virol* 1992; 66:2865–2874.

50 Ahmed R, Hahn CS, Somasundaram T, et al. Molecular basis of organ-specific selection of viral variants during chronic infection. *J Virol* 1991;65:4242–4247.

51 Ahmed R, Oldstone MBA. Organ specific selection of viral variants during chronic infection. *J Exp Med* 1988;167:1719–1724.

52 Ahmed R, Salmi A, Butler LD, et al. Selection of genetic variants of lymphocytic choriomeningitis virus in spleens of persistently infected mice: role in suppression of cytotoxic T lymphocyte response and viral persistence. *J Exp Med* 1984;160:521–540.

53 King CC, de Fries R, Kolhekar SR, Ahmed R. *In vivo* selection of lymphocyte-tropic and macrophage-tropic variants of lymphocytic choriomeningitis virus during persistent infection. *J Virol* 1984;64:5611–5616.

54 Matloubian B, Somasundaram T, Kolhekar SR, et al. Genetic basis of viral persistence: single amino acid change in the viral glycoprotein affects ability of lymphocytic choriomeningitis virus to persist in adult mice. *J Exp Med* 1990;172:1043–1048.

55 Salvato M, Borrow P, Shimomaye E, Oldstone MBA. Molecular basis of viral persistence: a single amino acid change in the glycoprotein of lymphocytic choriomeningitis virus is associated with suppression of the antiviral cytotoxic T-lymphocyte response and establishment of persistence. *J Virol* 1991; 65:1863–1869.

56 Villarete L, Somasundaram T, Ahmed R. Tissue-mediated selection of viral variants: correlation between glycoprotein mutation and growth in neuronal cells. *J Virol* 1994; 68:7490–7496.

57 Evans CF, Borrow P, de la Torre JC, Oldstone MBA. Virus-induced immunosuppression: kinetic analysis of the selection of a mutation associated with viral persistence. *J Virol* 1994; 68:7367–7373.

58 Matloubian M, Kolhekar SR, Somasundaram T, Ahmed R. Molecular determinants of macrophage-tropism and viral persistence: importance of single amino acid changes in the polymerase and glycoprotein of lymphocytic choriomeningitis virus. *J Virol* 1993; 67:7340–7349.

59 Dockter J, Evans CF, Tishon A, Oldstone MBA. Competitive selection *in vivo* by a cell for one variant over another: implications for RNA virus quasispecies *in vivo*. *J Virol* 1996;70:1799–1803.

60 Cheng-Mayer C, Seto D, Levy JA. Altered host range of HIV-1 after passage through various human cell types. *Virology* 1991;181:288–294.

61 Epstein LG, Kuiken C, Blumberg BM, et al. HIV-1 V3 domain variation in brain and spleen of children with AIDS: tissue-specific evolution within host-determined quasi-species. *Virology* 1991;180:583–590.

62 de la Torre JC, Rall G, Oldstone C, et al. Replication of lymphocytic choriomeningitis virus is restricted in terminally differentiated neurons. *J Virol* 1993;67:7350–7359.

63 Ehrnst A. Growth phase related loss of measles virus surface-associated antigens and cytotoxic susceptibility in persistently infected cells. *J Gen Virol* 1979;5:547–556.

64 Miller CA, Carrigan DR. Reversible repression and activation of measles virus infection in neural cells. *Proc Natl Acad Sci USA* 1982;79:1629–1633.

65 Zimmerman J, Glaser R, Rapp F. Effect of dibutyryl cyclic AMP on the induction of Epstein-Barr virus in hybrid cells. *J Virol* 1973;12:1442–1445.

66 Jacobsen H, Krause D, Friedman RM, Silverman RH. Induction of ppp(A2′p)nA-dependent RNase in murine JLS-V9R cells during growth inhibition. *Proc Natl Acad Sci USA* 1983;80:4954–4958.

67 Stark G, Dower WJ, Schimke R, et al. 2-5A Synthetase: assay, distribution and variation with growth hormone status. *Nature (London)* 1979;278:471–473.

68 Chebath J, Benech P, Revel M, Vigneron M. Constitutive expression of (2′-5′) oligo A synthetase confers resistance to picornavirus infection. *Nature (London)* 1987;330:587–588.

69 Kumar R, Choubey D, Lengyel P, Sen GC. Studies on the role of the 2′-5′-oligoadenylate synthetase-RNase L pathway in beta interferon-mediated inhibition of encephalomyocarditis virus replication. *J Virol* 1988; 62:3175–3182.

70 Streilein JW. Immune privilege as the result of local tissue barriers and immunosuppressive microenvironments. *Curr Opin Immunol* 1988;5:428–432.

71 Wekerle H, Sun D, Oropeza-Wekerle RL, Meyermann R. Immune reactivity in the nervous system: modulation of T lymphocyte activation by glial cells. *J Exp Biol* 1987; 32:43–57.

72 Oldstone MBA, Southern PJ. Trafficking of activated CTL into the central nervous system: use of a transgenic model. *J Neuroimmunol* 1993;46:25–31.

73 Joly E, Mucke L, Oldstone MBA. Viral persistence in neurons explained by a lack of MHC class I expression. *Science* 1991; 253:1283–1285.

74 Lawrence JM, Morris RJ, Wilson DJ, Raisman G. Mechanisms of allograft rejection in the rat brain. *Neuroscience* 1990;37:431–462.

75 Mucke L, Oldstone MBA. The expression of MHC class I antigens in the brain differs markedly in acute and persistent infections with lymphocytic choriomeningitis virus. *J Neuroimmunol* 1992;36:193–198.

76 Massa PT, Ozato K, McFarlin DE. Cell type specific regulation of major histocompatibility complex (MHC) class I gene expression in astrocytes, oligodendrocytes and neurons. *Glia* 1993;8:201–207.

77 Lampson L, Fisher C. Weak HLA and β-2 microglobulin expression of neuronal cell lines can be modulated by interferon. *Proc Natl Acad Sci USA* 1984;81:6476–6480.

78 Keane RW, Tallent MW, Podack ER. Resistance and susceptibility of neural cells to lysis by cytotoxic lymphocytes and by cytolytic granules. *Transplantation* 1992;54:520–526.

79 Rall GF, Mucke L, Oldstone MBA. Consequences of cytotoxic T lymphocyte interaction with major histocompatibility complex-expressing neurons in vivo. *J Exp Med* 1995;182:1201–1212.

80 Oldstone MBA, Blount P, Southern PJ, Lampert PW. Cytoimmunotherapy for persistent viral infection reveals a unique clearance pattern from the central nervous system. *Nature* 1986;321:239–243.

81 Fazakerley JK, Southern PJ, Bloom FE, Buchmeier MJ. High resolution *in situ* hybridization to determine the cellular distribution of LCMV RNA in the tissues of persistently infected mice: relevance to arenavirus disease and mechanisms of viral persistence. *J Gen Virol* 1991;72:1611–1625.

82 Guidotti LG, Ando K, Hobbs MV, et al. Cytotoxic T lymphocytes inhibit hepatitis B virus gene expression by a noncytolytic mechanism in transgenic mice. *Proc Natl Acad Sci USA* 1994;91:3764–3768.

83 Hseuh F, Walker C, Blackbourn D, Levy J. Suppression of HIV replication by CD8+ cell clones derived from HIV-infected and uninfected individuals. *Cell Immunol* 1994; 159:271–279.

84 Griffin DE, Levine B, Ubol S, Hardwick JM. The effects of alphavirus infection on neurons. *Ann Neurol* 1994;35:S23–S27.

85 Levine B, Hardwick JM, Trapp BD, *et al.* Antibody-mediated clearance of alphavirus infection from neurons. *Science* 1991;254:856–860.

86 Levine B, Griffin DE. Persistence of viral RNA in mouse brains after recovery from acute alphavirus encephalitis. *J Virol* 1992; 66:6429–6435.

87 Lipkin WI, Battenberg ELF, Bloom FE, Oldstone MBA. Viral infection of neurons can depress neurotransmitter mRNA levels without histologic injury. *Brain Res* 1988;451:333–339.

88 Lampert PW, Sims JK, Kniazeff AJ. Mechanisms of demyelination in JHM virus encephalomyelitis. Electron microscopic studies. *Acta Neuropathol (Berl)* 1973;24:76–85.

89 Weiner LP. Pathogenesis of demyelination induced by a mouse hepatitis virus (JHM virus). *Acta Neurol* 1973;18:298–303.

90 Rodriguez M, Leibowitz JL, Lampert PW. Persistent infection of oligodendrocytes in Theiler's virus-induced encephalomyelitis. *Ann Neurol* 1983;13:426–433.

91 Lipton HL, Dal Canto MC. Contrasting effects of immunosuppression on Theiler's virus infection in mice. *Infect Immun* 1977; 15:903–909.

92 Borrow P, Welsh CJR, Nash AA. Study of the mechanisms by which CD4+ T cells contribute to protection in Theiler's murine encephalomyelitis. *Immunology* 1993;80:502–506.

93 Gerety SJ, Rundell MK, Dal Canto MC, Miller SD. Class II-restricted T cell responses in Theiler's murine encephalomyelitis virus-induced demyelinating disease: VI. Potentiation of demyelination with and characterization of an immunopathologic CD4+ T cell line specific for an immunodominant VP2 epitope. *J Immunol* 1994;152:919–929.

94 Clatch RJ, Melvold RW, Miller SD, et al. Theiler's murine encephalomyelitis virus (TMEV)-induced demyelinating disease in mice is influenced by the H-2D region: correlation with TMEV specific delayed type hypersensitivity. *J Immunol* 1985;135:1408–1414.

95 Rodriguez M, Leibowitz J, David CS. Susceptibility to Theiler's virus-induced demyelination. Mapping of the genes with the H-2D region. *J Exp Med* 1986;163:620–631.

96 Rodriguez M, Dunkel AJ, Thiemann RL, et al. Abrogation of resistance to Theiler's virus-induced demyelination in H-2^b mice deficient in b2-microglobulin. *Neurology* 1992; 42(suppl 3):300.

97 Fiette L, Aubert C, Brahic M, et al. Theiler's virus infection of beta 2-microglobulin-deficient mice. *J Virol* 1993;67:589–592.

98 Borrow P, Tonks P, Welsh CJR, Nash AA. The role of $CD8^+$ T cells in the acute and chronic phases of Theiler's murine encephalomyelitis virus-induced disease in mice. *J Gen Virol* 1992;73:1861–1865.

99 Rodriguez M, Dunkel AJ, Thiemann RL, et al. Abrogation of resistance to Theiler's virus-induced demyelination in H-2^b mice deficient in β2-microglobulin. *J Immunol* 1993;151:266–276.

100 Ter Meulen V, Stephenson JR, Kreth HW. Subacute sclerosing panencephalitis. *Compr Virol* 1983;8:105–159.

101 Naniche D, Varior-Krishnen G, Cervoni F, et al. Human membrane cofactor protein (CD46) acts as a cellular receptor for measles virus. *J Virol* 1993;67:6025–6032.

102 Manchester M, Liszewski MK, Atkinson JP, Oldstone MBA. Multiple isoforms of CD46 (membrane cofactor protein) serve as receptors for measles virus. *Proc Natl Acad Sci USA* 1994;91:2161–2165.

103 Liszewski MK, Post TW, Atkinson JP. Membrane cofactor protein (MCP or CD46): newest member of the regulators of complement activation gene cluster. *Annu Rev Immunol* 1991;9:431–455.

104 Rall G, Manchester M, Callahan E, et al. A transgenic mouse model of measles virus infection of the brain. *Proc Natl Acad Sci* (in press).

18 The Neuropathogenesis of HIV-1-Associated Dementia

HOWARD E. GENDELMAN
ANUJA GHORPADE
YURI PERSIDSKY

OVERVIEW

Twenty percent of the adults and half of the children with the acquired immunodeficiency syndrome (AIDS) ultimately develop one or more neurologic illnesses directly attributable to human immunodeficiency virus type 1 (HIV-1) infection of the central nervous system (CNS) (1–3). These are collectively termed the *HIV-1–associated cognitive/motor complex* or *HIV-associated dementia.* Clinical sequelae of HIV-1 infection of the brain include cognitive, motor, and sensory defects. Initially, clinical neurologic findings are subtle and include mental and physical slowing. These symptoms can progress, usually in months, to forgetfulness and behavioral changes. Frank memory loss, difficulties with carrying out simple day-to-day tasks, apathy, and loss of spontaneity usually follow. Inevitably there are personality changes, social withdrawal, and a significant inability to perform even the simplest daily living tasks (including dressing, eating, and walking) (4). These can occur in the absence of opportunistic infections and neoplasms. Progression to the most florid dementia with incontinence, hallucinations, and then coma is common at or near the time of death. Unlike other viral encephalitides (where a nearly exclusive viral tropism occurs for neurons or is linked to autoimmune reactions (e.g., herpes simplex virus types 1 and 2 and measles virus infections, respectively), HIV-1 infection of the CNS revolves around selective viral growth in cells of the macrophage lineage (microglia, brain macrophages, and macrophage-derived multinucleated giant cells (MGCs)) (5–7). In HIV-1 encephalitis, the distribution of infected macrophages/microglia is archetypal, with viral predilection for cerebral white matter, deep gray matter (basal ganglia and thalamus), and the brainstem (8). Neurons, astrocytes, endothelial cells, and oligodendroglia are infected infrequently. Their role in this disease complex remains uncertain. In attempts to elucidate HIV-1 neuropathogenic mechanisms, laboratory and animal model (cellular neuroimmune) systems that mimic CNS disease were developed in our laboratories (9–12). The works, in toto, led to the discovery and mode of regulation of several biologically relevant HIV-1–induced neurotoxins and suggested that both HIV-1 infection and brain macrophage/microglial activation are required to initiate neural injury. New therapeutic strategies that are now being developed in our laboratories and elsewhere utilizing unique animal model and laboratory systems may ultimately lead to the abrogation of neurotoxic activities produced following HIV-1 infection of the brain. These include those targeted against the virus, the inflammatory neurotoxic activities of the brain macrophage/microglia, and those that protect neurons against the viral and cellular factors known to elicit brain injury.

CLINICAL, PATHOLOGICAL, AND BIOLOGICAL ASPECTS OF HIV-1 INFECTION OF THE BRAIN

The most severe forms of HIV-1–associated cognitive/motor complex manifest pathologically in an MGC encephalitis (also called *HIV-1 encephalitis*) and in vacuolar myelopathy. Such pathologic findings were described more than a decade ago (13). The neuropathologic manifestations of HIV-1 encephalitis consist of both an accumulation and an infiltration of astrocytes (termed *astrocytosis*) and monocytic cells (consisting of microglia, macrophages, and MGCs) in brain tissue. Reactive astrocytosis, with an increase in both the number and the size of astrocytes, usually accompanies the high levels of macrophage parenchymal infiltration. Nonspecific white matter pallor and variable degrees of vacuolation of myelin can also be common pathologic findings in affected brain tissue. Neuronal injury and cell dropout usually (but not always) follow the high levels of HIV replication (14–17). HIV-1 is selectively localized within perivascular and infiltrated parenchymal blood-derived brain macrophages and microglia. A pathologic hallmark of HIV-1 encephalitis is the presence of macrophage-derived MGCs (18–20) that arise from cell fusion events between infected or uninfected cells. When infection is demonstrated in astrocytes, it is highly restricted, and occurs at any significant level only in pediatric subjects (21,22). Virtually all demented patients with HIV-1 infection and advanced immunosuppression have high levels of virus in their brain. Although there is 100% correlation between neurologic disease and HIV expression, the converse is not always true (23). Indeed, high level viral gene expression does not always correlate with clinical manifestations of neurologic impairment. These findings underlie the molecular complexity of HIV-1 neuropathogenesis (Fig 18-1).

Viral infection of brain macrophages and microglia is accompanied by neuronal loss in white matter, deep gray matter, and cortex. Pathologic examinations of the frontal lobes of AIDS patients show an 18% loss of neurons and a 31% reduction of the perikaryon volume. Morphometric studies revealed a 30% to 50% decrease in the number of large neurons in the frontal, parietal, and temporal cortex of encephalitic AIDS brain tissue accompanied by a 20% reduction in neocortical width (14–17). Neuronal dysfunction likely underlies clinical cognitive and motor impairments seen as a consequence of HIV dementia.

Although microglia remain the primary cell type infected by HIV-1, the precise mechanism of infection of these cells remains incompletely understood. This is in part due to their low levels of CD4 expression (24). Nevertheless, in vitro HIV-1 infection of microglia can be blocked by antibodies to CD4 or with soluble CD4, indicating the

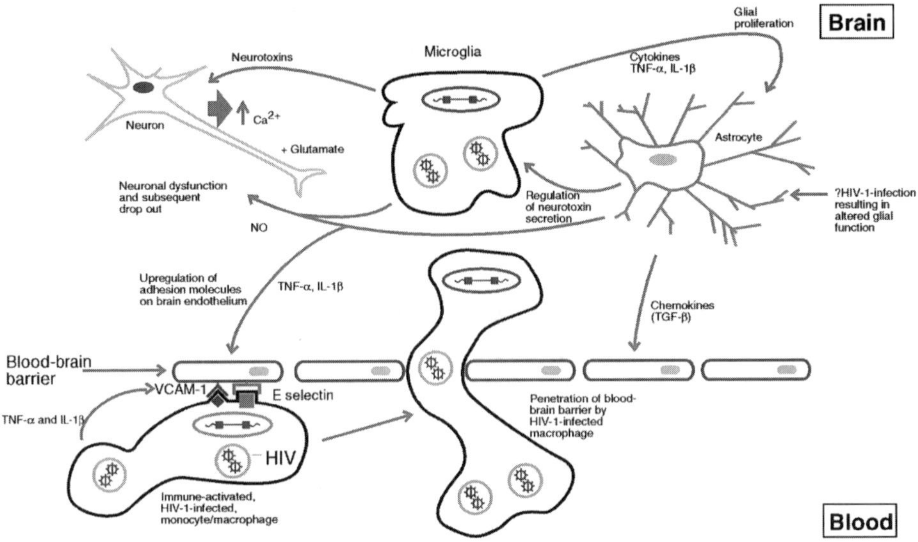

Figure 18-1. Overview of the pathobiologic events in HIV-1 encephalitis. Immune-activated HIV-infected blood monocytes/macrophages overexpress tumor necrosis factor (TNF)-α and interleukin (IL)-1β, and therefore induce high levels of E-selectin and vascular cell adhesion molecule-1 (VCAM-1) on brain endothelium. Both adhesion molecules mediate *trans*endothelial migration of the virus-infected macrophages. Release of virions from these cells results in infection of microglia. Activated brain macrophages and microglia induce astrogliosis through cytokine production and secrete high levels of neurotoxins. These toxins cause neuronal damage by inducing an excessive Ca^{2+} influx mediated through *N*-methyl-D-aspartate (NMDA) receptors. The levels of neurotoxicity are regulated by astrocytes. These cells initially suppress neurotoxicity but this effect might be lost when the viral load in the CNS increases. HIV-1 infection and activation of the CNS result in the production of transforming growth factor (TGF)-, endothelial adhesion molecule expression, and chemokines that favor selective entry of increasing numbers of monocytes/macrophages into the CNS. NO = nitric oxide. (Reprinted by permission of the publisher from Nottet HSLM, Gendelman HE. Unraveling the neuroimmune mechanisms for the HIV-1 associated cognitive/motor complex. *Immunol Today* 1996;16:441–448. Elsevier Trends Journal, Tarrytown, NY.)

dependence of infection on this receptor (25). HIV-1–induced CNS inflammation may result in the upregulation of CD4 in microglia following neuroimmune activation (26,27). This could increase the cells' susceptibility to infection and expand the viral reservoir in brain. Microglia also express high-affinity Fc receptors for immunoglobulins, suggesting that antibody-mediated viral uptake may be an additional means for HIV-1 infection (28,29). Recently, it has been shown that microglia express the β chemokine receptors CCR3 and CCR5 that are utilized as co-receptors for HIV-1 infection, thus, adding yet another dimension to the complexities of microglia HIV-1 interactions (30).

Monocyte tropic HIV-1 isolates lead to productive infection of microglia in vitro (31–33). HIV-1–infected microglia will form MGCs. Several groups demonstrated productive infection by HIV-1 in microglia, using either mixed or purified populations of human fetal, infant, and adult glia (34–37). They found cytopathic effects similar to those obtained upon infection of monocyte-derived macrophages. Infected microglia harbor viral particles intracellularly, which is consistent with the hypothesis that these cells carry a virus reservoir in the brain. Such morphologic findings have been demonstrated in patients with HIV-1 encephalitis (38). Importantly, the stage of maturation or gestational development may play a critical role in the susceptibility of human microglia to HIV-1 infection. This notion is supported by the fact that differential effector cell responses have been observed in microglia isolated from first- as compared to second-trimester and to adult human brain (33,39) (Ghorpade A, Gendelman HE, unpublished observations).

But how do HIV-1–infected, immunologically competent microglia/microphages produce disease? This question is only beginning to be answered. First, they are the primary cell type to respond to injury. Microglial activation in response to a stimulus includes proliferation, recruitment, and differentiation of phagocytic cells. Second, activated microglia express major histocompatibility complex (MHC) class I and II antigens and adhesion molecules, and secrete a myriad of cytokines, immunomodulatory molecules, and reactive oxygen intermediates. It is these abilities that permit microglial cells to play a unique role in brain injury and inflammatory responses (40–46).

HIV-1 is selectively localized within perivascular and infiltrated parenchymal blood-derived brain macrophages and microglia (47). This implies that the macrophage (as well as the virus) first enters the brain hematogenously. Moreover, virtually all demented patients with HIV-1 infection and advanced immunosuppression have detectable levels of virus in their brain. However, high levels of viral gene expression do not always correlate with clinical manifestations of disease (23,48). The absolute numbers of immunologically competent brain macrophages and microglia in the CNS are a better predictor for neurologic impairment than is viral gene expression per se (49). These findings support the importance of the immune-activated macrophage in disease pathogenesis.

Several lines of evidence support the theory that both microglial/macrophage viral infection and cellular activation drive the clinical and pathologic manifestations of HIV-1 dementia (as described already) (50–54). First, the major target cell for HIV-1 in brain (as mentioned) is the macrophage. Second, viral infection of brain macrophages and microglia within the CNS is accompanied by neuronal loss (16,17,55). Third, several studies suggested that HIV-1 enters the CNS shortly after infection either during the acute seroconversion reaction or during the time of subclinical infection (56). Fourth, a discrepancy between the numbers and localization of HIV-infected cells and the severity of neurologic abnormalities supports the notion that diffusable factors (e.g., cytokines) produced from virus-infected macrophages induce brain pathology (53,54). Cytokines can have a differential effect on HIV infection, depending on the nature of the molecule, the cell type producing it, the stimulus eliciting the response, and the stage of the viral life cycle (54). Moreover, it is the interplay of the various molecules being synthesized by the different cell types and the intercellular interactions that eventually determine effects on viral replication (57). Cytokines may also induce a variety of paracrine cellular amplification responses necessary for the generation of cellular and viral toxins that result in brain tissue injury and sustained viral infection (53,54). There is ample evidence for diffuse CNS activation in HIV-1–associated neurologic impairments (10,11,58,59). Fifth, HIV primes macrophages (10,11), and secondary factors such as brain-specific transcriptional/regulatory elements or opportunistic infections and neoplasms are required to trigger the high levels of neurotoxin production required to sustain clinical CNS disease (54). Thus, the pathogenesis of the HIV-1–associated encephalopathy revolves around productive viral replication in brain macrophages. But by what mechanism (or mechanisms) does the brain macrophage perform its deadly work in the brain? The likely requirements are HIV-1 infection and cellular activation. In support of this idea is the detection of significantly increased numbers of MHC class II antigen, TNF-α, and interleukin (IL)-1β–positive macrophages in CNS tissue during disease (59). An animal model system for HIV dementia was developed where virus-infected monocytes were inoculated into the brains of mice with severe combined immunodeficiency (SCID) (12,60). Such direct cell inoculation resulted in the reproduction of the major aspects of disease (virus-infected macrophages, astrocytosis, microglial activation, and neuronal damage). Thus, interplays between viral and host factors produced from HIV-1–infected macrophages likely predict the development and progression of HIV-1–associated cognitive and motor dysfunctions.

In laboratory studies, HIV infection primes monocytes for activation and as a consequence, virus-infected monocytes overexpress a variety of potential neurotoxins (e.g., eicosanoids, platelet-activating factor (PAF), TNF-α, and nitric oxide (NO)) following immune activation (10,11,61,62). These molecules are potent neuromodulators and overexpression may result in altered neuronal function and inevitably neuronal dropout. For example, NO can precipitate severe neuronal degeneration depending on its redox state. PAF and leukotrienes (e.g., leukotriene B_4 (LTB_4), LTD_4, and lipoxin A_4 (LXA_4) have excitatory effects on neurons (63,64). Indeed, PAF, NO, and arachidonic acid increase intracellular neuronal Ca^{2+} levels, which leads to enhanced neurotransmission (65–67). Although the rise in intracellular Ca^{2+} may not by itself cause neuronal injury, the prevention of a rise in intracellular Ca^{2+} leads to an abrogation of neuronal death (68).

Macrophage-produced neurotoxins could participate in HIV-1–associated neural injury in several ways (69–75). TNF-α may contribute to neural damage by increasing voltage-dependent Ca^{2+} currents (76). TNF-α together with IL-1β stimulates astrocytosis, a prominent neuropathologic finding in HIV encephalitis. TNF-α also can upregulate NO in HIV-infected macrophages. Human fetal microglia, when immune stimulated with lipopolysaccharide, produce high levels of TNF-α, IL-1β, and IL-6 (72,77). Multiple roles for TNF-α have been suggested, based on studies performed on cultured human adult microglia. TNF-α leads to enhancement of viral replication, myelin damage, and oligodendrocyte damage (73–75). TNF-α production by microglia is inhibited when cells are treated with either pentoxifylline, dexamethasone, or thalidomide

(78,79). Addition of TNF-α antibodies, soluble TNF-α, or pentoxifylline significantly reduces HIV-1 replication in microglial cultures. Conditioned medium from microglia results in oligodendrocyte death, which is blocked by TNF-α inhibitors (39). TNF-α and reactive superoxides can also stimulate manganese-dependent superoxide dismutase, which may be protective against superoxide radicals (80). In addition, microglia express both the TNF-R1 and -R2 receptors for TNF-α. TNF-R1 is a suicidal receptor that, when ligated, leads to intracellular signaling and cell death (79). TNF-α also leads to release of bioactive transforming growth factor (TGF)-β (81). Interferon (IFN)-γ can regulate macrophage activation and induce quinolinate (an *N*-methyl-D-aspartate (NMDA)–like agonist) and PAF production from macrophages (82). In conjunction with IL-1β, IFN-γ can induce NO synthase (NOS) expression with consequent NO production in astrocytes. HIV replication in microglial/brain macrophages may play a central role in the production of high levels of β_2-microglobulin, neopterin, PAF, TNF-α, and NO observed during advanced viral infection of the CNS (53,54). Cytokine-induced production of NO· may potentiate NMDA receptor–mediated neurotoxicity, although NO· itself does not appear to be directly neurotoxic (77). Rather, NO· reacts with superoxide anion (O_2^-) to yield a neurotoxic substance, probably in the form of peroxynitrite or one of its breakdown products (83). It is likely that cytokine stimulation of the inducible form of NOS in macrophages as well as astrocytes may contribute to HIV-related neurotoxicity. The role of reactive oxygen intermediates in mediating neurotoxicity is well established. CNS tissue is highly susceptible to oxidative damage, as it contains a high amount of iron and fatty acids susceptible to conversion. TNF-α modulates Ca^{2+} currents in neurons (76). Neuronal dropout is a hallmark of progressive HIV dementia, and neurotoxicity resulting through oxidative damage is thought to be critical. Activated microglia are known to produce superoxide anions as a result of respiratory burst activity (84).

Several groups have begun to validate the pathobiologic importance of HIV-1–associated neurotoxins by monitoring their levels in the cerebrospinal fluid (CSF) and brain tissue of patients with progressive CNS disease. For example, the levels of TNF-α, IL-1β, IFN-γ, PAF, inducible NOS, quinolinate, and eicosanoids are elevated in the CSF and brain tissue of AIDS patients with neurologic impairments (53,54). Results of reconstitution studies carried out in vitro with cultivated neurons support a biologic role for TNF-α and PAF in neuronal dropout in vivo. We have begun to investigate the effects of diverse anti-inflammatory drugs on neurotoxin production by activated HIV-infected macrophages. These studies should lead to the elucidation of the exact composition of neurotoxins and the mechanisms for CNS dysfunction in AIDS.

HIV-1 AND THE BLOOD-BRAIN BARRIER

Results of several studies suggest that HIV-1 might enter the CNS shortly after infection, either during the acute seroconversion reaction or during the time of subclinical infection. Despite such an early viral invasion of the CNS, the clinical neurologic manifestations of cognitive and motor impairments occur relatively late in disease. It is likely that the blood-brain barrier (BBB) poses a strong and elaborate barrier to entry of inflammatory macrophages, a prerequisite for clinical disease. However, in select patients, the BBB becomes compromised, leading to a reseeding of the brain by HIV, an expansion of the viral CNS load, the subsequent generation of brain chemokine or cytokine inflammatory responses, and the transendothelial migration of macrophages into the CNS. This serves to further expand the CNS viral reservoir and to both initiate and sustain neurologic disease. Indeed, the levels of HIV-1 in the brains of demented patients are usually high whereas lower amounts of virus often are found in the brains of subjects without neurologic impairments.

Theoretically, HIV can enter the brain through several different mechanisms, each of which is not mutually exclusive. First, HIV-1 might enter brain tissue by direct infection of cells that form the BBB—the brain microvascular endothelial cells (BMVECs). Second, HIV-1 might gain entry into brain tissue via a "Trojan horse" mechanism inside infected lymphocytes or monocytes. Third, HIV-infected monocytes may induce the expression of adhesion molecules on the BMVECs (85) that allow binding and infiltration of immunologically competent HIV-infected or uninfected monocytes into the CNS; these same cells might also damage and disrupt the BBB through their secretion of metalloproteinases (86,87) or other inflammatory molecules. Our recent studies found limited evidence for direct infection of BMVECs. On balance, work by other investigators demonstrated infection of BMVECs by lymphotropic HIV-1 (88). However, the pathobiologic significance of these findings awaits further investigation as brain-derived viral strains are almost uniformly macrophage tropic. Moreover, BMVEC infection in vivo during HIV-1 encephalitis has rarely been reported. Nevertheless, in simian immunodeficiency virus (SIV) infection of the brain, direct infection of BMVECs likely plays a more prominent role in viral neuropathogenesis (89a). Thus, the notion that virus is carried into the brain through $CD4^+$ T lymphocytes or monocytes is a plausible one. Although T cells clearly enter the brain during HIV encephalitis, such cells have not been unequivocally demonstrated to support viral replication within the CNS. Ample evidence exists for the transendothelial migration of monocytes through the BBB during progressive neurologic disease.

Our recent studies and those conducted in other laboratories investigated the adhesive interactions between immunocompetent monocytes and BMVECs. Such interactions, if present during disease, could prove important for the migration of inflammatory cells into the brain. These works revealed that mononuclear phagocytes have the capacity to induce expression of adhesion molecules on BMVECs and disrupt the underlying matrix, permitting the transendothelial migration of monocytes into the CNS (11). Immune activation of the HIV-infected monocytes induces E-selectin and vascular cell adhesion molecule-1 (VCAM-1) on BMVECs, much greater than what is seen with replicate uninfected similarly activated cells. As it is known that E-selectin or VCAM-1 or both mediate *trans*endothelial migration of monocytes, these data support the contention that immunocompetent HIV-infected monocytes have a selective advantage for entry into the CNS. To explore the in vivo relevance of these findings, the relationships between the expression of adhesion molecules, proinflammatory cytokines such as tumor necrosis TNF-α and IL-1β, and HIV were analyzed in HIV-1–infected brain tissue. Levels of TNF-α and IL-1β were sought as they are known to induce adhesion molecule expression on BMVECs. TNF-α and IL-1β gene expression in brain closely paralleled HIV-1 and endothelial E-selectin levels and to a lesser degree, VCAM-1 in affected tissue. Both adhesion molecule proteins were detected in brain endothelial cells of subjects who died of HIV-1 encephalitis but not in control brains without neurologic disease. By contrast, expression of intercellular adhesion molecule-1 (ICAM-1) in encephalitic brain tissue was not exclusively localized to BMVECs and correlated poorly with HIV-1 and cytokine RNA levels. Similar results were obtained from encephalitic brains of SIV-infected macaques (89). Here, VCAM-1 antigens were readily detected on BMVECs in association with virus-infected monocytes around small venules. Also, soluble VCAM-1 concentrations in CSF from encephalitic animals were increased approximately 20-fold above those from animals without encephalitis, and monocyte adhesion to brain tissue of encephalitic animals could be partially blocked by anti–VCAM-1 antibodies. In addition to a role for VCAM-1 in macrophage infiltration in human brain, E-selectin may be involved in the CNS penetration of HIV-infected macrophages. E-selectin promotes endothelial adhesion to monocytes as well as to polymorphonuclear cells and memory T cells, whereas VCAM-1 mediates monocyte, lymphocyte, basophil, and eosinophil attachment. This, together with other findings, suggests that factors other than adhesion molecules are involved in the specific recruitment of monocytes into the brain during HIV-1 encephalitis. First, the chemokine β peptides, macrophage inflammatory proteins 1α and 1β (MIP-1α and MIP-1β), are induced in human monocytes after infection with HIV-1 (90). Moreover, HIV infection significantly alters the pattern of β chemokine expression induced by TNF, itself an important proinflammatory cytokine upregulated during the course of progressive viral infection. Second, activated HIV-infected monocytes overexpress leukotrienes, molecules that increase BBB permeability (10). Third, transforming growth factor (TGF)-β is present in brain tissue of AIDS patients, but not in uninfected tissue. This cytokine has potent chemotactic activity for monocytes and can induce migration of these cells at very low (femtomolar) concentrations. Fourth, human endothelial cells activated by cytokines secrete monocyte chemotactic protein (MCP). Fifth, there is as yet no evidence that other low-molecular-weight chemoattractants that affect the ability of T cells to penetrate the BBB, including members of the IL-8 and RANTES (regulated upon activation T cell expressed and secreted) families, are operative in HIV encephalitis. Lastly, in an artificial BBB system constructed in our laboratories, immune activation of monocytes produced a profound increase (up to 10-fold) in the numbers of migrating cells (through the endothelial matrix, the astrocyte component of this BBB model system) (91). This artificial structure consisted of a matrix-coated membrane with BMVECs on one side and astrocytes on the other. Astrocyte end-feet contacted the monolayer of BMVECs, forming tight junctions. Virus-infected monocytes with or without immune activation were placed onto the upper chamber of the BBB model system. Interestingly, viral infection did not enhance migration. Thus, several factors may affect the selective entry of monocytes into brain tissues of HIV-1–infected subjects. These data taken together suggest that a major impetus for the transendothelial migration of monocytes into the brain during HIV encephalitis is immune activation.

ANIMAL MODELS FOR HIV DEMENTIA

Tissue culture systems described have limitations in adequately reflecting the complexities of cell-to-cell communications in the CNS or for measuring behavioral consequences of viral infection within the brain. Indeed, the neuropathogenesis of virus-induced dementia can only be comprehensively studied (other than in humans) in animal model systems. This is most important in attempts to answer the central unresolved question of HIV dementia: How do relatively small numbers of infected macrophages/microglia produce such widespread devastating neurologic dysfunction in a subset of individuals? To these ends, several animal model systems mimicking HIV infection of the CNS have been proposed (92–98). We review one such system developed in our laboratory where HIV-1–infected monocytes are placed into areas of a SCID mouse brain commonly affected in humans with disease. The idea for such a small animal model was initially developed by William Tyor (60). The model utilizes SCID mice lacking functional B and T cells due to a defect in T-cell receptor and immunoglobulin variable-chain rearrangement. This allows the animals to accept human xenografts without rejection. Importantly, neuropathologic reactions induced following the introduction of virus-infected, immunologically competent macrophages into the CNS can be studied without the overlying complexities of T- and B-cell reactions. However, the initial work was limited in scope (60). We have now extended our initial findings by demonstrating that this animal system can reproducibly and quantitatively mimic several important aspects of HIV-1 encephalitis (12). In these experiments, highly purified human monocyte–derived macrophages were infected with HIV-1_{ADA} (a macrophage tropic viral isolate) in vitro and then stereotactically inoculated into the brains (caudate and putamen) of 4-week-old SCID mice. The results obtained were relevant to the neuropathogenesis of HIV-1 encephalitis and were demonstrated consistently in the recipient animals assayed in six independent experiments. First, HIV-infected human monocytes remained functional and expressed HIV-1 antigens in SCID mouse brain tissue up to 5 weeks following human cell inoculations. These results paralleled what was previously seen in tissue culture assays of virus-infected cells. Second, human monocytes became immunologically activated in mouse CNS and expressed HLA-DR, IL-1β, IL-6, and TNF-α. Third, monocytes in mouse brain were mobile and traveled as far as 300 μm from the site of injection. This mobility allowed the induction of pathologic alterations in brain tissue distant from the initial site of injury. Fourth, a significant proportion of the inoculated human cells were located perivascularly in the mouse brains. Fifth, a progressive development of neural inflammatory cell responses began soon after monocytes were inoculated into the brains (within 3 days) and continued weeks after the cell inoculations. Murine inflammatory reactions developed in response to human monocyte activation. Indeed, activation of murine microglia/macrophages (morphologic signs, IL-1β and IL-6 expression) and endothelial cells (VCAM-1) corresponded to monocyte infiltration. Sixth, a progressive astrogliosis was observed qualitatively and semiquantitatively throughout the inoculated hemisphere in response to the virus-infected monocytes. The range of astrocyte responses exceeded the inoculation site. Although present in brains with uninfected monocytes, it was significantly more pronounced in virus-infected tissue (by computer-assisted image analyses and enzyme-linked immunosorbent assay for glial fibrillary acidic protein) than in brains containing uninfected control cells. Seventh, neuronal damage was shown at 3 days and at later time points after inoculation and was more prominent in areas around HIV-infected cells. Morphologic alterations were compatible with apoptosis as detected by an in situ labeling technique terminal deoxynucleotidyl transferase-mediated dUTP nick end labeling (TUNEL). Furthermore, vacuolation of neuropil and dystrophic changes were also found in nerve cells by immune labeling for neuronal markers. In toto, this animal model of HIV encephalitis pathologically resembles several important aspects of the disease, including widespread astrogliosis, apoptosis of neurons and other CNS cells, and macrophage/microglial activation in response to a relatively small amount of HIV-1–infected macrophages and MGCs located in the basal ganglia, internal capsule, and cortex. Reproducibility is a critical validation criterion for any animal model used to study human disease. In this regard, we were able to detect equal numbers of human monocytes (infected and uninfected) and the development of astrocytosis in targeted regions of the brain in 90% of the animals inoculated. A significant correlation was shown between the number of virus-infected human cells detected in brain tissue, astrocytosis, and the degree of neuronal damage in affected animals. Because of its reproducibility, the fact that it mirrors many of the pathologic features of HIV-1 encephalitis in humans, and its relative inexpense, the model should serve as an important means to test potential therapies designed to ameliorate neurologic dysfunction in infected humans.

THERAPEUTIC STRATEGIES

As described above, HIV-1–infected brain macrophages/microglia initiate an inflammatory cascade in brain leading to neuronal dysfunction. Therefore, it is important that any therapeutic strategy include antiretroviral agents designed to decrease the CNS viral load as well as anti-inflammatory and neuroprotective compounds. The later two are designed to diminish macrophage neurotoxin secretions as well as to protect neurons against such inflammatory factors. Nevertheless, combined antiretroviral therapies in sufficient doses may alone produce clinical improvement in mental function in HIV-infected subjects. Indeed, zidovudine administered transiently in monotherapy improves clinical neurocognitive function in children with significant virus-induced neurologic symptoms. This is coincident with a decline in CSF quinolinate and β_2-microglobulin. Newer proposed therapies are aimed at reducing inflammation in HIV-1 encephalitis by preventing the production of specific (or groups of) macrophage-generated neurotoxins or by protecting neurons from toxic injury. However, the successful alteration of immune function in brain tissue could secondarily affect the progression of HIV infection outside the CNS. For example, corticosteroids (e.g., dexamethasone and prednisone) that inhibit arachidonic acid metabolism may have untoward effects in overall immune function and in viral replication within the periphery. This is compounded when treating patients with an already severe immunodeficiency and opportunistic infections. More specific drugs that block PAF or leukotrienes are likely to be of greater benefit and are now in development.

Strategies to protect neurons from a final common pathway of excitotoxic injury appear promising. NMDA receptor antagonists might be useful in therapy of a diverse set of neurologic diseases, including HIV encephalitis. The NMDA receptor is one of three receptors for glutamate, the principal excitatory neurotransmitter in the brain involved in long-term neural potentiation and depression, thus affecting memory and learning. Antagonists of voltage-dependent Ca^{2+} channels, such as nimodipine, can ameliorate NMDA receptor–mediated neurotoxicity by decreasing the calcium burden of neurons. Putative HIV-induced neurotoxins are blocked by NMDA receptor antagonists. Taken together, therapeutic strategies directed against the instigator of the disease process, HIV, the prevention of brain macrophage/microglia neurotoxin secretion, and protection of neurons from the final common pathways of excitotoxic injury should prove helpful in combination therapies designed to combat the mental deterioration found commonly after HIV infection of the CNS.

REFERENCES

1 Price R, Brew B, Sindtis J, et al. The brain and AIDS: central nervous system HIV-1 infection and AIDS dementia complex. *Science* 1988; 239:586–592.

2 Janssen RS, Cornblath DR, Epstein LG, et al. Nomenclature and research case definitions for neurological manifestations of human immunodeficiency virus type-1 (HIV-1) infection. *Neurology* 1991;41:778–785.

3 Price RW. Understanding the AIDS dementia complex (ADC). The challenge of HIV and its effects on the central nervous system. In: Price R, Perry S, eds. *HIV, AIDS and the brain.* New York: Raven, 1994:1–45.

4 Navia BA, Jordan BD, Price RW. The AIDS dementia complex: I. Clinical features. *Ann Neurol* 1986;19:517–524.

5 Koening S, Gendelman HE, Orenstein JM, et al. Detection of AIDS virus in macrophages in brain tissue from AIDS patients with encephalopathy. *Science* 1986;233:1089–1093.

6 Wiley CA, Schrier RD, Nelson JA, et al. Cellular localization of human immunodeficiency virus infection within brains of acquired immune deficiency syndrome patients. *Proc Natl Acad Sci USA* 1986; 83:7089–7093.

7 Vazeux R, Brousse N, Jarry A, et al. AIDS subacute encephalitis. Identification of HIV-infected cells. *Am J Pathol* 1987;126:403–410.

8 Budka H. Neuropathology of human immunodeficiency virus infection. *Brain Pathol* 1991;1:163–175.

9 Genis P, Jett M, Bernton EW, et al. Cytokines and arachidonic metabolites produced during human immunodeficiency virus (HIV)-infected macrophage-astroglia interactions: implications for the neuropathogenesis of HIV disease. *J Exp Med* 1992;172:1703–1718.

10 Nottet HSLM, Jett M, Flanagan CR, et al. A regulatory role for astrocytes in HIV-1 encephalitis. An overexpression of eicosanoids, platelet-activating factor, and tumor necrosis factor-α by activated HIV-1 infected monocytes is attenuated by primary human astrocytes. *J Immunol* 1995;154:3567–3581.

11 Nottet HSLM, Persidsky Y, Sasseville VG, et al. Mechanisms for transendothelial migration of HIV-1-infected monocytes into brain. *J Immunol* 1996;156:1284–1295.

12 Persidsky Y, Limoges J, McComb R, et al. Human immunodeficiency virus encephalitis in SCID mice. *Am J Pathol* 1996; 149:1027–1053.

13 Navia BA, Chao EW, Petito CK, Price RW. The AIDS dementia complex: II. Neuropathology. *Ann Neurol* 1986;19:525–535.

14 Everall I, Luthbert P, Lantos P. Neuronal loss in

the frontal cortex in HIV infection. *Lancet* 1991;337:1119–1121.

15 Ketzler S, Weis S, Haug H, Budka H. Loss of neurons in the frontal cortex in AIDS brains. *Acta Neuropathol (Berl)* 1990;80:92–94.

16 Wiley CA, Masliah E, Morey M, et al. Neocortical damage during HIV infection. *Ann Neurol* 1991;29:651–657.

17 Masliah E, Ge N, Morey M, et al. Cortical dendritic pathology in human immunodeficiency virus encephalitis. *Lab Invest* 1992;66: 285–291.

18 Sharer LR, Cho E, Epstein LG. Multinucleated giant cells and HTLV-III in AIDS encephalopathy. *Hum Pathol* 1985;16:170–176.

19 Budka H. Multinucleated giant cells in the brain: a hallmark of the acquired immunodeficiency syndrome (AIDS). *Acta Neuropathol (Berl)* 1986;69:253–256.

20 Dickson DW. Multinucleated giant cells in acquired immunodeficiency syndrome: origin from endogenous microglia? *Acta Pathol Lab Med* 1986;110:967–968.

21 Saito Y, Sharer LR, Epstein LG, et al. Overexpression of nef as a marker for restricted HIV-1-infection of astrocytes in post mortem pediatric central nervous tissues. *Neurology* 1994;44:474–481.

22 Tornatore C, Chandra R, Berger JR, Major EO. HIV-1 infection of subcortical astrocytes in the pediatric central nervous system. *Neurology* 1994;44:481–487.

23 Wiley CA, Achim C. Human immunodeficiency virus encephalitis is the pathological correlate of dementia in acquired immunodeficiency syndrome. *Ann Neurol* 1994; 36:673–676.

24 Funke F, Hauh A, Rieber EP, et al. The cellular receptor (CD4) for the human immunodeficiency virus is expressed on neurons and glial cells in human brain. *J Exp Med* 1987; 165:1230–1235.

25 Jordan CA, Watkins BA, Kufta C, Dubois-Dalcq M. Infection of brain microglial cells by human immunodeficiency virus type I CD4 dependent. *J Virol* 1991;65:736–742.

26 Perry VH, Gordon S. Modulation of CD4 antigen on macrophages and microglia in the rat brain. *J Exp Med* 1987;166:1138–1143.

27 Glenn JA, Ward SA, Stone CR, et al. Characterization of ramified microglial cells: detailed morphology, morphological plasticity and proliferative capacity. *J Anat* 1992;182:109–118.

28 Dickson DW, Mattiace LA, Katsuhiro K, et al. Biology of disease. Microglia in human disease, with an emphasis on acquired immune deficiency syndrome. *Lab Invest* 1991;64:135–156.

29 Akiyama H, McGeer PL. Brain microglia constitutively express β2 integrins. *J Neuroimmunol* 1990;30:81–93.

30 He J, Chen Y, Farzan M, et al. *Nature* 1997; 385:645–649.

31 Watkins BA, Dorn HH, Kelly WB, et al. Specific tropism of HIV-1 for microglial cells in primary human brain cultures. *Science* 1990; 249:549–553.

32 Peudenier S, Hery C, Montagnier L, Tardieu M. Human microglial cells: characterization in cerebral tissue and in primary culture, and study of their susceptibility to HIV-1 infection. *Ann Neurol* 1991;29:152–161.

33 Lee SC, Hatch WC, Liu W, et al. Productive infection of human fetal microglia by HIV-1. *Am J Pathol* 1993;143:1032–1039.

34 Ioannidis JPA, Reichlin S, Skolnik PR. Long-term productive human immunodeficiency virus-1 infection in human infant microglia. *Am J Pathol* 1995;147:1200–1206.

35 Sharpless NE, O'Brien WA, Verdin E, et al. Human immunodeficiency virus tropism for brain microglial cells is determined by a region of the env glycoprotein that also controls macrophage tropism. *J Virol* 1992;66:2588–2593.

36 Dubois-Dalcq M, Jordan CA, Kelly WB, Watkins BA. Understanding HIV-1 infection of the brain: a challenge for neurobiologists. *AIDS* 1990;4:567–576.

37 Brinkmann R, Schwinn A, Narayan O, et al. Human immunodeficiency virus infection in microglia: correlation between cells infected in the brain and cells cultured from infectious brain tissue. *Ann Neurol* 1992;31:361–365.

38 Sharer L, Epstein LG, Cho ES, et al. Pathologic features of AIDS encephalopathy in children: evidence for LAV/HTLV-III infection of brain. *Hum Pathol* 1986;17:271–284.

39 Wilt SG, Milward E, Zhou JM, et al. In vitro evidence for a dual role of tumour necrosis factor-α in human immunodeficiency virus type I encephalopathy. *Ann Neurol* 1995;37:381–394.

40 Sedgewick JD, Schwender S, Gregersen R, et al. Resident macrophages (ramified microglia) of the adult brown Norway rat central nervous system are constitutively major histocompatibility complex positive. *J Exp Med* 1993; 177:1145–1152.

41 Mauerhoff T, Pujol-Borrell R, Mirakian R, Battazo GF. Differential expression and regulation of major histocompatibility complex (MHC) products in neural and glial cells of the human fetal brain. *J Neuroimmunol* 1988;18:271–289.

42 Gehrmann J, Matsumoto Y, Kreutzberg GW. Microglia: intrinsic immune effector cell of the brain. *Brain Res Rev* 1995;20:269–287.

43 Streit WJ, Graeber MB, Kreutzberg GW. Functional plasticity of microglia: a review. *Glia* 1988;1:301–307.

44 Perry VH, Gordon S. Macrophages and microglia in the nervous system. *Trends Neurosci* 1988;11:273–277.

45 Ling EA, Wong DC. The origin and nature of ramified and amoeboid microglia: a historical review and current concepts. *Glia* 1993;7:9–18.

46 Perry VH, Lawson LJ, Reid DM. Biology of the mononuclear phagocyte system of the central nervous system and HIV infection. *J Leukoc Biol* 1994;56:399–406.

47 Kure K, Weidenheim KM, Lyamn WD, Dickson DW. Morphology and distribution of HIV-1 positive microglia in subacute AIDS encephalitis: pattern of involvement resembling a multisystem degeneration. *Acta Neuropathol (Berl)* 1990;80:393–400.

48 Takahashi K, Wesselingh SL, Griffin DE, et al. Localization of HIV-1 in human brain using polymerase chain reaction/in situ hybridization and immunocytochemistry. *Ann Neurol* 1996;39:705–711.

49 Glass JD, Fedor H, Wesselingh, SL, McArthur JC. Immunocytochemical quantitation of human immunodeficiency virus in the brain: correlations with dementia. *Ann Neurol* 1995; 38:755–762.

50 Brew BJ, Wesselingh SL, Gonzales M, et al. How HIV leads to neurological disease. *Med J Aust* 1996;164:233–234.

51 Spencer DC, Price RW. Human immunodeficiency virus and the central nervous system. *Annu Rev Microbiol* 1992;46:655–693.

52 Tyor WR, Wesselingh ST, Griffin JW, et al. Unifying hypothesis for the pathogenesis of HIV-associated dementia complex, vacuolar myelopathy, and sensory neuropathy. *J Acquir Immune Defic Syndr Hum Retrovirol* 1995;9:379–388.

53 Gendelman HE, Lipton S, Tardieu M, et al. The neuropathogenesis of HIV-1 infection. *J Leukol Biol* 1994;56:389–399.

54 Lipton SA, Gendelman HE. Dementia associated with the acquired immunodeficiency syndrome. *N Engl J Med* 1995;332:934–940.

55 Masliah E, Ge N, Achim CL, et al. Patterns of neurodegeneration in HIV encephalitis. *NeuroAIDS* 1996;1:161–173.

56 Resnick L, Berger JR, Shapshak P, Tourtellotte WW. Early penetration of the blood-brain-barrier by HIV. *Neurology* 1988;38:9–14.

57 Fauci AS, Pantaleo G, Stanley S, Weissman D. Immunopathogenesis of HIV infection. *Ann Intern Med* 1996;124:654–663.

58 Griffin DE, Wesselingh SL, McArthur JC. Elevated central nervous system prostaglandins in human immunodeficiency virus-associated dementia. *Ann Neurol* 1994;35:592–597.

59 Tyor WR, Glass JD, Griffin JW, et al. Cytokine expression in the brain during the acquired immunodeficiency syndrome. *Ann Neurol* 1992; 31:349–360.

60 Tyor WR, Power C, Gendelman HE, Markham RB. A model of human immunodeficiency virus encephalitis in SCID mice. *Proc Natl Acad Sci USA* 1993;90:8658–8662.

61 Bukrinsky M, Nottet HSLM, Schmidtmayerova H, et al. Regulation of nitric oxide synthase activity in human immunodeficiency virus type 1 (HIV-1)-infected monocytes: implications for HIV-associated neurological disease. *J Exp Med* 1995;181:735–745.

62 Gelbard HA, Nottet HSLM, Swindells S, et al. Platelet-activating factor: a candidate human immunodeficiency virus type 1-induced neurotoxin. *J Virol* 1994;68:4628–4635.

63 Clark GD, Happel LT, Zorumski CF, Bazan NG. Enhancement of hippocampal excitatory synaptic transmission by platelet-activating factor. *Neuron* 1992;9:1211–1216.

64 Kato K, Clark GD, Bazan NG, Zorumski CF. Platelet-activating factor as a potential retrograde messenger in CA1 hippocampal long-term potentiation. *Nature* 1994;367:175–179.

65 Kornecki E, Ehrlich YH. Neuroregulatory and neuropathological actions of ether-phospholipid platelet-activating factor. *Science* 1988; 240:1792–1794.

66 Miller B, Sarantis M, Traynelis SF, Attwell D. Potentiation of NMDA receptor currents by arachidonic acid. *Nature* 1992;355:722–725.

67 Khurana G, Bennett MR. Nitric oxide and arachidonic acid modulation of calcium currents in postganglionic neurones of avian cultured ciliary ganglia. *Br J Pharmacol* 1993;480–485.

68 Lipton SA. HIV-related neuronal injury. Potential therapeutic intervention with calcium channel antagonists and NMDA receptors. *Mol Neurobiol* 1994;8:181–196.

69 Chao CC, Hu S, Sheng WS, Peterson PK. Tumour necrosis factor-alpha production by human fetal microglial cells: regulation by other cytokines. *Dev Neurosci* 1995;17:97–105.

70 Selmaj KW, Raine CS. Tumor necrosis factor mediates myelin and oligodendrocyte damage in vitro. *Ann Neurol* 1988;23:339–346.

71 Dickson DW, Lee SC, Mattiace LA, et al. Mi-

croglia and cytokines in neurological disease, with special reference to AIDS and Alzheimer's disease. *Glia* 1993;7:75–83.

72 Lee SC, Liu W, Dickson DW, et al. Cytokine production by human fetal microglia and astrocytes: differential induction by lipopolysaccharide and IL-β. *J Immunol* 1993; 150:2659–2667.

73 Courad PO. Interactions between lymphocytes, macrophages and central nervous system. *J Leukoc Biol* 1994;56:407–415.

74 Vitkovic L, da Cunha A, Tyor WR. Cytokine expression and pathogenesis in AIDS brain. In: Price RW, Perry SW, eds. *HIV, AIDS and the brain.* New York: Raven, 1994:203–222.

75 McGeer PL, McGeer EG. The inflammatory response system of brain: implications for therapy of Alzheimer and other neurodegenerative diseases. *Brain Res Rev* 1995;21:195–218.

76 Soliven B, Albert J. Tumor necrosis factor modulate Ca^{2+} currents in cultured sympathetic neurons. *J Neurosci* 1992;12:2665–2671.

77 Koka P, He K, Zack JA, et al. Human immunodeficiency virus 1 envelope proteins induce interleukin-1, tumour necrosis factor-α, and nitric oxide in glial cultures derived from fetal, neonatal and adult human brain. *J Exp Med* 1995;182:941–952.

78 Chao CC, Hu S, Close K, et al. Cytokine release from microglia: differential inhibition by pentoxifylline and dexamethasone. *J Infect Dis* 1992;166:847–853.

79 Peterson PK, Hu S, Sheng WS, et al. Thalidomide inhibits tumour necrosis factor-α production by lipopolysaccharide and lipoarabinomannan-stimulated human microglial cells. *J Infect Dis* 1995;172:1137–1140.

80 Wong GHW, Elwell JH, Oberley LW, Goeddel DV. Manganous superoxide dismutase is essential for cellular resistance to cytotoxicity of tumour necrosis factor. *Cell* 1989;58:923–931.

81 Chao CC, Hu S, Sheng WS, et al. Tumour necrosis factor-α mediates the release of bioactive transforming growth factor-β in murine microglial cell cultures. *Clin Immunol Immunopathol* 1995;77:358–365.

82 Heyes MP, Rubinow D, Lane C, Markey SP. Cerebrospinal fluid quinolinic acid correlations are increased in acquired immune deficiency syndrome. *Ann Neurol* 1989;26:275–277.

83 Janabi N, Chabrier S, Tardieu M. Endogenous nitric oxide activates prostaglandin F2α production in human microglia cells but not in astrocytes. A study of interactions between eicosanoids, nitric oxide, and superoxide anion (O_2^-) regulatory pathways. *J Immunol* 1996; 157:2129–2135.

84 Colton CA, Gilbert DL. Microglia, an in vivo source of reactive oxygen intermediate species in the brain. *Adv Neurol* 1993;59:321–326.

85 Hurwitz AA, Berman JW, Lyman WD. The role of the blood-brain barrier in HIV infection of the central nervous system. *Adv Neuroimmunol* 1994;4:249–256.

86 Woessner JF Jr. Matrix metalloproteinases and their inhibitors in connective tissue remodeling. *FASEB J* 1991;5:21450–21454.

87 Romanic AM, Madri JA. Extracellular matrix-degrading proteinases in the nervous system. *Brain Pathol* 1994;4:145–156.

88 Moses AV, Bloom FE, Pauza D, Nelson JA. Human immunodeficiency virus infection of human brain capillary endothelial cells occurs via a CD4/galactosylceramide-independent mechanism. *Proc Natl Acad Sci USA* 1993; 90:10474–10478.

89 Sasseville VG, Newman W, Brodie SS, et al. Monocyte adhesion to endothelium in simian immunodeficiency virus-induced AIDS encephalitis is mediated by vascular cell adhesion molecule-1/α4β1 integrin interaction. *Am J Pathol* 1994;144:27–40.

89a Manlowski JL, Spelman JP, Resseter HG, et al. Neurovirulent simian immunodeficiency virus replicates productively in endothelial cells of the central nervous system *in vivo* and *in vitro*. *J Virol* 1994;68:8202–8208.

90 Schmidmaerova H, Nottet HSLM, Nuovo G, et al. Human immunodeficiency virus type 1 infection alters chemokine β peptide expression in human monocytes: implication for recruitment of leukocytes into brain and lymph nodes. *Proc Natl Acad Sci USA* 1996;93:700–704.

91 Persidsky Y, Stins M, Way D, et al. A model for monocyte migration through the blood-brain barrier during HIV-1 encephalitis. *J Immunol* 1997;158:3499–3510.

92 Toggas SM, Mucke L. Transgenic models in the study of AIDS dementia complex. *Curr Top Microbiol Immunol* 1996;206:223–241.

93 Toggas SM, Masliah E, Rockenstein EM, et al. Central nervous system damage produced by expression of the HIV-1 coat protein gp120 in transgenic mice. *Nature* 1994;367:188–193.

94 Chiang C-S, Powell HC, Gold LH, et al. Macrophage/microglial-mediated primary demyelination and motor disease induced by the central nervous system production of interleukin-3 in transgenic mice. *J Clin Invest* 1996;97:1512–1524.

95 Thomas FP, Chalk C, Lalonde R, et al. Expression of human immunodeficiency virus type I in the nervous system of transgenic mice

leads to neurological disease. *J Virol* 1994; 68:7099–7107.

96 Desrosiers RC. The simian immunodeficiency virus. *Annu Rev Immunol* 1990;8:557–576.

97 Dow SW, Poss ML, Hoover EA. Feline immunodeficiency virus: a neurotropic lentivirus. *J Acquir Immune Defic Syndr Hum Retrovirol* 1990;3:658–668.

98 Persidsky Y, Nottet HSLM, Sasseville VG, et al. The development of animal model systems for HIV-1 encephalitis and its associated dementia. *J Neurovirol* 1995;1:229–243.

19

Viral-Induced Demyelination Leading to Progressive Multifocal Leukoencephalopathy: The Involvement of Both Immune and Nervous System Target Cells

EUGENE O. MAJOR
BLANCHE L. CURFMAN

CHARACTERISTICS OF PROGRESSIVE MULTIFOCAL LEUKOENCEPHALOPATHY AND ITS ETIOLOGIC AGENT, JC VIRUS

Clinical Features of Progressive Multifocal Leukoencephalopathy

Progressive multifocal leukoencephalopathy (PML) is a viral-induced demyelinating disease in the human central nervous system occurring almost exclusively in immunodeficient individuals. Initially described as a series of histopathologic features (1), PML became a fully recognized clinical disease in 1958 (2,3), with a known viral etiology described a few years later (4,5). The clinical profile of a patient with PML frequently includes gait disturbances and muscle weakness leading to hemiparesis, cognitive abnormalities, and sensory and visual impairments (6). The neuroradiologic findings reflect the varied clinical signs. Magnetic resonance images (MRIs) and computed tomography (CT) scans show subcortical white matter lesions, most frequently in the cerebral hemispheres in the frontal, temporal, occipital, and parietal regions but also in the posterior fossa in the cerebellum and brainstem. The non-contrast-enhancing lesions usually are at the gray-white matter junction but may appear deeper in gray matter as well (7). PML lesions have characteristic histopathologic features of demyelination, enlarged hyperchromatic oligodendroglial cells, bizarre astrocytes, and macrophages. Perivascular infiltrates can also be a pathologic feature of PML. The presence of virus in these lesions is necessary for the confirmation of PML.

Although PML can occur at any age (it was recently described in children (8)), most patients are diagnosed during the fourth and fifth decades. Once an individual is diagnosed with PML, the life expectancy ranges from 6 months to several years. However, a number of patients have lived many years with little progression of clinical disease and even some sign of regression of the demyelinated lesions (9).

For the reported cases of PML up to the mid 1980s, lymphoproliferative diseases were the most common underlying immune deficit. Other immune disorders in PML included myeloproliferative disorders, neoplastic diseases, and granulomatous and inflammatory diseases such as sarcoidosis (10). From the mid 1960s to early in the 1980s, PML was considered rare, with only several hundred cases reported in the United States per year. Now, with human immunodeficiency virus type 1 (HIV-1) infection and acquired immunodeficiency syndrome (AIDS) increasing the numbers of immune-suppressed individuals, PML is found in 5% of all AIDS patients, may even be the AIDS-defining illness, and has been recognized with increasing frequency in allograft recipients and leukemia and lymphoma patients (11). Certainly, with the advent of AIDS, the number of PML cases reported worldwide has increased dramatically. This has created more interest and extensive investigations into the pathogenesis of viral-induced demyelination.

Virologic Characteristics of JC Virus

The human polyomavirus JC virus (JCV) is the etiologic agent for PML. It was isolated in 1971 from the brain tissue of a Hodgkin's lymphoma patient whose initials were JC (5). The virus was identified in cultures derived from human fetal brain which showed characteristics of the family *Papovaviridae* and genus *Polyomavirus*. This family includes another human polyomavirus, BK virus (BKV), which is associated with renal allografts. In allograft recipients, BKV infection results in rejection, hemorrhagic cystitis, and urinary stenosis (11). Other members of the family are the simian virus 40 (SV40) and the mouse polyomavirus. JCV is a small DNA-containing, icosahedral virus with a double-stranded, supercoiled DNA, 5.13 kb, encoding two nonstructural proteins and three capsid proteins. Transcripts made prior to DNA replication code for the early large T and small t proteins from one DNA strand using differential splicing of the messenger RNA (mRNA). Transcripts made from the opposite DNA strand in the opposite direction to the early mRNA follow DNA replication and code for the three virion structural proteins VP1, VP2, and VP3 (12). The virion is 40 nm in diameter. Viral replication and assembly occur in the nucleus of the target cells. Consequently, viral DNA and early and late protein antigens are detected only in the nucleus. There is little cell lysis evident in vitro, but JCV is cytolytic in susceptible human cells. For example, the infected, myelin-producing oligodendrocyte in PML lesions dies as a direct result of JCV infection. There is less evidence that astrocytes are lytically infected in PML but they do allow viral DNA replication (13). Human astrocytes in culture are very susceptible to JCV lytic infection and are able to produce high titers of virus (11).

Tissue and Cellular Host Range of JC Virus

Unlike many pathogenic viruses in the population, the host range for JCV is not dependent on a specific cell receptor to initiate infection. JCV attaches to the plasma membrane glycoproteins using the VP1 capsid protein. Treatment of cells with neuraminidase inhibits virus attachment. Presumably, virions are internalized by pinocytosis, with uncoating taking place in the cytoplasm near the nuclear membrane. JCV has the ability to agglutinate human type O erythrocytes, which is still the basis for viral quantitative measurement. Based on seroepidemiologic studies, JCV has a worldwide distribution and is a common infectious agent, with more than 80% of the population maintaining serum antibodies tested by hemagglutination inhibition.

The feature of JCV biology that is paradoxical is its prevalence in the human population worldwide yet it infects such a highly specialized and sequestered target cell, the myelinating oligodendrocyte in the brain. For many years since its isolation, JCV was thought to be strictly neurotropic, replicating and multiplying only in glial cells of human origin. It has been described routinely as having a very restricted host range. However, other cells in the body must be susceptible to initial JCV infection in order to initiate and sustain a humoral immune response, establish sites of latency, and permit reactivation during states of immunodeficiency.

Host cell susceptibility is now recognized as the sole property of the viral regulatory DNA sequences that lie between the mRNA start sites for the early and late transcripts. The regulatory sequences most frequently found in PML brain tissue and used for in vitro experiments exist as 98-bp, direct tandem repeats. These nucleotide structures contain the sites for initiation of DNA replication and binding of nuclear proteins that control JCV transcription. Cellular host range is determined at the transcriptional level while replication is at the species level (14). For viral infection to take place, the host cell must possess the appropriate nuclear DNA binding proteins that allow T protein synthesis, which initiates DNA replication.

JCV may be unique as a human viral pathogen, as its host range is determined by noncoding regulatory sequences approximately 200 bp long.

Alterations in these sequences, as expected, can lead to altered host range (15). Although the regulatory sequences associated with JCV found in PML lesions exist in direct tandem repeats, the regulatory sequences of JCV excreted in urine from PML and normal individuals do not. The urine-derived regulatory sequences, termed the *archetype sequences*, differ in their lack of repeats and inclusion of 23-bp and 66-bp inserts into the prototype JCV genome. The biologic significance of the difference between the two DNA arrangements is not clear. It has been suggested that archetype sequences can be deleted, rearranged, and duplicated to arrive at the regulatory region nucleotides of JC virions in PML brain tissue (16,17). As yet there is no evidence that an archetype regulatory region linked to the protein coding sequences is able to form progeny, infectious particles (18). Virions with the archetype sequences are found nearly exclusively in the urine. Without information on the biologic potential of these virions, what role they play in events leading up to central nervous system infection is not known.

The host range for JCV remains restricted to humans and mostly to human-derived cells in culture. However, over the last several years, evidence for cell types able to support JCV multiplication yielding infectious, mature virions indicates that JCV is not strictly neurotropic. JCV is now known to infect many different cell types. The most surprising finding has been its association with cells of the immune system (19). Table 19-1 lists the currently known tissues and cells that are susceptible to JCV infection resulting in DNA replication or virus multiplication. The table includes 16 different cell types that were not known to be susceptible to JCV prior to investigations reported in the late 1980s.

The expansion of the host range has advanced our understanding of the pathogenesis of JCV, which causes PML.

Table 19-1. Identification of Human Cells or Tissues Susceptible to JC Virus

Cell or Tissue Type	*Viral Product Detected*[a]	*Result*
Human fetal glia		
Oligodendrocyte precursor	Virions	Lytic
Astrocyte	Virions	Lytic
Schwann	Virions	Lytic
Astrocyte lines		
SVG	Virions	Lytic
POJ	Virions	Lytic
POS	Virions	Lytic
Neuroblastoma lines		
IMR	Virions	Lytic
SH-EP	Virions	Lytic
Human embryonic kidney	Few virions	Poorly lytic
Human uroepithelium	Few virions	Poorly lytic
Human B lymphocytes		
B-JAB	Few virions	Poorly lytic
Namalwa	Few virions	Poorly lytic
B cells ($CD19^+$)	Few virions	Poorly lytic
Human hematopoietic stem cells	Few virions	Poorly lytic
KG-1a	Few virions	Poorly lytic
$CD34^+$	Few virions	Poorly lytic
Brain		
Oligodendrocyte	Virus	Lytic
Astrocyte	Virus	Lytic
Bizarre astrocyte	DNA[b]	Unknown
B lymphocyte	DNA[b]	Unknown
Kidney (urine)		
Transitional epithelium (presumptive)	Virus DNA[c]	Presumed latent
Bone marrow		
B lymphocyte	DNA[b]	Presumed latent
Spleen		
B lymphocyte	DNA[b]	Presumed latent
Blood		
Peripheral blood lymphocytes	DNA[c]	Unknown
B lymphocytes ($CD19^+$)	DNA	Unknown
Tonsil		
Stromal cells	Virions	Lytic
Liver		
Not identified	DNA[d]	Unknown
Lymph node		
Not identified	DNA[d]	Unknown
Lung		
Not identified	DNA[d]	Unknown

[a]Virions: readily detectable amounts of infectious virus are produced in a permissive infection; few virions: barely detectable amounts of virus are produced.
[b]Viral DNA detected by in situ DNA-DNA hybridization, using biotin-labeled probe.
[c]Viral DNA detected by polymerase chain reaction.
[d]Viral DNA detected by blot hybridization using a radiolabeled probe.

DETECTION OF JC VIRUS DNA AND PROTEINS IN TISSUES AND CELLS

Central Nervous System Biopsy and Autopsy Tissue

The confirmatory diagnosis of PML still requires demonstration of either viral DNA, antigens, or virion particles in demyelinated lesions. Consequently, stereotactic brain biopsy is frequently performed and the tissue analyzed by laboratory assays. Immunocytochemical tests using antibody to an SV40, cross-reacting viral capsid protein can be routinely done. Viral proteins have been identified in the swollen nucleus of infected oligodendrocytes. Biotin-labeled DNA probes for in situ DNA hybridization also have been used extensively (13,20). These DNA probes are specific to JCV DNA, not cross-reacting with either SV40 or BKV, and are able to detect JCV infection in astrocytes and other cell types as well as oligodendrocytes (8,11,13). Figure 19-1 shows a human fetal astrocyte that is actively replicating viral DNA. In this cell, damage to the nuclear membrane allows leakage of viral DNA into the cytoplasm. Detection of viral antigen is a measure of late viral multiplication, whereas detection of viral DNA is a measure of viral replication that occurs earlier in the viral life cycle (12,14) and may identify infected cells that do not go directly to capsid protein synthesis. In situ DNA hybridization may be a more sensitive assay than immunocytochemistry for formalin-fixed, paraffin-embedded tissues as well as frozen sections (21).

Extraneural Sites of JC Virus Infection

With the increased occurrence of PML due to AIDS, many more tissues have been available for virologic studies. Although Table 19-1 lists several tissues with evidence of viral components, lymphoid tissue seems to correlate best with the presence of JCV in the brain. First recognized in bone marrow and spleen in 1987, JCV has been identified principally in $CD45R^+$ and $CD19^+$ lymphocytes (19,22). After it was observed that virus can replicate its DNA in these cell types in PML patients, cell cultures next confirmed that B lymphocytes were able to minimally support JCV multiplication. If JCV does reside in lymphoid tissues, then JCV may also be found in the peripheral circulation at some time during the course of disease.

JC Virus in Peripheral Blood and Cerebrospinal Fluid

Gene amplification techniques have been applied to the detection of viral genome sequences, with remarkable findings. When polymerase chain reaction (PCR) was used on peripheral blood mononuclear cells (PBMCs), JCV DNA was found in more than 75% of PML patients, in a surprisingly high number of HIV-1 seropositive individuals, and in others with immunocompromised backgrounds such as renal transplant recipients and patients with neoplasms (23,24). Viral DNA is also found in a high percentage of normal healthy individuals, as expected from the virus's epidemiology as a widespread global infectious agent. Flow cytometry was used to separate CD4 and CD19/20 cells, which allowed detection of JCV DNA in the CD19 population only.

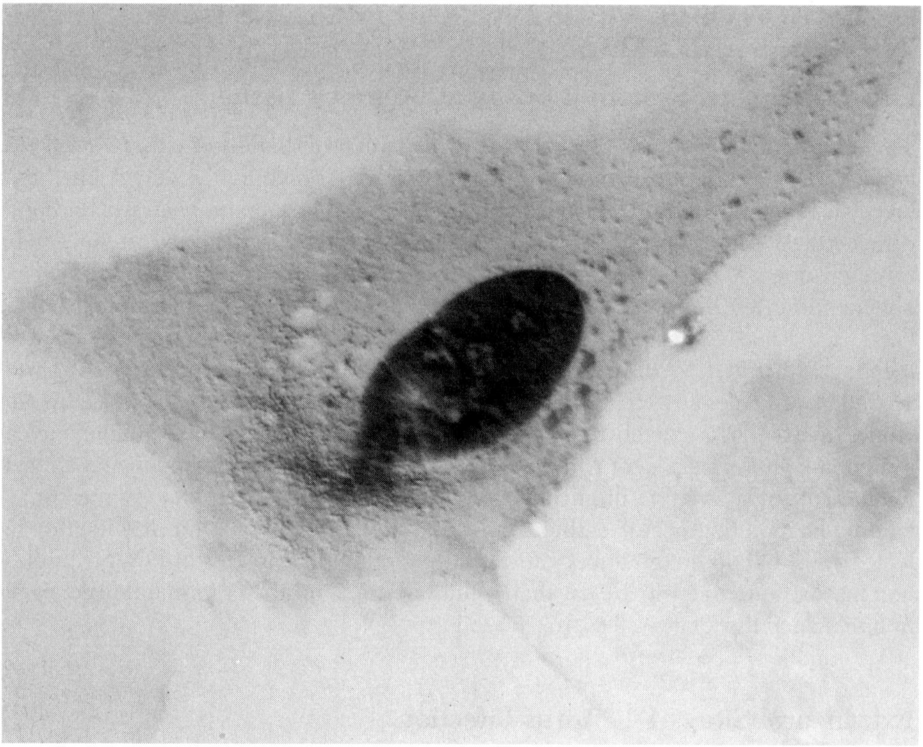

Figure 19-1. Identification of JC virus DNA in an infected human fetal astrocyte using in situ DNA hybridization. A biotin-labeled viral DNA probe was hybridized to cells grown on glass coverslips and fixed with 4% paraformaldehyde. The hybridization signal was developed using strepavidin-biotin-peroxidase in the presence of hydrogen peroxide and diaminobenzidene. A positive signal is demonstrated by the development of a brown precipitate in the nucleus of the cell in which viral DNA is replicating.

PCR analysis of cerebrospinal fluid (CSF), however, shows much greater specificity. Viral DNA is detected in 80% to 92% of patients with PML confirmed by biopsy, with a very high sensitivity of only several copies of the viral genome per 100 μL of CSF (25,26). Viral DNA is only rarely detected in the CSF of patients without PML, which may be interpreted as a false-positive finding. It is not likely that JCV appears in the CSF except from infection in the brain.

It should also be noted that PCR of urine from normal individuals as well as patients with PML indicates that JCV is frequently excreted. In some studies from Japan, as many as 75% of the hundreds of adults tested shed virus in the urine. The DNA clones analyzed for their nucleotide sequence showed an archetype regulatory region in nearly all of the samples (27). However, with little exception, the nucleotide sequence of JCV DNA found in PML brain tissue contains the direct, tandem repeat structure.

These observations suggest two important sites of latency for JCV: lymphoid tissues such as bone marrow and spleen, and the kidney. Considering that PML occurs almost exclusively in immunodeficient patients, activation of latent infection from lymphoid tissues becomes an attractive possibility.

MECHANISMS OF JC VIRUS PATHOGENESIS: IMMUNE AND NERVOUS SYSTEMS

Initial Infection

Virtually nothing is known about the initial, acute infection with JCV in the population. Since seroconversion takes place early in life, at ages 5 to 8 years, and occurs worldwide, it is assumed that JCV can cause an asymptomatic infection through a common route. There is no evidence, however, that the virus can infect the epithelial cells of the respiratory lining, nor is there evidence of virus stability that could survive a gastric infection. JCV actually is quite labile, is not acid stable, and must be stored at ultracold temperatures in a cryoprotective medium.

In vitro data showing JCV infection in B lymphocytes prompted experiments in which the susceptibility of stromal cells to infection was tested. These cells contribute to the architecture of lymph nodes and tonsil tissue, interact with recirculating lymphocytes, and are susceptible to BKV as well as Epstein-Barr virus. Stromal cells also produce a proliferative factor, interleukin (IL)-6, which promotes B-lymphocyte viability and growth. Human tonsillar stromal cells can be infected with JCV either by direct virus adsorption or by cocultivation with infected B cells (22). Several human tonsil tissues were also examined by PCR and demonstrated JCV DNA. A more thorough survey of human tonsil tissue is needed before stromal cells are considered an initial site of JCV infection. However, because of their susceptibility to JCV and interaction with circulating lymphocytes, potentially passing virus into B cells, stromal cells become an important target for future studies.

Establishment of Viral Latency

Although the initial site of JCV infection is not certain, virus does persist in the kidney (28,29). Healthy individuals as well as PML patients excrete JCV in their urine, indicating the kidney as a site of virus multiplication. Until JCV was identified in lymphoid tissues, the kidney was thought to be the principal site for viral latency. However, it is not known how reactivation of JCV in the kidney can take place in the severely immunocompromised host. Also, the viral DNA sequences of the regulatory region are different from those sequences normally found in brain lesions of PML patients. Although this observation suggests that DNA rearrangements and deletions occur during viral replication in the kidney or brain, the DNA sequences in the kidney do not appear to have biologic activity (18).

JCV DNA has been identified in the bone marrow and spleen of patients with PML, suggesting lymphoid tissues as another site of viral latency. JCV was found in cells that contained JCV DNA in the nucleus, and the presence of κ chain immunoglobulin on the cell surface identified these cells as B lymphocytes. Similar cells were found in the brain tissues of several PML patients (30). In vitro experiments revealed that JCV could infect the human B-cell lines BJAB and Namalwa (31) and normal human B lymphocytes. JCV could also infect human $CD34^+$ cells derived from human fetal liver and a $CD34^+$ stem cell line, KG-1a. When treated with phorbol ester, however, which will differentiate the KG-1a cells to a monocyte/macrophage, the KG-1 cells are not susceptible to JCV infection (22).

Figure 19-2 shows JCV-infected cells in the bone marrow, B lymphocytes, and brain tissue of PML patients detected by in situ DNA hybridization. Figure 19-2 also shows B lymphocytes sorted by flow cytometry and PCR analysis of a DNA template derived from peripheral blood from a PML patient. The PCR signal using primers from the highly conserved, T protein coding region of the JCV genome comes from the B-lymphocyte template. The occurrence of JCV DNA by PCR analysis of blood and CSF from PML, HIV-infected, and normal individuals is indicated in the graph.

The presence of virus in extraneural sites has provided insight into the cellular pathway of JCV infection. However, nothing is known about the relationship between viral latency and immune suppression. There has been only one report of a cell-mediated immune response to JCV (32). Whether there is a loss of specific T cells during immune suppression that correlates with viral reactivation or failure to control an acute infection is not known. Nor is it understood why some immunocompromised individuals with detectable JCV DNA in their peripheral blood develop PML while others with a similar viral burden do not. Because 85% of the population is exposed to JCV and develops antibodies, serum antibody levels may not play a significant role in limiting JCV infection (6,33). Intrathecal antibody synthesis tested in the CSF of PML patients was reported recently. Presence of antibody in the CSF may only be helpful for diagnosis once central nervous system infection has occurred (34).

Traffic of JC Virus to the Brain and Initiation of Infection

There are no animal models for the JCV-induced demyelination that leads to the clinical disease PML. Attempts to produce acute infection in nonhuman primates resulted in viral-caused malignant glioblastoma multiforme (35). Transgenic mice that express the JCV T protein were also produced. The founder mice developed multiple tumors of neuroectodermal origin and a dysmyelination (36). The pathology characteristic of PML was never observed. Consequently, the only evidence for JCV entry into the human brain comes from PML patients. In situ DNA hybridization of brain tissue has shown many infected cells surrounding vessels, suggesting a hematogenous route of infection (19). The multifocal nature of PML lesions also supports this observation of virus distribution in the cerebral hemispheres. Although not documented, virus may directly enter the brain through a viremia.

Another possible pathway of virus entry involves JCV-infected B lymphocytes, which have been identified in several PML brain samples (30). Since lymphocytes are able to cross an intact blood-brain-barrier, JCV may be delivered to the brain using an intracellular route. Whether T lymphocytes are infected is not clear. However, activated T

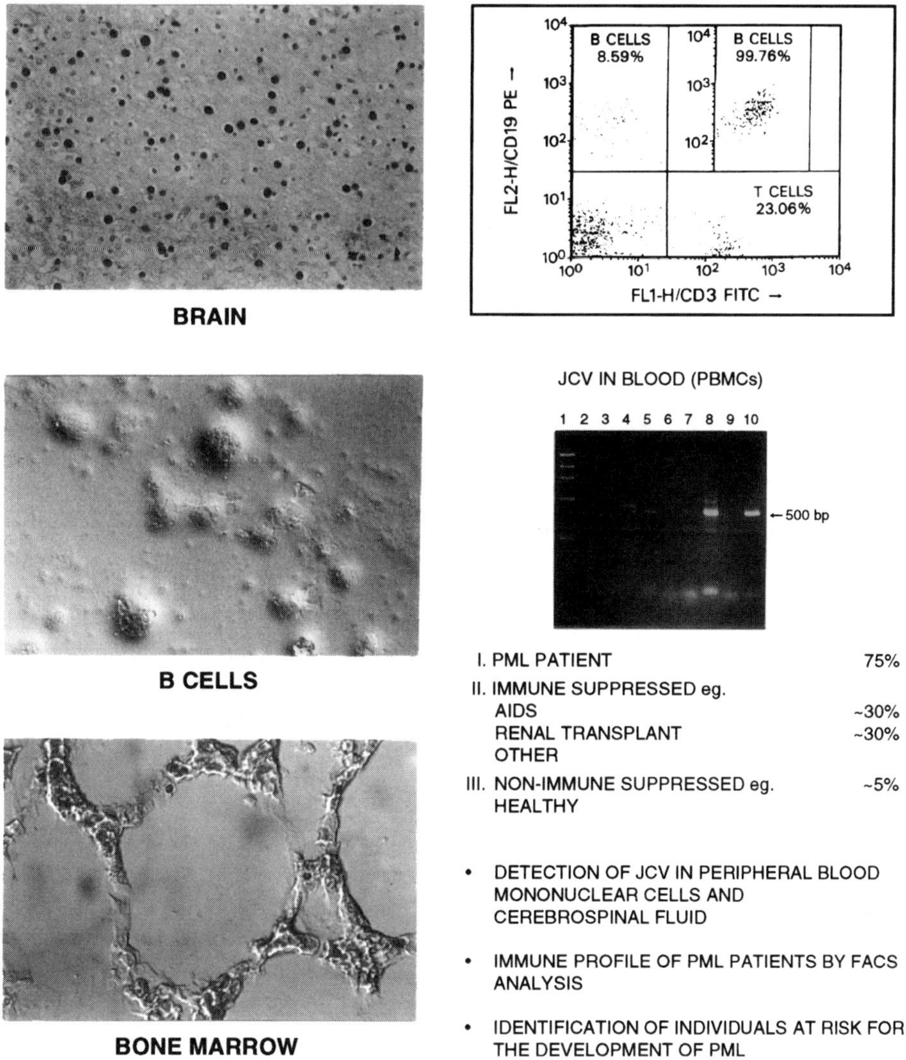

Figure 19-2. Detection of JC virus (JCV) genome in tissues. JCV DNA is detected in progressive multifocal leukoencephalopathy (PML) brain, B lymphocytes, and bone marrow (photomicrographs) using in situ DNA hybridization. Fluorescence-activated cell sorting (FACS) analysis is used to separate T and B cells to pure populations. DNA templates are made from these cells and used in polymerase chain reactions whose amplified products are identified by gel electrophoresis. The number of individuals with or without PML with JCV DNA present in their peripheral circulation is shown as a percentage of the samples tested. Gel electrophoresed PCR products derived from templates prepared from PML patient lymphocytes are shown in lanes 2, 5, 7, and 8 (template from B cells sorted by flow cytometry as shown above). Templates from non-PML, AIDS patients are in lanes 4 and 6. Lane 1 is nucleotide markers, lane 3 contains only primers, lane 9 is nontemplate control and lane 10 is JCV DNA positive control. Bullet statements indicate the important features of PML that are necessary to further document.

cells in culture secrete a factor that suppresses JCV DNA replication, making T cells an unlikely viral carrier (37). B lymphocytes also can adhere to endothelial cells with expression of adhesion molecules and potentially pass infection to the astrocytes that participate in the architecture of the blood-brain barrier. Although astrocytes are very susceptible to JCV infection, there is little evidence of JCV-infected, glial fibrillary acidic protein (GFAP)–positive cells along cerebral vasculature.

Once JCV enters the brain, it predominantly infects the oligodendrocyte, with minor infection of astrocytes. There is no evidence that JCV infects neurons, macrophages, microglia, or endothelial cells. It appears to be restricted to macroglial cells in the central nervous system.

MOLECULAR REGULATION OF JC VIRUS INFECTION

Tissue and Cell Type Specificity

One of the most intriguing aspects of the biology of JCV is its limited host range for transcription and replication. It is generally accepted that viral tropism is governed by the regulatory sequences that exist as direct tandem repeats approximately 98 bp long. Transcription is regulated in a cell type–specific manner; early mRNA for T protein is made most efficiently in glial cells. Viral DNA replication is regulated in a species manner where T protein functions in concert with primate host cell DNA polymerases (14,38,39). To dissect the molecular control of JCV gene expression, the regulatory region sequences of the prototype Mad-1 strain has been used as the model.

Figure 19-3 graphically demonstrates the DNase footprint pattern of nuclear proteins from glial cells that bind on specific nucleotides of the Mad-1 genome sequences (12). The regions that demonstrate nuclease protection, shown on the top of the figure, have been designated A, B, Z, C, and D (reviewed extensively elsewhere (38)). There are a minimum of 10 proteins identified to date that show specific DNA binding patterns. Eight of these proteins bind on nucleotides found in the first 50 bp in each of the tandem repeats. This region includes the TATA binding domain that binds multiple proteins, the TATA binding complex, and also the Tst-1 POU domain protein (40). Just upstream from this location is a pentanucleotide that binds the Purα and YB-1 proteins. Directly adjacent is the recognition site for the nuclear factor (NF)-1 transcription factor, which is found in all isolates of JCV DNA from PML brain tissues. NF-1 proteins exist as a family of DNA binding proteins that recognize a common binding site at their amino terminal end. However, the carboxyl terminal end of the protein differs for each of four classes and acts as the transcriptional activator site. Human fetal glial cells that are highly susceptible to JCV infection express increased levels of the NF-1 class D factor, whereas the nonsusceptible HeLa cells express high levels of class C. Current Northern blot analysis of many cell types (e.g., glial and B lymphocytes) shows that expression of NF-1 class D correlates with susceptibility to JCV infection (41). However, NF-1 class D protein by itself may be necessary for transcription but is not the sole factor for permissive infection. There are cell types (e.g., neuroblastomas) that express high amounts of this protein but do not transcribe or replicate JCV DNA. This observation

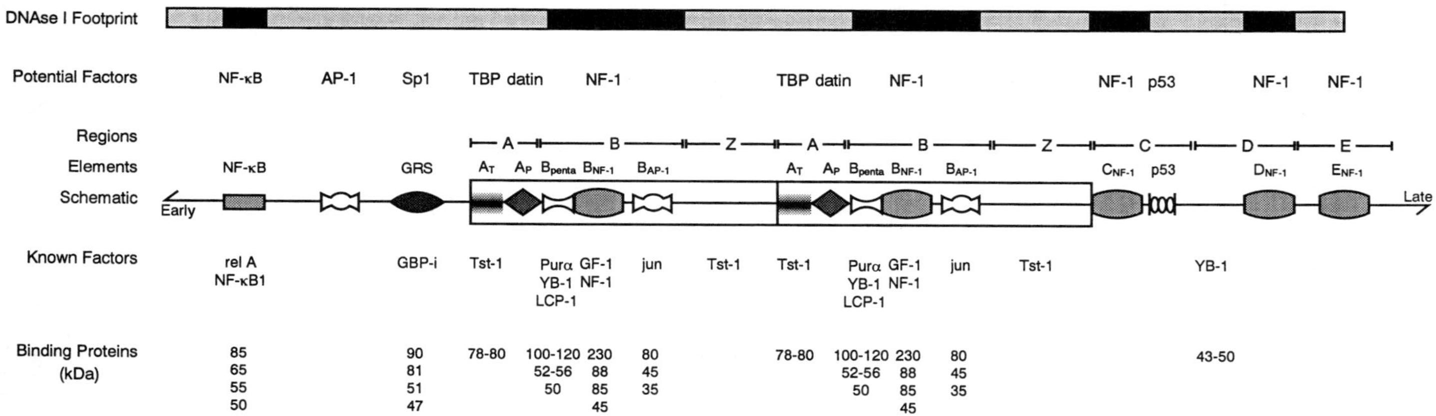

Figure 19-3. Structural organization of the JC virus (JCV) transcriptional control region. The schematic in the center of the figure illustrates the structure of the JCV promoter region, with boxed 98-bp repeats and motifs representing binding sites for potential and known transcription factors. The DNAse I footprint pattern is cumulative and depicts areas of protection as darkly shaded regions between the lighter boxes representing unprotected regions. Potential transcription factor binding sites are derived from computer-aided analyses, utilizing the Signal Scan software program from GenBank. Transcription factors that have been shown to bind to the viral promoter are identified as "known factors" while those known only by their sizes are depicted as "binding factors" with the size, in kilodaltons, indicated. (Reproduced by permission from Raj GV, Khalili K. Transcriptional regulation: lessons from the human neurotropic polyomavirus, JCV. *Virology* 1995;213:283–291.)

suggests that factors may bind this or other nucleotides on the regulatory sequences that block or negatively regulate JCV expression (39).

The NF-1 binding site is also important (42,43) as it is juxtaposed directly with the c-jun or AP-1 binding site. This configuration of NF-1/c-jun appears in many neural-related gene promoters including human GFAP, myelin basic protein, and the proenkephalin genes (44). The significance of these two cellular transcriptional protein binding regions occurring in the nervous system is not known but is the focus of intense investigation.

It does appear that the A and B domains contain protein binding sites that predominate the transcriptional control of the JCV genome. Unlike the closely related primate SV40 virus, the JCV origin of DNA replication occurs within the tandem repeats overlapping the TATA binding sites. Host polymerases are used and interact with the viral T protein to initiate replication. The limited tropism of JCV for its replication function is associated with cellular polymerases (45) that are present in primate but not rodent cells. For example, T protein can be made in mouse or hamster glial cells but replication will not proceed.

The nucleotides upstream of the B domain, labeled in Figure 19-3 as the Z region, do not seem to contain protein binding sites. Originally thought to be analogous with the SV40 enhancer sequences (12), it is unclear what regulatory function these sequences may possess. It is possible that these sequences contribute a *cis*-acting function in binding factors to the A and B sites or act as transcriptional enhancers. The C and D regions outside of the tandem repeat sequences also bind cellular factors. The NF-1 and c-jun proteins, the cell cycle–related p53 protein, and the GBP-i glial binding protein also have binding sites outside the tandem repeat structures. There is also an NF-κB binding site in the coding sequences for the early T protein which has been described as activating basal and activated levels of both early and late transcription (38). NF-κB is an important cellular transcription factor that responds to cytokine and other signal transduction pathways and consequently regulates many cell functions. However, its role in JCV regulation is not certain but warrants further investigation.

Noncellular Factors Influence JC Virus Regulation

Role of Human Immunodeficiency Virus Because of the high incidence of PML in AIDS patients, it is thought that HIV-1 influences JCV multiplication. With the occurrence of JCV infection in lymphocytes and stromal cells, the opportunity for direct or indirect contact of these two viruses is certain but has not been directly shown in situ. However, the HIV-1 transactivating protein tat can activate JCV late promoter transcription by interacting with two regions of the JCV regulatory region (46). Tat may also induce cellular factors, which in turn can activate JCV infection. Because HIV-1 and JCV are able to infect human astrocytes, cell culture models are available to ask these specific questions. HIV-1 establishes a latent infection in these cells that can be reactivated by the cytokines tumor necrosis factor (TNF)-α and interleukin (IL)-1β. Both of these cytokines are upregulated by the HIV-1 tat protein. JCV infection in astrocytes is productive but has a slow time course typical of JCV infection in PML patients. Molecular interactions between these two human viral pathogens are under investigation.

Role of Herpesvirus Family A member of the human herpesvirus family also can upregulate JCV expression. Cytomegalovirus (CMV), a prominent organism causing infection in immunosuppressed individuals, is able to allow JCV replication in fibroblasts (47). CMV infection in fibroblasts can induce replication of plasmids carrying the JCV replication origin sequences. Whether CMV also supports viral expression leading to virion multiplication has not been demonstrated yet. However, these observations of JCV interaction with other human viral pathogens that are also prevalent in the human population and cause severe disease in immunocompromised individuals may explain viral persistence and activation.

TRIAL THERAPIES

PML was once considered a rare disease before HIV-1 infection and AIDS caused a dramatic increase in the immunosuppressed population. Diagnosis of PML was not made frequently and possible treatment regimens were undertaken sporadically. The numbers of patients did not allow a formal, large study to evaluate drug effectiveness or delivery. However, two aspects of this disease have changed the prospects for investigating therapies against viral infection and for treatment for PML.

One is the increased incidence of PML, which has created a more urgent need to examine drugs that may show antiviral activity. The other factor is the advances made in understanding the pathogenesis of PML, including its association with infection in lymphoid tissues. This observation has prompted the use of gene amplification techniques, PCR, to identify virus in the blood and CSF. With PCR, it is now possible to track quantitatively the presence of virus during a treatment trial. It may also be possible to use PCR analysis for diagnosis, to detect JCV DNA in CSF, although the standards and data evaluation for this technique have yet to be determined (26).

Two antiviral drugs have been tested in vitro against JCV infection, cytosine arabinoside (ARA-C) and topotecan.

Nucleoside Analogues

Nucleoside analogues that block DNA replication have been used as antineoplastic drugs for many years. For example, ARA-C has been used against myeloproliferative diseases. It also has been periodically used in the treatment of PML, with no consistent evidence of its effectiveness (11). Cell culture experiments of JCV-infected human fetal glial cells showed that ARA-C can inhibit JCV replication at doses that are not toxic to the host cells. Table 19-2 shows that ARA-C introduced into JCV-infected cultures at 25 μg/mL of culture medium reduced the amount of virions assayed over a 5-week period. There was also a reduction in the number of infected cells actively replicating JCV DNA as tested by in situ DNA hybridization. A phase II national trial conducted through the AIDS Clinical Trial Group (ACTG) is currently evaluating ARA-C's effectiveness in 65 AIDS patients with biopsy-proved PML (48). The drug is delivered either intravenously or intrathecally for a 3-month period. The conclusions of this study are currently being evaluated since the trial's end in late 1996. ARA-C was found not to be

Table 19-2. Inhibition of JC Virus Infection in Cytosine Arabinoside (ARA-C)–Treated Human Fetal Glial Cell Cultures

	Days After Infection			
Sample	***14***	***21***	***28***	***35***
Control	< 2	< 2	< 2	< 2
No Ara-C	< 2	1024[a]	> 4906	2048
Ara-C[b]	< 2	< 2	< 2	< 2
Ara-C	< 2	< 2	< 2	< 2

[a]Titer (50 μL/mL) expressed as the reciprocal of the highest dilution resulting in hemagglutination of human type O erythrocytes.
[b]Ara-C at 25 μg/mL of culture medium; added fresh every 3 days.
The cells in all cultures survived well and were able to plate out and undergo mitosis during Ara-C treatment at this concentration.
The Hemagglutination (HA) titer shows the effectiveness of Ara-C. The Ara-C–treated flasks did not demonstrate any virus multiplication by HA assay, while the non–Ara-C–treated cells showed viral cytopathic effect and a large number of hybridization-positive cells.

effective in reversing the course of PML. However, this protocol demonstrated the ability now to evaluate such a complex, clinical disease with laboratory support during therapy. Analysis of other antiviral drugs as well as better delivery of these drugs to the central nervous system at the site of PML lesions may be possible in the future.

Topoisomerase Inhibitors

Because of the circular, supercoiled structure of the JCV genome DNA, its replication requires nicking and untwisting of the parental strands. The viral T protein provides helicase activity to assist in DNA replication, but to complete the synthesis of daughter strands of DNA, cellular topoisomerase, DNA topoisomerase 1, activity is also required. Topotecan and its derivatives possess topoisomerase inhibitory activity. One of these derivatives, camptothecin, effectively blocks JCV DNA replication in glial cells (49). To be effective, camptothecin was added in pulse treatments of cells but was not toxic. The drug did not interfere with the transcription of DNA topoisomerase 1. The family of topoisomerase inhibitors, including camptothecin and 9-topotecan, may be useful in treating PML. Future clinical trials are being designed to evaluate these drugs.

EPILOGUE

New technologies exemplified by PCR allow highly sensitive detection of viral genetic information in any organ and cell in the body. Such methods have advanced our understanding of the pathogenesis and, particularly, the molecular mechanisms that underlie virus-induced diseases of the nervous system. Determining the route of JCV infection through lymphoid tissues and peripheral blood to the central nervous system is only one example of the application of these methods. This observation has possibly solved the difficult problem of understanding how a virus that is widespread in the world's population could find a highly specialized and sequestered cell in the white matter of the brain. But with new information coming from clinics and laboratories, another set of problems arise and need to be addressed in the future. We have identified individuals with immunosuppressive illness who do not have PML but who do carry virus in the peripheral blood. We need now to understand the correlation of the immune deficits with the onset of PML. What are the risk factors for the development of PML? Is there a specific loss of T-cell subsets whose absence leads to viral reactivation from latency? If PML occurs in 5% of AIDS patients, what circumstances promote the onset of this neurologic disease in these patients but not others? It is necessary to identify individuals who are at risk for the development of PML and to design therapies and methods for therapeutic delivery that could prevent the disease and treat affected patients.

Recently JCV was implicated for the first time in genetic and neoplastic pathologies in humans. This virus is now associated serologically with populations who demonstrate chromosomal aberrations (50) and with the occurrence of an oligoastrocytoma in an immunocompetent individual (51). Investigating the importance of these observations and their implications on the risks of JCV-induced diseases takes on new emphasis and will require more intensive clinical and basic studies.

REFERENCES

1 Hallervorden J. Eigennartige und nicht rubriziebare Prozesse. In: Bumke O, ed. *Handbuch der Geiteskranheiten, Die Anatomie der Psychosen*. Vol. 2. Berlin: Springer, 1930.

2 Astrom K-E, Mancall EL, Richardson EP Jr. Progressive multifocal leukoencephalopathy. *Brain* 1958;81:93–127.

3 Richardson EP Jr. Progressive multifocal leukoencephalopathy. *N Engl J Med* 1961;265:815–823.

4 ZuRhein GM. Association of papovavirions with a human demyelinating disease (progressive multifocal leukoencephalopathy). *Prog Med Virol* 1969;11:185–247.

5 Padgett BL, ZuRhein G, Walker D, et al. Cultivation of papova-like virus from human brain with progressive multifocal leucoencephalopathy. *Lancet* 1971;1:1257–1260.

6 Brooks BR, Walker DL. Progressive multifocal leukoencephalopathy. *Neurol Clin* 1984;2:299–313.

7 Whiteman ML, Post MJ, Berger JR, et al. Progressive multifocal leukoencephalopathy in 47 HIV-seropositive patients: neuroimaging with clinical and pathologic correlation. *Radiology* 1993;187:233–240.

8 Berger JR, Scott G, Albrecht J, et al. Progressive multifocal leukoencephalopathy in HIV-1 infected children. *AIDS* 1992;6:837–841.

9 Berger JR, Mucke L. Prolonged survival and partial recovery in AIDS-associated progressive multifocal leukoencephalopathy. *Neurology* 1988;38:1060–1065.

10 Major EO, Ault GS. Progressive multifocal leukoencephalopathy: clinical and laboratory observations on a viral induced demyelinating disease in the immunodeficient patient. *Curr Opin Neurol* 1995;8:184–190.

11 Major EO, Amemiya K, Tornatore CS, et al. Pathogenesis and molecular biology of progressive multifocal leukoencephalopathy, the JC virus-induced demyelinating disease of the human brain. *Clin Microbiol Rev* 1992;5:49–73.

12 Frisque RJ, Bream GL, Cannella MT. Human polyomavirus JC virus genome. *J Virol* 1984; 51:458–469.

13 Aksamit AJ, Mourrain P, Sever JL, Major EO. Progressive multifocal leukoencephalopathy: investigation of three cases using in situ hybridization with JC virus biotinylated DNA probe. *Ann Neurol* 1985;18:490–496.

14 Feigenbaum L, Khalili K, Major EO, Khoury

G. Regulation of the host range of human papovavirus JCV. *Proc Natl Acad Sci USA* 1987; 84:3695–3698.

15 Vacante DA, Traub R, Major EO. Extension of JC virus host range to monkey cells by insertion of a simian virus 40 enhancer into the JC virus regulatory region. *Virology* 1989;170:353–361.

16 Iida T, Kitamura T, Guo J, et al. Origin of JC polyomavirus variants associated with progressive multifocal leukoencephalopathy. *Proc Natl Acad Sci USA* 1993;90:5062–5065.

17 Ault GS, Stoner GL. Human polyomavirus JC promoter/enhancer rearrangement patterns from progressive multifocal leukoencephalopathy brain are unique derivatives of a single archetypal structure. *J Gen Virol* 1993;74:1499–1507.

18 Daniel AM, Swenson JJ, Reddy Mayreddy RP, et al. Sequences within the early and late promoters of archetype JC virus restrict viral DNA replication and infectivity. *Virology* 1996;216: 90–101.

19 Houff SA, Major EO, Katz DA, et al. Involvement of JC virus infected mononuclear cells from the bone marrow and spleen in the pathogenesis of progressive multifocal leukoencephalopathy. *N Engl J Med* 1988;318:301–305.

20 Houff SA, Katz D, Kufta C, Major EO. A rapid method for in situ hybridization for viral DNA in brain biopsies from patients with AIDS. *AIDS* 1989;3:843–845.

21 Aksamit AJ, Sever JL, Major EO. Progressive multifocal leukoencephalopathy: JC virus detection by in situ hybridization compared with immunocytochemistry. *Neurology* 1986;36:499–504.

22 Monaco MCG, Atwood WJ, Gravell M, et al. JC virus infection of hematopoietic progenitor cells, primary B lymphocytes, and tonsillar stromal cells: implications for viral latency. *J Virol* 1996;70:7004–7012.

23 Tornatore CS, Berger JR, Houff SA, et al. Detection of JC virus DNA in peripheral lymphocytes from patients with and without progressive multifocal leukoencephalopathy. *Ann Neurol* 1992;31:454–462.

24 Dorries K, Vogel E, Gunther S, Czub S. Infection of human polyomavirus JC and BK in peripheral blood leukocytes from immunocompetent individuals. *Virology* 1994;198:59–70.

25 McGuire D, Barhite S, Hollander H, Miles M. JC virus DNA in cerebrospinal fluid of human immunodeficiency virus-infected patients: predictive value for progressive multifocal leukoencephalopathy. *Ann Neurol* 1995;37:395–399.

26 Weber T, Turner RW, Frye S, et al. Progressive multifocal leukoencephalopathy diagnosed by amplification of JC virus-specific DNA from cerebrospinal fluid. *AIDS* 1994;8:49–57.

27 Yogo Y, Kitamura T, Sugimoto C, et al. Isolation of a possible archetypal JC virus DNA sequence from nonimmunocompromised individuals. *J Virol* 1990;64:3139–3143.

28 Flaegstad T, Sundsfjord A, Arthur RR, et al. Amplification and sequencing of the control regions of BK and JC virus from human urine by polymerase chain reaction. *Virology* 1991;180: 553–560.

29 Kitamura T, Aso Y, Kuniyoshi N, et al. High incidence of urinary JC virus excretion in nonimmunosuppressed older patients. *J Infect Dis* 1990;161:1128–1133.

30 Major EO, Amemiya K, Elder G, Houff SA. Glial cells of the human developing brain and B cells of the immune system share a common DNA binding factor for recognition of the regulatory sequences of the human polyomavirus, JCV. *J Neurosci Res* 1990;27:461–471.

31 Atwood WJ, Amemiya K, Traub R, et al. Interaction of the polyomavirus JC virus, with human B-lymphocytes. *Virology* 1992;190:716–723.

32 Willoughby ER, Price W, Padgett BL, et al. Progressive multifocal leukoencephalopathy (PML): in vitro cell-mediated immune responses to mitogens and JC virus. *Neurology* 1980; 30:256–262.

33 Knowles WA, Gibson PE, Hand JF, Brown DWG. An M-antibody capture radioimmunoassay (MACRIA) for detection of JC virus-specific IgM. *J Virol Methods* 1992;40:95–106.

34 Weber T, Trebst C, Frye S, et al. Intra-blood-brain-barrier synthesis of antibodies to JC virus in patients with progressive multifocal leukoencephalopathy. *J Infect Dis* 1997 (in press).

35 London WT, Houff SA, Madden DL, et al. Brain tumors in owl monkeys inoculated with a human polyomavirus (JC virus). *Science* 1978; 201:1246–1249.

36 Small JA, Khoury G, Jay G, et al. Early regions of JC virus and BK virus induce distinct and tissue-specific tumors in transgenic mice. *Proc Natl Acad Sci USA* 1986;83:8288–8292.

37 Chang DF, Otte J, Kerr DA, et al. Evidence that the soluble factors secreted by activated immune cells suppress replication of the human neurotropic JC virus DNA in glial cells. *Virology* 1996;221:226–231.

38 Raj GV, Khalili K. Transcriptional regulation: lessons from the human neurotropic polyomavirus, JCV. *Virology* 1995;213:283–291.

39 Tada H, Lashgari M, Rappaport J, Khalili K. Cell type-specific expression of JC virus early promoter is determined by positive and negative regulation. *J Virol* 1989;63:463–466.

40 Wegner M, Droplet DW, Rosenfeld MG. Regulation of JC virus by the POU-domain transcription factor Tst-1: implications for progressive multifocal leukoencephalopathy. *Proc Natl Acad Sci USA* 1993;90:4743–4747.

41 Sumner C, Shinohara T, Durham L, et al. Expression of multiple classes of the nuclear factor-1 family in the developing human brain: differential expression of two classes of NF-1 genes. *J Neurovirol* 1996;2:87–100.

42 Sock E, Wegner M, Grummt F. DNA replication of human polyomavirus JC is stimulated by NF-1 in vivo. *Virology* 1991;182:298–308.

43 Renner K, Leger H, Wegner M. The POU domain protein Tst-1 and papovaviral large tumor antigen function synergistically to stimulate glia-specific gene expression of JC virus. *Proc Natl Acad Sci USA* 1994;91:6433–6437.

44 Amemiya K, Traub R, Durham L, Major EO. Adjacent nuclear factor-1 and activator protein binding sites in the enhancer of the neurotropic JC virus. A common characteristic of many brain-specific genes. *J Biol Chem* 1992;267: 14204–14211.

45 Walker DL, Frisque RJ. The biology and molecular biology of JC virus. In: Salzman NP, ed. *The papovaviridae*. New York: Plenum, 1986: 327–377.

46 Tada H, Rappaport J, Lashgari MS, et al. Transactivation of the JC virus late promoter by the tat protein of type 1 human immunodeficiency virus in glial cells. *Proc Natl Acad Sci USA* 1990;87:3479–3483.

47 Heilbronn R, Albrecht I, Stephan S, et al. Human cytomegalovirus induces JC virus DNA replication in human fibroblasts. *Proc Natl Acad Sci USA* 1993;90:11406–11410.

48 AIDS Clinical Trial Group. A phase II multicenter study comparing antiretroviral therapy alone to antiretroviral therapy plus cytosine arabinoside (ARA-C) for the treatment of progressive multifocal leukoencephalopathy (PML) in human immunodeficiency virus (HIV) infected subjects sponsored by The National Institute of Allergy and Infectious Diseases. Twenty Second AIDS Clinical Trials Group Meeting (ACTG); Protocol A243, Washington, D.C., 1996.

49 Kerr DA, Chang CF, Gordon J, et al. Inhibition of human neurotropic virus (JCV) DNA replication in glial cells by camptothecin. *Virology* 1993;196:612–618.

50 Neel JV, Major EO, Awa AA, et al. Rogue type chromosomal damage in lymphocytes is associated with infection with the human polyomavirus JCV: an hypothesis. *Proc Natl Acad Sci USA* 1996;93:2690–2695.

51 Rencic A, Gordon J, Otte J, et al. Detection of JC virus DNA sequence and expression of the viral oncoprotein, tumor antigen, in brain of immunocompetent patient with oligoastrocytoma. *Proc Natl Acad Sci USA* 1996;93:7352–7357.

20

Molecular Pathogenesis of Genetic and Infectious Prion Diseases

STANLEY B. PRUSINER

Prions cause a group of human and animal neurodegenerative diseases that are now classified together because their etiology and pathogenesis involve modification of the prion protein (PrP) (1). Prion diseases are manifest as infectious, genetic, and sporadic disorders. These diseases can be transmitted among mammals by the infectious particle designated *prion* (2). Despite intensive searches over the past three decades, no nucleic acid has been found within prions (3,4), yet a modified isoform of the host-encoded PrP, designated *PrP^{Sc}*, is essential for infectivity (1,5–7). In fact, considerable experimental data argue that prions are composed exclusively of PrP^{Sc}. Earlier terms used to describe the prion diseases include *transmissible encephalopathies, spongiform encephalopathies*, and *slow virus diseases* (8). The human prion disorders include kuru, Creutzfeldt-Jakob disease (CJD), Gerstmann-Sträussler-Scheinker (GSS) syndrome, and fatal familial insomnia (FFI).

Studies of the prion diseases have taken on new significance with the recent report of atypical CJD in three teenagers and nine young adults (9,10). All but one of these cases have been reported from Great Britain where more than 160,000 cattle have died of bovine spongiform encephalopathy (BSE), or mad cow disease as it is often called (11,12). It now seems possible that bovine prions pass to humans through the consumption of tainted beef products. The number of cases of atypical CJD caused by bovine prions that may occur in the years ahead is unknown.

The experimental transmissions of CJD and kuru from humans to apes ushered in an exciting period of neurologic research that focused first on kuru—a disease of epidemic proportions centered in the Fore region of the New Guinea highlands—and subsequently on CJD and GSS syndrome (8). Upon transmission of kuru to apes in 1966, the possibility that kuru was transmitted among the New Guinea natives by ritualistic cannibalism was no longer remote. Such transmission studies were stimulated by the insightful suggestion of Hadlow (13) that the neuropathology of kuru resembled that of scrapie, and thus that the disease might be transmissible after intracerebral inoculation of brain extracts into apes following a prolonged incubation time.

Scrapie of sheep and goats possesses an equally fascinating history. For many years,

British scientists had argued about whether natural scrapie was a genetic or an infectious disease (14). Scrapie, like kuru and CJD, caused death of the host without any sign of an immune response to a "foreign infectious agent." Debate about scrapie was heightened in 1967, when Tikvah Alper et al. (3) reported the extraordinary resistance of the scrapie agent to inactivation by ionizing and ultraviolet (UV) irradiation. Speculation about the composition of the scrapie agent increased over the following decade.

ORIGIN OF THE PRION CONCEPT

Once an effective protocol was developed for preparation of partially purified fractions of scrapie agent from hamster brain, investigators could demonstrate that procedures modifying or hydrolyzing proteins diminish scrapie infectivity (2,15). At the same time, tests done in search of a scrapie-specific nucleic acid did not demonstrate any dependence of infectivity on a polynucleotide (2), in agreement with earlier studies reporting the extreme resistance of infectivity to UV irradiation at 254 nm (3). Based on these findings, the term *prion* was introduced to distinguish the proteinaceous infectious particles that cause scrapie, CJD, GSS, and kuru from both viroids and viruses (2). It now seems likely that the scrapie agent may be composed only of a protein that adopts an abnormal conformation (16,17).

PRION PROTEINS

After it was established that scrapie prion infectivity in partially purified fractions depended on protein (15), the search for a scrapie-specific protein intensified. While the insolubility of scrapie infectivity made purification problematic, my colleagues and I took advantage of this property along with its relative resistance to degradation by proteases to extend the degree of purification. In subcellular fractions from Syrian hamster (SHa) brain enriched for scrapie infectivity, a protease-resistant PrP of 27 to 30 kd, designated *PrP 27-30*, was identified and found to be absent in control animals (18–20). Radioiodination of partially purified fractions revealed a protein unique to preparations from scrapie-infected brains (18,19).

Purification of PrP 27-30 to homogeneity allowed determination of its NH_2-terminal amino acid sequence (21). This permitted the synthesis of an isocoding mixture of oligonucleotides that was subsequently used to identify PrP complementary DNA (cDNA) clones (22–25). It was found that PrP is encoded by a chromosomal gene and not by a nucleic acid within the infectious scrapie prion particle (22,24). Levels of PrP messenger RNA (mRNA) remain unchanged throughout the course of scrapie infection—an observation that led to the identification of the normal PrP gene product, a protein of 33 to 35 kd, designated *PrP*^{C} (22,24). PrP^{C} is protease sensitive, while PrP 27-30 is the protease-resistant core of a 33- to 35-kd disease-specific protein, designated *PrP*^{Sc} (24,26). At the same time, it was found that the brains of normal and scrapie-infected hamsters express similar levels of PrP mRNA and a protease-sensitive PrP designated *PrP*^{C} (24). PrP^{C} or a subset of PrP molecules is the substrate for PrP^{Sc}.

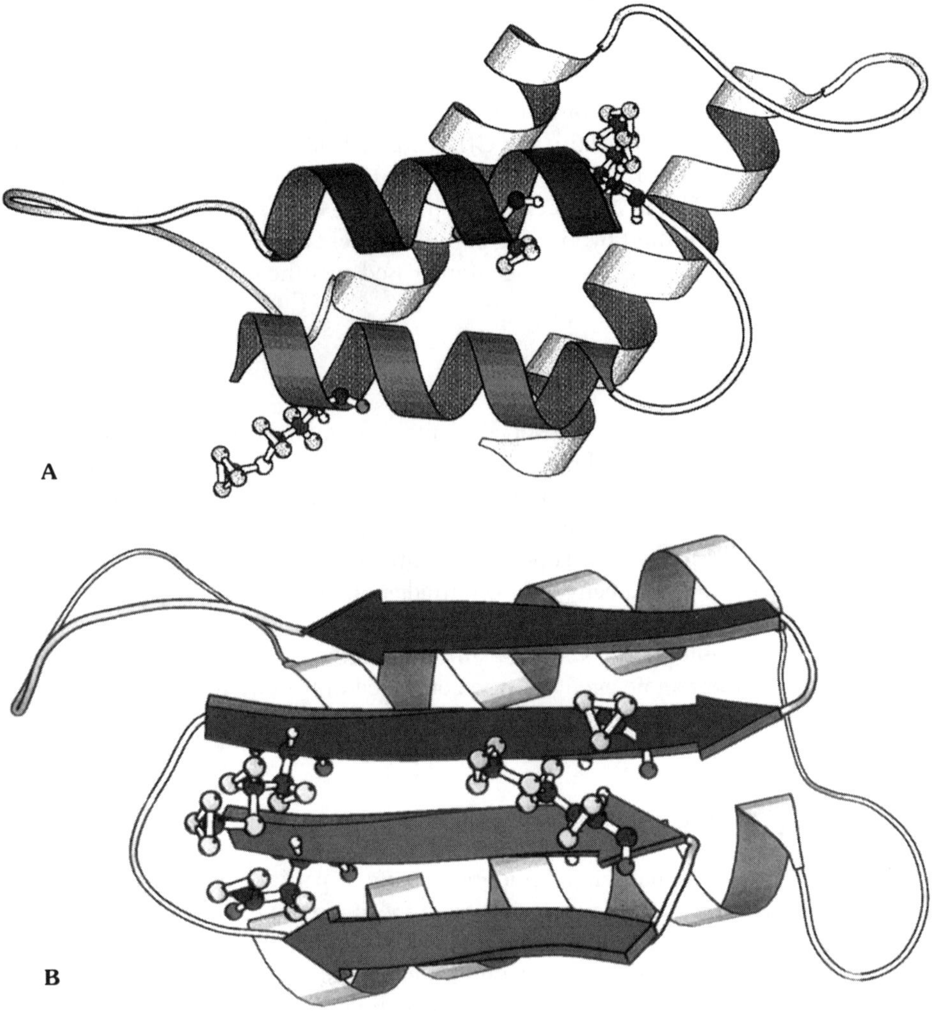

Figure 20-1. Plausible models for the tertiary structures of PrP^{Sc} and PrP^{C}. (A) The proposed three-dimensional structure of PrP^{C} (35). Helix 1 is on the bottom while helix 2 is on the top. We believe that helices 1 and 2 are converted into β-sheet structure during the formation of PrP^{Sc}. The H2-H3 loop corresponding to the S2b-H3 loop in PrP^{Sc} is shown on the left. Four residues (Asn-108, Met-112, Met-129, and Ala-133) implicated in the species barrier as noted above are shown in the ball-and-stick model. (B) The proposed three-dimensional structure of PrP^{Sc} (36). This structure was chosen from the six penultimate models of PrP^{Sc} because it appeared to correlate best with genetic data on residues involved in species barrier. It contains a four-strand mixed β-sheet with two α-helices packed against one face of the sheet. Strands 1a and 1b (on the bottom) correspond to the helix 1 in PrP^{C} while strands 2a and 2b (on the top) correspond to the helix 2. Helices 3 and 4 in this model remain unchanged from the PrP^{C} model (35). Four residues (Asn-108, Met-112, Met-129, and Ala-133) implicated in the species barrier (107) are shown in the ball-and-stick model. They cluster on the solvent accessible surface of the β-sheet, which might provide a plausible interface for the PrP^{Sc}-PrP^{C} interaction. The

Cell Biology of PrP^{Sc} Formation

In scrapie-infected cells, PrP^{C} molecules destined to become PrP^{Sc} exit to the cell surface prior to conversion into PrP^{Sc} (27–30). Like other GPI-anchored proteins, PrP^{C} appears to re-enter the cell through a subcellular compartment bounded by cholesterol-rich, detergent-insoluble membranes that might be caveolae or early endosomes (31). Within this cholesterol-rich, nonacidic compartment, GPI-anchored PrP^{C} can be either converted into PrP^{Sc} or partially degraded (31). PrP^{Sc} is trimmed at the N-terminus in an acidic compartment in scrapie-infected cultured cells to form PrP 27-30 (30,32). In contrast, N-terminal trimming of PrP^{Sc} is minimal in the brain, where little PrP 27-30 is found (33).

STRUCTURES OF PRION PROTEIN ISOFORMS

In a search for a posttranslational chemical modification that might explain the differences in the properties of these two PrP isoforms, PrP^{Sc} was analyzed by mass spectrometry and gas phase sequencing. The amino acid sequence was the same as that deduced from the translated open reading frame (ORF) of the PrP gene, and no modifications that might differentiate PrP^{C} from PrP^{Sc} were found (16). These findings forced consideration of the possibility that conformation distinguishes the two PrP isoforms.

Molecular Modeling

By comparing the amino acid sequences of 11 mammalian and one avian PrP, structural analyses using a neural network algorithm predicted four α-helical regions (Fig 20-1) (34–36). Interestingly, the four putative α-helical domains of PrP designated *H1*, *H2*, *H3*, and *H4* (34) showed both strong helix preference in the α/α class prediction and strong β-sheet preference in the β/β class prediction. These results are consistent with the hypothesis that some of these domains undergo conformational changes from α-helices to β-sheets during the formation of PrP^{Sc} (36).

Spectroscopy

PrP^{C} and PrP^{Sc} were purified using nondenaturing procedures (17,37). Fourier transform infrared (FTIR) spectroscopy and circular dichroism (CD) demonstrated that PrP^{C} has a high α-helix content (42%) and no β-sheet (3%) (17). In contrast, the β-sheet

---

S2b-H3 loop connecting the β-sheet and helix 3 is implicated in the species barrier and is shown at the upper left hand side of the figure. This conformationally flexible loop could come into contact with PrP^{C} during the formation of the PrP^{Sc}-PrP^{C} complex. Therefore, the specific molecular recognition during prion replication might involve both the β-sheet as the primary binding site and the S2b-H3 loop as an additional site for interaction.

content of PrP^{Sc} was 43% and the α-helix content was 30% as measured by FTIR (17) and CD spectroscopy (38,39). Denaturation of N-terminally truncated PrP^{Sc} (PrP 27-30) under conditions that reduced scrapie infectivity resulted in a concomitant diminution of β-sheet content (40,41).

We and others suggested that the conversion of PrP^{C} into PrP^{Sc} may proceed through a metastable or partially unfolded intermediate designated *PrP** (42,43). Intermediates in the refolding of PrP 27-30 from a denatured state have been identified by fluorescence and CD spectroscopy (44). Results of experiments with immunoprecipitated [^{35}S-]Met–labeled $SHaPrP^{C}$ and a more than 50-fold excess of purified $SHaPrP^{Sc}$ have been interpreted as showing that PrP^{C} becomes protease resistant under these conditions (45). Using a similar protocol, we showed that synthetic peptides can induce protease resistance in PrP^{C} but no scrapie infectivity was found under these conditions (46).

Nuclear magnetic resonance (NMR) studies have provided evidence supporting the molecular models described above. Chemical shift measurements of a 56 polymer (mer) synthetic peptide spanning H1 and H2 show that these regions, particularly H1, can form α-helices (47). An *Escherichia coli*–derived polypeptide of 111 residues was found to contain H3 and H4, which were stabilized by the single disulfide bond found in PrP (48). Another putative helix within this polypeptide that was not predicted by the model was reported; whether this helix will be found in longer *E. coli*–derived polypeptides remains to be determined (49).

TRANSGENETICS AND GENE TARGETING

Species Barrier

To test the hypothesis that differences in PrP gene sequences might be responsible for the species barrier, Tg mice expressing SHaPrP were constructed (50). The PrP genes of Syrian hamsters and mice (Mo) encode proteins differing at 16 positions. Inoculation of Tg(SHaPrP) mice with SHa prions demonstrated abrogation of the species barrier resulting in abbreviated incubation times due to a nonstochastic process (50). The length of the incubation time after inoculation with SHa prions was inversely proportional to the level of $SHaPrP^{C}$ in the brains of Tg(SHaPrP) mice (50). Bioassays of brain extracts from clinically ill Tg(SHaPrP) mice inoculated with Mo prions revealed that only Mo prions but no SHa prions were produced. Conversely, inoculation of Tg(SHaPrP) mice with SHa prions led to the synthesis of SHa prions only.

Modeling Gerstmann-Sträussler-Scheinker Syndrome

The codon 102 point mutation found in GSS patients was introduced into the MoPrP gene, and Tg(MoPrP-P101L)H mice were created expressing high levels of the mutant transgene product. Five lines of Tg(MoPrP-P101L) mice developed central nervous system (CNS) degeneration indistinguishable from experimental murine scrapie, with neuropathology consisting of widespread spongiform morphology and astrocytic gliosis and PrP amyloid plaques (51). Brain extracts prepared from spontaneously ill Tg(Mo-

PrP-P101L) mice transmitted CNS degeneration to Tg196 mice (51,52). Crossing Tg196 mice to mice in which the PrP gene has been ablated ($Prnp^{0/0}$) (53) reduced the incubation time to approximately 200 days (52). The Tg196 mice express low levels of the mutant transgene product $MoPrP^{C}$ (P101L) but do not develop spontaneous disease. These findings as well as the transmission of prions from patients who died of GSS syndrome to apes and monkeys (54) and Tg(MHu2M-P102L) mice (55) argue persuasively that prions are devoid of nucleic acid.

Prion Protein–Deficient Mice

Ablation of the PrP gene in mice did not affect the development of these animals (53,56). Two different lines of $Prnp^{0/0}$ mice remained healthy up to the age of 2 years but one study reported that these mice display abnormal sleep-wake cycles and circadian rhythms (57). Another line of $Prnp^{0/0}$ mice showed loss of Purkinje cells in the cerebellum after the age of 70 weeks (58). $Prnp^{0/0}$ mice are resistant to scrapie (6) and do not propagate prions (7,59,60).

Hippocampal slices from $Prnp^{0/0}$ mice reportedly show abnormalities in γ-aminobutyric acid (GABA)–mediated synaptic transmission and diminished long-term potentiation (LTP) (61,62). However, our attempts to reproduce these findings were unsuccessful (63). Also notable are studies on cerebellar slices in which neurotransmission was found to be similar in $Prnp^{0/0}$ and untargeted control animals (64).

Transmission of Human Prions to Transgenic Mice

Because our initial transgenetic studies had shown that the "species barrier" between mice and Syrian hamster for the transmission of prions can be abrogated by expression of a SHaPrP transgene in mice, Tg mice expressing human (Hu) PrP were constructed. These Tg(HuPrP)FVB mice inoculated with Hu prions failed to develop CNS dysfunction more frequently than non-Tg control animals (65). Faced with this apparent dichotomy, we constructed mice expressing a chimeric Hu/Mo PrP transgene designated *MHu2M* (66). HuPrP differs from MoPrP at 28 of 254 positions while MHu2M differs at nine residues. We found that mice expressing the MHu2M transgene are susceptible to human prions and exhibit abbreviated incubation times (65).

When Tg(HuPrP) mice were crossed with $Prnp^{0/0}$ mice, they were rendered susceptible to Hu prions. These findings suggested that Tg(HuPrP)FVB mice were resistant to Hu prions because $MoPrP^{C}$ inhibited the conversion of $HuPrP^{C}$ into PrP^{Sc}; once $MoPrP^{C}$ was removed by gene ablation, then the inhibition was abolished (55). While earlier studies argued that PrP^{C} forms a complex with PrP^{Sc} during the formation of nascent PrP^{Sc} (50), these findings suggested that PrP^{C} also binds to another macromolecule during the conversion process. We provisionally designated this second macromolecule *protein* X. Like the binding of PrP^{C} to PrP^{Sc}, which is most efficient when the two isoforms have the same sequence (50), the binding of PrP^{C} to protein X seems to exhibit the highest affinity when these two proteins are from the same species. Whether protein X is a chaperone involved in catalyzing the conformational changes that feature in the formation of PrP^{Sc} (17) remains to be established.

INHERITED PRION DISEASES

The recognition that approximately 10% of cases of prion diseases are familial led to the suspicion that genetics plays a role in these diseases (67). The discovery of the PrP gene and its linkage to scrapie incubation times in mice (68) raised the possibility that mutation might feature in the hereditary human prion diseases. A proline→leucine mutation at codon 102 was shown to be linked genetically to development of GSS syndrome with a log of odds (LOD) score exceeding 3 (Fig 20-2) (69). This mutation has been found in 10 different families in nine different countries including the original GSS family.

An insert of 144 bp containing six octarepeats at codon 53 was documented in patients with CJD from four families residing in southern England (70). Genealogic investigations showed that all four families are related, arguing for a single founder born more than two centuries ago. The LOD score for this extended pedigree exceeds 11. Studies from several laboratories demonstrated that two, four, five, six, seven, eight, or nine octarepeats in addition to the normal five are found in individuals with inherited CJD.

Many families with CJD have a point mutation at codon 178 resulting in an aspartic acid→arginine substitution (71). FFI, which presents with insomnia, is genetically linked to the D178N mutation with a LOD score exceeding 5 (72). The neuropathology in these patients with FFI is restricted to selected nuclei of the thalamus. It appears that the allele with the D178N mutation encodes an M at position 129 in FFI while a V is encoded at position 129 in familial CJD (73). The discovery that FFI is an inherited prion disease clearly widens the clinical spectrum of these disorders and raises the possibility that many other degenerative diseases of unknown etiology may be caused by prions.

PRION DIVERSITY

For many years, studies of experimental scrapie were performed exclusively with sheep and goats. The disease was first transmitted by intraocular inoculation (74) and later by intracerebral, oral, subcutaneous, intramuscular, and intravenous injections of brain extracts from sheep developing scrapie. Incubation periods of 1 to 3 years were common and often many of the inoculated animals failed to develop disease (75). Different breeds of sheep exhibited markedly different susceptibilities to scrapie prions inoculated subcutaneously, suggesting that the genetic background might influence host permissiveness (76).

The diversity of scrapie prions was first appreciated in goats inoculated with "hyper" and "drowsy" isolates (77). The lengths of the incubation times have been used to distinguish prion strains inoculated into sheep, goats, mice, and hamsters (78).

The discovery that incubation times are controlled by the relative dosage of *Prnp*^{a} and *Prnp*^{b} alleles (Table 20-1) (79) was foreshadowed by studies of Tg(SHaPrP) mice in which the length of the incubation time after inoculation with SHa prions was inversely proportional to the transgene product, SHaPrP^C (50). Not only the PrP gene dose, but also the passage history of the inoculum, particularly in *Prnp*^{b} mice, determine the

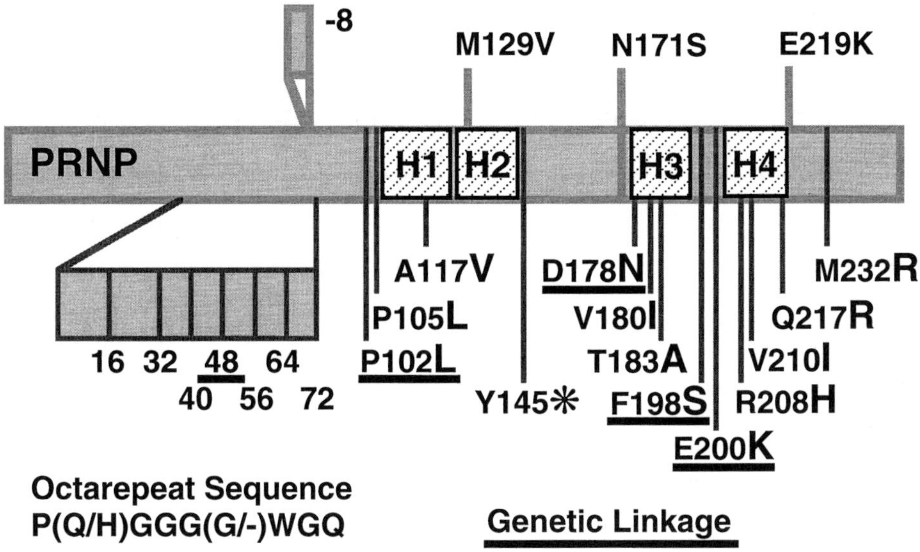

Figure 20-2. Human prion protein gene (*PRNP*). The open reading frame (ORF) is denoted by the large gray rectangle. Human *PRNP* wild-type coding polymorphisms are shown above the rectangle while mutations that segregate with the inherited prion diseases are depicted below. The wild-type human PrP gene contains five octarepeats [P(Q/H)GGG(G/-)WGQ] from codons 51 to 91 (108). Deletion of a single octarepeat at codon 81 or 82 is not associated with prion disease (109–111); whether this deletion alters the phenotypic characteristics of a prion disease is unknown. There are common polymorphisms at codons 117 (Ala→Ala) and 129 (Met→Val); homozygosity for methionine or valine at codon 129 appears to increase susceptibility to sporadic Creutzfeldt-Jakob disease (CJD) (112). Additional polymorphisms have been found at codons 171 (Asn→Ser) and 219 (Glu→Lys) (113,114). Octarepeat inserts of 16, 32, 40, 48, 56, 64, and 72 amino acids at codon 67, 75, or 83 are designated by the small rectangle below the ORF. These inserts segregate with familial CJD, and genetic linkage has been demonstrated where sufficient specimens from family members are available (115–122). Point mutations are designated by the wild-type amino acid preceding the codon number and the mutant residue follows (e.g., P102L). These point mutations segregate with the inherited prion diseases and significant genetic linkage (underlined mutations) has been demonstrated where sufficient specimens from family members are available. Mutations at codons 102 (Pro→Leu), 117 (Ala→Val), 198 (Phe→Ser), and 217 (Gln→Arg) are found in patients with Gerstmann-Sträussler-Scheinker (GSS) syndrome (69,120,123–130). Point mutations at codons 178 (Asp→Asn), 200 (Glu→Lys), 208 (Arg→,His), and 210 (Val→Ile) are found in patients with familial CJD (71,99,100,131–133). Point mutations at codons 198 (Phe→Ser) and 217 (Gln→Arg) are found in patients with GSS syndrome who have PrP amyloid plaques and neurofibrillary tangles (134,135). Additional point mutations at codons 145 (Tyr→Stop), 105 (Pro→Leu), 180 (Val→Ile), and 232 (Met→Arg) have been recently reported (136,137). Single letter codes for amino acids are as follows: A = Ala; D = Asp; E = Glu; F = Phe; I = Ile; K = Lys; L = Leu; M = Met; N = Asn; P = Pro; Q = Gln; R = Arg; S = Ser; T = Thr; V = Val; Y = Tyr.

Table 20-1. Mouse PrP-A Expression Is a Major Determinant of Incubation Times in Mice Inoculated with the RML Scrapie Prions[a]

Mice	*Prnp Genotype (copies)*	*Prnp Transgenes (copies)*	*Alleles a*	*Alleles b*	*Incubation Time[a] (days ± SEM)*	*n*
Prn-p$^{0/0}$	0/0	—	0	0	> 600	4
Prn-p$^{+/0}$	a/0	—	1	0	426 ± 18	9[a]
B6.I-1	b/b	—	0	2	360 ± 16	7
B6.I-2	b/b	—	0	2	379 ± 8	10
B6.I-3	b/b	—	0	2	404 ± 10	20
(B6 × B6.I-1)F1	a/b	—	1	1	268 ± 4	7
B6 .I-1 × Tg(MoPrP-B$^{0/0}$)15	a/b	—	1	1	255 ± 7	11[b]
B6.I-1 × Tg(MoPrP-B$^{0/0}$)15	a/b	—	1	1	274 ± 3	9[c]
B6.I-1 × Tg(MoPrP-B$^{+/0}$)15	a/b	bbb/0	1	4	166 ± 2	11[b]
B6.I-1 × Tg(MoPrP-B$^{+/0}$)15	a/b	bbb/0	1	4	162 ± 3	8[c]
C57BL/6J (B6)	a/a	—	2	0	143 ± 4	8
B6.I-4	a/a	—	2	0	144 ± 5	8
Non-Tg(MoPrP-B$^{0/0}$)15	a/a	—	2	0	130 ± 3	10
Tg(MoPrP-B$^{+/0}$)15	a/a	bbb/0	2	3	115 ± 2	18
Tg(MoPrP-B$^{+/+}$)15	a/a	bbb/bbb	2	6	111 ± 5	5
Tg(MoPrP-B$^{+/0}$)94	a/a	>30b	2	>30	75 ± 2	15
Tg(MoPrP-A$^{+/0}$)B4053	a/a	>30a	>30	0	50 ±	16

[a]Data from (79).
[b]The homozygous Tg(MoPrP-B$^{+/+}$)15 mice were maintained as a distinct subline selected for transgene homozygosity two generations removed from the (B6 × LT/Sv)F2 founder. Hemizygous Tg(MoPrP-B$^{+/0}$)15 mice were produced by crossing the Tg(MoPrP-B$^{+/+}$)15 line with B6 mice.
[c]Tg(MoPrP-B$^{+/0}$)15 mice were maintained by repeated backcrossing to B6 mice.

length of the incubation time (79). The PrP^{Sc} allotype in the inoculum produced the shortest incubation times when it was the same as that of PrP^{C} in the host.

Patterns of PrP^{Sc} Deposition

Besides measurements of the length of the incubation time, profiles of spongiform degeneration have also been used to characterize different prion strains (80). Comparisons of PrP^{Sc} accumulation on histoblots with histologic sections showed that PrP^{Sc} deposition preceded vacuolation and only those regions with PrP^{Sc} underwent degeneration (81). Microdissection of individual brain regions confirmed the conclusions of the histoblot studies: Those regions with high levels of PrP 27-30 had intense vacuolation (82). Thus, we concluded that the deposition of PrP^{Sc} is responsible for the neuropathologic changes found in the prion diseases.

While studies with both mice and Syrian hamster established that each isolate has a specific signature as defined by a specific pattern of PrP^{Sc} accumulation in the brain

(79,81), comparisons must be done on an isogenic background (51,66). Variations in the patterns of PrP^{Sc} accumulation were found to be equally as great as those seen between two strains when a single strain is inoculated in mice expressing different PrP genes.

Are Prion Strains Different PrP^{Sc} Conformers?

Explaining the problem of multiple distinct prion isolates might be accommodated by multiple PrP^{Sc} conformers that act as templates for the folding of de novo synthesized PrP^{Sc} molecules during prion "replication." Although it is clear that passage history can be responsible for the prolongation of incubation time when prions are passed between mice expressing different PrP allotypes or between species (50), many scrapie strains show distinct incubation times in the same inbred host (83).

Although the proposal for multiple PrP^{Sc} conformers is unorthodox, we already know that PrP can assume at least two profoundly different conformations: PrP^{C} and PrP^{Sc} (17). Of note, two different isolates from mink dying of transmissible mink encephalopathy exhibit different sensitivities of PrP^{Sc} to proteolytic digestion, supporting the suggestion that isolate-specific information might be carried by PrP^{Sc} (84). How many conformations PrP^{Sc} can assume is unknown. The molecular size of a PrP^{Sc} homodimer is consistent with the ionizing radiation target size of 55,000 ± 9000 daltons as determined for infectious prion particles independent of their polymeric form (85). If prions are oligomers of PrP^{Sc}, which seems likely, then this offers another level of complexity, which in turn generates additional diversity.

In FFI, the protease-resistant fragment of PrP^{Sc} after deglycosylation has a relative molecular size of 19 kd, whereas the size of that from other inherited and sporadic prion diseases is 21 kd (86). Extracts from the brains of FFI patients transmitted disease to Tg mice expressing the chimeric MHu2M PrP gene approximately 200 days after inoculation and induced formation of the 19-kd PrP^{Sc}, whereas familial (E200K) and sporadic CJD produced the 21-kd PrP^{Sc} in these mice (87,119). Our findings argue that PrP^{Sc} acts as a template for the conversion of PrP^{C} into nascent PrP^{Sc} and provides a mechanism for replication of prion strains.

BOVINE SPONGIFORM ENCEPHALOPATHY

Beginning in 1986, an epidemic of a previously unknown prion disease named *bovine spongiform encephalopathy* or *mad cow disease* appeared in cattle in Great Britain (88); protease-resistant PrP was found in the brains of the ill cattle (89,90). It has been proposed that BSE represents a massive common-source epidemic that has caused more than 160,000 cases to date (11,12). Dairy cows were routinely fed meat and bone meal (MBM) prepared by rendering the offal of sheep and cattle as a nutritional supplement. Since 1988, the practice of using dietary protein supplements for domestic animals derived from rendered sheep or cattle offal has been banned. Recent statistics argue that the epidemic is now under control as a result of the 1988 food ban (Fig 20-3).

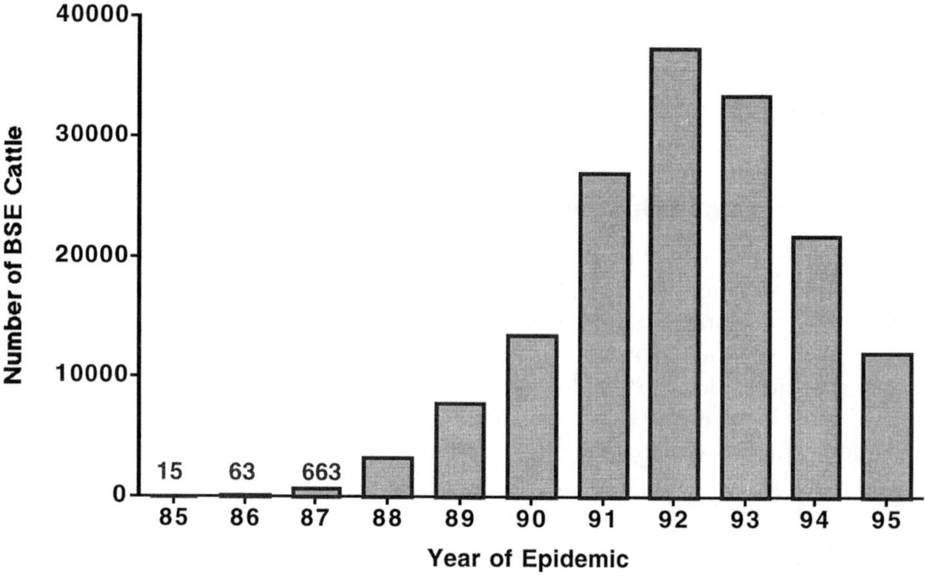

FIGURE 20-3. Bovine spongiform encephalopathy (BSE) epidemic in Great Britain. The number of annual cases of BSE in cattle is plotted for the past decade. (Data compiled by Dr. John Wilesmith from the Central Veterinary Laboratory, Weybridge, England (12). Reprinted with permission of Macmillan Magazines Ltd.)

Brain extracts from BSE cattle transmit disease to mice, cattle, sheep, and pigs after intracerebral inoculation (91,92). Transmissions to mice and sheep suggest that cattle preferentially propagate a single "strain" of prions (93). Of particular significance is the transmission of BSE to the marmoset after intracerebral inoculation and more recently, to the macaque (94,95). Recent cases of atypical CJD in three teenagers and nine young adults in the Great Britain and France raise the possibility of transmission of BSE to humans (9,10).

Our experience with Tg(HuPrP)FVB mice expressing both human and mouse PrP^C (55,65) contrasts with that reported for a case of iatrogenic CJD. When Tg(HuPrP)FVB mice were inoculated with Hu prions from the patient with iatrogenic CJD, the mice developed CNS dysfunction approximately 300 days later (96). When this same inoculum was injected into Tg(HuPrP)$Prnp^{0/0}$ mice, the incubation time was reduced to approximately 200 days, which is similar to that reported by us for other Hu prions (55). Based on the susceptibility of Tg(HuPrP) mice to Hu prions from this iatrogenic CJD patient and the resistance of these mice to bovine prions from cattle dying of BSE, the authors concluded that BSE prions are unlikely to be pathogenic for humans (96). This conclusion seems contrary to recent reports describing atypical CJD in more than 10 teenagers and young adults.

It is notable that bovine PrP is more homologous with HuPrP than is sheep PrP in the region between codons 96 and 167, which feature in the species barrier in the transmission of Hu prions into mice, as demonstrated by the susceptibility of Tg(MHu2M) mice to Hu prions (55,65). Whether the differences in the amino acid sequence between bovine and sheep PrP in this central domain are responsible for the apparent differential susceptibility of humans to bovine and sheep prions remains to be established. It is notable that epidemiologic studies over nearly three decades have failed to establish convincing evidence for transmission of sheep prions to humans (97). Of interest is the high incidence of CJD among Libyan Jews that was initially attributed to the consumption of lightly cooked sheep brain (98); however, subsequent studies showed that this geographic cluster of CJD is due to an E200K mutation of the PrP gene (see Fig 20-2) (87,99,100).

CONCLUSIONS

Prions Are Not Viruses

The study of prions has taken several unexpected directions over the past few years. The discovery that prion diseases in humans are uniquely both genetic and infectious has greatly strengthened and extended the prion concept. To date, 19 different mutations in the human PrP gene that cause the inherited prion diseases have been found. Yet, the transmissible prion particle is composed largely, if not entirely, of PrP^{Sc} (1). These findings and many others argue that prions differ from all known microorganisms as well as viruses and viroids.

Do Prions Exist in Lower Organisms?

In *Saccharomyces cerevisiae*, ure2 and [URE3] mutants can grow on ureidosuccinate under conditions of nitrogen repression such as glutamic acid and ammonia (101). Mutants of ure2 exhibit mendelian inheritance, whereas [URE3] is cytoplasmically inherited (102). The [URE3] phenotype can be induced by UV irradiation and by overexpression of ure2p, the gene product of ure2; deletion of ure2 abolishes [URE3]. The function of ure2p is unknown but it has substantial homology with glutathione-S-transferase; attempts to demonstrate this enzymic activity with purified ure2p have not been successful (103). Whether the [URE3] protein is a posttranslationally modified form of ure2p that acts on unmodified ure2p to produce more of itself remains to be established.

Another possible yeast prion is the [PSI] phenotype (102). [PSI] is a nonmendelian inherited trait that can be induced by expression of the PNM2 gene (104). The [PSI] phenotype requires moderate levels of expression of heat shock protein 104 (Hsp104); ablation of the HSP104 gene or overexpression prevents [PSI] (105). In the filamentous fungus *Podospora anserina*, the het-s locus controls the vegetative incompatibility; conversion from the S^s to the s state seems to be a posttranslational, autocatalytic process (106).

Future Studies

The knowledge accrued from the study of prion diseases may provide an effective strategy for defining the etiologies and dissecting the molecular pathogenesis of the more common neurodegenerative disorders such as Alzheimer's disease, Parkinson's disease, and amyotrophic lateral sclerosis. Since people at risk for inherited prion diseases can now be identified decades before neurologic dysfunction is evident, the development of an effective therapy is imperative.

Tg mice expressing foreign or mutant PrP genes now permit virtually all facets of prion diseases to be studied and have created a framework for future investigations. Furthermore, the structure and organization of the PrP gene suggest that PrP^{Sc} is derived from PrP^{C} or a precursor by a posttranslational process. Studies with scrapie-infected cultured cells have provided much evidence that the conversion of PrP^{C} to PrP^{Sc} is a posttranslational process that probably occurs within a subcellular compartment bounded by cholesterol-rich membranes. The molecular mechanism of PrP^{Sc} formation remains to be elucidated, but chemical and physical studies showed that the conformations of PrP^{C} and PrP^{Sc} are profoundly different.

The study of prion biology and diseases is a new and emerging area of biomedical investigation. While prion biology has its roots in virology, neurology, and neuropathology, its relationships to the disciplines of molecular and cell biology as well as protein chemistry have become evident only recently. Learning how prions multiply and cause disease will certainly open up new vistas in biochemistry and genetics.

REFERENCES

1 Prusiner SB. Molecular biology of prion diseases. *Science* 1991;252:1515–1522.

2 Prusiner SB. Novel proteinaceous infectious particles cause scrapie. *Science* 1982;216:136–144.

3 Alper T, Cramp WA, Haig DA, Clarke MC. Does the agent of scrapie replicate without nucleic acid? *Nature* 1967;214:764–766.

4 Riesner D, Kellings K, Meyer N, et al. Nucleic acids and scrapie prions. In: Prusiner SB, Collinge J, Powell J, Anderton B, eds. *Prion diseases of humans and animals*. London: Ellis Horwood, 1992:341–358.

5 Prusiner SB, McKinley MP, Bowman KA, et al. Scrapie prions aggregate to form amyloid-like birefringent rods. *Cell* 1983;35:349–358.

6 Büeler H, Aguzzi A, Sailer A, et al. Mice devoid of PrP are resistant to scrapie. *Cell* 1993;73:1339–1347.

7 Prusiner SB, Groth D, Serban A, et al. Ablation of the prion protein (PrP) gene in mice prevents scrapie and facilitates production of antiPrP antibodies. *Proc Natl Acad Sci USA* 1993;90:10608–10612.

8 Gajdusek DC. Unconventional viruses and the origin and disappearance of kuru. *Science* 1977;197:943–960.

9 Will RG, Ironside JW, Zeidler M, et al. A new variant of Creutzfeldt-Jakob disease in the UK. *Lancet* 1996;347:921–925.

10 Chazot G, Broussolle E, Lapras CI, et al. New variant of Creutzfeldt-Jakob disease in a 26-year-old French man. *Lancet* 1996;347:1181.

11 Wells GAH, Wilesmith JW. The neuropathology and epidemiology of bovine spongiform encephalopathy. *Brain Pathol* 1995;5:91–103.

12 Anderson RM, Donnelly CA, Ferguson NM, et al. Transmission dynamics and epidemiology of BSE in British cattle. *Nature* 1996;382:779–788.

13 Hadlow WJ. Scrapie and kuru. *Lancet* 1959;2:289–290.

14 Parry HB. Recorded occurrences of scrapie from 1750. In: Oppenheimer DR, ed. *Scrapie disease in sheep*. New York: Academic, 1983:31–59.

15 Prusiner SB, McKinley MP, Groth DF, et al. Scrapie agent contains a hydrophobic protein. *Proc Natl Acad Sci USA* 1981;78:6675–6679.

16 Stahl N, Baldwin MA, Teplow DB, et al. Structural analysis of the scrapie prion protein using mass spectrometry and amino acid sequencing. *Biochemistry* 1993;32:1991–2002.

17 Pan K-M, Baldwin M, Nguyen J, et al. Conversion of α-helices into β-sheets features in the formation of the scrapie prion proteins.

Proc Natl Acad Sci USA 1993;90:10962–10966.

18 Bolton DC, McKinley MP, Prusiner SB. Identification of a protein that purifies with the scrapie prion. *Science* 1982;218:1309–1311.

19 Prusiner SB, Bolton DC, Groth DF, et al. Further purification and characterization of scrapie prions. *Biochemistry* 1982;21:6942–6950.

20 McKinley MP, Bolton DC, Prusiner SB. A protease-resistant protein is a structural component of the scrapie prion. *Cell* 1983;35:57–62.

21 Prusiner SB, Groth DF, Bolton DC, et al. Purification and structural studies of a major scrapie prion protein. *Cell* 1984;38:127–134.

22 Basler K, Oesch B, Scott M, et al. Scrapie and cellular PrP isoforms are encoded by the same chromosomal gene. *Cell* 1986;46:417–428.

23 Locht C, Chesebro B, Race R, Keith JM. Molecular cloning and complete sequence of prion protein cDNA from mouse brain infected with the scrapie agent. *Proc Natl Acad Sci USA* 1986;83:6372–6376.

24 Oesch B, Westaway D, Wälchli M, et al. A cellular gene encodes scrapie PrP 27-30 protein. *Cell* 1985;40:735–746.

25 Chesebro B, Race R, Wehrly K, et al. Identification of scrapie prion protein-specific mRNA in scrapie-infected and uninfected brain. *Nature* 1985;315:331–333.

26 Meyer RK, McKinley MP, Bowman KA, et al. Separation and properties of cellular and scrapie prion proteins. *Proc Natl Acad Sci USA* 1986;83:2310–2314.

27 Stahl N, Borchelt DR, Hsiao K, Prusiner SB. Scrapie prion protein contains a phosphatidylinositol glycolipid. *Cell* 1987;51:229–240.

28 Borchelt DR, Scott M, Taraboulos A, et al. Scrapie and cellular prion proteins differ in their kinetics of synthesis and topology in cultured cells. *J Cell Biol* 1990;110:743–752.

29 Caughey B, Raymond GJ. The scrapie-associated form of PrP is made from a cell surface precursor that is both protease- and phospholipase-sensitive. *J Biol Chem* 1991;266:18217–18223.

30 Taraboulos A, Raeber AJ, Borchelt DR, et al. Synthesis and trafficking of prion proteins in cultured cells. *Mol Biol Cell* 1992;3:851–863.

31 Taraboulos A, Scott M, Semenov A, et al. Cholesterol depletion and modification of COOH-terminal targeting sequence of the prion protein inhibit formation of the scrapie isoform. *J Cell Biol* 1995;129:121–132.

32 Caughey B, Raymond GJ, Ernst D, Race RE. N-Terminal truncation of the scrapie-associated form of PrP by lysosomal protease(s): implications regarding the site of conversion of PrP to the protease-resistant state. *J Virol* 1991;65:6597–6603.

33 McKinley MP, Meyer R, Kenaga L, et al. Scrapie prion rod formation *in vitro* requires both detergent extraction and limited proteolysis. *J Virol* 1991;65:1440–1449.

34 Gasset M, Baldwin MA, Lloyd D, et al. Predicted α-helical regions of the prion protein when synthesized as peptides from amyloid. *Proc Natl Acad Sci USA* 1992;89:10940–10944.

35 Huang Z, Gabriel J-M, Baldwin MA, et al. Proposed three-dimensional structure for the cellular prion protein. *Proc Natl Acad Sci USA* 1994;91:7139–7143.

36 Huang Z, Prusiner SB, Cohen FE. Scrapie prions: a three-dimensional model of an infectious fragment. *Folding Design* 1996;1:13–19.

37 Turk E, Teplow DB, Hood LE, Prusiner SB. Purification and properties of the cellular and scrapie hamster prion proteins. *Eur J Biochem* 1988;176:21–30.

38 Safar J, Roller PP, Gajdusek DC, Gibbs CJ Jr. Conformational transitions, dissociation, and unfolding of scrapie amyloid (prion) protein. *J Biol Chem* 1993;268:20276–20284.

39 Caughey BW, Dong A, Bhat KS, et al. Secondary structure analysis of the scrapie-associated protein PrP 27-30 in water by infrared spectroscopy. *Biochemistry* 1991;30:7672–7680.

40 Gasset M, Baldwin MA, Fletterick RJ, Prusiner SB. Perturbation of the secondary structure of the scrapie prion protein under conditions associated with changes in infectivity. *Proc Natl Acad Sci USA* 1993;90:1–5.

41 Safar J, Roller PP, Gajdusek DC, Gibbs CJJ. Thermal-stability and conformational transitions of scrapie amyloid (prion) protein correlate with infectivity. *Protein Sci* 1993;2:2206–2216.

42 Jarrett JT, Lansbury PT Jr. Seeding "one-dimensional crystallization" of amyloid: a pathogenic mechanism in Alzheimer's disease and scrapie? *Cell* 1993;73:1055–1058.

43 Cohen FE, Pan K-M, Huang Z, et al. Structural clues to prion replication. *Science* 1994;264:530–531.

44 Safar J, Roller PP, Gajdusek DC, Gibbs CJ Jr. Scrapie amyloid (prion) protein has the conformational characteristics of an aggregated molten globule folding intermediate. *Biochemistry* 1994;33:8375–8383.

45 Kocisko DA, Come JH, Priola SA, et al. Cell-free formation of protease-resistant prion protein. *Nature* 1994;370:471–474.

46 Kaneko K, Peretz D, Pan K-M, et al. Prion protein (PrP) synthetic peptides induce cellular PrP to acquire properties of the scrapie isoform. *Proc Natl Acad Sci USA* 1995;32: 11160–11164.

47 Zhang H, Kaneko K, Nguyen JT, et al. Conformational transitions in peptides containing two putative α-helices of the prion protein. *J Mol Biol* 1995;250:514–526.

48 Riek R, Hornemann S, Wider G, et al. NMR structure of the mouse prion protein domain PrP(121-231). *Nature* 1996;382:180–182.

49 Mehlhorn I, Groth D, Stöckel J, et al. High-level expression and characterization of a purified 142-residue polypeptide of the prion protein. *Biochemistry* 1996;35:5528–5537.

50 Prusiner SB, Scott M, Foster D, et al. Transgenetic studies implicate interactions between homologous PrP isoforms in scrapie prion replication. *Cell* 1990;63:673–686.

51 Hsiao KK, Groth D, Scott M, et al. Serial transmission in rodents of neurodegeneration from transgenic mice expressing mutant prion protein. *Proc Natl Acad Sci USA* 1994;91:9126–9130.

52 Telling GT, Haga T, Torchia M, et al. Interactions between wild-type and mutant prion proteins modulate neurodegeneration in transgenic mice. *Genes Dev* 1996;10:1736–1750.

53 Büeler H, Fischer M, Lang Y, et al. Normal development and behaviour of mice lacking the neuronal cell-surface PrP protein. *Nature* 1992;356:577–582.

54 Masters CL, Gajdusek DC, Gibbs CJ Jr. Creutzfeldt-Jakob disease virus isolations from the Gerstmann-Sträussler syndrome. *Brain* 1981;104:559–588.

55 Telling GC, Scott M, Mastrianni J, et al. Prion propagation in mice expressing human and chimeric PrP transgenes implicates the interaction of cellular PrP with another protein. *Cell* 1995;83:79–90.

56 Manson JC, Clarke AR, Hooper ML, et al. 129/Ola mice carrying a null mutation in PrP that abolishes mRNA production are developmentally normal. *Mol Neurobiol* 1994;8:121–127.

57 Tobler I, Gaus SE, Deboer T, et al. Altered circadian activity rhythms and sleep in mice devoid of prion protein. *Nature* 1996;380:639–642.

58 Sakaguchi S, Katamine S, Nishida N, et al. Loss of cerebellar Purkinje cells in aged mice homozygous for a disrupted PrP gene. *Nature* 1996;380:528–531.

59 Manson JC, Clarke AR, McBride PA, et al. PrP gene dosage determines the timing but not the final intensity or distribution of lesions in scrapie pathology. *Neurodegeneration* 1994;3: 331–340.

60 Sakaguchi S, Katamine S, Shigematsu K, et al. Accumulation of proteinase K-resistant prion protein (PrP) is restricted by the expression level of normal PrP in mice inoculated with a mouse-adapted strain of the Creutzfeldt-Jakob disease agent. *J Virol* 1995;69:7586–7592.

61 Collinge J, Whittington MA, Sidle KC, et al. Prion protein is necessary for normal synaptic function. *Nature* 1994;370:295–297.

62 Manson JC, Hope J, Clarke AR, et al. PrP gene dosage and long term potentiation. *Neurodegeneration* 1995;4:113–114. Letter.

63 Lledo P-M, Tremblay P, DeArmond SJ, et al. Mice deficient for prion protein exhibit normal neuronal excitability and synaptic transmission in the hippocampus. *Proc Natl Acad Sci USA* 1996;93:2403–2407.

64 Herms JW, Kretzschmar HA, Titz S, Keller BU. Patch-clamp analysis of synaptic transmission to cerebellar Purkinje cells of prion protein knockout mice. *Eur J Neurosci* 1995; 7:2508–2512.

65 Telling GC, Scott M, Hsiao KK, et al. Transmission of Creutzfeldt-Jakob disease from humans to transgenic mice expressing chimeric human-mouse prion protein. *Proc Natl Acad Sci USA* 1994;91:9936–9940.

66 Scott M, Groth D, Foster D, et al. Propagation of prions with artificial properties in transgenic mice expressing chimeric PrP genes. *Cell* 1993;73:979–988.

67 Meggendorfer F. Klinische und genealogische Beobachtungen bei einem Fall von spastischer Pseudosklerose Jakobs. *Z Ges Neurol Psychiatr* 1930;128:337–341.

68 Carlson GA, Kingsbury DT, Goodman PA, et al. Linkage of prion protein and scrapie incubation time genes. *Cell* 1986;46:503–511.

69 Hsiao K, Baker HF, Crow TJ, et al. Linkage of a prion protein missense variant to Gerstmann-Sträussler syndrome. *Nature* 1989;338: 342–345.

70 Poulter M, Baker HF, Frith CD, et al. Inherited prion disease with 144 base pair gene insertion. 1. Genealogical and molecular studies. *Brain* 1992;115:675–685.

71 Goldfarb LG, Haltia M, Brown P, et al. New mutation in scrapie amyloid precursor gene (at codon 178) in Finnish Creutzfeldt-Jakob kindred. *Lancet* 1991;337:425.

72 Petersen RB, Tabaton M, Berg L, et al. Analysis of the prion protein gene in thalamic dementia. *Neurology* 1992;42:1859–1863.

73 Goldfarb LG, Petersen RB, Tabaton M, et al. Fatal familial insomnia and familial Creutzfeldt-Jakob disease: disease phenotype determined by a DNA polymorphism. *Science* 1992;258:806–808.

74 Cuillé J, Chelle PL. Experimental transmission of trembling to the goat. *C R Seances Acad Sci* 1939;208:1058–1060.

75 Dickinson AG, Stamp JT. Experimental scrapie in Cheviot and Suffolk sheep. *J Comp Pathol* 1969;79:23–26.

76 Gordon WS. Variation in susceptibility of sheep to scrapie and genetic implications. In: *Report of scrapie seminar, ARS 91-53*. Washington, DC: US Department of Agriculture, 1966:53–67.

77 Pattison IH, Millson GC. Scrapie produced experimentally in goats with special reference to the clinical syndrome. *J Comp Pathol* 1961;71:101–108.

78 Dickinson AG, Meikle VMH, Fraser H. Identification of a gene which controls the incubation period of some strains of scrapie agent in mice. *J Comp Pathol* 1968;78:293–299.

79 Carlson GA, Ebeling C, Yang S-L, et al. Prion isolate specified allotypic interactions between the cellular and scrapie prion proteins in congenic and transgenic mice. *Proc Natl Acad Sci USA* 1994;91:5690–5694.

80 Fraser H. Neuropathology of scrapie: the precision of the lesions and their diversity. In: Prusiner SB, Hadlow WJ, eds. *Slow transmissible diseases of the nervous system*. Vol. 1. New York: Academic, 1979:387–406.

81 Hecker R, Taraboulos A, Scott M, et al. Replication of distinct prion isolates is region specific in brains of transgenic mice and hamsters. *Genes Dev* 1992;6:1213–1228.

82 Casaccia-Bonnefil P, Kascsak RJ, Fersko R, et al. Brain regional distribution of prion protein PrP27-30 in mice stereotaxically microinjected with different strains of scrapie. *J Infect Dis* 1993;167:7–12.

83 Bruce ME, McConnell I, Fraser H, Dickinson AG. The disease characteristics of different strains of scrapie in *Sinc* congenic mouse lines: implications for the nature of the agent and host control of pathogenesis. *J Gen Virol* 1991;72:595–603.

84 Bessen RA, Marsh RF. Identification of two biologically distinct strains of transmissible mink encephalopathy in hamsters. *J Gen Virol* 1992;73:329–334.

85 Bellinger-Kawahara CG, Kempner E, Groth DF, et al. Scrapie prion liposomes and rods exhibit target sizes of 55,000 Da. *Virology* 1988;164:537–541.

86 Monari L, Chen SG, Brown P, et al. Fatal familial insomnia and familial Creutzfeldt-Jakob disease: different prion proteins determined by a DNA polymorphism. *Proc Natl Acad Sci USA* 1994;91:2839–2842.

87 Gabizon R, Rosenmann H, Meiner Z, et al. Mutation and polymorphism of the prion protein gene in Libyan Jews with Creutzfeldt-Jakob disease. *Am J Hum Genet* 1993;33:828–835.

88 Wells GAH, Scott AC, Johnson CT, et al. A novel progressive spongiform encephalopathy in cattle. *Vet Rec* 1987;121:419–420.

89 Hope J, Reekie LJD, Hunter N, et al. Fibrils from brains of cows with new cattle disease contain scrapie-associated protein. *Nature* 1988;336:390–392.

90 Prusiner SB, Fuzi M, Scott M, et al. Immunologic and molecular biological studies of prion proteins in bovine spongiform encephalopathy. *J Infect Dis* 1993;167:602–613.

91 Fraser H, McConnell I, Wells GAH, Dawson M. Transmission of bovine spongiform encephalopathy to mice. *Vet Rec* 1988;123:472.

92 Dawson M, Wells GAH, Parker BNJ, Scott AC. Primary parenteral transmission of bovine spongiform encephalopathy to the pig. *Vet Rec* 1990;127:338.

93 Bruce M, Chree A, McConnell I, et al. Transmission of bovine spongiform encephalopathy and scrapie to mice: strain variation and the species barrier. *Philos Trans R Soc Lond B Biol Sci* 1994;343:405–411.

94 Baker HF, Ridley RM, Wells GAH. Experimental transmission of BSE and scrapie to the common marmoset. *Vet Rec* 1993;132:403–406.

95 Lasmézas CI, Deslys J-P, Demaimay R, et al. BSE transmission to macaques. *Nature* 1996; 381:743–744.

96 Collinge J, Palmer MS, Sidle KC, et al. Unaltered susceptibility to BSE in transgenic mice expressing human prion protein. *Nature* 1995; 378:779–783.

97 Cousens SN, Harries-Jones R, Knight R, et al. Geographical distribution of cases of Creutzfeldt-Jakob disease in England and Wales 1970-84. *J Neurol Neurosurg Psychiatry* 1990;53:459–465.

98 Kahana E, Milton A, Braham J, Sofer D. Creutzfeldt-Jakob disease: focus among Libyan Jews in Israel. *Science* 1974;183:90–91.

99 Goldfarb L, Korczyn A, Brown P, et al. Muta-

tion in codon 200 of scrapie amyloid precursor gene linked to Creutzfeldt-Jakob disease in Sephardic Jews of Libyan and non-Libyan origin. *Lancet* 1990;336:637–638.

100 Hsiao K, Meiner Z, Kahana E, et al. Mutation of the prion protein in Libyan Jews with Creutzfeldt-Jakob disease. *N Engl J Med* 1991;324:1091–1097.

101 Lacroute F. Non-mendelian mutation allowing ureidosuccinic acid uptake in yeast. *J Bacteriol* 1971;106:519–522.

102 Wickner RB. [URE3] as an altered URE2 protein: evidence for a prion analog in *Saccharomyces cerevisiae*. *Science* 1994;264:566–569.

103 Coschigano PW, Magasanik B. The *URE2* gene product of *Saccharomyces cerevisiae* plays an important role in the cellular response to the nitrogen source and has homology to glutathione S-transferases. *Mol Cell Biol* 1991;11:822–832.

104 Cox BS, Tuite MF, McLaughlin CS. The psi factor of yeast: a problem in inheritance. *Yeast* 1988;4:159–178.

105 Chernoff YO, Lindquist SL, Ono B, et al. Role of the chaperone protein Hsp104 in propagation of the yeast prion-like factor [psi^+]. *Science* 1995;268:880–884.

106 Deleu C, Clavé C, Bégueret J. A single amino acid difference is sufficient to elicit vegetative incompatibility in the fungus *Podospora anserina*. *Genetics* 1993;135:45–52.

107 Schätzl HM, Da Costa M, Taylor L, et al. Prion protein gene variation among primates. *J Mol Biol* 1995;245:362–374.

108 Kretzschmar HA, Stowring LE, Westaway D, et al. Molecular cloning of a human prion protein cDNA. *DNA* 1986;5:315–324.

109 Puckett C, Concannon P, Casey C, Hood L. Genomic structure of the human prion protein gene. *Am J Hum Genet* 1991;49:320–329.

110 Vnencak-Jones CL, Phillips JA. Identification of heterogeneous PrP gene deletions in controls by detection of allele-specific heteroduplexes (DASH). *Am J Hum Genet* 1992;50: 871–872.

111 Laplanche J-L, Chatelain J, Launay J-M, et al. Deletion in prion protein gene in a Moroccan family. *Nucleic Acids Res* 1990;18:6745.

112 Palmer MS, Dryden AJ, Hughes JT, Collinge J. Homozygous prion protein genotype predisposes to sporadic Creutzfeldt-Jakob disease. *Nature* 1991;352:340–342.

113 Fink JK, Peacock ML, Warren JT, et al. Detecting prion protein gene-mutations by denaturing gradient gel-electrophoresis. *Hum Mutat* 1994;4:42–50.

114 Kitamoto T, Tateishi J. Human prion diseases with variant prion protein. *Philos Trans R Soc Lond B Biol Sci* 1994;343:391–398.

115 Owen F, Poulter M, Lofthouse R, et al. Insertion in prion protein gene in familial Creutzfeldt-Jakob disease. *Lancet* 1989;1:51–52.

116 Owen F, Poulter M, Shah T, et al. An in-frame insertion in the prion protein gene in familial Creutzfeldt-Jakob disease. *Mol Brain Res* 1990;7:273–276.

117 Collinge J, Harding AE, Owen F, et al. Diagnosis of Gerstmann-Sträussler syndrome in familial dementia with prion protein gene analysis. *Lancet* 1989;2:15–17.

118 Collinge J, Owen F, Poulter H, et al. Prion dementia without characteristic pathology. *Lancet* 1990;336:7–9.

119 Telling GC, Parchi P, DeArmond SJ, et al. Evidence for the conformation of the pathologic isoform of the prion protein enciphering and propagating prion diversity. *Science* 1996; 274:2079–2082.

120 Goldfarb LG, Brown P, Goldgaber D, et al. Creutzfeldt-Jakob disease and kuru patients lack a mutation consistently found in the Gerstmann-Sträussler-Scheinker syndrome. *Exp Neurol* 1990;108:247–250.

121 Goldfarb LG, Brown P, McCombie WR, et al. Transmissible familial Creutzfeldt-Jakob disease associated with five, seven, and eight extra octapeptide coding repeats in the *PRNP* gene. *Proc Natl Acad Sci USA* 1991;88: 10926–10930.

122 Palmer MS, Mahal SP, Campbell TA, et al. Deletions in the prion protein gene are not associated with CJD. *Hum Mol Genet* 1993; 2:541–544.

123 Goldgaber D, Goldfarb LG, Brown P, et al. Mutations in familial Creutzfeldt-Jakob disease and Gerstmann-Sträussler-Scheinker's syndrome. *Exp Neurol* 1989;106:204–206.

124 Doh-ura K, Tateishi J, Sasaki H, et al. Pro→ Leu change at position 102 of prion protein is the most common but not the sole mutation related to Gerstmann-Sträussler syndrome. *Biochem Biophys Res Commun* 1989;163: 974–979.

125 Goldfarb LG, Mitrova E, Brown P, et al. Mutation in codon 200 of scrapie amyloid protein gene in two clusters of Creutzfeldt-Jakob disease in Slovakia. *Lancet* 1990;336:514–515.

126 Goldfarb L, Brown P, Goldgaber D, et al. Identical mutation in unrelated patients with Creutzfeldt-Jakob disease. *Lancet* 1990;336: 174–175.

127 Hsiao KK, Doh-ura K, Kitamoto T, et al. A prion protein amino acid substitution in ataxic

Gerstmann-Sträussler syndrome. *Ann Neurol* 1989;26:137.

128 Hsiao KK, Cass C, Schellenberg GD, et al. A prion protein variant in a family with the telencephalic form of Gerstmann-Sträussler-Scheinker syndrome. *Neurology* 1991;41:681–684.

129 Hsiao K, Prusiner SB. Inherited human prion diseases. *Neurology* 1990;40:1820–1827.

130 Tateishi J, Kitamoto T, Doh-ura K, et al. Immunochemical, molecular genetic, and transmission studies on a case of Gerstmann-Sträussler-Scheinker syndrome. *Neurology* 1990;40:1578–1581.

131 Gabizon R, Meiner Z, Cass C, et al. Prion protein gene mutation in Libyan Jews with Creutzfeldt-Jakob disease. *Neurology* 1991; 41:160.

132 Ripoll L, Laplanche J-L, Salzmann M, et al. A new point mutation in the prion protein gene at codon 210 in Creutzfeldt-Jakob disease. *Neurology* 1993;43:1934–1938.

133 Mastrianni JA, Iannicola C, Myers R, Prusiner SB. Identification of a new mutation of the prion protein gene at codon 208 in a patient with Creutzfeldt-Jakob disease. *Neurology* 1995;45(suppl):201. Abstract.

134 Hsiao K, Dlouhy S, Farlow MR, et al. Mutant prion proteins in Gerstmann-Sträussler-Scheinker disease with neurofibrillary tangles. *Nat Genet* 1992;1:68–71.

135 Dlouhy SR, Hsiao K, Farlow MR, et al. Linkage of the Indiana kindred of Gerstmann-Sträussler-Scheinker disease to the prion protein gene. *Nat Genet* 1992;1:64–67.

136 Kitamoto T, Iizuka R, Tateishi J. An amber mutation of prion protein in Gerstmann-Sträussler syndrome with mutant PrP plaques. *Biochem Biophys Res Commun* 1993;192: 525–531.

137 Kitamoto T, Ohta M, Doh-ura K, et al. Novel missense variants of prion protein in Creutzfeldt-Jakob disease or Gerstmann-Sträussler syndrome. *Biochem Biophys Res Commun* 1993;191:709–714.

Index

Note: Page numbers with an *f* indicate figures; those with a *t* indicate tables.